Let's Code It! ICD-10-CM

Shelley C. Safian, PhD, RHIA
*MAOM/HSM/HI, CCS-P, COC, CPC-I,
AHIMA-Approved ICD-10-CM/PCS Trainer*

Mary A. Johnson, MBA-HM-HI, CPC
Central Carolina Technical College

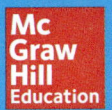

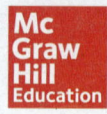

LET'S CODE IT! ICD-10-CM

Published by McGraw-Hill Education, 2 Penn Plaza, New York, NY 10121. Copyright © 2019 by McGraw-Hill Education. All rights reserved. Printed in the United States of America. No part of this publication may be reproduced or distributed in any form or by any means, or stored in a database or retrieval system, without the prior written consent of McGraw-Hill Education, including, but not limited to, in any network or other electronic storage or transmission, or broadcast for distance learning.

Some ancillaries, including electronic and print components, may not be available to customers outside the United States.

This book is printed on acid-free paper.

1 2 3 4 5 6 7 8 9 LMN 21 20 19 18

ISBN 978-1-260-03994-8
MHID 1-260-03994-3

Senior Portfolio Manager: *William Mulford*
Senior Product Developer: *Michelle Flomenhoft*
Product Developer: *Michelle Gaseor*
Executive Marketing Manager: *Roxan Kinsey*
Senior Content Project Managers: *Sherry Kane/Brent dela Cruz*
Senior Buyer: *Laura Fuller*
Senior Design: *Tara McDermott*
Lead Content Licensing Specialist: *Beth Thole*
Cover Image: *©Ingram Publishing*
Compositor: *SPi Global*

All credits appearing on page or at the end of the book are considered to be an extension of the copyright page.

Library of Congress Cataloging-in-Publication Data

Names: Safian, Shelley C., author. | Johnson, Mary A. (Medical record coding program manager), author.
Title: Let's code it! / Shelley C. Safian, PhD, RHIA, MAOM/HSM, CCS-P, CPC-H, CPC-I, AHIMA-Approved ICD-10-CM/PCS Trainer, Mary A. Johnson, CPC, Central Carolina Technical College.
Description: First edition. | New York, NY : McGraw-Hill Education, [2019] | Includes index. Contents: v. 1. ICD-10 CM: The complete medical coding solution — v. 2. ICD-10 CM/PCS: The complete medical coding solution — v. 3. Procedure: The complete medical coding solution.
Identifiers: LCCN 2017032194| ISBN 9781260039948 (v. 1 : alk. paper) | ISBN 9781260031997 (v. 2 : alk. paper) | ISBN 9781260031577 (v. 3 : alk. paper)
Subjects: LCSH: Medicine—Terminology—Code numbers. | Nosology—Code numbers.
Classification: LCC R123 .S185 2019 | DDC 610.1/4—dc23 LC record available at https://lccn.loc.gov/2017032194

The Internet addresses listed in the text were accurate at the time of publication. The inclusion of a website does not indicate an endorsement by the authors or McGraw-Hill Education, and McGraw-Hill Education does not guarantee the accuracy of the information presented at these sites.

mheducation.com/highered

ABOUT THE AUTHORS

Shelley C. Safian

Shelley Safian has been teaching medical coding and health information management for more than 15 years, at both on-ground and online campuses. In addition to her regular teaching responsibilities at University of Central Florida and Berkeley College Online, she often presents seminars sponsored by AHIMA and AAPC, writes regularly about coding for the *Just Coding* newsletter, and has written articles published in AAPC's *Healthcare Business Monthly, SurgiStrategies,* and *HFM* (Healthcare Financial Management) magazine. Safian is the course author for multiple distance education courses on various coding topics, including ICD-10-CM, ICD-10-PCS, CPT, and HCPCS Level II coding.

Safian is a Registered Health Information Administrator (RHIA) and a Certified Coding Specialist–Physician-based (CCS-P) from the American Health Information Management Association and a Certified Outpatient Coder (COC) and a Certified Professional Coding Instructor (CPC-I) from the American Academy of Professional Coders. She is also a Certified HIPAA Administrator (CHA) and has earned the designation of AHIMA-Approved ICD-10-CM/PCS Trainer.

Safian completed her Graduate Certificate in Health Care Management at Keller Graduate School of Management. The University of Phoenix awarded her the Master of Arts/Organizational Management degree and a Graduate Certificate in Health Informatics. She earned her Ph.D. in Health Care Administration with a focus in Health Information Management.

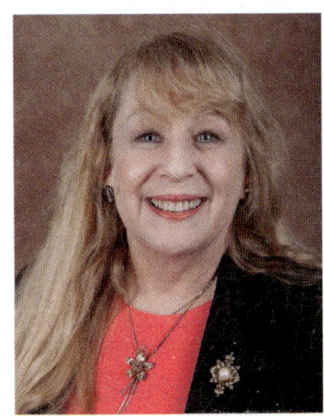

Courtesy of Shelley C. Safian

Mary A. Johnson

Mary Johnson is currently the Medical Record Coding Program Director at Central Carolina Technical College, Sumter, South Carolina. Her background includes corporate training as well as on-campus and online platforms. Johnson also designs and implements customized coding curricula. Johnson received her Bachelor of Arts dual degree in Business Administration and Marketing from Columbia College, and earned a Masters of Business Administration with a dual focus in Healthcare Management and Health Informatics from New England College. Johnson is a Certified Professional Coder (CPC) credentialed through the American Academy of Professional Coders and is ICD-10-CM proficient.

Acknowledgments

—This book is dedicated to all of those who have come into my life sharing encouragement and opportunity to pursue work that I love; for the benefit of all of my students: past, present, and future.—*Shelley*

—This book is dedicated in loving memory of my parents, *Dr. and Mrs. Clarence J. Johnson Sr.,* for their love and support. Also, to those students with whom I have had the privilege to work and to those students who are beginning their journey into the world of medical coding.—*Mary*

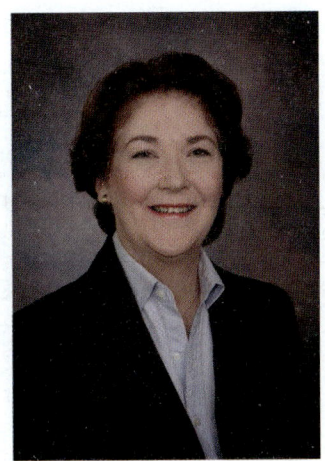

Courtesy of Mary A. Johnson

BRIEF CONTENTS

Guided Tour xii
Preface xvi

PART I: Medical Coding Fundamentals 1

1 Introduction to the Languages of Coding 2
2 Abstracting Clinical Documentation 22
3 The Coding Process 39

PART II: Reporting Diagnoses 53

4 Introduction to ICD-10-CM 54
5 Coding Infectious Diseases 101
6 Coding Neoplasms 145
7 Coding Conditions of the Blood and Immunological Systems 173
8 Coding Endocrine Conditions 198
9 Coding Mental, Behavioral, and Neurological Disorders 228
10 Coding Dysfunction of the Optical and Auditory Systems 263
11 Coding Cardiovascular Conditions 294
12 Coding Respiratory Conditions 329
13 Coding Digestive System Conditions 356
14 Coding Integumentary Conditions 382
15 Coding Muscular and Skeletal Conditions 406
16 Coding Injury, Poisoning, and External Causes 429
17 Coding Genitourinary, Gynecology, Obstetrics, Congenital, and Pediatrics Conditions 470
18 Factors Influencing Health Status (Z Codes) 519
19 Inpatient (Hospital) Diagnosis Coding 541
20 Diagnostic Coding Capstone 568

PART VI: Reimbursement, Legal, and Ethical Issues 1155

39 Reimbursement 1156
40 Introduction to Health Care Law and Ethics 1185

Appendix 1216
Glossary 1218
Index 1229

> **Let's Code It!** ICD-10-CM is part of the comprehensive Let's Code It! series. This product was specifically chosen for your course, and you will notice that Parts III-V are not included, along with the corresponding chapters and pages. This is intentional and please know that you are not missing any content.

End-of-Chapter Reviews

Most chapters end with the following assessment types to reinforce the chapter learning outcomes: Let's Check It! Terminology; Let's Check It! Concepts; Let's Check It! Guidelines; Let's Check It! Rules and Regulations; and You Code It! Basics.

YOU CODE IT! Practice

Using the techniques described in this chapter, carefully read through the case studies and determine the most accurate ICD-10-CM code(s) and external cause code(s), if appropriate, for each case study.

1. George Donmoyer, a 58-year-old male, presents today with a sore throat, persistent cough, and earache. Dr. Selph completes an examination and appropriate tests. The blood-clotting parameters, the thyroid function studies, as well as the tissue biopsy confirm a diagnosis of malignant neoplasm of the extrinsic larynx.
2. Monica Pressley, a 37-year-old female, comes to see Dr. Wheaten today because she has been having diarrhea and abdominal cramping and states her heart feels like its quavering. The MRI scan confirms a diagnosis of benign pancreatic islet cell adenoma.
3. Suber Wilson, a 57-year-old male, was diagnosed with a malignant neoplasm of the liver metastasized from the prostate; both sites are being addressed in today's encounter.
4. William Amerson, a 41-year-old male, comes in for his annual eye examination. Dr. Leviner notes a benign right conjunctiva nevus.
5. Edward Bakersfield, a 43-year-old male, presents with shortness of breath, chest pain, and coughing up blood. After a thorough examination, Dr. Benson notes stridor and orders an MRI scan. The results of the MRI confirm the diagnosis of bronchial adenoma.
6. Elizabeth Conyers, a 56-year-old female, presents with unexplained weakness, weight loss, and dizziness. Dr. Amos completes a thorough examination and does a work-up. The protein electrophoresis (SPEP) and quantitative immunoglobulin results confirm the diagnosis of Waldenström's macroglobulinemia.
7. James Buckholtz, a 3-year-old male, is brought in by his parents. Jimmy has lost his appetite and is losing weight. Mrs. Buckholtz tells Dr. Ferguson that Jimmy's gums bleed and he seems short of breath. Dr. Ferguson notes splenomegaly and admits Jimmy to Weston Hospital. After reviewing the blood tests, MRI scan, and bone marrow aspiration results, Jimmy is diagnosed with acute lymphoblastic leukemia.
8. Kelley Young, a 39-year-old female, presents to Dr. Clerk with the complaints of sudden blurred vision, dizziness, and numbness in her face. Kelley states she feels very weak and has headaches. Dr. Clerk admits Kelley to the hospital. After reviewing the MRI scan, her hormone levels from the blood workup, and urine tests, Kelley is diagnosed with a primary malignant neoplasm of the pituitary gland.
9. Ralph Bradley, a 36-year-old male, comes to see Dr. Harper because he is weak, losing weight, and vomiting and has diarrhea with some blood showing. Ralph was diagnosed with HIV 3 years ago. Dr. Harper completes an examination noting paleness, tachycardia, and tachypnea. Ralph is admitted to the hospital. The biopsied tissue from an endoscopy confirms a diagnosis of Kaposi's sarcoma of gastrointestinal organ.

YOU CODE IT! Application

The following exercises provide practice in abstracting physician documentation from our health care facility, Prader, Bracker, & Associates. These case studies are modeled on real patient encounters. Using the techniques described in this chapter, carefully read through the case studies and determine the most accurate ICD-10-CM code(s) for each case study. Remember to include external cause codes, if appropriate.

PRADER, BRACKER, & ASSOCIATES
A Complete Health Care Facility
159 Healthcare Way • SOMEWHERE, FL 32811 • 407-555-6789

PATIENT: Kassandra, Kelly
ACCOUNT/EHR #: KASSKE001
DATE: 09/16/18
Attending Physician: Oscar R. Prader, MD

S: Pt is a 19-year-old female who has had a sore throat and cough for the past week. She states that she had a temperature of 101.5 F last night. She also admits that it is painful to swallow. No OTC medication has provided any significant relief.

O: Ht 5'5". Wt. 148 lb. R 20. T 101 F. BP 125/82. Pharynx is inspected, tonsils enlarged. There is pus noted in the posterior pharynx. Neck: supple, no nodes. Chest: clear. Heart: regular rate and rhythm without murmur.

A: Acute pharyngitis

P: 1. Send pt for Strep test
2. Recommend patient gargle with warm salt water and use OTC lozenges to keep throat moist
3. Rx if needed once results of Strep test come back
4. Return in 2 weeks for follow-up

ORP/pw D: 9/16/18 09:50:16 T: 9/18/18 12:55:01

Determine the most accurate ICD-10-CM code(s).

WESTON HOSPITAL
629 Healthcare Way • SOMEWHERE, FL 32811 • 407-555-6541

PATIENT: DAVIS, HELEN
ACCOUNT/EHR #: DAVIHE001
DATE: 10/21/18
Attending Physician: Renee O. Bracker, MD

CHAPTER 39 REVIEW
Reimbursement

Let's Check it! Terminology

Match each term to the appropriate definition.

Part I

1. LO 39.2 A physician, typically a family practitioner or an internist, who serves as the primary care physician for an individual. This physician is responsible for evaluating and determining the course of treatment or services, as well as for deciding whether or not a specialist should be involved in care.
2. LO 39.1 A type of health insurance coverage that controls the care of each subscriber (or insured person) by using a primary care provider as a central health care supervisor.
3. LO 39.2 A type of health insurance that uses a primary care physician, also known as a gatekeeper, to manage all health care services for an individual.
4. LO 39.2 A policy that covers loss or injury to a third party caused by the insured or something belonging to the insured.
5. LO 39.1 The total management of an individual's well-being by a health care professional.
6. LO 39.3 An insurance company pays a provider one flat fee to cover the entire course of treatment for an individual's condition.
7. LO 39.2 The agency under the Department of Health and Human Services (DHHS) in charge of regulation and control over services for those covered by Medicare and Medicaid.
8. LO 39.3 Payment agreements that outline, in a written fee schedule, exactly how much money the insurance carrier will pay the physician for each treatment and/or service provided.
9. LO 39.3 An extra reduction in the rate charged to an insurer for services provided by the physician to the plan's members.
10. LO 39.1 The amount of money, often paid monthly, by a policyholder or insured, to an insurance company to obtain coverage.
11. LO 39.2 Auto accident liability coverage will pay for medical bills, lost wages, and compensation for pain and suffering for any person injured by the insured in an auto accident.
12. LO 39.3 Agreements between a physician and a managed care organization that pay the physician a predetermined amount of money each month for each member of the plan who identifies that provider as his or her primary care physician.
13. LO 39.2 A plan that reimburses a covered individual a portion of his or her income that is lost as a result of being unable to work due to illness or injury.
14. LO 39.2 Individuals who are supported, either financially or with regard to insurance coverage, by others.

A. Automobile Insurance
B. Capitation Plans
C. Centers for Medicare & Medicaid Services (CMS)
D. Dependents
E. Disability Compensation
F. Discounted FFS
G. Episodic Care
H. Fee-for-Service (FFS) Plans
I. Gatekeeper
J. Health Care
K. Health Maintenance Organization (HMO)
L. Insurance Premium
M. Liability Insurance
N. Managed Care

CHAPTER 39 | REIMBURSEMENT 1181

Real Abstracting Practice with You Code It! Practice, You Code It! Application, and Capstone Case Studies Chapters

Gain real-world experience by using actual patient records (with names and other identifying information changed) to practice ICD-10-CM, ICD-10-PCS, CPT, and HCPCS Level II coding for both inpatients and outpatients. *You Code It! Practice* exercises give students the chance to practice coding with short coding scenarios. *You Code It! Application* exercises give students the chance to review and abstract physicians' notes documenting real patient encounters in order to code those scenarios. Both of these types of exercises can be found at the end of most chapters. *Capstone Chapters* come at the end of Parts II–V and include 15 additional real-life outpatient and inpatient case studies to help students synthesize and apply what they have learned through hands-on coding practice with each code set.

In addition, all of the exercises in the Chapter Review can be assigned through Connect. Of particular note are the *You Code It! Practice* exercises, which offer our unique **CodePath** option. In Connect, students are presented with a series of questions to guide them through the critical thinking process to determine the correct code.

ix

PREFACE

Welcome to *Let's Code It!* This product is part of a multipart series that instructs students on how to become proficient in medical coding—a health care field that continues to be in high demand. The Bureau of Labor Statistics notes the demand for health information management professionals (which includes coders) will continue to increase incredibly through 2024 and beyond.

Let's Code It! provides a 360-degree learning experience for anyone interested in the field of medical coding, with strong guidance down the path to coding certification. Theory is presented in easy-to-understand language and accompanied by lots of examples. Hands-on practice is included with real-life physician documentation, from both outpatient and inpatient facilities, to promote critical thinking analysis and evaluation. This is in addition to determination of accurate codes to report diagnoses, procedures, and ancillary services. All of this is assembled to support the reader's development of a solid foundation upon which to build a successful career after graduation.

The Safian/Johnson Medical Coding series includes the following products:

Let's Code It!
Let's Code It! ICD-10-CM
Let's Code It! ICD-10-CM/PCS
Let's Code It! Procedure
You Code It! Abstracting Case Studies Practicum, 3e

The different solutions are designed to fit the most common course content selections. *Let's Code It!* is the comprehensive offering with coverage of ICD-10-CM, ICD-10-PCS, CPT, and HCPCS Level II.

These products are further designed to give your students the medical coding experience they need in order to pass their first medical coding certification exams, such as the CCS/CCS-P or CPC/COC. The products offer students a variety of practice opportunities by reinforcing the learning outcomes set forth in every chapter. The chapter materials are organized in short bursts of text followed by practice—keeping students active and coding! These products were developed based on the 2017 code sets, with 2018 updates implemented as much as possible prior to publication. Updates will be made to the answer keys and Connect exercises on an annual basis.

Here's What You Can Expect from *Let's Code It!*

- Each of the six parts of this product includes an Introduction to provide students with an overview of the information within that part and how they can use this knowledge.
  - Part I: Medical Coding Fundamentals
  - Part II: Reporting Diagnoses
  - Part III: Reporting Physicians Services and Outpatient Procedures
  - Part IV: DMEPOS & Transportation
  - Part V: Inpatient (Hospital) Reporting
  - Part VI: Legal, Ethical, and Reimbursement Issues
- **Part I: Medical Coding Fundamentals** helps students build a strong theoretical foundation regarding the various code sets. The chapters teach students how and when each code set is used and how to abstract documentation. These chapters also teach them how to use a solid coding process, including the importance of queries, how to write a legal query, exposure to the Official Guidelines, and confirmation of medical necessity.

- **Part II: Reporting Diagnoses** provides students with an incremental walkthrough of the ICD-10-CM code set.
- **Part III: Reporting Physicians Services and Outpatient Procedures** provides students with a progressive learning experience for using CPT® procedure codes.
- **Part IV: DMEPOS & Transportation** gives students insight into, and hands-on practice using, the HCPCS Level II code set to report the provision of durable medical equipment, prosthetics, orthotics, and other medical supplies.
- **Part V: Inpatient (Hospital) Reporting** shows students how to build an accurate ICD-10-PCS code to report inpatient procedures, services, and treatments.
- The coding chapters in Parts II–V all include real-life scenarios, as well as physician documentation mainly in the form of procedure notes and operative reports (both inpatient and outpatient) for students to practice abstracting and coding.
  - *Let's Code It! Scenarios* provide step-by-step instruction so students can learn to use their critical-thinking skills throughout the coding process to determine the correct code.
  - *You Code It! Case Studies* provide students with hands-on practice coding scenarios and case studies throughout each chapter.
  - *You Interpret It!* questions present additional opportunities for students to use critical-thinking skills to identify details required for accurate coding.
  - *Chapter Reviews* include assessments of chapter concepts:
    - Let's Check It! Terminology
    - Let's Check It! Concepts
    - Let's Check It! Guidelines
    - Let's Check It! Rules and Regulations
    - You Code It! Basics
    - You Code It! Practice Case Studies
    - You Code It! Application Case Studies
- *Examples* are included throughout each chapter to help students make the connection between theoretical and practical coding.
- *Coding Bites* highlight key concepts and tips to further support understanding and learning.
- *Guidance Connection* features point to the specific Official Guideline applicable for the concept being discussed.
- *Capstone Chapters* come at the end of Parts II–V with 15 additional real-life outpatient and inpatient case studies to help students synthesize and apply what they have learned through hands-on coding practice with each code set.
- **Part VI: Legal, Ethical, and Reimbursement Issues** provides a concise overview connecting these broad topics to a professional coding specialist's job requirements.
- *Examples* again take students through real-life scenarios to help them understand how they will use this information.
- *Coding Bites* provide tips and highlight key concepts.
- This part also includes material to teach students how to access credible resources on the Internet.
- *Codes of Ethics* from both AHIMA and AAPC are included as well as information on compliance plans.
- *You Interpret It!* questions present students with opportunities to use critical-thinking skills to identify details required for accurate job performance.
- *Chapter Reviews* include assessments of chapter concepts:
  - Let's Check It! Terminology
  - Let's Check It! Concepts
  - Let's Check It! Which Type of Insurance?
  - Let's Check It! Rules and Regulations
  - You Code It! Application Case Studies

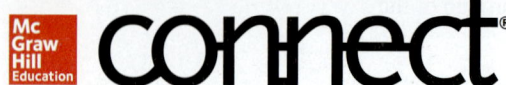

McGraw-Hill Connect® is a highly reliable, easy-to-use homework and learning management solution that utilizes learning science and award-winning adaptive tools to improve student results.

Homework and Adaptive Learning

- Connect's assignments help students contextualize what they've learned through application, so they can better understand the material and think critically.
- Connect will create a personalized study path customized to individual student needs through SmartBook®.
- SmartBook helps students study more efficiently by delivering an interactive reading experience through adaptive highlighting and review.

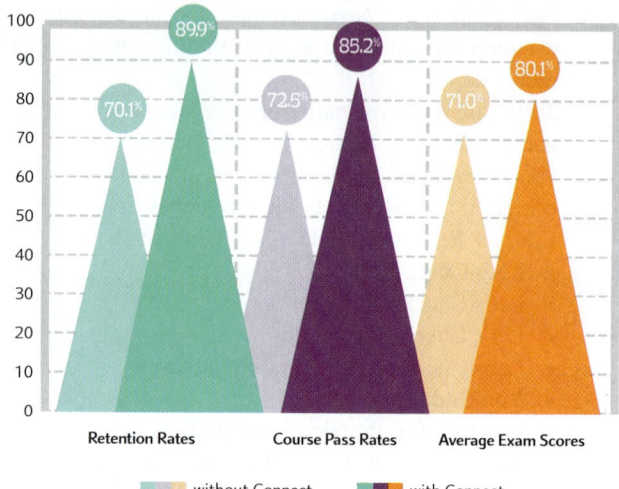

Connect's Impact on Retention Rates, Pass Rates, and Average Exam Scores

Using **Connect** improves retention rates by **19.8** percentage points, passing rates by **12.7** percentage points, and exam scores by **9.1** percentage points.

Over **7 billion questions** have been answered, making McGraw-Hill Education products more intelligent, reliable, and precise.

Quality Content and Learning Resources

- Connect content is authored by the world's best subject matter experts, and is available to your class through a simple and intuitive interface.
- The Connect eBook makes it easy for students to access their reading material on smartphones and tablets. They can study on the go and don't need internet access to use the eBook as a reference, with full functionality.
- Multimedia content such as videos, simulations, and games drive student engagement and critical thinking skills.

73% of instructors who use **Connect** require it; instructor satisfaction **increases** by 28% when **Connect** is required.

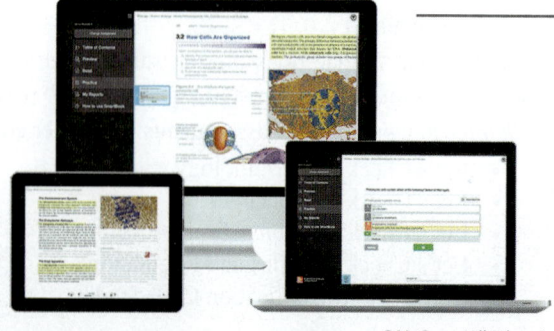

©McGraw-Hill Education

Robust Analytics and Reporting

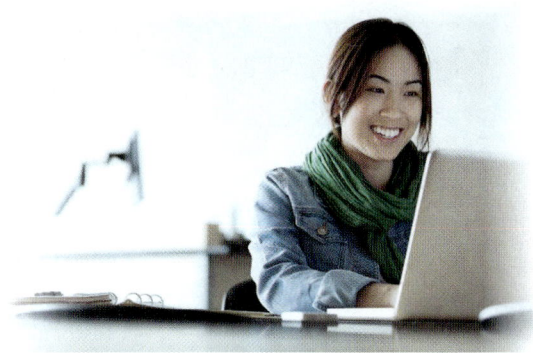
©Hero Images/Getty Images

- Connect Insight® generates easy-to-read reports on individual students, the class as a whole, and on specific assignments.
- The Connect Insight dashboard delivers data on performance, study behavior, and effort. Instructors can quickly identify students who struggle and focus on material that the class has yet to master.
- Connect automatically grades assignments and quizzes, providing easy-to-read reports on individual and class performance.

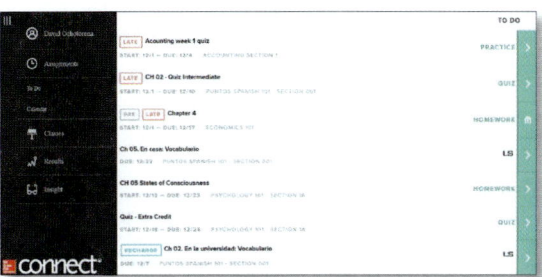

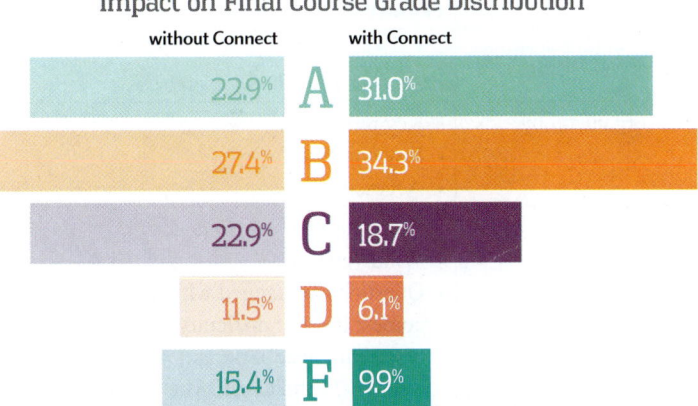

Impact on Final Course Grade Distribution

	without Connect	with Connect
A	22.9%	31.0%
B	27.4%	34.3%
C	22.9%	18.7%
D	11.5%	6.1%
F	15.4%	9.9%

More students earn **As** and **Bs** when they use **Connect**.

Trusted Service and Support

- Connect integrates with your LMS to provide single sign-on and automatic syncing of grades. Integration with Blackboard®, D2L®, and Canvas also provides automatic syncing of the course calendar and assignment-level linking.
- Connect offers comprehensive service, support, and training throughout every phase of your implementation.
- If you're looking for some guidance on how to use Connect, or want to learn tips and tricks from super users, you can find tutorials as you work. Our Digital Faculty Consultants and Student Ambassadors offer insight into how to achieve the results you want with Connect.

www.mheducation.com/connect

CONNECT FOR YOU CODE IT!

McGraw-Hill Connect for You Code It! will include:

- All end-of-chapter questions
- CodePath versions of You Code It! practice questions, in which students are presented with a series of questions to guide them through the critical thinking process to determine the correct code
- Interactive Exercises, such as Matching, Sequencing, and Labeling activities
- Testbank questions
- Lecture-style videos, which will provide additional guidance on challenging coding questions

INSTRUCTORS' RESOURCES

You can rely on the following materials to help you and your students work through the material in the book; all are available in the Instructor Resources under the Library tab in *Connect* (available only to instructors who are logged in to *Connect*).

Supplement	Features
Instructor's Manual (organized by Learning Outcomes)	• Lesson plans • Answer keys for all exercises
PowerPoint Presentations (organized by Learning Outcomes)	• Key terms • Key concepts • Accessible
Electronic Testbank	• Computerized and *Connect* • Word version • Questions are tagged with learning outcomes; level of difficulty; level of Bloom's taxonomy; feedback; and ABHES, CAAHEP, and CAHIIM competencies.
Tools to Plan Course	• Correlations by learning outcomes to accrediting bodies such as ABHES, CAAHEP, and CAHIIM • Sample syllabi • Asset map—recap of the key instructor resources as well as information on the content available through *Connect*

Want to learn more about this product? Attend one of our online webinars. To learn more about them, please contact your McGraw-Hill learning technology representative. To find your McGraw-Hill representative, go to www.mheducation.com and click "Contact," then "Contact a Sales Rep."

Need help? Contact the McGraw-Hill Education Customer Experience Group (CXG). Visit the CXG website at www.mhhe.com/support. Browse our frequently asked questions (FAQs) and product documentation and/or contact a CXG representative.

ACKNOWLEDGMENTS

Board of Advisors

A select group of instructors participated in our Coding Board of Advisors. They provided timely and focused guidance to the author team on all aspects of content development. We are extremely grateful for their input on this project.

Christine Cusano, CMA (AAMA), CPhT,
Lincoln Technical Institute

Gerry Gordon, BA, CPC, CPB,
Daytona College

Shalena Jarvis, RHIT, CCS

Jan Klawitter, AS, CPC, CPB, CPC-I,
San Joaquin Valley College

Tatyana Pashnyak, CHTS-TR,
Bainbridge State College

Patricia Saccone, MA, RHIA, CCS-P,
Waubonsee Community College

Stephanie Scott, MSHI, RHIA, CDIP, CCS, CCS-P, Moraine Park Technical College

Reviews

Many instructors reviewed the manuscript while it was in development and provided valuable feedback that directly affected the product's development. Their contributions are greatly appreciated.

Julie Alles-Grice, MSCTE, RHIA

Alicia Alva, AS, San Joaquin Valley College

Kelly Berge, MSHA, CPC, CCS-P, Berkeley College

Valerie Brock, EdS, MBA, RHIA, CDIP, CPC, Tennessee State University

William Butler, MHA, UNC Healthcare

Heather Copen, RHIA, CCS-P, Ivy Tech Community College

Gerard Cronin, MS, DC, Salem Community College

Christine Cusano, CMA (AAMA), CPhT, Lincoln Technical Institute

Patti Fayash, CCS, ICD-10-CM/PCS AHIMA Approved Trainer, Luzerne County Community College

Rashmi Gaonkar, BS, MS, MHA/Informatics, ASA College

Savanna Garrity, MPA, CPC, Madisonville Community College

Deborah Gilbert, RHIA, MBA, CMA, Dalton State College

Terri Gilbert, MS, ECPI University

Gerry Gordon, BA, CPC, CPB, Daytona College

Michelle A. Harris, CPC, CPB, CPC-I, Bossier Parish Community College

Susan Hernandez, B.S.B.A., San Joaquin Valley College

Judith Hurtt, MEd, East Central Community College

Beverlee Jackson, BA, RHIT, CCS, AHIMA Ambassador, Central Oregon Community College

Shalena Jarvis, RHIT, CCS

Mary Z. Johnston, RN, BSN, RHIA, CPC, CPC-H, CPC-I, Ultimate Medical Academy

Jan Klawitter, AS, CPC, CPB, CPC-I, San Joaquin Valley College

Jennifer Lamé, MPH, RHIT, Southwest Wisconsin Technical College

Jorell Lawrence, MSA, CPC, Stratford University

Tracey Lee, MSA, CPC, Vista College

Angela Leuvoy, AAS, CMA, CPT, CBCS, Fortis College

Glenda Lloyd, MBA, BS, RHIA, Rasmussen College, Vista College

Lynnae Lockett, RN, RMA, CMRS, MSN, Bryant & Stratton College

Marta Lopez, MD, BXMO, RMA, Miami Dade College

JanMarie Malik, MBA, RHIA, CCS-P, National University

Barbara Marchelletta, BS, CMA (AAMA), CPT, CPC, AHI, Beal College

David Martinez, MHSA, RHIT, RMA, University of Phoenix

Jillian McDonald, BS, RMA (AMT), EMT, CPT(NPA)

Cheryl Miller, MBA/HCM, Westmoreland County Community College

Robin Moore, CPC, CCMA, Davis College

Lisa Nimmo, CPC, CFPC, Central Carolina Technical College

Melissa Oelfke, RHIA, HIT Program Coordinator, Rasmussen College

Barbara Parker, CPC, CCS-P, CMA (AAMA), Olympic College

Brenda Parks-Brown, MHS, HCA, CCS, CMA, Miller-Motte Technical College

Tatyana Pashnyak, CHTS-TR, Bainbridge State College

Staci Porter, AA, San Joaquin Valley College

Terri Randolph, MBA/HCM, CAHI, CBCS, CEHRS, Eagle Gate College

Lisa Riggs, CPC, CPC-I, Ultimate Medical Academy

Rolando Russell, MBA, RHIA, CPC, CPAR, Ultimate Medical Academy

Patricia Saccone, MA, RHIA, CCS-P, Waubonsee Community College

Georgina Sampson, RHIA, Anoka Technical College

Stephanie Scott, MSHI, RHIA, CDIP, CCS, CCS-P, Moraine Park Technical College

Mary Jo Slater, MS, MIE, Community College of Beaver County

Karen K. Smith, MEd, RHIA, CDIP, CPC, University of Arkansas for Medical Sciences

Kameron Stutzman, MEd, CMBS, IBMC College

Stephanie Vergne, MAEd, RHIA, CPC, Hazard Community & Technical College

Technical Editing/Accuracy Panel

A panel of instructors completed a technical edit and review of all content in the page proofs to verify its accuracy.

Amber Capell, BS, CPC, CPC-I, Ultimate Medical Academy

Savanna Garrity, MPA, CPC, Madisonville Community College

Susan Holler, MSEd, CPC, CMRS, Bryant & Stratton College

Katurah M. Jones, MPA, MBA, RHIA, AHI, CPC, CPB, Hunter College, New York University

Janis A. Klawitter, AS, CPC, CPB, CPC-I, San Joaquin Valley College

Tracey Lee MSA, CPC, Vista College

Ajay Mehra, BSc, RT(R), CCS-P, RHIT, Rochester Community & Technical College

Corina Miranda, CMPC-I, CMRS, CPC, Northwest Vista College/Alamo Community Colleges

Robin Moore, CPC, CCMA, Davis College

Barbara Parker, CPC, CCS-P, CMA (AAMA), Olympic College

Jerri Rowe, MBA, CFE, RHIA, CPC, CRC, Allen School of Health Sciences

Kathy J Ware, MCLS, RHIT, CPC, CPB, CPC-I, Lord Fairfax Community College

Deborah Zenzal, RN, MSHIM, MS, CPC, CCS-P, RMA

Digital Tool Development

Special thanks to the instructors who helped with the development of Connect and SmartBook.

Tammy L. Burnette, PhD, CPC, CPB, Tyler Junior College

Denise DeDeaux, MBA, Fayetteville Technical College

Judith Hurtt, MEd, East Central Community College

Shalena Jarvis, RHIT, CCS

Shauna Phillips, RMA, CCMA, AHI

Lisa Riggs, CPC, CPC-I, Ultimate Medical Academy

Patricia A. Saccone, MA, RHIA, CCS-P, Waubonsee Community College

PART I

MEDICAL CODING FUNDAMENTALS

INTRODUCTION

Coding is not like anything you have ever studied before. No courses that you experienced in elementary, middle, or high school have prepared you for learning this skill. Biology and your science classes began your education that your anatomy and physiology class continued. Other courses you are taking as part of this program also typically connect to something, in some way, you have previously learned.

As you begin this educational journey, you will use your critical thinking skills as well as some experiences you may have had as a patient yourself (or as the loved one of a patient). For the most part, though, this will be different, so prepare yourself for a new learning experience.

In Part I, the chapters Introduction to the Languages of Coding, Abstracting Clinical Documentation, and The Coding Process share an overview of the concepts and skills you will apply in the chapters that follow. You will be introduced to the tools you have and will need to use as a professional coding specialist. Together, these three chapters create the foundation, the first layer, of a multilayered approach to learning coding. Then, the remaining Parts will share with you, one by one, the best practices for how to use each of these tools correctly. You will then be given many opportunities for hands-on practice so that you can build your skills and reinforce the knowledge you have obtained.

1 Introduction to the Languages of Coding

Key Terms

Classification Systems
Condition
Diagnosis
Eponym
External Cause
Inpatient
Medical Necessity
Nonessential Modifiers
Outpatient
Procedure
Reimbursement
Services
Treatments

Learning Outcomes

After completing this chapter, the student should be able to:

LO 1.1 Explain the four purposes of medical coding.
LO 1.2 Identify the structure of the ICD-10-CM diagnosis coding manual.
LO 1.3 Differentiate between the types of procedures and the various procedure coding manuals.
LO 1.4 Examine the HCPCS Level II coding manual used to report the provision of equipment and supplies.

CODING BITES

We use the concept of *"languages"* to help you relate medical coding—and its code sets—to an idea you already understand. In the health care industry, however, the various code sets, such as ICD-10-CM or HCPCS Level II, are referred to as **Classification Systems**.

Classification Systems
The term used in health care to identify ICD-10-CM, CPT, ICD-10-PCS, and HCPCS Level II code sets.

CODING BITES

A **diagnosis** explains WHY the patient requires the attention of a health care provider and a **procedure** explains WHAT the physician or health care provider did for the patient.

1.1 The Purpose of Coding

Around the world, languages exist to enable clear and accurate communication between individuals in similar groups or working together in similar functions. The purpose of using health care coding languages is to enable the sharing of information, in a specific and efficient way, between all those involved in health care.

Coding languages are constructed of individual codes that are more precise than words. (You will discover this as you venture through this textbook.) By communicating using codes rather than words, you can successfully convey to others involved (1) exactly what happened during a provider-patient encounter and (2) why it occurred. You, as the professional coding specialist, have the responsibility to accurately interpret health care terms and definitions (medical terminology) into numbers or number-letter combinations (alphanumeric codes) that specifically convey **diagnoses** and **procedures**.

Why is it so critical to code diagnoses and procedures accurately? The coding languages, known as **classification systems**, communicate information that is key to various aspects of the health care system, including

- Medical necessity
- Statistical analyses
- Reimbursement
- Resource allocation

Medical Necessity

The diagnosis codes that you report explain the justification for the procedure, service, or treatment provided to a patient during his or her encounter. Every time a health care professional provides care to a patient, there must be a valid medical reason. Patients certainly want to know that health care professionals performed procedures or provided care for a specific, justified purpose, and so do third-party payers! This is referred to as **medical necessity**. Requiring medical necessity ensures that health care providers are not performing tests or giving injections without a good medical reason. Diagnosis codes explain *why* the individual came to see the physician and support the physician's decision about *what* procedures to provide.

Medical necessity is one of the reasons why it is so very important to code the diagnosis accurately and with all the detail possible. If you are one number off in your code selection, you could accidentally cause a claim to be denied because the diagnosis, identified by your incorrect code, does not justify the procedure.

Let's analyze an example:

> **EXAMPLE**
> Dr. Justini performs a colonoscopy on Shoshanna because a lab test identified that she had blood in her feces (melena).

A colonoscopy involves the insertion of a camera, with surgical tools, into the patient's anus, rectum, and up through the large intestine. If you are Shoshanna, or if you are the one paying for this procedure, you want to make certain that this colonoscopy was done to support Shoshanna's good health and not any other reason. This is clearly communicated when you report the code: K92.1 Melena (the presence of blood in feces). Now, whether for resource allocation or reimbursement, it is understood that Dr. Justini was caring properly for Shoshanna and her good health.

Statistical Analyses

Research organizations and government agencies statistically analyze the data provided by codes to develop programs, identify research areas, allocate funds, and write public health policies that will best address areas of concern for the health of our nation. For example, we can only know that a disease such as Alzheimer's needs diagnostic tests, treatments, and possibly a vaccine or a cure by studying statistics to see what individual signs and symptoms are being identified and treated around the country and around the world.

Reimbursement

In most cases, there are three parties involved in virtually every encounter: the health care provider, the patient, and the person or organization paying for the care provided (frequently, a health care insurance company). However, the insurance company is not always an actual insurance company, so the broader term "third-party payer" is used. Third-party payers use our coding data to determine how much they should pay health care professionals for the attention and services they provide patients. This is the role that coding plays in the **reimbursement** process. The codes make it easier for the organizations involved to evaluate and manage all their data.

Resource Allocations

Whether a health care facility is a one-physician office or a large hospital, there are not unlimited resources available. Administrators and managers must ensure that all resources are employed in the most efficient and effective manner. Computer programs can easily and quickly organize data (the codes) to identify the largest patient population's diagnoses and the most frequently provided treatments and services. With these details, staff members, equipment, and money can be directed to those patients and locations that need them the most.

Diagnosis
A physician's determination of a patient's condition, illness, or injury.

Procedure
Action taken, in accordance with the standards of care, by the physician to accomplish a predetermined objective (result); a surgical operation.

Medical Necessity
The determination that the health care professional was acting according to standard practices in providing a particular procedure for an individual with a particular diagnosis. Also referred to as medically necessary.

CODING BITES
The WHY justifies the WHAT.

Reimbursement
The process of paying for health care services after they have been provided.

CODING BITES
In most cases, there are three parties involved in reimbursement:
- The health care provider = First party
- The patient = Second party
- The insurance company or other organization financially responsible = Third-party payer

1.2 Diagnosis Coding

When a person goes to see a health care provider, he or she must have a reason—a health-related reason. After all, as much as you might like your physician, you probably wouldn't make an appointment, sit in the waiting room, and go through all the paperwork just to say, "hello." Whether the reason is a checkup, a flu shot, or something more serious, there is always a reason *why*. The physician will create notes, either written or dictated, recounting the events of the visit. The diagnosis, or diagnostic statement, in these notes will explain the reason *why* the patient was seen and treated.

The physician's notes explain, in writing, the reasons *why* the encounter occurred. The notes may document a specific condition or illness, the signs or symptoms of a yet-unnamed problem, or another reason for the encounter, such as a preventive service. As a coding specialist, it is your job to translate this explanation into a diagnosis code (or codes) so that everyone involved will clearly understand the issues of a particular patient at a particular time.

The International Classification of Diseases – 10th Revision – Clinical Modification (ICD-10-CM) code book contains all of the codes from which you will choose to report the reason *why* the health care professional cared for the patient during a specific encounter.

Overview of the International Classification of Diseases – 10th Revision – Clinical Modification (ICD-10-CM) Code Book Sections

The ICD-10-CM code book (whether paper or electronic) is made up of several sections. Here is an overview of its parts and how you will utilize the information in these sections to determine the most accurate code or codes to report the reasons *why* an encounter occurred.

Index to Diseases and Injuries [aka Alphabetic Index]

The Alphabetic Index [Index to Diseases and Injuries] lists, in alphabetic order, the terms used by the physician to describe the reasons why the patient required attention from a health care professional.

The Alphabetic Index lists all diagnoses and other reasons to provide health care by their basic description alphabetically from A to Z (see Figure 1-1). Diagnostic descriptions are listed by

- **Condition** (e.g., infection, fracture, and wound)
- **Eponym** (e.g., Epstein-Barr syndrome and Cushing's disease)
- Other descriptors (e.g., personal history, family history)

CODING BITES

This is just an overview to help you orient yourself to the structure of the code book. You will learn, in depth, how to use the ICD-10-CM code set to report any and all of the reasons *why* a patient needs the care of a health care professional in *Part II: Reporting Diagnoses*.

Condition
The state of abnormality or dysfunction.

Eponym
A disease or condition named for a person.

Abnormal, abnormality, abnormalities (*see also* Anomaly)

- acid-based balance (mixed) E87.4
- albumin R77.0
- alphafetoprotein R77.2
- alveolar ridge K08.9
- anatomical relationship Q89.9
- apertures, congenital, diaphragm Q79.1
- auditory perception H93.29-
-- diplacusis — *see* Diplacusis
-- hyperacusis — *see* Hyperacusis
-- recruitment — *see* Recruitment, auditory
-- threshold shift — *see* Shift, auditory threshold
- autosomes Q99.9

FIGURE 1-1 ICD-10-CM Alphabetic Index, partial listing under main term Abnormal

So, whichever type of words you read in the documentation, you should be able to find them in the Alphabetic Index in one form or another.

The Alphabetic Index can only suggest a possible code to report the patient's diagnosis, and you will use this suggestion to guide you to the correct page or subsection in the Tabular List (see the next subsection of this text, *Tabular List of Diseases and Injuries*). The Official Guidelines require you to always find a suggested code in the Tabular List to confirm it is accurate, or to find another code that might be better.

Tabular List of Diseases and Injuries

The Tabular List provides you with each and every available code in the ICD-10-CM code book, in order of the code characters—alphanumeric order. You need to carefully read the descriptions, beginning at the top of the three-character code category. When you begin reading at this point, you can make certain that you find the best code, to the highest level of specificity, according to the physician's documentation.

You will find that the Tabular List section shows all ICD-10-CM codes, first in alphabetic order and then in numeric order: A00 through Z99.89 (see Figure 1-2), along with additional details (notations and symbols) that guide you to the accurate code.

Ancillary Sections of ICD-10-CM

Neoplasm Table

The Neoplasm Table (Figure 1-3) itemizes all of the anatomical sites in the human body that may develop a tumor (neoplasm). Columns in this table further describe the type of neoplasm and suggest a code that may be accurate. As with other codes suggested by the Alphabetic Index, you will need to go to the Tabular List to look up any code found on the Neoplasm Table to confirm accuracy, additional characters required, and other details before you can determine the accurate code to report.

You will learn how to use the Neoplasm Table to report diagnoses of benign, malignant, and other types of neoplasms in the *Coding Neoplasms* chapter.

Table of Drugs and Chemicals

The Table of Drugs and Chemicals (Figure 1-4) lists pharmaceuticals and chemicals that may cause poisoning or adverse effects in the human body. The multiple columns in this table categorize the intent of how or why the patient became ill from the drug or chemical to suggest a possible code. As with all of these, this suggested code must

> **CODING BITES**
>
> Notations in the Tabular List help make your coding process more accurate and a bit easier. For example, as you can see in Figure 1-2, the condition represented by code category B67 is Echinococcosis. Now, read the INCLUDES note directly below B67; it reads . . . INCLUDES hydatidosis. This notation lets you know that, if the physician wrote "echinococcosis" or "hydatidosis" in the documentation, this is the correct code category.
>
> In ICD-10-CM, the INCLUDES note provides you with alternative words or phrases that the physician might use that mean the same condition. In English, they are known as synonyms. In ICD-10-CM, they are known as **nonessential modifiers**.
>
> You will learn more about notations in the *Introduction to ICD-10-CM* chapter.

B67 Echinococcosis

   INCLUDES hydatidosis

   B67.0 Echinococcus granulosus infection of liver

   B67.1 Echinococcus granulosus infection of lung

   B67.2 Echinococcus granulosus infection of bone

   B67.3 Echinococcus granulosus infection, other and multiple sites

      B67.31 Echinococcus granulosus infection, thyroid gland

      B67.32 Echinococcus granulosus infection, multiple sites

      B67.39 Echinococcus granulosus infection, other sites

   B67.4 Echinococcus granulosus infection, unspecified

      Dog tapeworm (infection)

FIGURE 1-2 ICD-10-CM Tabular List, partial list of codes included in code category B67 Echinococcosis

---

Nonessential Modifiers
Descriptors whose inclusion in the physician's notes are not absolutely necessary and that are provided simply to further clarify a code description; optional terms.

	Malignant Primary	Malignant Secondary	Ca in situ	Benign	Uncertain Behavior	Unspecified Behavior
Neoplasm, neoplastic	C80.1	C79.9	D09.9	D36.9	D48.9	D49.9
-abdomen, abdominal	C76.2	C79.8-	D09.8	D36.7	D48.7	D49.89
--cavity	C76.2	C79.8-	D09.8	D36.7	D48.7	D49.89
--organ	C76.2	C79.8-	D09.8	D36.7	D48.7	D49.89
--viscera	C76.2	C79.8-	D09.8	D36.7	D48.7	D49.2
--wall—see also Neoplasm, abdomen, wall, skin	C44.509	C79.2-	D04.5	D23.5	D48.5	D49.2
---connective tissue	C49.4	C79.8-	-	D21.4	D48.1	D49.2
---skin	C44.509					
----basal cell carcinoma	C44.519	-	-	-	-	-
----specified type NEC	C44.599	-	-	-	-	-
----squamous cell carcinoma	C44.529	-	-	-	-	-

FIGURE 1-3 The Neoplasm Table from ICD-10-CM, listings for abdominal neoplasms

Substance	Poisoning, Accidental (Unintentional)	Poisoning, Intentional Self-harm	Poisoning, Assault	Poisoning, Undetermined	Adverse Effect	Underdosing
Acefylline piperazine	T48.6X1	T48.6X2	T48.6X3	T48.6X4	T48.6X5	T48.6X6
Acemorphan	T40.2X1	T40.2X2	T40.2X3	T40.2X4	T40.2X5	T40.2X6
Acenocoumarin	T45.511	T45.512	T45.513	T45.514	T45.515	T45.516
Acenocoumarol	T45.511	T45.512	T45.513	T45.514	T45.515	T45.516
Acepifylline	T48.6X1	T48.6X2	T48.6X3	T48.6X4	T48.6X5	T48.6X6
Acepromazine	T43.3X1	T43.3X2	T43.3X3	T43.3X4	T43.3X5	T43.3X6
Acesulfamethoxypyridazine	T37.0X1	T37.0X2	T37.0X3	T37.0X4	T37.0X5	T37.0X6
Acetal	T52.8X1	T52.8X2	T52.8X3	T52.8X4	—	—
Acetaldehyde (vapor)	T52.8X1	T52.8X2	T52.8X3	T52.8X4	—	—
- liquid	T65.891	T65.892	T65.893	T65.894	—	—
P-Acetamidophenol	T39.1X1	T39.1X2	T39.1X3	T39.1X4	T39.1X5	T39.1X6
Acetaminophen	T39.1X1	T39.1X2	T39.1X3	T39.1X4	T39.1X5	T39.1X6

FIGURE 1-4 The Table of Drugs and Chemicals from ICD-10-CM, listings from Acefylline piperazine to Acetaminophen
Source: *ICD-10-CM Official Guidelines for Coding and Reporting,* The Centers for Medicare and Medicaid Services (CMS) and the National Center for Health Statistics (NCHS)

be reviewed in the Tabular List to ensure completeness and accuracy before you can report it.

You will learn how to use the Table of Drugs and Chemicals in the chapter *Coding Injury, Poisoning, and External Causes.*

Index to External Causes

External Cause
An event, outside the body, that causes injury, poisoning, or an adverse reaction.

The Index to **External Causes** (Figure 1-5) lists the causes of injury and poisoning. These codes are used to explain *how* a patient got injured and *where* (place of occurrence) he or she was when the injury happened.

As with the other content in the Alphabetic Index, the code or codes shown here are only suggestions and must be confirmed in the Tabular List before you are permitted to report them. You will learn about the importance of reporting these codes as you

> **Abandonment** (causing exposure to weather conditions) (with intent to injure or kill) NEC X58
>
> **Abuse** (adult) (child) (mental) (physical) (sexual) X58
>
> **Accident** (to) X58
> - aircraft (in transit) (powered) — *see also* Accident, transport, aircraft
> -- due to, caused by cataclysm — *see* Forces of nature, by type
> - animal-rider — *see* Accident, transport, animal-rider
> - animal-drawn vehicle — *see* Accident, transport, animal-drawn vehicle occupant
> - automobile — *see* Accident, transport, car occupant
> - bare foot water skier V94.4
> - boat, boating — *see also* Accident, watercraft
> -- striking swimmer
> -- powered V94.11
> -- unpowered V94.12
> - bus — *see* Accident, transport, bus occupant
> - cable car, not on rails V98.0

FIGURE 1-5 The Index to External Causes, first listings including main terms Abandonment, Abuse, and Accident

progress through your learning experience, particularly in the chapter *Coding Injury, Poisoning, and External Causes*.

The Format of ICD-10-CM Codes

A complete, valid ICD-10-CM code will always begin with a 3-character code category: a letter of the alphabet followed by a minimum of 2 characters (either letters or numbers).

E54	Ascorbic acid deficiency (scurvy)
O9A	Maternal malignant neoplasms, traumatic injuries, and abuse

A majority of the codes will require additional characters to communicate more specific information about the patient's condition. When an additional character is needed to complete the code, a symbol to the left of the code in the Tabular List will identify that additional characters are necessary. The symbol may be a bullet ● or it may be a box with a check mark ☑4, depending upon the publisher of your code book. You will find a legend to explain the meaning of each symbol at the bottom of the page in your code book. As you evaluate the options available for the additional character, make certain to place a dot (period) between the third and fourth characters.

Let's take a look at an example together:

☑4 **M17 Osteoarthritis of knee**
   M17.0 Bilateral primary osteoarthritis of knee

The symbol to the left of code M17 alerts you that this code requires a 4th character. In looking at the second line of this example (M17.0), you can see that this fourth character shares additional, important information about the patient's condition. It is not enough to communicate that the patient has been diagnosed with osteoarthritis of the knee. You must explain the specific location (from our example, bilateral = both knees) and specific type of condition (from our example, primary osteoarthritis).

ICD-10-CM codes can be as short as three (3) characters and can add additional characters containing more specificity about the patient's condition . . . up to a total of seven (7) characters. These additional characters ensure that as much detail as possible about the patient's condition is communicated accurately and completely.

> **CODING BITES**
>
> When additional characters are required, those codes with fewer characters are invalid. The need for additional characters is mandatory, not a suggestion.

CODING BITES

You will learn many more details about reporting diagnoses in *Part II: Reporting Diagnoses,* with more in-depth introduction to ICD-10-CM as well as details by body system.

EXAMPLE

The Tabular List shows you which details to abstract from the documentation. All you have to do is keep reading. The portion of the ICD-10-CM Tabular List below shows options for additional characters and the information these characters convey.

S43.3 Subluxation and dislocation of other and unspecified parts of shoulder girdle

  S43.30 Subluxation and dislocation of unspecified parts of shoulder girdle
   Dislocation of shoulder girdle NOS
   Subluxation of shoulder girdle NOS

  S43.301 Subluxation of unspecified parts of right shoulder girdle
  S43.302 Subluxation of unspecified parts of left shoulder girdle
  S43.303 Subluxation of unspecified parts of unspecified shoulder girdle
  S43.304 Dislocation of unspecified parts of the right shoulder girdle
  S43.305 Dislocation of unspecified parts of the left shoulder girdle
  S43.306 Dislocation of unspecified parts of unspecified shoulder girdle

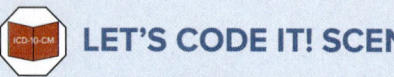

LET'S CODE IT! SCENARIO

MCGRAW GENERAL HOSPITAL

DATE OF ADMISSION: 05/27/18

DATE OF DISCHARGE: 05/28/18

PATIENT: YOUNG, MATTHEW JAMES

HISTORY: Neonate is male, delivered 05/27/2018 at 1915 hours by C-section due to previous C-section. Mother is:

- gravida 2, para 2, AB 1
- blood type B positive
- GBS negative
- hepatitis B surface antigen negative
- rubella immune
- VDRL nonreactive

VITAL SIGNS:
Weight: 6 pounds 9 ounces
Height: 10-1/2 inches
Head circumference: 14 inches

GENERAL:
APGAR = 10 @1 min., 10 @5 min
SKIN: Portwine nevus on right ankle
NEUROLOGIC: Alert, vigorous cry, good tone, nonfocal

DISPOSITION:
The neonate was discharged to his mother. I instructed the mother to phone me PRN. I told her that I want to see both in my office in 10 days for a follow-up.

Let's Code It!

Dr. Michaels delivered Matthew James Young and examined him. Being born is the confirmed reason why the baby needed Dr. Michael's time and expertise. You need to translate the reason *why* into an ICD-10-CM diagnosis code. So, begin in the Alphabetic Index of your ICD-10-CM manual. What should you look up? Matthew needed to be examined right after being born, so let's look up:

Birth . . . nothing here that matches.
Next, try: Newborn. We have a match!
Newborn (infant) (liveborn) (singleton) Z38.2   *pg. 233 in index*

Turn in the Tabular List to this code and begin by reading at the three-character code category:

☑4 Z38 Liveborn infants according to place of birth and type of delivery

> NOTE: This category is for use as the principal code on the initial record of a newborn baby. It is to be used for the initial birth record only. It is not to be used on the mother's record.

You know that Matthew was just born, so this note confirms you are in the right place in the code book. Notes, notations, symbols, and other marks in the code book are there to help point you in the right direction and to support your determination of the correct code.

Our next step is to look at the mark to the left of the code . . . it may be a box with a check mark ☑4, it may be a dot ●, or the following lines may just be indented. However your copy of the code book alerts you, it is clear . . . this code needs an additional character. And this is not a suggestion; it is mandatory.

There are three options for a fourth character:

☑5 Z38.0 Single liveborn infant, born in hospital
Z38.1 Single liveborn infant, born outside hospital
Z38.2 Single liveborn infant, unspecified as to place of birth

You can see in the record above that Matthew was born in McGraw General Hospital and, therefore, Z38.0 is the most accurate.

But we aren't done yet. There is a symbol to the left of code Z38.0. It is telling you that an additional character is required. Let's look at the two options:

Z38.00 Single liveborn infant, delivered vaginally
Z38.01 Single liveborn infant, delivered by cesarean   *pg. 1227*

Go back to the documentation and read the information provided by the doctor. He noted that Matthew was born via a C-section (the C stands for cesarean).

There are no more symbols or notations here in the Tabular List. Next, double-check the **Official Guidelines, Section 1C. Chapter 21, subsection 12) Newborns and Infants** as well as **Chapter 16, subsection 6) Code all clinically significant conditions.** It appears that there are no further details or codes needed . . . so this is the code.

Good job! You were able to determine that code Z38.01 most accurately reports Matthew's birth. You did it!

1.3 Procedure Coding

Once the physician has determined the patient's condition or problem, he or she can then establish a treatment plan. Generally, there are three terms used to describe actions that the physician can take to support a patient's good health or to improve a current condition:

Procedures are actions, or a series of actions, taken to accomplish an objective (result). For example, surgically removing a mole or resectioning the small intestine.

Services are actions that will most often involve counseling, educating, and advising the patient, such as discussing test results or sharing recommendations for risk reduction.

Treatments are typically an application of a health care service, such as radiation treatments for tumor reduction or acupuncture.

Services
Spending time with a patient and/or family about health care situations.

Treatment
The provision of medical care for a disorder or disease.

These actions provided by the physician, or other health care professional, are done for one of three reasons:

Diagnostic tests or procedures are performed to provide the physician with additional information required to determine a confirmed diagnosis.

Preventive procedures and services are provided to keep a healthy patient healthy. In other words . . . to avoid illness or injury. These also include early detection testing, known as screenings.

Therapeutic procedures, treatments, and services are performed with the intention of removing, correcting, or repairing an abnormality or condition.

There are three different code sets available for you to use to translate health care procedures, services, and treatments into codes. These three code sets are

- *Current Procedural Terminology* (CPT)
- *International Classification of Diseases – 10th Revision – Procedure Coding System* (ICD-10-PCS)
- *Healthcare Common Procedure Coding System* (HCPCS) Level II

Current Procedural Terminology (CPT)

CPT codes are used to describe procedures performed by a physician in any location. These services range from speaking with a patient about test results to performing surgery or determining a treatment plan. In addition, CPT codes are used to report the contribution made by **outpatient** facilities (a physician's office, a clinic, an ambulatory surgical center, or the emergency department of a hospital) such as a sterile procedure room, trained nursing and support staff, etc.

The Organization of the CPT Code Book

The CPT book has two parts, which in turn have many sections.

The CPT book (see Figure 1-6) has six sections, which are generally presented in numeric order by code number:

- Evaluation and Management: 99201–99499
- Anesthesia: 00100–01999 and 99100–99140
- Surgery: 10021–69990
- Radiology: 70010–79999
- Pathology and Laboratory: 80047–89398
- Medicine: 90281–99199, 99500–99607

The second part of the CPT book also contains several sections, including

- *Category II codes:* used for supplemental tracking of performance measurements. These codes are not reimbursable but support research on specific physician actions taken on behalf of a patient's health.
- *Category III codes:* temporary codes used to report emerging technological procedures. Technology and health care are innovating and improving every day. These codes enable tracking physician adoption and the frequency of use to identify what should stay and what will be deleted.
- Appendixes A–M: modifiers and other relevant additional information.
- Alphabetic Index: all the CPT codes in alphabetical order by code description, presented in four types of entries (see Figure 1-7):
  a. Procedures or services, such as bypass, decompression, insertion.
  b. Anatomical site or organ, such as brain stem, spinal cord, lymph nodes.
  c. Condition, such as pregnancy, fracture, abscess.
  d. Eponyms, synonyms, or abbreviations, such as Potts-Smith Procedure or EEG.

Outpatient
An **outpatient** is a patient who receives services for a short amount of time (less than 24 hours) in a physician's office or clinic, without being kept overnight. An **outpatient facility** includes a hospital emergency room, ambulatory care center, same-day surgery center, or walk-in clinic.

CODING BITES

CPT codes and sections run, generally, in numeric order; however, there are exceptions throughout. Bottom line . . . *read carefully and completely.*

CODING BITES

More information about Category II and Category III codes will be covered in the chapter *Introduction to CPT.*

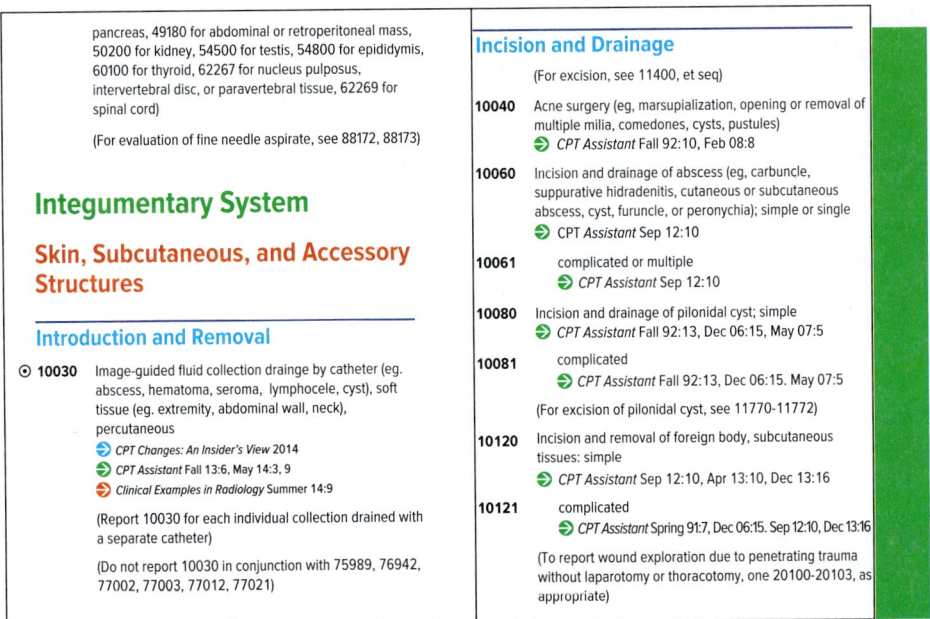

FIGURE 1-6 CPT main section, showing codes 10030–10121 Source: American Medical Association, *CPT Professional Manual*

The Formats of CPT Codes

The codes listed in the various CPT sections each have different structures:

CPT codes (Category I codes) are five-digit codes. They have all numbers (no letters, no punctuation). Example: 51100 Aspiration of bladder; by needle.

Category II codes are five-character codes, with four numbers followed by the letter "F." Example: 2001F Weight recorded.

Category III codes are five-character codes. These codes also have four numbers; however, Category III codes are followed by the letter "T." Example: 0208T Pure tone audiometry (threshold), automated; air only.

Modifiers (listed in Appendix A of your CPT code book) are two characters: two numbers, two letters, or one letter and one number. Modifiers are appended to CPT

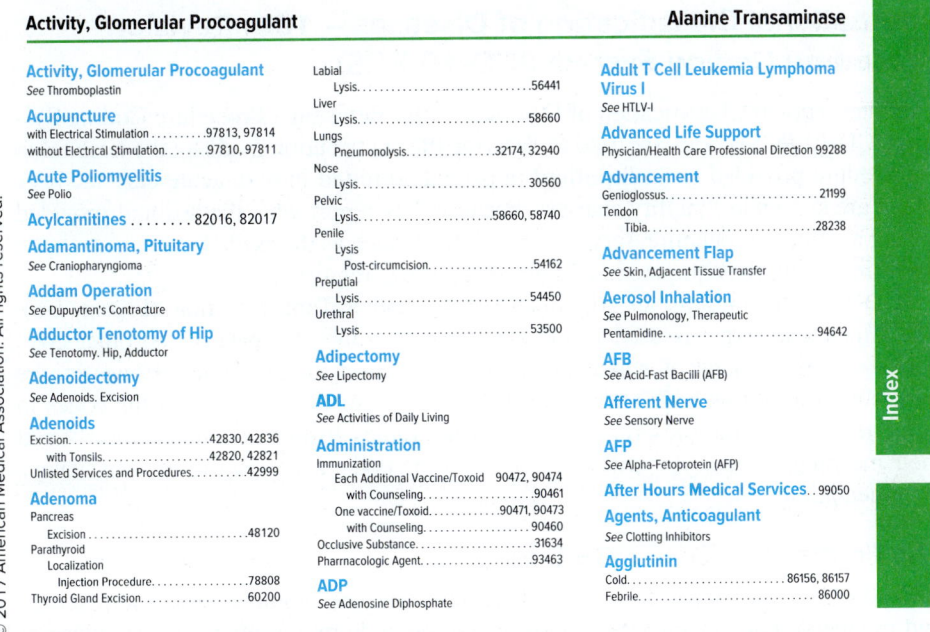

FIGURE 1-7 CPT Alphabetic Index, partial listings from Activity, Glomerular Procoagulant to Agglutinin Source: American Medical Association, *CPT Professional Manual*

CHAPTER 1 | INTRODUCTION TO THE LANGUAGES OF CODING 11

LET'S CODE IT! SCENARIO

Corey Carter, a 55-year-old male, came to the McGraw Ambulatory Surgery Center, an outpatient facility, so Dr. Lucano could perform a percutaneous core needle biopsy on his thyroid. Corey's primary care physician referred him to Dr. Lucano after noting a lump on his thyroid during an annual physical.

Let's Code It!

Open your CPT book to the Alphabetic Index. Which term should you look up? Let's dissect the scenario:

Biopsy = the procedure
Percutaneous core needle = the type of biopsy
Thyroid = the anatomical site

Let's begin by finding Biopsy in the Alphabetic Index:

Biopsy
See Brush Biopsy; Needle Biopsy
Abdomen 49000, 49321

Notice that Abdomen is the beginning of a long list of anatomical sites on which a biopsy can be done. Read down the list to find:

Thyroid 60100

Now, turn into the Main Section of CPT to find code 60100. You can see:

60100 Biopsy thyroid, percutaneous core needle

This matches Dr. Lucano's documentation perfectly—you can report this procedure code with confidence!

CODING BITES

You will learn many more details about reporting procedures in *Part III: Reporting Physicians Services and Outpatient Procedures.*

inpatient
A patient admitted into a hospital for an overnight stay or longer.

codes under special circumstances, such as the use of unusual anesthesia, two surgeons working on the same patient at the same time, or a multipart procedure performed over time. When required, a modifier is added after the main CPT code with a hyphen. Example: 47600-54 Cholecystectomy, surgical care only.

International Classification of Diseases – 10th Revision – Procedure Coding System (ICD-10-PCS)

The International Classification of Diseases – 10th Revision – Procedure Coding System (ICD-10-PCS) codes are used to describe the contribution made by the hospital to a procedure provided to an **inpatient** (a patient admitted into an acute care facility). These are known as "facility charges" because they report what the hospital provided during a specific procedure, service, or treatment, such as the skilled nursing staff, the operating room, the equipment, and whatever else is required.

ICD-10-PCS contains an Alphabetic Index and a Tables section (Figure 1-8). The Alphabetic Index is used in the same way you use this part of the other code books—to get an idea of where in the Tables section to find codes. However, the Tables section of this code set is very different. Rather than a listing of the codes in numeric or alphanumeric order, you will find Tables listing various characters and their meanings. Then, you will actually build the code, according to the physician's documentation.

The Format of ICD-10-PCS Codes

ICD-10-PCS codes have seven (7) characters and are alphanumeric (both letters and numbers). Each of the seven positions in the code represents a specific piece of information relating to a procedure, service, or treatment provided. These meanings

Section	0	Medical and Surgical
Body System	2	Heart and Greater Vessels
Operation	5	Destruction: Physical eradication of all or a portion of a body part by the direct use of energy, force, or a destructive agent

Body Part	Approach	Device	Qualifier
4 Coronary Vein 5 Atrial Septum 6 Atrium, Right 8 Conduction Mechanism 9 Chordae Tendineae D Papillary Muscle F Aortic Valve G Mitral Valve H Pulmonary Valve J Tricuspid Valve K Ventricle, Right L Ventricle, Left M Ventricular Septum N Pericardium P Pulmonary Trunk Q Pulmonary Artery, Right R Pulmonary Artery, Left S Pulmonary Vein, Right T Pulmonary Vein, Left V Superior Vena Cava W Thoracic Aorta	0 Open 3 Percutaneous 4 Percutaneous Endoscopic	Z No Device	Z No Qualfier
7 Atrium, Left	0 Open 3 Percutaneous 4 Percutaneous Endoscopic	Z No Device	K Left Atrial Appendage Z No Qualifier

FIGURE 1-8 Table 025, one of the tables from ICD-10-PCS Tables section

change for each section of the codebook. But don't worry. No memorization is required . . . the code book provides you with what you need to know. All you have to do is read carefully.

For example, in the Medical and Surgical Section, each character reports the:

1. *Section* of the ICD-10-PCS code set.
2. *Body system* upon which the procedure or service was performed.
3. *Root operation,* which explains the category or type of procedure.
4. *Body part,* which identifies the specific anatomical site involved in the procedure.
5. *Approach,* which reports which method was used to perform the service or treatment.
6. *Device,* which reports, when applicable, what type of device was involved in the service or procedure.
7. *Qualifier,* which adds any additional detail.

> **EXAMPLE**
> 0DQ48ZZ Repair of the esophagogastric junction, via natural opening endoscopic
> 0RRJ0J6 Replacement of shoulder joint humeral surface with synthetic substitute, right side, open approach

Whereas in the Imaging Section, each character reports the:

1. *Section* of the ICD-10-PCS code set.
2. *Body system* upon which the procedure or service was performed.
3. *Root type,* which explains the type of imaging, such as MRI or CT scan.
4. *Body part,* which identifies the specific anatomical site imaged and recorded.
5. *Contrast,* which reports if contrast materials were used in the imaging process
6. *Qualifier,* which adds any additional detail.
7. *Qualifier,* which adds any additional detail.

> **EXAMPLE**
> B31M110 Intraoperative fluoroscopy of the spinal arteries, low osmolar contrast, laser
> BB24ZZZ Bilateral CT scan of lungs, no contrast

LET'S CODE IT! SCENARIO

Marlena Takamoto, a 37-year-old female, contracted hepatitis seven years ago. The disease severely damaged her liver. She was admitted to Carolina Brookdale Hospital today so Dr. Lewis and his team can perform a liver transplantation, open approach. The liver donor was killed in a car accident early this morning.

Let's Code It!

The physicians will transplant a liver, using an open approach, from the donor to Marlena. The coder who works for Dr. Lewis will use CPT codes to report his services provided to Marlena. You work as the coder for Carolina Brookdale Hospital, so you need to use ICD-10-PCS to report the hospital's contribution in this surgery (the operating room, the support staff [surgical nurses, technicians, etc.], and other equipment).

The procedure is a transplant, so let's start by looking in the Alphabetic Index in ICD-10-PCS for transplant. In the index, we find

Transplantation
Liver 0FY00Z-

In this particular case, the Alphabetic Index provides you with the first six of the required seven characters. In other cases, you may find the Alphabetic Index will only provide you with three or four characters. Regardless, you must find this Table in the Tables section to complete the seven (7) characters. Using the first three characters provided by the Alphabetic Index, turn in the Tables section to the Table that begins with **0FY** (see below):

Section	0	Medical and Surgical
Body System	F	Hepatobiliary System and Pancreas
Operation	Y	Transplantation: Putting in or on all or a portion of a living body part taken from another individual or animal to physically take the place and/or function of all or a portion of a similar body part

14 PART I | MEDICAL CODING FUNDAMENTALS

Body Part	Approach	Device	Qualifier
0 Liver	**0** Open	**Z** No Device	**0** Allogeneic
G Pancreas			**1** Syngeneic
			2 Zooplastic

Now, with all of this information, let's build the correct code:

1. *Section of the ICD-10-PCS code set = Medical and Surgical 0*
2. *Body system upon which the procedure was performed = Hepatobiliary F*

    Remember, the liver is an organ that is part of the Hepatobiliary System.

3. *Root operation: the type of procedure = Transplantation Y*
4. *Body part: the specific anatomical site involved in the procedure = Liver 0*
5. *Approach: method used to perform the transplant = Open 0*
6. *Device, when applicable = No Device Z*
7. *Qualifier: any additional detail = Allogeneic 0*

Before reporting this code... check the **Official Guidelines,** specifically **B3.16 Transplantation vs. Administration.** This confirms that you used the correct root operation term of Transplantation.

Good job! Now you have built the ICD-10-PCS code for this procedure: **0FY00Z0.**

It would not be unusual for one patient encounter, for a patient admitted into the hospital, to ultimately require interpretation into all three coding languages: ICD-10-CM, CPT, and ICD-10-PCS.

EXAMPLE

Injured in an accident, Terence McCarthy was admitted into McGraw General Hospital with a major contusion of the spleen. Terence was brought into the operating room, he was placed in the supine position, and general anesthesia was administered by Dr. London. Dr. Berring performed a total splenectomy.

Together, let's review all of the codes that will be reported for this surgical procedure:

- The professional coding specialist for Dr. Berring, the surgeon, will report:

    S36.021A   Major contusion of spleen, initial encounter
    38100   Splenectomy; total

- The professional coding specialist for Dr. London, the anesthesiologist, will report:

    S36.021A   Major contusion of spleen, initial encounter
    00790-P1   **Anesthesia for intraperitoneal procedures in upper abdomen including laparoscopy; not otherwise specified**

- The professional coding specialist for McGraw General Hospital, the facility, will report:

    S36.021A   **Major contusion of spleen, initial encounter**
    07TP0ZZ   **Splenectomy, open approach**

HCPCS Level II Procedure Codes

In some cases, you might determine that the CPT code set does not contain a code that accurately and completely reports a procedure or service. It is possible that a HCPCS Level II code may do the job.

> **CODING BITES**
>
> Use a medical dictionary whenever you do not know the meaning of a term:
>
> *Allogeneic* means coming from a different individual of the same species.
>
> *Syngeneic* means coming from a genetic identical, such as from an identical twin.
>
> *Zooplastic* means the tissue or organ is coming from a donor of another species into a human.

> **CODING BITES**
>
> You will learn many more details about reporting inpatient procedures in *Part V: Inpatient (Hospital) Reporting.*

HCPCS (pronounced "hick-picks") is the abbreviation for Healthcare Common Procedure Coding System.

- **HCPCS Level I codes are actually called CPT codes.** While CPT codes are maintained by the American Medical Association (AMA), this code set was adopted by our industry as the first level of HCPCS.
- HCPCS Level II codes are referred to as HCPCS Level II codes.

For the most part, health care services are listed in the HCPCS Level II section titled Procedures/Professional Services (Temporary) G0008–G0151 [but not exclusively, so be certain to check the Alphabetic Index first]. As always, reading carefully and completely is required. However, as you scan the codes and their descriptions in this section of HCPCS Level II, you may find some are very close to CPT code descriptions. But . . . not exactly. Let's look at the simple repair of a 2.1 cm superficial laceration on the patient's left hand being repaired with tissue adhesive.

In CPT, under REPAIR (CLOSURE), the in-section guidelines state: *"Use the codes in this section to designate wound closure utilizing sutures, staples, or tissue adhesives, either singly or in combination with each other or in combination with adhesive strips."*

The definition in CPT of a simple repair includes *". . . requires simple one layer closure."* With this scenario, this would lead to code

12001	Simple repair of superficial wounds of scalp, neck, axillae, external genitalia, trunk and/or extremities (including hands and feet); 2.5 cm or less

Compare this with the most appropriate HCPCS Level II code:

G0168	Wound closure utilizing tissue adhesive(s) only

Which code reports the repair more accurately? You must go back to the documentation and read carefully, looking for the additional details included in the definition of Simple Repair in CPT. Was a one-layer closure performed? Was local anesthesia used? Was anything else done by the physician in addition to the application of the tissue adhesive?

If the answer to any of these questions is Yes, then you need to report the CPT code 12001. If the answers to all of these questions are No, then report G0168.

Let's look at an example that is perhaps a bit less complex. Compare and contrast these two codes, both of which are used for reporting speech therapy services:

92507	Treatment of speech, language, voice, communication, and/or auditory processing disorder; individual
S9128	Speech therapy, in the home, per diem

These two codes report similar services: speech therapy provided to an individual. However, they differ with regard to location, length of the session, and possibly the professional providing the therapy. Be certain to read the CPT in-section Guidelines related to the reporting of 92507 (and other codes in this subsection) before you decide. And, of course, you need to carefully abstract the details within the documentation from which you are coding and compare the specifics to each of the code descriptions, and perhaps to any others available. Then, and only then, can you determine which code to report.

Don't worry . . . one item, one detail, one concept at a time. It will take time, but we are confident you will be able to understand, learn, and master coding for health care services.

1.4 Equipment and Supplies

A large number of components of health care extend beyond what are usually referred to as procedures, services, and treatments you learned about earlier in Section 1.3

CODING BITES

Learn about the other types of HCPCS Level II codes in the section *Equipment and Supplies* in this chapter.

And learn more about the HCPCS Level II code set in the chapter *HCPCS Level II*.

of this chapter. This includes equipment that is provided for a patient's use at home, supplies that are not already included in other codes, and transportation services not described in the CPT book at all. HCPCS Level II also contains codes you can use to report them.

HCPCS Level II codes cover specific aspects of health care services, including

- Durable medical equipment (e.g., a wheelchair or a humidifier).
- Pharmaceuticals administered by a health care provider (e.g., a saline solution or a chemotherapy drug).
- Medical supplies provided for the patient's home use (e.g., an eye patch or gradient compression stockings).
- Dental services (e.g., all services provided by a dental professional).
- Transportation services (e.g., ambulance services).
- Vision and hearing services (e.g., trifocal spectacles or a hearing aid).
- Orthotic and prosthetic procedures (e.g., scoliosis brace or prosthetic arm).

HCPCS Level II codes are listed in sections, grouped by the type of service, the type of supply item, or the type of equipment they represent. However, you should not assume that a particular item or service is located in a specific section. Use the Alphabetic Index (Figure 1-9) to direct you to the correct section or subsection in the Alphanumeric Listing of the code book. One type of service or procedure might be located under several different categories depending upon the details.

Medicare and Medicaid want you to use HCPCS Level II codes; however, not all insurance carriers accept these codes. It is your responsibility, as a coding specialist, to find out whether each third-party payer with which your facility works will permit the reporting of HCPCS Level II codes on a claim form. If not, you should ask for the payer's policies on reporting the services and supplies covered by HCPCS Level II so you don't have a claim delayed or denied.

The Format of HCPCS Level II Codes

The codes listed in the HCPCS Level II code book are all structured the same way: one letter followed by four numbers. No dots, no dashes (Figure 1-10).

A0225	Ambulance service, neonatal transport, base rate, emergency transport, one way
E0130	Walker, rigid (pickup), adjustable or fixed height
J3480	Injection, potassium chloride, per 2 mEq
L0130	Cervical, flexible, thermoplastic collar, molded to patient
V5050	Hearing aid, monaural, in the ear

Cyclosporine, J7502, J7515, J7516
Cytarabine, J9100
Cytarabine liposome, J9098
Cytomegalovirus immune globulin (human), J0850

D

Dacarbazine, J9130
Daclizumab, J7513
Dactinomycin, J9120

FIGURE 1-9 HCPCS Level II Alphabetic Index, partial listing from Cyclosporine to Dactinomycin

FIGURE 1-10 One page from the HCPCS Level II Alphanumeric Listing, showing codes J7512–J7628 Center for Medicare and Medicaid Services (CMS)

CODING BITES

You will learn many more details about using the HCPCS Level II code set in *Part IV: DMEPOS & Transportation*.

LET'S CODE IT! SCENARIO

Rita Widden, a 92-year-old female, was being transferred from Hampton Medical Center to the Sunflower Nursing Home across town. Cosentti Ambulance Service provided nonemergency transportation prepared with basic life support (BLS) services.

Let's Code It!

Cosentti Ambulance Service provided nonemergency BLS (basic life support) transportation for Rita. After looking carefully in your CPT and ICD-10-PCS code books, you find that this type of service is not represented. Therefore, you need to look in the HCPCS Level II code set.

Begin in the Alphabetic Index, and find:

> **Transportation**
> Ambulance, A0021–A0999

This code set often will require some patience as you read through all of the code options, which were suggested by the Alphabetic Index, until you find the one that matches the services for which you are reporting:

> **A0428** Ambulance service, basic life-support, nonemergency transport, (BLS)

Good work! You got it!

Chapter Summary

Essentially, the process of coding begins with the physician's documentation stating why the patient needed care and what was done for this patient during this visit. As a professional coding specialist, you will interpret the documentation in the patient's record from medical terminology into codes: diagnosis codes to explain *why*, along with *how* and *where* if the patient is injured; and procedure codes to report *what* the physician or facility did for the patient during this encounter. You will need to confirm that the diagnosis code or codes support medical necessity for the procedures, services, and treatments provided. As you proceed through this textbook, read carefully and completely. Coding is like nothing you have experienced before, and you want to learn how to be proficient.

CODING BITES

ICD-10-CM ... Diagnosis Codes
- Used by all health care providers and facilities
- Report WHY the patient needed care [medical necessity]
- ICD-10-CM diagnosis codes = A12.3K5A (up to 7 alphanumeric)

CPT ... Procedure Codes
- Used by physicians to report services provided at any/all facilities
- Also used by outpatient care facilities [i.e., ambulatory surgery centers, hospital emergency rooms, hospital outpatient surgery centers, etc.]
- Report WHAT was done for the patient
- CPT procedure codes = 12345 (five numbers always)

ICD-10-PCS ... Procedure Codes
- Used only by hospitals for reporting facility services to inpatients
- ICD-10-PCS procedure codes = 012B4LZ (seven characters always)

HCPCS Level II ... Services and Supplies Codes
- Used to report services and supplies not already represented by a code in CPT [i.e., transportation, drugs administered by a health care professional, durable medical equipment, etc.]
- Used by any facility or provider
- Not all third-party payers accept the use of HCPCS Level II codes
- HCPCS Level II codes = A1234 (one letter, four numbers always)

All review ?'s correct

CHAPTER 1 REVIEW
Introduction to the Languages of Coding

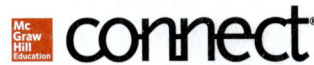

Enhance your learning by completing these exercises and more at connect.mheducation.com!

Let's Check It! Terminology

Match each key term to the appropriate definition.

1. LO 1.3 The provision of medical care for a disorder or disease. C
2. LO 1.2 The state of abnormality or dysfunction. B

A. Classification System
B. Condition
C. Diagnosis
D. Eponym
E. External Causes

CHAPTER 1 REVIEW

3. LO 1.1 The determination that the health care professional was acting according to standard practices in providing a particular procedure for an individual with a particular diagnosis. G
4. LO 1.1 The process of paying for health care services after they have been provided. J
5. LO 1.2 The explanation of how a patient became injured or poisoned, as well as other necessary details about the event; a health concern caused by something outside of the body. E
6. LO 1.1 A physician's determination of a patient's condition, illness, or injury. C
7. LO 1.1 Action taken, in accordance with the standards of care, by the physician to accomplish a predetermined objective (result); a surgical operation. I
8. LO 1.1 The category term used in health care to identify ICD-10-CM, CPT, ICD-10-PCS, and HCPCS Level II code sets. A
9. LO 1.3 A patient admitted into a hospital for an overnight stay or longer. F
10. LO 1.3 Spending time with a patient and/or family about health care situations. K
11. LO 1.3 Health care services provided to individuals without an overnight stay in the facility. H
12. LO 1.2 A disease or condition named for a person. D

F. Inpatient
G. Medical Necessity
H. Outpatient
I. Procedure
J. Reimbursement
K. Services
L. Treatment

Let's Check It! Concepts

Choose the most appropriate answer for each of the following questions.

1. LO 1.1 Coding languages communicate information that is key to which of the following aspect(s) of the health care system?
   a. medical necessity   b. reimbursement   c. resources allocation   **d. all of these**
2. LO 1.1 Coding is accurately interpreting health care terms and definitions into _____ that specifically convey diagnoses and procedures.
   a. letter combinations
   b. number combinations
   c. number-letter combinations
   d. numbers or number-letter combinations
3. LO 1.1 A diagnosis explains
   a. what the provider did for the patient.
   b. who the policyholder is.
   c. why the patient requires attention of the provider.
   d. where the patient was seen by the provider.
4. LO 1.1 A procedure explains
   a. where the patient was seen by the provider.
   b. what the provider did for the patient.
   c. why the patient requires attention of the provider.
   d. who the policyholder is.
5. LO 1.2 Which code book contains all of the codes to report the reason why the health care provider cared for the patient during a specific encounter?
   a. ICD-10-CM code book
   b. ICD-10-PCS code book
   c. CPT code book
   d. HCPCS Level II code book
6. LO 1.2 What part of the ICD-10-CM code book do you use to confirm that a diagnostic code is accurate?
   a. the Alphabetic Index
   b. the Index to External Causes
   c. the Tabular List
   d. the Neoplasm Table
7. LO 1.2 Diagnostic descriptions are listed by
   a. conditions such as fractures.
   b. eponyms such as Epstein-Barr syndrome.
   c. other descriptors such as family history.
   d. all of these.
8. LO 1.2 Which of the following would be an example of an eponym?
   a. infections
   b. wounds
   c. Arnold-Chiari disease
   d. family history

20 PART I | MEDICAL CODING FUNDAMENTALS

9. LO 1.2 The Index to External Causes lists the causes of
   a. injuries and poisoning
   b. diseases and syndromes
   c. injuries
   d. poisoning
10. LO 1.2 An example of an ICD-10-CM code is
   a. H2031
   b. 85460
   c. H61.022
   d. 08NTXZZ
11. LO 1.1 When ICD-10-CM codes support medical necessity, this means that
   a. there was a valid medical reason to provide care.
   b. a preexisting condition was treated.
   c. the patient was seen in a hospital.
   d. a licensed health care professional was involved.
12. LO 1.1 The why justifies the
   a. who
   b. where
   c. what
   d. when
13. LO 1.3 Surgical removal of a skin tag is an example of a
   a. treatment
   b. procedure
   c. service
   d. diagnosis
14. LO 1.3 _____ tests or procedures are performed to provide the physician with additional information to support the determination of a confirmed diagnosis.
   a. Diagnostic
   b. Preventive
   c. Therapeutic
   d. Conditional
15. LO 1.3 The code set(s) available for the coding specialist to use to translate health care procedures, services, and treatments into codes is/are
   a. CPT code book.
   b. ICD-10-PCS code book.
   c. HCPCS level II code book.
   d. all of these.
16. LO 1.3 The main body of the CPT book has _____ sections.
   a. 5
   b. 6
   c. 7
   d. 8
17. LO 1.3 An example of a Category II code is
   a. 89398
   b. 1134F
   c. V95.9
   d. 0241T
18. LO 1.3 The code set used for hospital facility reporting of procedures, services, and treatments provided to a patient who has been admitted as an inpatient is
   a. ICD-10-CM code book.
   b. CPT code book.
   c. ICD-10-PCS code book.
   d. HCPCS Level II code book.
19. LO 1.4 HCPCS Level II codes are presented as
   a. five numbers.
   b. one letter followed by four numbers.
   c. four numbers followed by two letters.
   d. one letter, a dash, and four numbers.
20. LO 1.4 An example of a HCPCS Level II code is
   a. J3285
   b. D7056ZZ
   c. 58940
   d. T84.010D

Let's Check It! Rules and Regulations

Please answer the following questions from the knowledge you have gained after reading this chapter.

1. LO 1.1 Explain what is meant by a third-party payer.
2. LO 1.2 Describe the Tabular List of Diseases and Injuries, including its format and why it is important.
3. LO 1.3 Explain the difference between diagnostic testing, preventive procedures, and therapeutic procedures.
4. LO 1.1 Discuss medical necessity and its importance.
5. LO 1.4 Do all insurance carriers accept HCPCS Level II codes and what is the responsibility of the coding specialist in regards to billing third-party payers?

2 Abstracting Clinical Documentation

Key Terms

Abstracting
Assume
Co-morbidity
Demographic
Interpret
Manifestation
Query
Sequela
Signs
Symptoms

Learning Outcomes

After completing this chapter, the student should be able to:

LO 2.1 Identify which health care professional for whom you are coding.

LO 2.2 Describe the process of abstracting physician documentation and operative notes.

LO 2.3 Recognize the terms used to describe diagnoses in documentation.

LO 2.4 Distinguish between co-morbidities, manifestations, and sequelae.

LO 2.5 Determine those conditions that require external cause codes to be reported.

LO 2.6 Recognize the terms used to describe procedures, services, and treatments provided.

LO 2.7 Create a legal query to obtain documentation about a missing, ambiguous, or contradictory component in the existing documentation.

2.1 For Whom You Are Reporting

Most people do not realize how many coders are involved in reporting one patient's surgical procedure or other type of encounter. Let's look at a scenario and dissect it:

Carly Camden, a 27-year-old female, was admitted into the hospital to have surgery on her broken leg.

- The surgeon will have a coder to report what he does for Carly.
- The anesthesiologist will have a coder to report administration of anesthesia.
- The facility will have a coder to report what the hospital did for Carly (providing the nursing and other support staff, equipment, and room, etc.). In this case, the facility is an acute care hospital. In other cases, the facility may be a same day surgery center, a skilled nursing facility, an imaging center, or another health care organization.
- The radiologist will have a coder to report for any imaging (e.g., x-rays, MRI, CT scan, etc.).
- The pathologist will have a coder to report for any blood work or lab tests provided.

Therefore, the first question you, as the professional coder, will need to ask is . . . for whom are you reporting? Only then will you know which key terms to look for as you abstract the operative notes, the physician's notes, and the reports.

There may also be many professionals providing different types of care for one patient for different reasons. For example . . .

> *Allen Davidson, a 59-year-old male, was admitted to the hospital due to a myocardial infarction (heart attack). Allen has type 2 diabetes mellitus.*
> - A cardiologist (heart specialist) will diagnose and treat Allen's heart problem.
> - An endocrinologist will diagnose and treat Allen's diabetes mellitus.
> - The facility, such as a hospital, will provide care for Allen and all of his health concerns.

For all professionals involved in the care of a patient, the reason or reasons *why* (diagnosis code or codes) care was required are critical to establishing medical necessity for the *what* (specific procedures, services, and treatments) provided. Yet, in a location, such as an acute care facility (hospital), there may be many issues for you to evaluate and connect.

2.2 The Process of Abstracting

You are learning that documentation about the encounter between physician and patient will be your primary source for details that you will use to determine the most accurate codes to report. Physicians, though, do not write their documentation solely for coding; therefore, there will be pieces of information included that you will not use in your coding process. Reading the entire patient record and pulling out the details necessary for determining the correct codes is known as **abstracting**.

Assume or Interpret

Always keep in mind the professional coding specialists' motto: *"If it isn't documented, it didn't happen. If it didn't happen, you can't code it!"*

If it is documented appropriately, there is no reason for you to **assume** any details; you only need to **interpret** what is documented.

One of the most challenging aspects of coding is the very fine line between assuming and interpreting. Yes, professional coding specialists must interpret the physician's documentation. This does not include assuming in any way. Assuming is making up details, filling in the blanks with your own specifics, guessing, or substituting your own knowledge for missing facts. Interpreting is an exact science; it involves changing information from one language to another. Just like *casa* = house (Spanish-to-English), fine needle aspiration = 10021 (medical terminology-to-CPT). This is why coding can be so challenging. We are responsible for not only translating from one language (medical terminology) to another (medical codes) but also for accurately figuring out into *which* language (CPT or ICD-10-CM or ICD-10-PCS or HCPCS Level II) medical terminology must be translated. Another major factor is that no one is a natural-born speaker of medical terminology, so you are required to learn a new language to understand the languages of medical coding. Imagine if you were born speaking English, but you had to learn to speak French before achieving your ultimate goal of interpreting French words into Spanish.

Source Documents

The patient's health care record is at the center of health information management in general as well as the primary focus for you, as the professional coding specialist. Within this record, whether it is written on paper or typed into an electronic health record (EHR), are several important components that you will use to gather details necessary to determine the correct code or codes.

CODING BITES

Patient = *Who* is provided with care

Physician = *Who* is the health care provider you are representing

Diagnosis = *Why* the provider is caring for this individual during this encounter

External Cause = *How* and *Where* the patient became injured

Procedure = *What* the provider did for the individual

Facility = *Where* the services were provided

Abstracting
Identifying the key words or terms needed to determine the accurate code.

Assume
Suppose to be the case, without proof; guess the intended details.

Interpret
Explain the meaning of; convert a meaning from one language to another.

CODING BITE

Keep a medical dictionary by your side so that the minute you come upon a word you don't understand for an absolute fact, you can look it up right away. If you don't understand what you are reading, you will not be able to interpret it accurately.

EXCELLENT RESOURCE: *MedlinePlus,* an online medical dictionary and encyclopedia, is an excellent and reliable source created and maintained by the US National Library of Medicine.

Virtually every patient record should include all, or most, of these pages or sections:

- *Patient's Registration Form:* This document or section includes the patient's **demographic** information, as well as health insurance policy numbers and the name of the individual who will be financially responsible for the patient's care.
- *Referral Authorization Form:* If another physician or health care provider referred this patient for a consultation, you will need to know this to determine the correct evaluation and management code.
- *Physician's Notes/Operative Reports:* Written documentation of what occurred during the encounter between physician and patient is also known as clinical documentation. The physician's notes or operative reports are your most important source for details required to determine the most accurate code or codes. Your job is to interpret the words—medical terminology—into codes. Your ability to interpret accurately is dependent upon your knowledge of anatomy and physiology, as well as medical terminology.
- *Pathology and Laboratory Reports:* Results of testing performed on blood, tissue, and other specimens hold important keys to the patient's condition. The results can provide you with important details necessary for you to determine a specific, accurate code.
- *Imaging Reports:* Similar to pathology reports, these are reports written by a radiologist containing his or her interpretations of images taken of the patient [e.g., x-ray, CT scan, MRI, etc.].
- *Medication Logs:* If the facility is residential, such as an acute care hospital, skilled nursing facility, long-term care facility, etc., the nursing staff must record every time they administer a medication to a patient, including the drug name, dosage, time administered, and route used for administration. All data must be reported.
- *Allergy List:* This list is included for the patient's safety so health care professionals can avoid giving the patient any substance to which he or she may be allergic.
- *History and Physical (H&P):* Essentially, this document, written by the admitting physician, explains the background and current issues used to make the decision to admit the patient into the hospital.
- *Consultations Reports:* When a specialist is asked by an attending physician to evaluate a patient's condition, a report is written and sent over to be included in the patient's medical record in the requesting physician's files, as well as those belonging to the consulting physician.
- *Discharge Summary:* At the time a patient is released from a facility, such as a hospital, the Discharge Summary provides the conclusions and results of the patient's stay in the facility in addition to follow-up advice.

Demographic
Demographic details include the patient's name, address, date of birth, and other personal details, not specifically related to health.

> **CODING BITE**
>
> **Principles of Documentation for Medical Records**
> *Adapted from the Centers for Medicare and Medicaid Services*
>
> 1. The documentation of each patient encounter should include:
>   - the date;
>   - the reason for the encounter;
>   - appropriate history and physical exam in relationship to the patient's chief complaint;
>   - review of lab, x-ray data, and other ancillary services, where appropriate;
>   - assessment; and
>   - a plan for care (including discharge plan, if appropriate).
> 2. Past and present diagnoses should be accessible.

3. The reasons for—and results of—x-rays, lab tests, and other ancillary services should be documented or included in the medical record.
4. Relevant health risk factors should be identified.
5. The patient's progress, including response to treatment, change in treatment, change in diagnosis, and patient noncompliance, should be documented.
6. The written plan for care should include, when appropriate:
   - treatments and medications, specifying frequency and dosage;
   - any referrals and consultations;
   - patient/family education; and
   - specific instructions for follow-up.
7. The documentation should support the intensity of the patient evaluation and/or the treatment, including thought processes and the complexity of medical decision making as it relates to the patient's chief complaint for the encounter.
8. All entries to the medical record should be dated and authenticated.
9. The CPT/ICD-10-CM/ICD-10-PCS/HCPCS Level II codes reported on the claim form should be supported by the documentation in the medical record.

Abstracting the Documentation

Abstracting is the first step in the coding process. You must read all clinical documentation related to the specific encounter all the way through, slowly and carefully. Whether the encounter was a short visit in a physician's office, an hours-long surgical procedure documented in operative reports, or a five-day stay in a hospital, you cannot expect that one sentence will give you a clear and complete picture of *what* occurred (the procedures or services) and *why* they were provided (the diagnosis or diagnoses). You learned about understanding the *why* and *what* in the *Introduction to the Languages of Coding* chapter. You are required to code all conditions documented to be relevant during this encounter or hospital stay, not just those in the official diagnostic statement. The same stands for the procedures.

Reasons That Are Not Illness; Procedures That Are Not Actions

There are times when an individual comes to see a health care provider without having a particular illness or injury. In such cases, you might assign a diagnosis code that explains *why* the patient was seen that is not a current health condition or injury. A healthy person might go to see a physician for preventive care, for routine and administrative exams, or for monitoring care and screenings for someone with a personal history or family history of a condition. As you read through the documentation, you may discover that the reason *why* the encounter was necessary may be wellness, rather than illness or injury.

In the same fashion, the description of *what* the physician provided may not be a procedure, service, or treatment. It may be advice or a second opinion. The physician and patient may meet to discuss previously done test results, a recommendation for a specific treatment plan, suggestions for risk-factor reduction (e.g., stop smoking), or a referral to another physician or facility.

2.3 Deconstructing Diagnostic Statements

Diagnosis codes, for either reimbursement or statistical purposes, will report only those conditions addressed by the provider during a specific encounter and not the patient's entire health history. When there is no confirmed diagnosis to provide

> **CODING BITE**
> One suggestion is to use scrap paper so you can jot down details as you read them, which may point toward *why* the patient required the attention of the physician (e.g., signs, symptoms, confirmed diagnoses), as well as *what* was provided (e.g., specific procedures, services, and treatments).

> **CODING BITE**
> Every health care professional/patient encounter must have at least one reportable [codeable] reason *why* and at least one reportable [codeable] explanation of *what*.

medical necessity for a procedure, service, or treatment performed, determining the diagnosis code to report will vary slightly, depending on whether you are coding for an inpatient or outpatient encounter.

- In an outpatient encounter, if there is no confirmed diagnostic statement, you will code the patient's **signs** and/or **symptoms** that led to the physician's decision for the next step in care.
- When an inpatient (admitted into the hospital) is being discharged without a confirmed diagnosis, you will code the suspected conditions listed on the discharge summary as if they were confirmed. You will not code the signs and symptoms.

Signs
Measurable indicators of a patient's health status.

Symptoms
A patient's subjective description of feeling.

Dissect the Diagnostic Statement

Now that you have identified all of the statements in the documentation that explain *why* the patient was cared for, take each statement apart to determine which word identifies the disease, illness, condition, or primary reason for the visit (also known as the "main term"). Separate this term from any words that may simply describe the type of condition or the location of the condition (anatomical site/body site). Keep a medical dictionary close by so you can look up any terms you don't clearly understand. Remember, if you do not completely understand the terms, how can you possibly interpret them?

Why is the physician caring for the patient? Many diagnostic statements are made up of multiple words, with each providing additional information. As you analyze the examples below, dissect the condition for which the physician is seeing the patient and separate out those terms used to provide more detail about that condition.

- *Herpes zoster* . . . The disease is "herpes" and "zoster" is the type of herpes.
- *Acute bronchospasm* . . . The condition is a "spasm" (muscle contraction) of the bronchus (a part of the lungs) and the term "acute" (which means severe) describes what type of bronchospasm the patient has.
- *Personal history of lung cancer* . . . The issue of concern is "history"—why the patient is being seen. The type of history is "personal" and the secondary descriptor is "malignant neoplasm of the lung (lung cancer)" to explain "a history of what?"
- *Myocardial infarction* . . . The condition is "infarction" (area of dead tissue) and "myocardial" (heart muscle) is the anatomical site of the infarction.
- *Congenital pneumothorax* . . . The condition is "pneumothorax" (air in the chest cavity) and the term "congenital" (present at birth) describes the cause of the condition.
- *Family history of renal failure* . . . The issue of concern is "history"—why the patient is being seen. The type of history is "family" and the secondary descriptor is "renal failure" (loss of function of the kidneys) to explain "a history of what?"

CODING BITE

A diagnostic term might have a suffix like:

Dermatitis	*derma* = skin + *-itis* = inflammation (a condition)
Acrophobia	*acro* = heights + *-phobia* = fear (a condition)

A procedural term might have a suffix like:

Pancreatectomy	*pancreat* = pancreas + *-ectomy* = to surgically remove (an action)
Conjunctivoplasty	*conjunctivo* = conjunctiva (part of the eye) + *-plasty* = to repair (an action)

LET'S CODE IT! SCENARIO

Dr. Olivera diagnosed Kathleen Belsara with ulcerative blepharitis of the right upper eyelid. He treated her with an injection of gentamicin 80mg, IM and gave her a prescription for gentamicin ointment 0.3% q.i.d. for 7 to 10 days.

Let's Code It!

Why did Dr. Olivera care for Kathleen? *ulcerative blepharitis of the right upper eyelid.*

The condition is: *blepharitis*

The type of blepharitis: *ulcerative*

Anatomical site affected: *right upper eyelid*

NOTE: These first three steps will get you started when it comes to determining the correct diagnosis code in ICD-10-CM. You will learn more about this beginning in the chapter *Introduction to ICD-10-CM*.

Also . . .

What did Dr. Olivera do for Kathleen? *an injection of gentamicin 80mg, IM*

The drug: *gentamicin*

The dosage: *80mg*

The route of administration: *IM (intramuscular) injection*

NOTE: These first three steps will get you started when it comes to determining the correct drug code in HCPCS Level II. You will learn more about this beginning in the chapter *HCPCS Level II*.

Recognize Inclusive Signs and Symptoms

As you abstract the documentation, you will need to identify any signs and symptoms that are already part of the description of a confirmed diagnosis. Physicians are trained in medical school to add all of the data (history, signs, symptoms, test results, etc.) together, almost like a math equation, to arrive at a diagnosis. This sign + that symptom = this diagnosis. These equations are based on the standards of care accepted by the health care industry around the world.

Think about it: *John comes to see Dr. Finch. John complains of chest congestion, runny nose, sneezing, headaches, being achy all over. Dr. Finch examines John, does a quick lab test, and tells John he has the flu.*

It is a fact that "chest congestion, runny nose, sneezing, headaches, being achy all over" are signs and symptoms of the flu. Therefore, when you report the code for the flu, there is no reason to also code the signs and symptoms of the flu . . . it is redundant.

GUIDANCE CONNECTION

Read the ICD-10-CM Official Guidelines for Coding and Reporting, section **I. Conventions, General Coding Guidelines and Chapter Specific Guidelines;** subsections

- **B.4** *Signs and Symptoms*
- **B.5** *Conditions that are an integral part of a disease process*
- **B.6** *Conditions that are not an integral part of a disease process*

LET'S CODE IT! SCENARIO

Ralph Carbonna, a 61-year-old male, came into the Emergency Department of McGraw General Hospital. Earlier in the day, Ralph felt lightheaded and a little dizzy. In addition, he complained that his heart was beating so wildly that he thought he may have had a heart attack. When interviewed by the nurse, Ralph revealed his previous diagnosis of type 1 diabetes mellitus, prompting Dr. Geller to order a blood glucose test. Dr. Geller also ordered an EKG (ECG) to check Ralph's heart. After getting the results of the tests, Dr. Geller determined that Ralph's lightheadedness and dizziness were a result of his abnormal glucose level. He spoke with Ralph about how to bring his diabetes mellitus under control and informed Ralph that the EKG was negative [normal], meaning there were no signs of a heart attack.

Let's Code It!

Dr. Geller confirmed that Ralph's *type 1 diabetes mellitus,* specifically his abnormal glucose level, caused his feelings of dizziness. Diabetes seems to be the only confirmed diagnosis in Dr. Geller's notes. You can report this with confidence, and this condition justifies performing the blood glucose test.

Dr. Geller also ordered an EKG (ECG). A diagnosis for diabetes does not provide any medical rationale for doing an EKG. In addition, the test was negative and, therefore, provided no diagnosis.

You still need a diagnosis code to report that there was a medical necessity to run the EKG. Why did Dr. Geller order the EKG? Because Ralph complained of a *rapid heartbeat.* A rapid heartbeat provides the medical necessity for performing the EKG.

Before you confirm any codes, be certain to read all notations and symbols and check the Official Guidelines. Now, you can continue with confidence.

For the encounter, you have one confirmed diagnosis (the diabetes) and one symptom unrelated to the confirmed diagnosis (rapid heartbeat).

GUIDANCE CONNECTION

Read the ICD-10-CM Official Guidelines for Coding and Reporting, section I. Conventions, General Coding Guidelines and Chapter Specific Guidelines; subsection **B.18. Use of Sign/Symptom/Unspecified Codes.** *"If a definitive diagnosis has not been established by the end of the encounter, it is appropriate to report codes for sign(s) and/or symptoms in lieu of a definitive diagnosis."*

Section **II. Selection of Principal Diagnosis,** subsection **H. Uncertain Diagnosis.** *"If the diagnosis documented at the time of discharge is qualified as 'probable', 'suspected', 'likely', 'questionable', 'possible', or 'still to be ruled out', or other similar terms indicating uncertainty, code the condition as if it existed or was established."* NOTE: This guideline is applicable only to inpatient admissions to short-term, acute, long-term care, and psychiatric hospitals.

2.4 Identifying Manifestations, Co-morbidities, and Sequelae

Manifestations

Manifestation
A condition that develops as the result of another, underlying condition.

There are some diseases (also known as *underlying conditions*) that actually cause patients to develop other conditions. This second condition, directly the result of the first condition, is known as a **manifestation**. In these cases, scientific evidence proves that the patient would not have the manifested disease or problem if the first condition had not already been present. The cause-and-effect relationship between the two conditions must be documented by the physician and supported by medical research to be coded as a manifestation.

A manifestation is a second condition CAUSED by a first condition. Let's use diabetes mellitus as an example. Diabetes is known to cause problems with patients' eyes. The physician determined that the patient has diabetic retinopathy with macular edema. This documentation confirms that diabetes CAUSED the retinopathy to develop. You will often find combination codes in ICD-10-CM. These codes report both the underlying condition and the manifestation. In our example, the combination code is

E11.351   **Type 2 diabetes mellitus with proliferative diabetic retinopathy with macular edema**

This one code, E11.351, tells the whole story about this patient's condition. However, not all conditions and their manifestations have combination codes from which to choose. When an appropriate combination code is not available, you will need to select two codes (or more) to clearly communicate the complete story of a patient's diagnosis. One example is a patient who is admitted to the hospital with pulmonary histoplasmosis, a documented manifestation of the patient's HIV-positive status. In this case, there is no combination code, so two codes are needed to tell the whole story of this patient's condition.

B20   **Human immunodeficiency virus**

B39.0   **Acute pulmonary histoplasmosis capsulati**

> **CODING BITES**
> The underlying condition is known as the etiology—the original source or cause for the development of a disease or condition.

Co-morbidities

A **co-morbidity** is a condition that is present in the same body at the same time as another problem or disease, but the two conditions are unrelated—there is no documented cause-and-effect relationship. These "other diagnoses" may be referred to in the physician's documentation. However, only those conditions that the physician has specifically evaluated, treated, or ordered additional testing for or those requiring additional monitoring, nursing care, or more time in the hospital should be reported with a code.

> **Co-morbidity**
> A separate diagnosis existing in the same patient at the same time as an unrelated diagnosis.

EXAMPLE
Lindsey, 28 weeks pregnant, fell and broke her leg. So, the pregnancy and the fracture are co-morbidities—they are two conditions present in the same patient at the same time. You know that being pregnant does not cause a fracture and a fracture does not cause pregnancy.

Which code will you report first? The code that is the reason for the encounter with the physician. You are coding for Dr. Kessler, an orthopedist, and Lindsey comes in because her leg hurts. Dr. Kessler confirms her leg is fractured, so the fracture will be reported first because this is Dr. Kessler's primary concern—caring for the fracture. However, Dr. Kessler MUST take the pregnancy into consideration because pregnancy is a systemic condition and will impact the treatment plan for the fracture. The pregnancy code will also be reported (after the fracture code).

EXAMPLE
Mary-Ellen's history includes asthma. She is here to see the dermatologist to have a benign mole removed from her arm. Dr. Callen does not ask about Mary-Ellen's asthma. The asthma does not have any relationship at all to the benign mole or the care/treatment of the mole. You will only determine the correct diagnosis code for the benign mole. The asthma will NOT be reported at all.

CHAPTER 2 | ABSTRACTING CLINICAL DOCUMENTATION

> **GUIDANCE CONNECTION**
>
> Read the ICD-10-CM Official Guidelines for Coding and Reporting, section **III. Reporting Additional Diagnoses.**

> **EXAMPLE**
>
> Paul's history includes asthma. He is here to see Dr. Hannah, his family physician, for his annual checkup. Dr. Hannah asks Paul about his asthma and writes a prescription for a refill for his inhaler. In addition to the annual exam code, you will also need to report the code for the asthma because the physician paid attention to it during this encounter.

Sequela
A cause-and-effect relationship between an original condition that has been resolved with a current condition; also known as a late effect.

Sequelae

A **sequela** is the residual impact of a previous condition or injury that may need the attention of a physician. When the patient has come to see the health care professional for the treatment of a sequela (also known as a late effect), you must code the particular problem as a sequela only in the following situations:

- Scarring
- Nonunion of a fracture
- Malunion of a fracture
- When the connection is specifically documented by the physician or health care professional confirming the new condition as a sequela (a late effect) of a previous condition

Coding a sequela requires at least two codes, in the following order:

1. The sequela condition, which is the condition that resulted and is being treated, such as a scar or paralysis.
2. The sequela (late effect) or original-condition code with the seventh character "S."

> **EXAMPLE**
>
> Jenna Malaletto, an 18-year-old female, was using a hydrofluoric acid mixture to etch glass for an art class last spring and got some on her left forearm, causing a corrosion burn of the third degree. She came in today to see Dr. Rosen to discuss treatment options for the adherent scarring.
>
> Dr. Rosen is discussing treatment options of the scars that were left behind after the third-degree corrosion burn had healed. This is known as a sequela, and it is the reason for this encounter. However, as you learned, you will also need to report what caused the scar—the corrosion burn.
>
> L90.5   Scar conditions and fibrosis of skin (adherent scar)
> T22.712S Corrosion of third degree of left forearm, sequela

> **CODING BITES**
>
> You will learn a lot more about reporting co-morbidities, manifestations, and sequelae in *Part II: Reporting Diagnoses*.

2.5 Reporting External Causes

You learned in the *Introduction to the Languages of Coding* chapter that in addition to the *why* and the *what*, if a patient is injured, you will need to abstract details about *how* and *where* the patient became injured. As you learn more about determining external cause codes, you will discover that a simple statement such as "the patient was hurt in a car accident" does not contain enough information to determine the accurate external cause code. The details of the accident are very important. For example:

- Was the patient the driver, a passenger, or outside of the vehicle?
- Was the vehicle a car, a pick-up truck, a van, or a heavy transport vehicle?
- Did the vehicle collide with another vehicle, a nonmotor vehicle, or a stationary object?
- Was this a traffic accident or a nontraffic accident?

LET'S CODE IT! SCENARIO

Victor Lamza, a 13-year-old male, was brought into the Emergency Department complaining of pain after he banged his head. Dr. Farxia diagnosed him with a contusion of the scalp. When asked by Dr. Farxia what he was doing immediately before he got hurt, he reluctantly admitted that he had made a bet with his friends at Space Camp. They wanted to see who could stay the longest in the weightlessness simulator; Victor was in there for 6 hours.

Let's Code It!

Dr. Farxia documented that Victor's staying too long in the weightlessness simulator caused the contusion of his scalp. You will need to code *why* Dr. Farxia cared for Victor (his injury), *how* he became injured, and *where* he was when the injury occurred.

S00.03XA	Contusion of scalp, initial encounter
X52.XXXA	Prolonged stay in weightless environment, initial encounter
Y92.838	Other recreation area as the place of occurrence of the external cause
Y93.89	Activity, other specified
Y99.8	Other external cause status (recreation or sport)

There are thousands of different ways a patient can become injured, and there is a different code for almost every incident: the typical, the silly, the unusual, and the surprising.

ICD-10-CM provides a separate *Index to External Causes,* usually found between the Index to Diseases and Injuries (Alphabetic Index) and the beginning of the Tabular List. This index will point you to the correct subsection in the Tabular List, within the code range of V00–Y99.

You will learn more details about how to code external causes later in this textbook in the chapter *Coding Injury, Poisoning, and External Causes.*

2.6 Deconstructing Procedural Statements

In addition to abstracting the terms from the documentation related to the diagnosis code or codes, you will also need to identify those terms that relate to what was done for the patient.

Due to the structure of medical terminology, you might find that the word or term mentioned in the documentation describing what was done for the patient is a combination term identifying both the action taken and the anatomical site on which the action was performed.

EXAMPLES

i. Neuroplasty: *neuro* = nerves + *-plasty* = repair
ii. Thrombolysis: *thrombo* = blood clot + *-lysis* = dissolving
iii. Gastrectomy: *gastr* = stomach + *-ectomy* = surgical removal

Other times, the procedure will be identified by its name. This name may be

- a description of the action, such as ablation, debridement, or injection
- an eponym (named after the individual who invented it), such as Abbe-Estlander procedure, Swan-Ganz catheter, or Dupuy-Dutemps operation
- an abbreviation or acronym, such as ECG = electrocardiography; GTT = glucose tolerance test; PET = positron emission tomography; TAVR = transcatheter aortic valve replacement

CODING BITE

Only the procedures, services, and treatments actually provided during a specific encounter, by a specific physician, health care professional, or facility, will be coded.

Review and practice your medical terminology and keep a medical dictionary close at hand. As you gain more experience, the process of deconstructing the statements in the various types of documentation will become easier (not really easy, but easier). You learned about the part of this career that involves interpreting and you cannot interpret the words if you don't know what they mean.

Interpreting for Each Code Set

You will find that you not only need to understand medical terminology overall to interpret the physician's documentation into codes; each code set may require you to interpret them differently.

LET'S CODE IT! SCENARIO

McGRAW HILL HOSPITAL

DATE OF PROCEDURE: 08/18/2018

PATIENT: Christine Gordon

PREOPERATIVE DIAGNOSIS: Acute right lower abdominal pain.

POSTOPERATIVE DIAGNOSIS: Acute appendicitis.

OPERATION PERFORMED: Laparoscopic appendectomy.

SURGEON: Charles E. Manchester, MD

SEDATION: General endotracheal anesthetic.

PROCEDURE:

This 47-year-old female presented with signs and symptoms consistent with acute appendicitis. Preoperative CT scan indicates an inflamed appendix, rupture not probable. Patient signed written consent for a laparoscopic appendectomy.

Let's Code It!

The documentation created by Dr. Manchester clearly provides us with the details of what occurred during this encounter with this patient, Christine Gordon. She was having lower right side abdominal pain, which was determined to be appendicitis (*why* reported with ICD-10-CM code K35.80 Acute Appendicitis Not Otherwise Specified) and the doctor performed a surgical laparoscopic appendectomy (*what*). Seems very straightforward, doesn't it?

A good place to begin is the CPT Alphabetic Index; look up:

Appendectomy

Appendix Excision. 44950, 44955, 44960

Laparoscopic 44970

Turn to the Main Section of CPT to find code 44970 because Dr. Manchester specifically documented that the appendectomy was done laparoscopically. So, now you have found the correct code to report for Dr. Manchester's work:

44970   Laparoscopy, surgical, appendectomy

--*

Now, if you were the coder for the hospital at which the surgery occurred, you would need to report this same procedure using the ICD-10-PCS code set.

Dr. Manchester performed this surgical procedure on Christine Gordon in the hospital. The hospital provided the support staff (nurses, technicians, etc.), as well as the equipment, the room, etc. You learned earlier that the hospital's coder would use ICD-10-PCS codes to report their participation and care for this patient. Let's look at the documentation again . . .

"the doctor performed a surgical laparoscopic appendectomy"

In the ICD-10-PCS code book's Alphabetic Index, you will see:

Appendectomy
see Excision, Appendix 0DBJ
see Resection, Appendix 0DTJ

Which is correct? The ICD-10-PCS code book includes the definitions right in the front of the code book:

Excision: Cutting out or off, without replacement, a portion of a body part

Resection: Cutting out or off, without replacement, all of a body part

You learned in medical terminology class that appendectomy = surgical removal of the appendix. Therefore, you have documentation that the entire appendix was surgically removed, and this is called *"Resection"* by ICD-10-PCS. Terrific! Now we will turn to the 0DT Table in ICD-10-PCS.

First character: Section: **Medical and Surgical**

This is correct because this was a surgical procedure.

Second character: System: **Gastrointestinal System**

You know this is correct because you learned in anatomy class that the appendix is part of the gastrointestinal system.

Third character: Root Operation: **Resection**

You confirmed this by reading the root operation term definition for "resection" and comparing it with the physician's documentation.

Fourth character: Body Part: **Appendix**

The documentation clearly states the appendix is the body part that was removed.

Fifth character: Approach: **Percutaneous Endoscopic**

The documentation states that this procedure was performed laparoscopically. A laparoscope is an endoscope passed through the skin of the abdomen using small slits (percutaneously). Therefore, you know that this procedure was done using a percutaneous endoscopic approach.

Sixth character: Device: **None**

Seventh character: Qualifier: **None**

Great! So, if you were the coder for the hospital where Dr. Manchester performed surgery, you would report ICD-10-PCS code

0DTJ4ZZ Resection of the appendix, via percutaneous endoscope

Good work!

You can see how the two procedure code sets, CPT and ICD-10-PCS, use different terms to describe and report the same procedure. Use your resources, like a medical dictionary, and you will be able to interpret all of the terms correctly.

2.7 How to Query

Once you have completed abstracting the documentation, you may find that details needed to determine a specific code are not included. Should this happen, you should **query** the physician who wrote the documentation to ask him or her to provide clarification or additional specifics. Every day, coders and health information management specialists find documentation with information that is

- Missing or incomplete
  - for example, *What specific type of fracture?*
- Ambiguous or inconsistent
  - for example, *Procedure notes state a single lead pacemaker was inserted; however, the equipment list states the pacemaker was dual lead.*
- Contradictory
  - for example, *In first paragraph, notes state, "Patient denies any cough or chest congestion."; however, last paragraph states patient was prescribed Tessalon (a cough suppressant).*

In Section 2.2 *The Process of Abstracting*, you learned the difference between assuming and interpreting. Therefore, you will need to ask the physician to add the details you need to the patient's record so you can move forward and determine the correct code. This process is known as creating a query, and it must be done in a very specific manner so as not to break the law.

Writing the Query

Remember that one important use of codes is to determine reimbursement. Different codes are paid at different amounts. [You will learn more about this in the *Reimbursement* chapter.] When writing a query, the law does not permit you to prompt or promote a specific response so you don't inadvertently influence the physician to opt for the higher-paying detail rather than the truth. This means you must ask for the details in a nonleading manner. Asking open-ended questions or providing multiple options for the answer are the best approaches.

Query
To ask; an official request to the attending physician for more specific information related to a patient's condition or treatment.

> **EXAMPLE**
>
> *Dr. Osage saw Jose Ramirez and documented him to have a displaced fracture of the metatarsal bone of the right foot.*
>
> *After rereading the operative notes again, and reviewing the entire patient record, you discover that the detail of which specific bone was fractured is missing. Therefore, you need to query Dr. Osage.*
>
> **Open-ended query:**
>
> Which metatarsal bone was fractured?
>
> **Multiple-choice query:**
>
> Which metatarsal bone was fractured?
>
> A. First
> B. Second
> C. Third
> D. Fourth
> E. Fifth
>
> *-*-*

> Dr. Stabler performed a total hysterectomy on Melinda Blaudon.
>
> After rereading the operative notes again, and reviewing the entire patient record, you discover that the detail of which approach was used to perform the hysterectomy is missing. Therefore, you need to query Dr. Stabler.
>
> **Open-ended query:**
>
> What approach was used in the surgery?
>
> **Multiple-choice query:**
>
> What approach was used in the surgery?
>
> A. Open
> B. Percutaneous endoscopic [Laparoscopic]
> C. Via natural orifice

CODING BITE

Before using an unspecified diagnosis code, query the physician to gain the details needed to use a more specific code. Unspecified or NOS (not otherwise specified) codes should only be used as a last resort when the physician cannot be contacted.

The query you write to request the specific details needed should be accompanied by the pertinent clinical information from the patient's chart. You want to make it clear to the physician what you need clarified or supported with more details. There are many query templates available and often larger organizations have their own versions, already approved by attorneys.

Query Pathways

The specific details will need to be added to the chart in a time-efficient manner; therefore, the way you deliver the query to the physician is important. Most facilities have an existing process for delivering a query to the attending physician. Certainly, in a physician's office or small clinic, it may be easier than in a hospital to connect with the physician to ask a question or questions and obtain a response or responses.

Some electronic health record software programs include a query feature. Alternatively, using a secure, encrypted e-mail system can provide a swift route for asking for the details required as well as a written response. Remember our creed: *"If it's not documented, it didn't happen. If it didn't happen, you cannot code it!"* This reinforces the importance of obtaining those additional specifics in writing from the physician.

For those facilities still using paper patient records, query notes should be attached to the front of charts, so all relevant information about that patient, for that encounter, is at hand and easy for the physician to reference and annotate.

Chapter Summary

In preparation for you to learn the process of determining the specific code or codes, you must be able to gather the required information from the clinical documentation. You must read through the clinical documentation in the patient's record and understand everything you read so you can collect the specifics you need. If details are missing, ambiguous, or conflicting, you will need to query the physician to have the documentation amended. This is your responsibility and a critical part of the coding process.

CHAPTER 2 REVIEW
Abstracting Clinical Documentation

Let's Check It! Terminology

Match each key term to the appropriate definition.

1. LO 2.2 Suppose to be the case, without proof; guess the intended details.
2. LO 2.3 A patient's subjective description of feeling.
3. LO 2.7 To ask; an official request to the attending physician for more specific information related to a patient's condition or treatment.
4. LO 2.3 Measurable indicators of a patient's health status.
5. LO 2.2 The patient's name, address, date of birth, and other personal details, not specifically related to health.
6. LO 2.2 Explain the meaning of; convert a meaning from one language to another.
7. LO 2.4 A cause-and-effect relationship between an original condition that has been resolved with a current condition; also known as a late effect.
8. LO 2.4 A condition that develops as the result of another, underlying condition.
9. LO 2.2 Identifying the key words or terms needed to determine the accurate code.
10. LO 2.4 A separate condition or illness present in the same patient at the same time as another, unrelated condition or illness.

A. Abstracting 9
B. Assume 1
C. Co-morbidity 10
D. Demographic 5
E. Interpret 6
F. Manifestation 8
G. Query 3
H. Sequela 7
I. Signs 4
J. Symptoms 2

Let's Check It! Concepts

Choose the most appropriate answer for each of the following questions.

1. LO 2.1 The first question you, as the professional coder, will need to ask is
   a. does the patient have health insurance?
   b. is there a preexisting condition?
   c. for whom are you reporting?
   d. is this encounter to treat a sequela?

2. LO 2.1 The _____ will have a coder to report for any imaging procedures.
   a. anesthesiologist
   b. radiologist
   c. cardiologist
   d. pathologist

3. LO 2.1 Which of the following is an acute care facility?
   a. The physician's office
   b. A nursing facility
   c. A hospital
   d. An assisted living facility

4. LO 2.2 Converting a meaning from one language to another is called
   a. assuming.
   b. interpreting.
   c. querying.
   d. supposing.

5. LO 2.2 The most important source for details required for the coding specialist to determine the most accurate code or codes is found in which part of the patient's record?
   a. Patient's Registration Form
   b. Referral Authorization Form
   c. Physician's Notes/Operative Reports
   d. Imaging Reports

6. LO 2.2 What is the best way to begin abstracting clinical documentation?
   a. Listen to the nurse explain the encounter.
   b. Read all the way through the clinical documentation for the specific encounter.

    c. Talk to the technician.

    d. Read the patient's registration form.

7. **LO 2.2** Every patient encounter must have at least _____ reportable [codeable] reason *why* and at least _____ reportable [codeable] explanation of *what*.

    a. 1, 1   b. 2, 1   c. 1, 2   d. 3, 1

8. **LO 2.3** All of the following would be considered a diagnostic "main term" except

    a. herpes.   b. acute.   c. spasm.   d. infarction.

9. **LO 2.3** The patient has been diagnosed with hypersecretion of thyroid stimulating hormone. Identify the condition.

    a. hormone   b. thyroid   c. stimulating   d. hypersecretion

10. **LO 2.3** Which official guideline is concerned with conditions that are an integral part of a disease process?

    a. Section 1.B.4   b. Section 1.B.5   c. Section 1.B.6   d. Section 1.B.7

11. **LO 2.4** A manifestation is a _____ condition caused by the _____ condition.

    a. first, second   b. third, fourth   c. second, first   d. second, third

12. **LO 2.4** Coding a sequela requires at least _____ codes.

    a. 1   b. 2   c. 3   d. 4

13. **LO 2.5** External causes explain _____ and _____ the patient became injured.

    a. why, what   b. what, where   c. how, where   d. why, how

14. **LO 2.5** Which of the following would be an example of an external causes code?

    a. H26.053   b. M62.831   c. S00.03A   d. Y92.838

15. **LO 2.6** The suffix *-plasty* means

    a. to dissolve.   b. to repair.   c. to crush.   d. to remove.

16. **LO 2.6** The abbreviation *ECG* stands for

    a. electrocardiography.   b. electroencephalography.

    c. electroconvulsive therapy.   d. electrocautery.

17. **LO 2.7** When you find missing or incomplete information in the physician's notes, you should

    a. place the file at the bottom of the pile.

    b. figure out the information yourself; you should know what the doctor is thinking.

    c. ask a coworker.

    d. query the physician.

18. **LO 2.7** Before using an unspecified or NOS (not otherwise specified) code(s), you should

    a. code the case as unspecified and move to the next file.

    b. assume what the missing information is.

    c. query the physician to gain the details needed to use a more specific code.

    d. leave it for your coworker to do.

19. **LO 2.3** Tom is diagnosed with herpes zoster, conjunctivitis. Which ICD-10-CM diagnosis code would you assign?

    a. B02.9   b. B02.31   c. B02.0   d. B02.1

20. **LO 2.6** Judith presents for a unilateral mammography. Which procedural (CPT) code would you assign?

    a. 77053   b. 77054   c. 77065   d. 77066

Let's Check It! A Diagnosis or Procedure

First, identify the following statements as a diagnosis or a procedure, and then identify the main term.

Example: Factitial dermatosis:

   a. diagnosis or procedure: _diagnosis_   b. main term: _dermatosis_

1. LO 2.3 Sprained wrist, left, initial encounter:
   a. diagnosis or procedure: _diagnosis_   b. main term: _Sprain_
2. LO 2.6 Tympanic neurectomy:
   a. diagnosis or procedure: _proc_   b. main term: _neurectomy_
3. LO 2.3 Acute bronchitis:
   a. diagnosis or procedure: _diag_   b. main term: _bronchitis_
4. LO 2.6 Cerebral thrombolysis:
   a. diagnosis or procedure: _proc_   b. main term: _thrombolysis_
5. LO 2.3 Newborn circulatory failure:
   a. diagnosis or procedure: _diag_   b. main term: _failure_
6. LO 2.6 Laryngeal web laryngoplasty:
   a. diagnosis or procedure: _proc_   b. main term: _laryngoplasty_
7. LO 2.3 Cutaneous abscess of chest wall, initial encounter:
   a. diagnosis or procedure: _diag_   b. main term: _abscess_
8. LO 2.6 Planned tracheostomy:
   a. diagnosis or procedure: _proc_   b. main term: _tracheostomy_
9. LO 2.3 Stenosis of the esophagus:
   a. diagnosis or procedure: _diag_   b. main term: _Stenosis_
10. LO 2.6 Ulna osteomyelitis:
    a. diagnosis or procedure: _diag_   b. main term: _osteomyelitis_

Let's Check It! Rules and Regulations

Please answer the following questions from the knowledge you have gained after reading this chapter.

1. LO 2.2 What is the professional coding specialists' motto? pg. 23
2. LO 2.2 Explain the difference between assuming and interpreting.
3. LO 2.3 Explain the ICD-10-CM Official Guidelines concerning Signs and Symptoms—Section 1.B.4; include where the guideline directs you.
4. LO 2.4 Discuss the ICD-10-CM Official Guidelines concerning Sequela—Section 1.B.10; include where the guideline directs you.
5. LO 2.4 Discuss co-morbidity and the correct coding sequence for the encounter.

The Coding Process

Learning Outcomes

After completing this chapter, the student should be able to:

- **LO 3.1** Implement the six actions of the coding process.
- **LO 3.2** Locate main terms in the Alphabetic Index.
- **LO 3.3** Confirm the accurate code in the Tabular List, Main Section, or Tables.
- **LO 3.4** Apply the Official Guidelines to ensure accurate code determination.
- **LO 3.5** Analyze documentation and code selection to confirm medical necessity.

Key Terms

Alphabetic Index
Alphanumeric
Coding Process
Linking
Main Section
Notations
Official Guidelines
Symbols
Tables
Tabular List

Coding Process
The sequence of actions required to interpret physician documentation into the codes that accurately report what occurred during a specific encounter between health care professional and patient.

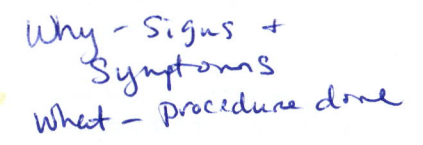

3.1 The Coding Process Overview

There are six specific actions that you should take as part of the **coding process**. As you gain experience, it will take you less time to go through these tasks. However, remember that time is not the number one consideration when coding—no matter what anyone says, accuracy is the most important factor. Following all of these actions every time you code will support your development of habits that will maintain accuracy throughout your career.

Action 1. Abstract the documentation

- Read completely through the documentation for the encounter, from beginning to end.
- Then, reread the documentation and identify the main words regarding the diagnoses (*why*) and procedures (*what*) of the encounter.
- Remember, if the patient was injured, you will need to identify the external causes (*how* and *where*) as well.

Action 2. Query, if necessary

- Make a list of any questions you have regarding unclear or missing information necessary to code the encounter. Query the health care provider who cared for the patient. Never assume or guess. You are only allowed to code what you know from actual documentation. *If it is not documented, it did not happen. If it didn't happen, you cannot code it!*
- Create a query using nonleading questions, with open-ended or multiple-option formatting, to have the physician amend the documentation, so you can use those added details to determine the accurate code or codes. NOTE: In school, your queries should go to your instructor.

Action 3. Code the diagnosis or diagnoses

- Code each diagnosis and/or appropriate signs or symptoms describing *why* the health care provider treated this patient during this encounter, as documented in the notes, to tell the whole story. Use the best, most accurate code or codes available based on that documentation.
- Read the symbols and notations around the code in the Tabular List.
- Go to the Official Guidelines to review any coding rules with which you must comply.

NOTE: Part II: Reporting Diagnoses of this textbook *will share with you everything you need to know to determine the accurate diagnosis code or codes.*

Action 4. Code the procedure or procedures

- Determine for whom you are reporting: physician, outpatient facility, or inpatient facility. This way, you will know which code set to use: CPT or ICD-10-PCS.
- Code each procedure, service, or treatment, as stated in the notes, describing what the provider did for the patient during this encounter. You should not code any procedures that are simply recommended, suggested, or ordered; you can only code those that have already been provided to the patient during the encounter for which you are reporting. Use the best, most accurate codes available based on the documentation.
- Read the symbols and notations around the code in the Main Section. Check for Guidelines (in front of this section as well as in the subsection) to review any coding rules with which you must comply.
- In some cases, you will also need to report a code or codes using the HCPCS Level II code set. You will learn more about this code set in *Part IV: DMEPOS & Transportation.*

NOTE: Part III: Reporting Physician Services and Outpatient Procedures *will share with you everything you need to know to determine the accurate procedure code or codes. This chapter is just an introduction.*

Action 5. Confirm medical necessity

- Ensure that each and every procedure code is supported by at least one diagnosis code to verify medical necessity.

Action 6. Double-check your codes

You, as the professional coding specialist, have a responsibility to ensure that you are submitting only accurate, truthful information, supported by the physician's documentation. Yet, we are all human and anyone can make a mistake. *Now* is the time to build the habit of double-checking your work before you hit that submit button.

- Go back into the code books you have used and reread the full descriptions, all notations, and symbols for the codes you have assigned. Compare these details, once more, with the original documentation—just to be certain you did not misread anything.
- Read carefully, one letter at a time, one number at a time, so you can catch and correct any typos before your work becomes official.

Taking action to code precisely will result in a greater number of your claims getting paid quickly and your reports will represent accurate data. You owe this to your facility, your patients, and yourself.

CODING BITES

One diagnosis code can provide the explanation of medical necessity for more than one procedure code. One procedure code may be provided to treat more than one diagnosis, but there must be at least one diagnosis code to explain why each procedure was medically necessary.

For inpatient settings, the admission into the facility must also be justified—explained by a diagnosis code or codes. You will learn more about this later in this chapter, subsection 3.5 *Confirming Medical Necessity*

CODING BITES

Begin to build the habit, right now, of reading slowly, carefully, and completely. There are so many times, when reviewing a coding error, we have heard, "*Oh, I can't believe I didn't read that!*" It is better for you to find and correct your own mistakes than have anyone else find your mistakes and suffer the consequences.

3.2 The Alphabetic Indexes

Once you have abstracted the main terms that describe the diagnosis (*why*) and the procedure (*what*) from within the physician documentation or operative reports, the next action is to determine the codes that accurately report these details. You will begin by matching those main terms to an entry in the appropriate code book's **Alphabetic Index**.

In the *Introduction to the Languages of Coding* chapter, you learned to connect the details you abstracted from the medical documentation to the correct code set:

- Diagnoses (*why*) = ICD-10-CM code set
- Physicians services (*what*) = CPT code set
- Outpatient facility services (*what*) = CPT code set
- Inpatient (hospital) facility services (*what*) = ICD-10-PCS code set
- Transportation, equipment, drugs (*what*) = HCPCS Level II code set

Each of these code set books includes a section, or part, that is called the Alphabetic Index. Each Alphabetic Index lists all of the main terms that are represented by codes within its set, in alphabetic order (A to Z). So . . .

In ICD-10-CM's Alphabetic Index, you will see terms such as:

Abscess
Carcinoma
Hyperemia
Pneumonia
Shock
Ulcer

In CPT's Alphabetic Index, you will see terms such as:

Angioplasty
Bypass
Discography
Insertion
Psychotherapy
Reconstruction

In ICD-10-PCS's Alphabetic Index, you will see terms such as:

Cannulation
Detachment
Extraction
Laryngoplasty
Repair
Supplement

In HCPCS Level II's Alphabetic Index, you will see terms such as:

Commode
IPPB machine
Nebulizer
Wheelchair

Once you find the main term that matches the word or words that you abstracted from the medical documentation, you may find an indented list containing adjectives providing more detail about that specific main term. It may be an additional description, such as chronic or laparoscopic, or it may be the anatomical site that was involved.

Alphabetic Index
The section of a code book showing all codes, from A to Z, by the short code descriptions.

> **EXAMPLES**
>
> **ICD-10-CM: ABDOMINAL ABSCESS**
> Abscess
>   Abdominal
>
> **CPT: INSERTION OF A GASTROSTOMY TUBE**
> Insertion
>   Gastrostomy Tube
>
> **ICD-10-PCS: REPAIR OF MAXILLA**
> Repair
>   Maxilla
>
> **HCPCS LEVEL II: NEBULIZER FILTER**
> Nebulizer
>   Filter

Often, you will find that further details will be necessary, and options will be provided in another list, indented from the previous indented list.

> **EXAMPLES**
>
> **ICD-10-CM: ABSCESS IN THE WALL OF THE ABDOMINAL CAVITY**
> Abscess
>   Abdominal
>   Cavity
>   Wall
>
> **CPT: PERCUTANEOUS INSERTION OF GASTROSTOMY TUBE**
> Insertion
>   Gastrostomy Tube
>   Laparoscopic
>   Percutaneous
>
> **ICD-10-PCS: REPAIR OF THE RIGHT MAXILLA**
> Repair
>   Maxilla
>   Left
>   Right
>
> **HCPCS LEVEL II: NON-DISPOSABLE NEBULIZER FILTER**
> Nebulizer
>   Filter
>   Disposable
>   Non-disposable

You are required to keep making choices, matching the documentation, all the way to the most specific detail. Once at the most specific level, you will see that the Alphabetic Index will suggest a code or codes.

> **EXAMPLES**
>
> **ICD-10-CM: ABSCESS IN THE WALL OF THE ABDOMINAL CAVITY**
> Abscess
>   Abdominal
>
> *(continued)*

> Cavity K65.1
> Wall L02.211
>
> **CPT: PERCUTANEOUS INSERTION OF GASTROSTOMY TUBE**
> Insertion
> Gastrostomy Tube
> Laparoscopic 43653
> Percutaneous 43246
>
> **ICD-10-PCS: REPAIR OF THE RIGHT MAXILLA**
> Repair
> Maxilla
> Left 0NQV
> Right 0NQT
>
> **HCPCS LEVEL II: NON-DISPOSABLE NEBULIZER FILTER**
> Nebulizer
> Filter
> Disposable A7013
> Non-disposable A7014

You are not done with the coding process yet. These codes will guide you to find the suggested code in the Main Section, Tabular List, or Tables of that code book. You are not permitted, by law, to report a code from the Alphabetic Index without first confirming that it is the best possible option in the Tabular List, Main Section, or Tables.

3.3 The Tabular List, Main Section, Tables, and Alphanumeric Section

Think of the Alphabetic Index as a very cheap GPS mapping app. You cannot count on it to give you accurate information because it is not designed to get you to your precise destination. Sometimes, yes, it will get you to the correct front door. Sometimes, however, it will mistakenly take you to the house down the block, and you will have to look at all of the houses and all of the addresses in the area to see which one is correct. You begin with a suggested code from the Alphabetic Index to get you to the correct neighborhood. However, you cannot report this code until you have confirmed it is correct and complete, using the ICD-10-CM's **Tabular List**, CPT's **Main Section**, ICD-10-PCS's **Tables** section, or HCPCS Level II's **Alphanumeric Section** of the appropriate code book.

These sections list all of the codes available in that code set, only this time, they are listed in numeric or **alphanumeric** order by the code first, followed by the words describing exactly what that code represents. Here, you will find several things to help you get to absolute accuracy.

Full Code Descriptions

In these sections, you will be able to read the full code description, not the shortened version used in the Alphabetic Index. Let's continue with our examples from the previous section, 3.2 *The Alphabetic Indexes:*

> **EXAMPLE**
>
> **ICD-10-CM**
> *The Alphabetic Index gave you:*
>
> Abscess, Abdominal, Cavity K65.1
> Abscess, Abdominal, Wall L02.211
>
> *(continued)*

CODING BITES

The Main Section and Tabular List of the code books all contain additional **symbols** and **notations** to help you determine the most accurate code. The book actually can help you determine the accurate code or codes!

More about these in chapters later in this book.

Symbols
Marks, similar to emojis, that provide additional direction to use codes correctly and accurately.

Notations
Alerts and warnings that support more accurate use of codes in a specific code set.

Tabular List of Diseases and Injuries
The section of the ICD-10-CM code book listing all of the codes in alphanumeric order.

Main Section
The section of the CPT code book listing all of the codes in numeric order.

Tables
The section of the ICD-10-PCS code book listing all of the codes in alphanumeric order, based on the first three characters of the code.

Alphanumeric Section
The section of the HCPCS Level II code book listing all of the codes in alphanumeric order.

alphanumeric
Containing both letters and numbers.

> *The Tabular List gives you:*
>
> > K65.1 Peritoneal abscess (mesenteric abscess)
> > L02.211 Cutaneous abscess of abdominal wall
>
> **CPT**
> *The Alphabetic Index gave you:*
>
> > Insertion, Gastrostomy Tube, Laparoscopic 43653
> > Insertion, Gastrostomy Tube, Percutaneous 43246
>
> *In the Main Section, you will read:*
>
> > 43653 Laparoscopy, surgical; gastrostomy, without construction of gastric tube (e.g. Stamm procedure)
> > 43246 Esophagogastroduodenoscopy, flexible, transoral; with directed placement of percutaneous gastrostomy tube
>
> **ICD-10-PCS**
> *The Alphabetic Index gave you:*
>
> > Repair, Maxilla, Left 0NQS
> > Repair, Maxilla, Right 0NQR
>
> *In the Tables Section, you must build the code out to seven (7) characters based on the additional details in the operative notes:*
>
> > 0NQS0ZZ Repair of maxilla, left side, open approach
> > 0NQRXZZ Repair of maxilla, right side, external approach
>
> **HCPCS LEVEL II**
> *The Alphabetic Index gave you:*
>
> > Nebulizer, Filter, Disposable A7013
> > Nebulizer, Filter, Non-disposable A7014
>
> *In the Alphanumeric List, you will read:*
>
> > A7013 Filter, disposable, used with aerosol compressor or ultrasonic generator
> > A7014 Filter, non-disposable, used with aerosol compressor or ultrasonic generator

Look at all the additional details provided in the complete code descriptions. As you can see with just our few examples, there are specifics that may require you to go back to the documentation to confirm these additional details are still accurate. While you are here, you also need to read the complete code descriptions for all of the other codes in this code category. It is not uncommon that you may find another code that is a better match for the documentation.

Conventions (Notations and Symbols)

In addition to full code descriptions, you will also find conventions (notations and symbols) in the Tabular List (ICD-10-CM) and Main Section (CPT) that include tips and hints pointing you toward the correct code. This section is a preview of more in-depth discussions about symbols that will come in future chapters. So, for now, just a little glance.

ICD-10-CM

In the Tabular List above K65.1 is a notation that states:
> *Use additional code* to identify infectious agent
> > K65.1 Peritoneal abscess (mesenteric abscess)

A "*Use additional code*" notation reminds you that you will need to include a second code reporting the detail identified in the notation. This notation helps you ensure you are reporting complete information about a patient's diagnosis that will support medical necessity for the appropriate treatment.

CPT

In the Main Section to the left of code 97803 is a star symbol:

★97803   Medical nutrition therapy; re-assessment and intervention, individual, face-to-face with the patient, each 15 minutes

Both at the bottom of the page in CPT and in the "Introduction" in the front of the CPT code book, you can see that this symbol ★ informs you, the coder, that if this service was provided using audio/video synchronous equipment (i.e., Skype, FaceTime), you will need to append modifier 95 to this code. This small symbol helps you avoid committing fraud.

ICD-10-PCS

The majority of the codes suggested in the Alphabetic Index of ICD-10-PCS are not complete codes. This fact will not let you forget that you have to go into the Tables section to build the code out to seven (7) characters (based on the additional details in the operative notes). To report a complete, valid code, you must go into the Tables section.

0NQS0ZZ Repair of maxilla, left side, open approach

0NQRXZZ Repair of maxilla, right side, external approach

NOTE: Even in those occasions when the Alphabetic Index provides you with all seven characters for the code, you still should go to the appropriate Table to confirm. It will only take a few seconds, and you can be certain you are reporting the complete and accurate code.

HCPCS LEVEL II

In the Alphanumeric Section, to the left of code J8705 is a symbol:

☑   J8705 Topotecan, oral, 0.25mg

The symbol ☑, in some versions of the HCPCS Level II book, alerts you that this code description includes a specific quantity. When seeing this, you should confirm the quantity documented with the quantity in the code description. The code may need to be reported multiple times.

> **CODING BITES**
> You will learn more about ICD-10-CM conventions, notations, and symbols in the chapter titled *Introduction to ICD-10-CM*.

> **CODING BITES**
> You will learn more about CPT conventions, notations, and symbols in the chapter titled *Introduction to CPT*.

> **CODING BITES**
> You will learn more about ICD-10-PCS conventions in the chapter titled *Introduction to ICD-10-PCS*.

> **CODING BITES**
> You will learn more about HCPCS Level II conventions, notations, and symbols in the chapter titled *HCPCS Level II*.

3.4 The Official Guidelines

With all these code sets and all these codes, you can see that the process to get from documentation to code is more complicated than simply finding a word here and a code there. Coding is important work, so you want to get it accurate every time. To accomplish this, it is essential to have help and support exactly when you need it. And you have that help right at your fingertips within each code set's book. Always there, just the turn of a few pages, is the guidance from those who created these code sets and who oversee their legal and correct use. These are the published **Official Guidelines** with which you must comply. You don't need to memorize them; you just need to remember they are there and refer to them every time you are working to determine a code.

Official Guidelines
A listing of rules and regulations instructing how to use a specific code set accurately.

ICD-10-CM

Usually in the front of this code book, you will find the section titled "***ICD-10-CM Official Guidelines for Coding and Reporting.***"

CPT

In the front of each individual main section, you will find the guidelines applicable to that part of the CPT codes. So, in front of the *Evaluation and Management (E/M) Services* codes are the pages containing the ***Evaluation and Management (E/M) Services Guidelines;*** in front of the *Anesthesia* code section are the ***Anesthesia Guidelines;*** etc.

In addition, it is important to note that the CPT book also includes official guidelines within the sections, at some subsections, with advice and direction for accurate coding of just those procedures, services, and treatments. This means you must get in the habit of reading from the beginning of each section *and* the beginning of the subsection before determining a code. It only takes a few seconds and it can make the difference between accuracy and fraudulent reporting.

ICD-10-PCS

Usually in the front of this code book, you will find the section titled "***ICD-10-PCS Official Guidelines for Coding and Reporting.***"

Guidance Connection

Throughout this book, you will see special boxes titled **GUIDANCE CONNECTION** that will point you to a specific guideline in that particular code set directly related to whatever concept or aspect is being discussed. Take a minute and turn to that Guideline in your personal code book and read it, think about it, and identify how you would apply this guideline to your work as a professional coding specialist. There is no need to memorize these details because they will always be there for you, right inside your code book, at your fingertips.

LET'S CODE IT! SCENARIO

DATE OF PROCEDURE: 08/18/2018
PATIENT: ARTHUR FERGUSON
PREOPERATIVE DIAGNOSIS: Acute upper abdominal pain
POSTOPERATIVE DIAGNOSIS: Liver tumor
OPERATION PERFORMED: Diagnostic laparoscopy; Laparoscopic ablation, using radiofrequency
SURGEON: Harrison Brusk, MD
SEDATION: General endotracheal anesthetic
ESTIMATED BLOOD LOSS: Minimal.
COMPLICATIONS: None.

INDICATIONS FOR PROCEDURE:

This 57-year-old male presented with signs and symptoms consistent with liver malfunction. Laparoscopic investigation to confirm suspected liver tumor, and if so, ablation. The informed consent form was signed.

DESCRIPTION OF OPERATION:

The patient was brought to the operating room and placed in a supine position on the operating table. After administration of general anesthetic, I prepped and draped the upper abdomen in the usual sterile fashion.

A small incision was made into the umbilicus through which a bladeless 11 mm trocar was inserted without difficulty. After the pneumo-peritoneum was established, the patient was moved into the Trendelenburg position. Two additional 5 mm trocar insertions were made. The liver was visualized and two tumors were identified, one on the

(continued)

distal portion of the liver and one on the proximal surface. The diagnostic laparoscopy was then converted to a surgical procedure so we could remove the tumors. Using radiofrequency techniques, both tumors were successfully ablated.

Let's Code It!

The documentation created by Dr. Brusk clearly provides us with the details of what occurred during this encounter with this patient, Arthur Ferguson. He was having upper abdominal pain that was determined to be two liver tumors (*why* reported with ICD-10-CM code *D13.4 Benign neoplasm of liver*) and the doctor performed a diagnostic laparoscopy, followed by a surgical laparoscopic ablation of liver tumors (*what*). Seems very straightforward, doesn't it?

A good place to begin: in the CPT Alphabetic Index, look up:

> **Ablation**
> Liver (Tumor)
> Cryosurgical.............................. 47381, 47383
> Laparoscopic 47370, 47371
> Radiofrequency....................... 47380-47382

Turn to the Main Section of CPT to find code 47370 because Dr. Brusk specifically documented that the ablation was done laparoscopically. Directly above code 47370 are some official guidelines that provide important direction:

"Surgical laparoscopy always includes diagnostic laparoscopy. To report a diagnostic laparoscopy (peritoneoscopy) (separate procedure), use 49320."

Without this direction, you might have gone to the trouble to report both 49320 and 47370. So, now you saved yourself some time and found the correct code to report for Dr. Brusk's work:

> **47370   Laparoscopy, surgical, ablation of 1 or more liver tumor(s); radiofrequency**

If you had reported both codes, this could constitute overcoding—which would be fraud.

See . . . the Guidelines help you code accurately, and legally.

Good work!

3.5 Confirming Medical Necessity

No one believes physicians or other health care professionals should be permitted to do whatever they want to a patient without a valid reason. In our industry, this valid reason is known as medical necessity, and you learned about it in the *Introduction to the Languages of Coding* chapter. The code or codes that you report to identify the reasons *why* the patient required the attention of a health care professional justify *what* the physician or health care professional did to the patient or for the patient . . . but only when they are in accordance with the standards of care.

Outpatient Settings

In an outpatient setting, once you have determined the accurate diagnosis codes and procedure codes, you must confirm that you are reporting at least one diagnosis code to identify medical necessity by **linking** it to at least one procedure code. Multiple procedure codes can link to one diagnosis code, and multiple diagnosis codes can link to one procedure code. But there must be at least one of each to support the encounter.

Linking
Confirming medical necessity by pairing at least one diagnosis code to at least one procedure code.

You must take this action to ensure that the diagnosis codes you are reporting accurately represent the documented reasons *why* the physician made the decisions he or she made and provided care to this patient, based on those reasons. You must make certain you did not miss anything in the documentation. You must make certain you did not jot down, or enter, the code incorrectly [a typo?].

LET'S CODE IT! SCENARIO

Ahmed Obodeh, a 23-year-old male, came in to see Dr. Starkey because he hit his head on a cabinet and has had a headache for 2 days nonstop. Dr. Starkey examined Ahmed and ordered an MRI of his brain to be taken. Just before the nurse took him down to imaging, Ahmed told Dr. Starkey that he also banged his left knee and was having pain when walking. So Dr. Starkey told the nurse to have radiology take an x-ray of his left knee while he was there. Afterwards, Dr. Starkey gave Ahmed instructions for care of a mild concussion, and suggested an ace bandage for his knee and over-the-counter pain relievers for 1 week.

Let's Code It!

Dr. Starkey diagnosed Ahmed with a mild concussion and provided an MRI of the brain and an x-ray of the left knee. Let's analyze this. The concussion is a traumatic impact of the brain and skull. This matches with the MRI of the brain. Perfect.

But there is no diagnosis to justify the x-ray of the knee. Did Dr. Starkey order an unnecessary test? Was he trying to cheat the insurance company and take advantage of Ahmed? No. He is a good doctor and he was doing a good job by ordering the x-ray of Ahmed's knee. How will you communicate that he was properly caring for his patient?

Go back to the documentation. What was written about Ahmed's knee? *"was having pain when walking"* The report of pain by a patient is a symptom and a valid reason for the provision of an x-ray. Therefore, you will determine the diagnosis code to explain that pain in the knee was the medical necessity.

Diagnosis		Procedure
Brain concussion [S06.0X0A]	–Links to–	MRI brain [70551]
Pain in left knee [M25.562]	–Links to–	X-ray of knee, left [73560-LT]

You are really learning!

Inpatient Setting

In an inpatient setting, the diagnosis code or codes reported must support the medical necessity for the patient to require acute care in a hospital setting—24-hour care from trained health care professionals.

For example, *uncomplicated mild intermittent asthma* [J45.20], occasional narrowing of the bronchi causing diminished breathing, relieved with a prescription inhaler, is not a reason to admit a patient into the hospital to receive round-the-clock care; however, *mild intermittent asthma with status asthmaticus* [J45.22], a life-threatening asthma attack that is not responding to normal treatments such as an inhaler or nebulizer, certainly might be.

LET'S CODE IT! SCENARIO

DATE OF ADMISSION: 09/18/2018
ADMITTING DIAGNOSIS: Suspected bowel obstruction
CHIEF COMPLAINT: Severe abdominal pain, vomiting, bloating

(continued)

> **HISTORY OF PRESENT ILLNESS:** Patient is a 29-year-old male with a history of Crohn's disease of the large intestine. The patient came to the ER for an episode of vomiting, continuous, 36 hours. Patient states crampy abdominal pain and bloating. Abdominal ultrasound shows thickening of the bowel wall resulting in acute stricture of the descending colon. Patient is admitted with suspected Crohn's disease with bowel obstruction. Consult with gastroenterology is requested.
>
> ### Let's Code It!
>
> The admitting diagnosis appears to be clear:
>
> **K50.112   Crohn's disease of large intestine with intestinal obstruction**
>
> You could see the problem getting reimbursed for this hospital stay if, by mistake, this code was reported:
>
> **K50.10   Crohn's disease of large intestine without complications**
>
> The little details are important!

Chapter Summary

In this chapter, you learned how to take the data culled from the physician's documentation and interpret the data into another language, a medical code (ICD-10-CM, CPT, HCPCS Level II, or ICD-10-PCS). Following each and every one of the six actions required will help you ensure that you are accurately interpreting what occurred between physician and patient during a specific encounter or during a patient's stay in a hospital. In the next part of this book, you will delve more deeply into diagnosis coding using the language of ICD-10-CM.

> ### CODING BITES
>
> Action 1. Abstract the documentation
> Action 2. Query, if necessary
> Action 3. Code the diagnosis or diagnoses
> Action 4. Code the procedure or procedures
> Action 5. Confirm medical necessity
> Action 6. Double-check your codes

CHAPTER 3 REVIEW
The Coding Process

Let's Check It! Terminology

Match each key term to the appropriate definition.

1. LO 3.2 The section of a code book showing codes, from A to Z, by the short code descriptions.
2. LO 3.3 The section of the ICD-10-PCS code book listing all of the codes in alphanumeric order, based on the first three characters of the code.
3. LO 3.1 The sequence of actions required to interpret physician documentation into the codes that accurately report what occurred during a specific encounter between health care professional and patient.
4. LO 3.3 A code consisting of both numbers and letters.
5. LO 3.5 Confirming medical necessity by pairing at least one diagnosis code to at least one procedure code.
6. LO 3.3 The section of the CPT code book listing all of the codes in numeric order.
7. LO 3.4 A listing of rules and regulations instructing how to use a specific code set accurately.
8. LO 3.2 Alerts and warnings that support more accurate use of codes in a specific code set.
9. LO 3.2 Marks, similar to emojis, that provide additional direction to use codes correctly and accurately.
10. LO 3.3 The section of the ICD-10-CM code book listing all of the codes in alphanumeric order.

A. Alphabetic Index — 1
B. Alphanumeric — 4
C. Coding Process — 3
D. Official Guidelines — 7
E. Linking — 5
F. Main Section — 6
G. Notations — 8
H. Symbols — 9
I. Tables — 2
J. Tabular List — 10

Let's Check It! Concepts

Choose the most appropriate answer for each of the following questions.

1. LO 3.1 There are _____ specific actions that you should take to construct your proper coding process.
    a. 3
    b. 4
    c. 5
    d. 6
2. LO 3.1 The most important factor in coding is
    a. speed of the coding process.
    b. accuracy of codes.
    c. level of codes
    d. quantity of codes.
3. LO 3.1 *Abstract the documentation* is Action _____ in the coding process.
    a. 1
    b. 2
    c. 3
    d. 4
4. LO 3.1 Action 5 in the coding process is to
    a. code the diagnosis or diagnoses.
    b. code the procedure or procedures.
    c. confirm medical necessity.
    d. double-check your codes.
5. LO 3.1 Every encounter between patient and health care professional must have at least _____ diagnosis code(s) and at least _____ procedure code(s).
    a. 2, 2
    b. 1, 2
    c. 1, 1
    d. 2, 1
6. LO 3.2 After abstracting the main terms, a coder will go next to the
    a. External cause codes.
    b. Tabular listings.
    c. Alphabetic Index.
    d. Appendix C.

50   PART I | MEDICAL CODING FUNDAMENTALS

7. **LO 3.2** Pneumonia would be an example of a term found in which Alphabetic Index?
   a. ICD-10-CM
   b. CPT
   c. ICD-10-PCS
   d. HCPCS Level II

8. **LO 3.2** IPPB machine would be an example of a term found in which Alphabetic Index?
   a. ICD-10-CM
   b. CPT
   c. ICD-10-PCS
   d. HCPCS Level II

9. **LO 3.2** The Main Section and Tabular List of the code books all contain additional _____ and _____ to help you determine the most accurate code.
   a. notations, modifiers
   b. symbols, notations
   c. figures, icons
   d. transformers, symbols

10. **LO 3.3** Which of the following code books lists the codes in numeric order?
    a. ICD-10-CM
    b. HCPCS Level II
    c. CPT
    d. ICD-10-PCS

11. **LO 3.3** Which of the following is a full code description?
    a. Carbuncle of trunk L02.23
    b. Furuncle of trunk L02.22
    c. Cutaneous abscess of chest wall L02.213
    d. Impetigo L01.0

12. **LO 3.3** In the ICD-10-CM Tabular List above code K70.31 there is a notation. What is the notation?
    a. Use additional code to identify alcohol abuse and dependence
    b. Code first underlying diseases
    c. Code also, if applicable, viral hepatitis
    d. Code first poisoning due to drug or toxin, if applicable

13. **LO 3.3** If you see this symbol ✚ in the CPT code book's main section beside a code, it tells you that
    a. the code is a revised code.
    b. moderate sedation is included in this code.
    c. the code is an add-on code.
    d. the code is a new code.

14. **LO 3.3** Which code set requires you, the coder, to build the code out to seven characters?
    a. ICD-10-CM
    b. HCPCS Level II
    c. CPT
    d. ICD-10-PCS

15. **LO 3.3** What is the correct ICD-10-PCS code for the Repair of maxilla, left side, open approach?
    a. 0NQT0ZZ
    b. 0NQRXZZ
    c. 0NQR0ZZ
    d. 0NQV0ZZ

16. **LO 3.3** What is the correct CPT code for a Laparoscopy, surgical; gastrostomy, without construction of gastric tube?
    a. 43246
    b. 43653
    c. 48001
    d. 43246

17. **LO 3.4** Official _____ are a listing of rules and regulations instructing you how to use a specific code set accurately.
    a. guidelines
    b. linking
    c. tables
    d. appendix

18. **LO 3.4** The official guidelines for ICD-10-CM can usually be found in the
    a. back of the code book.
    b. Alphabetic Index.
    c. Tabular List.
    d. front of the code book.

19. **LO 3.5** The why justifies the _____
    a. where.
    b. who.
    c. what.
    d. when.

20. LO 3.5 _____ confirm(s) medical necessity by pairing at least one diagnosis code to at least one procedure code.
  a. Tables
  b. Linking
  c. Guidelines
  d. Appendix

Let's Check It! Guidelines

Part I
Refer to the ICD-10-CM Official Guidelines and match each section number to the corresponding guideline.

1. Diagnostic Coding and Reporting Guidelines for Outpatient Services.
2. Selection of Principal Diagnosis.
3. Conventions, general coding guidelines and chapter specific guidelines.
4. Reporting Additional Diagnoses.

A. Section I 3
B. Section II 2
C. Section III 4
D. Section IV 1

Part II
Refer to the ICD-10-CM Official Guidelines and match each section number to the corresponding guideline.

1. LO 3.4 Sequela (Late Effects)
2. LO 3.4 Format and Structure
3. LO 3.4 Abbreviations – Tabular List abbreviations
4. LO 3.4 Etiology/manifestation convention ("code first", "use additional code" and "in diseases classified elsewhere" notes)
5. LO 3.4 "Code Also" note
6. LO 3.4 Conditions that are an integral part of a disease process
7. LO 3.4 Placeholder character
8. LO 3.4 Conditions that are not an integral part of a disease process
9. LO 3.4 Signs and symptoms
10. LO 3.4 Laterality

A. Section 1.A.2 2
B. Section 1.A.4 7
C. Section 1.A.6.b 3
D. Section 1.A.13 4
E. Section 1.A.17 5
F. Section 1.B.4 9
G. Section 1.B.5 6
H. Section 1.B.6 8
I. Section 1.B.10 1
J. Section 1.B.13 10

Let's Check It! Rules and Regulations

Please answer the following questions from the knowledge you have gained after reading this chapter.

1. LO 3.1 List the six Actions of the coding process and explain each action in your own words.
2. LO 3.2 Discuss the Alphabetic Index and the role it plays in the coding process.
3. LO 3.3 Explain the ICD-10-CM Tabular List, how the codes are listed, and why it is important.
4. LO 3.4 Describe what the Official Guidelines are, why they are important, where they are located, and if you are required to comply with these guidelines.
5. LO 3.5 Discuss the importance of linking a diagnosis code to a procedure code.

PART II

REPORTING DIAGNOSES

INTRODUCTION

For the second layer of your learning, you will focus on interpreting and reporting the key terms and details about the diagnoses, signs, and symptoms—the reasons *why* the physician provided care to the patient during a specific encounter. As you learned in Part I of this book, this is known as medical necessity.

The concept of medical necessity is as simple as it sounds—the determination that a medical procedure, service, or treatment needed to be provided to a patient because of an identified health care issue or concern. Overall, the industry uses the accepted standards of care by which to measure the rationale—the justification—for every action taken on behalf of an individual patient.

For example, atrial fibrillation [irregular heart beats in the upper chambers of the heart] may be a diagnosis that supports the insertion of a pacemaker; however, ventricular fibrillation [irregular heart beats in the lower chambers of the heart] does not. A diagnosis of dysphasia [problems with speech] justifies the provision of a speech evaluation; however, a diagnosis of dysphagia [problems with swallowing] does not. The physician's confirmation of a hydrocele [collection of fluid in tunica vaginalis, spermatic cord, or testis] can only be diagnosed in a male patient and the determination of a hematometra [accumulated blood in the uterus] can only be diagnosed in a female.

When you think about it—why would anyone pay for, or accept, the provision of medical treatment to patients who do not need treatment? The way you will explain that the physician's actions were reasonable and correct is by reporting the accurate diagnosis code or codes.

4 Introduction to ICD-10-CM

International Classification of Diseases - 10th Revision Clinical Modification

Key Terms

Acute
Adverse Effect
Alphabetic Index
Anatomical Site
Chronic
Condition
Confirmed
Differential Diagnosis
Eponym
External Cause
First-Listed
Index to External Causes
Inpatient Facility
Manifestation
Neoplasm Table
Nonessential Modifiers
Not Elsewhere Classifiable (NEC)
Not Otherwise Specified (NOS)
Other Specified
Outpatient Services
Principal Diagnosis
Sequela (Late Effect)
Systemic Condition
Table of Drugs and Chemicals
Tabular List of Diseases and Injuries
Underlying Condition
Unspecified

Learning Outcomes

After completing this chapter, the student should be able to:

LO 4.1 Explain the official conventions used in ICD-10-CM.
LO 4.2 Translate the Official Guidelines and how they impact the way codes are reported.
LO 4.3 Use the Alphabetic Index in ICD-10-CM properly.
LO 4.4 Employ the information within the Tabular List to determine the accurate code to report.
LO 4.5 Distinguish which conditions mentioned in the documentation to report.
LO 4.6 Utilize what you learned in this chapter to determine the correct diagnosis code to report.

STOP! Remember, you need to follow along in your ICD-10-CM code book for an optimal learning experience.

4.1 Introduction and Official Conventions

In the chapters *Introduction to the Languages of Coding* and *The Coding Process*, you were provided with a brief overview of the various code sets. Now, let's begin to dig deeper into the specifics of the ICD-10-CM code set and how to implement it as part of the coding process.

Introduction

In the very front of the ICD-10-CM code book is the *Introduction*. Here you can learn about the history of ICD-10-CM and how we got to this tenth revision. The use of codes to describe the reasons *why* a patient would need the care of a health care professional is an ever-evolving process. These codes, and coding overall, will continue to change throughout your career as a professional coder, so you will need to learn to adapt and change as the needs of health care progress.

ICD-10-CM Official Conventions

The Official Conventions are a very important part of the ICD-10-CM code set. You need to learn the specifics of how codes are presented, and what symbols and notations mean, so you can use them accurately.

Throughout the ICD-10-CM code book, directions, tips, symbols, and helpful notations are available to guide you to the accurate code for a patient encounter. Let's go through common notations and abbreviations, with examples, so you can develop a clear understanding of their meanings.

Punctuation

Punctuation in ICD-10-CM adds information and helps you further your quest for the best, most appropriate code.

Brackets [ ]

Found in the Tabular List, *brackets* will show you alternate terms, alternate phrases, and/or synonyms to provide additional detail or explanation to the description. In the following example, the provider may have diagnosed the patient with food-borne intoxication due to either *Clostridium perfringens* or *C. welchii*. In either case, A05.2 would be the correct code. The same for our other examples: If the documentation reads either "benign recurrent meningitis" or "Mollaret's," code G03.2 can be reported, and if either "third nerve palsy" or "palsy of the oculomotor nerve" is documented, code H49.02 is valid.

> **EXAMPLES**
> A05.2 Food-borne *Clostridium perfringens* [*Clostridium welchii*] intoxication
> G03.2 Benign recurrent meningitis [Mollaret]
> H49.02 Third [oculomotor] nerve palsy, left eye

Italicized or Slanted Brackets [ ]

Italicized, or *slanted*, *brackets*, used in the Alphabetic Index, will surround an additional code or codes (i.e., secondary codes) that *must* be included with the initial code. It is the Alphabetic Index's way of telling you that you may need to report more than one code, as well as in what order to sequence these codes.

The italic brackets tell you that if the patient has been diagnosed with schistosomiasis due to granuloma, you have to use two codes: first, B65.9 for the underlying condition (the schistosomiasis) and, second, G07 for the granuloma itself.

> **EXAMPLE**
> Granuloma L92.9
>   brain (any site) G06.0
>   schistosomiasis B65.9 *[G07]*

Parentheses ( )

Throughout the code set, *parentheses* show you additional terms or phrases that are also included in the description of a particular code. The additional terms are called **nonessential modifiers**. The modifiers can be used to provide additional definition but do not change the description of the condition. The additional terms are not required in the documentation, so if the provider did not use the additional term, the code description is still valid.

Take a look at the first example below. Whether the physician wrote the diagnosis as "malaria," "malarial," or "malarial fever," code B54 would still be a valid suggestion.

In the Tabular List example, code H18.52 would be valid for a diagnosis written by the physician as "epithelial corneal dystrophy" or "juvenile corneal dystrophy."

> **EXAMPLES**
> **In the Alphabetic Index:**
> Malaria, malarial (fever) B54
> Injury, thyroid (gland) NEC S19.84
>
> *(continued)*

CODING BITES

NOTE: This code set is maintained by the U.S. federal government; however, there are many different publishers. Each publisher may present the symbols and notations in its own way. Don't worry. The conventions section in the very front of your code book, in Section 1.A of the Official Guidelines, as well as the legend along the bottom of every page will always explain what means what. All you have to do is read.

Nonessential Modifiers Descriptors whose inclusion in the physician's notes are not absolutely necessary and that are provided simply to further clarify a code description; optional terms.

> **In the Tabular List:**
> H18.52 Epithelial (juvenile) corneal dystrophy
> H44.631 Retained (old) magnetic foreign body in lens, right eye

Colon :

A *colon* (two dots, one on top of the other), used in the Tabular List, emphasizes that one or more of the following descriptors are *required* to make the code valid for the diagnosis.

> **CODING BITES**
> Health care is an industry that uses many, many abbreviations and acronyms. Keep a medical dictionary close at hand so you can look up any with which you are not familiar.

> **EXAMPLE**
> venous embolism and thrombosis (of):
>   cerebral (I63.6, I67.6)
>   coronary (I21–I25)
> *You would read these as:*
>   venous embolism and thrombosis (of), cerebral (I63.6, I67.6)
>   venous embolism and thrombosis (of), coronary (I21–I25)

Abbreviations

NEC

Not Elsewhere Classifiable (NEC)
Specifics that are not described in any other code in the ICD-10-CM book; also known as *not elsewhere classified*.

Not elsewhere classifiable (NEC), or *not elsewhere classified,* indicates that the physician provided additional details of a condition but that the ICD-10-CM book did not include those extra details in any of the other codes in the book. NEC may appear in either the Alphabetic Index or the Tabular List, as you can see in our examples here.

Before reporting a code with NEC in its description, you want to check and double-check that there is not another code with a more complete description that matches the details documented in the physician's notes.

> **EXAMPLES**
>   K72.-   Hepatic failure, not elsewhere classified
> Infection, coronavirus NEC B34.2

NOS

Not Otherwise Specified (NOS)
The absence of additional details documented in the notes.

Not otherwise specified (NOS) means that the physician did not document any additional details that are identified in any of the other available code descriptions. On occasion, you may find an NOS in the Alphabetic Index, but most often, you will see these notations in the Tabular List.

Before reporting a code with NOS in the description, you need to reread the physician's documentation and complete patient chart to make certain the specifics you need to report a more complete code are not there. And, even then, you should query the physician to obtain the details, as you learned in the chapter *Abstracting Clinical Documentation.* An NOS code should be a very last resort to report.

> **EXAMPLES**
>   R10.811   Right upper quadrant abdominal tenderness NOS
>   Z30.09   Encounter for other general counseling and advice on contraception (Encounter for family planning advice NOS)

General Notes

Includes, Excludes1, and Excludes2

Let's begin the explanations of INCLUDES, EXCLUDES1, and EXCLUDES2 notations with an example. Turn, in the ICD-10-CM Tabular List, to code F31:

F31 Bipolar disorder

INCLUDES	manic-depressive illness
	manic-depressive psychosis
	manic-depressive reaction
EXCLUDES1	bipolar disorder, single manic episode (F30.-)
	major depressive disorder, single episode (F32.-)
	major depressive disorder, recurrent (F33.-)
EXCLUDES2	cyclothymia (F34.0)

> **GUIDANCE CONNECTION**
>
> Read the ICD-10-CM Official Guidelines for Coding and Reporting, section **I. Conventions, General Coding Guidelines and Chapter Specific Guidelines**, subsection **A. Conventions for the ICD-10-CM**, paragraph **6. Abbreviations**.

These notations are in the Tabular List to help you determine the correct code. They provide you with additional terms as well as alternate codes that you might find better match what the physician wrote. Notations are all designed to make the coding process easier and more accurate.

INCLUDES

The INCLUDES notation provides you with additional terms and diagnoses that are included in the above code (this code's description). These notations provide you with additional terms, and variations of descriptors, that expand the meaning of this code's description, making it easier to match what the physician wrote in the documentation. Take a look at our example: The INCLUDES notation explains to you that diagnoses of *bipolar disorder, manic-depressive illness, manic-depressive psychosis,* and *manic-depressive reaction* are all reported from code category F31.

EXCLUDES1

There are times when two diagnostic statements may be close to each other, yet actually conflict with each other. The EXCLUDES1 notation identifies codes that cannot be used together on the same health claim form with the originally listed code. The notation explains that the two codes

- Are contradictory to each other.
- Cannot coexist in the same person at the same time.
- Are redundant.

Using our example above, this notation tells you that F32 Major-depressive disorder, single episode is mutually exclusive to (cannot be reported with) F31 Bipolar disorder.

> **EXAMPLE**
>
> Turn in your ICD-10-CM code book, Tabular List, and find code:
> J99 Respiratory disorders in diseases classified elsewhere
>
> EXCLUDES1 *respiratory disorders in:*
>
> *amebiasis (A06.5)*
>
> *blastomycosis (B40.0–B40.2)*
>
> You would read the excluded diagnoses as . . .
>
> EXCLUDES1 respiratory disorders in ambeiasis (A06.5)
>
> EXCLUDES1 respiratory disorders in blastomycosis (B40.0–B40.2)

EXCLUDES2

An EXCLUDES2 notation is a warning to *Stop and Double-Check the Documentation* so you don't report the code above the notation when a code shown in the notation

> **GUIDANCE CONNECTION**
>
> Read the ICD-10-CM Official Guidelines for Coding and Reporting, section **I. Conventions, General Coding Guidelines and Chapter Specific Guidelines**, subsection **A. Conventions for the ICD-10-CM**, paragraphs **10. Includes notes; 11. Inclusion terms;** and **12. Excludes notes.**

may be more accurate. You will see specific conditions listed in the notation that are *not* a part of the code above and a suggestion for an alternate code that may be a more accurate match to the physician's notes. In some cases, the EXCLUDES2 notation may be alerting you that an additional code may be needed to complete telling the story about the patient's condition. Using our example, you can see that the EXCLUDES2 notation tells you that F34.0 Cyclothymia is not the same as F31 Bipolar disorder. Now you can go back to the physician's notes, double-check the information, and determine which is the more accurate code to report, or if you need to report both codes.

> **EXAMPLE**
>
> Turn in your ICD-10-CM Tabular List to:
>
> ✓4 **M66.1** Rupture of synovial cyst
>
> EXCLUDES2 rupture of popliteal cyst (M66.0)
>
> The EXCLUDES2 notation alerts you to STOP AND DOUBLE-CHECK THE DOCUMENTATION to confirm which type of cyst the physician documented. If the documentation states a synovial cyst, then continue determining the correct additional characters for **M66.1.** If the documentation states that the cyst was a popliteal cyst, then you need to report **M66.0** to be more accurate.

Code First

Certain conditions and diseases can cause other problems in the body. Individuals with diabetes, for example, are known to have problems with their eyes or circulation, just to name a few, as a direct result of having diabetes. Patients found to be HIV-positive are prone to conditions such as pneumonia, again as a direct result of the fact that they have human immunodeficiency virus infection. In these examples, diabetes and HIV are what are known as **underlying conditions**. The resulting conditions (e.g., circulation problems, pneumonia) are called **manifestations**.

The *Code first* notation is a reminder that you are going to need another code to identify the underlying disease that caused the diagnosed condition. This notation also tells you the sequence in which to report the two codes: the underlying condition first followed by the manifestation (see Figure 4-1). Often, the notation will reference the most common underlying diseases for a manifestation (along with their codes)! Cool!

Underlying Condition
One disease that affects or encourages another condition.

Manifestation
A condition caused or developed from the existence of another condition.

> **13. Etiology/manifestation convention ("code first", "use additional code", and "in diseases classified elsewhere" notes)**
>
> Certain conditions have both an underlying etiology and multiple body system manifestations due to the underlying etiology. For such conditions, ICD-10-CM has a coding convention that requires the underlying condition to be sequenced first, if applicable, followed by the manifestation. Wherever such a combination exists, there is a "use additional code" note at the etiology code, and a "code first" note at the manifestation code. These instructional notes indicate the proper sequencing order of the codes, etiology followed by manifestation.
>
> In most cases the manifestation codes will have the code title, "in diseases classified elsewhere." Codes with this title are a component of the etiology/manifestation convention. The code title indicates that it is a manifestation code. "In diseases classified elsewhere" codes are never permitted to be used as first-listed or principal diagnosis codes. They must be used in conjunction with an underlying condition code and they must be listed following the underlying condition. See category F02, Dementia in other diseases classified elsewhere, for an example of this convention.

PART II | REPORTING DIAGNOSES

> There are manifestation codes that do not have "in diseases classified elsewhere" in the title. For such codes, there is a "use additional code" note at the etiology code and a "code first" note at the manifestation code and the rules for sequencing apply.
>
> In addition to the notes in the Tabular List, these conditions also have a specific Alphabetic Index entry structure. In the Alphabetic Index both conditions are listed together with the etiology code first followed by the manifestation codes in brackets. The code in brackets is always to be sequenced second.
>
> An example of the etiology/manifestation convention is dementia in Parkinson's disease. In the Alphabetic Index, code G20 is listed first, followed by code F02.80 or F02.81 in brackets. Code G20 represents the underlying etiology, Parkinson's disease, and must be sequenced first, whereas codes F02.80 and F02.81 represent the manifestation of dementia in diseases classified elsewhere, with or without behavioral disturbance.
>
> "Code first" and "Use additional code" notes are also used as sequencing rules in the classification for certain codes that are not part of an etiology/manifestation combination.
>
> See Section I.B.7. Multiple coding for a single condition.

FIGURE 4-1 ICD-10-CM Convention I.A.13. Etiology/manifestation convention.
Source: CDEC.gov

The *Code first* notation is ICD-10-CM's way of informing you that

1. You may need to report another code in addition to the code above to accurately tell the whole story of a diagnosis.
2. This other code should be reported first, before the code above the *Code first* notation.

EXAMPLE

I26.01 Septic pulmonary embolism with acute cor pulmonale

Code first underlying infection

This notation tells you that

1. You need to report both code I26.01 and a code for an infection (see the physician's notes to determine the exact infection).
2. You need to report the code for the infection first, followed by I26.01.

Use Additional Code

Similar to the *Code first* notation, the *Use additional code* notation is ICD-10-CM's way of informing you that

1. You may need to report another code *in addition* to the code above to accurately tell the whole story of a diagnosis.
2. This extra (additional) code should be reported *after* the code above the *Use additional code* notation.

EXAMPLE

G00.2 Streptococcal meningitis

Use additional code to further identify the organism (B95.0–B95.5)

(continued)

CODING BITES

An underlying condition must come first and then a manifestation develops from it. Think of an underlying condition as the trunk of a tree and a manifestation as a branch that grows out from that trunk. If the tree trunk didn't exist, there would be no branch.

> This notation tells you that
> 1. You need to report both code G00.2 and a code from the range B95.0-B95.5 (as per the physician's notes).
> 2. You need to report G00.2 first, followed by the code from B95.0-B95.5.

Code Also

The *Code also* notation is similar to the *Code first* and *Use additional code* notations, just without the predetermination of sequencing. ICD-10-CM is alerting you that the physician's notes may contain some additional condition or issue that should be reported with a separate code, in addition to the code above this notation. This notation leaves it up to you to decide whether or not the additional code is needed to tell the whole story. If it is needed, you will need to use the Official Guidelines, Sections II and III, to determine the reporting order.

> **EXAMPLE**
>
> H18.041 Kayser-Fleischer ring, right eye
>
> *Code also* any associated Wilson's disease (E83.01)
>
> This *Code also* notation alerts you to check the documentation to see if there is a diagnosis of Wilson's disease mentioned in connection with the Kayser-Fleischer ring of the patient's right eye.
>
> If so, then . . .
>
> 1. You need to report both code H18.041 and code E83.01 (as per the physician's notes).
> 2. You need to determine from the physician's documentation, and using the **Official Guidelines, Section II. Selection of Principal Diagnosis, and Section III. Reporting Additional Diagnoses**, which code to report first.

Category Notes

Occasionally, you may see informational notes under the description of a three-character code or at the top of a subsection in the Tabular List. These notes share important information and clarifications that you need to know before you determine the code or codes to report.

> **EXAMPLES**
>
> I69 Sequelae of cerebrovascular disease
>
> **Note:** Category I69 is to be used to indicate conditions in I60–I67 as the cause of sequelae. The "**sequelae**" include conditions specified as such or as residuals that may occur at any time after the onset of the causal condition.
>
> *-*-*
>
> **Chapter 15. Pregnancy, Childbirth and the Puerperium (O00–O9A)**
>
> **Note:** Codes from this chapter are for use only on maternal records, never on newborn records. Codes from this chapter are for use for conditions related to or aggravated by the pregnancy, childbirth, or by the puerperium (maternal causes or obstetric causes).

GUIDANCE CONNECTION

Read the ICD-10-CM Official Guidelines for Coding and Reporting, section **I. Conventions, General Coding Guidelines and Chapter Specific Guidelines**, subsection **A. Conventions for the ICD-10-CM**, paragraph 17. "Code also note."

CODING BITES

Sometimes notations appear under the three-character code at the top of a category but are not repeated after each additional code in its section. This is another reason why it is important to start reading at the three-character code, even when the Alphabetic Index directs you to a code with more characters. You don't want to miss any important directives, such as INCLUDES, EXCLUDES, *Code first*, or *Use additional code* notations.

Sequela
A cause-and-effect relationship between an original condition that has been resolved with a current condition; also known as a late effect.

And

The guidelines for the accurate use of ICD-10-CM instruct you to interpret the use of the word *and* in a code description as "and/or." Therefore, if the physician's notes include only one part of a code description but not the other, the code may still be correct.

> **EXAMPLE**
>
> J38.01 Paralysis of vocal cords and larynx, unilateral
>
> You would be correct to report code J38.01 on the basis of physician's notes that confirm a diagnosis of paralysis of the vocal cords only, paralysis of the larynx only, or paralysis of both the vocal cords and larynx.

With

The term "with" can be seen in both the Alphabetic Index and the Tabular List, and you should read this as a connection **confirmed** by the physician. A phrase you may see in the physician's documentation is "associated with." To use a combination code containing "with," you do not need the physician to document the connection between the two diagnoses. The **Official Guidelines** direct us to avoid using a combination code when the physician's documentation specifies that the conditions are *not* related or associated with each other.

> **EXAMPLE**
>
> Lorrie Demming, a 31-year-old female, G1, P0, came to see Dr. Southland because of bleeding. She is in her third trimester and very worried about the baby. Dr. Southland confirmed the hemorrhage was associated with her placenta previa.
>
> O44.13 Placenta previa with hemorrhage, third trimester

Other Specified

The phrase **other specified** means the same thing as NEC: The physician specified additional information that the ICD-10-CM book doesn't have in any of the other codes in the category.

> **EXAMPLE**
>
> Dr. Josephs diagnosed Allen Halverson with portal cirrhosis of the liver. Turn to the ICD-10-CM Tabular List code category:
>
> ☑4 K74 Fibrosis and cirrhosis of liver
>
>   K74.3 Primary biliary cirrhosis
>
>   K74.4 Secondary biliary cirrhosis
>
> ☑5 K74.6 Other and unspecified cirrhosis of liver
>
>   K74.60 Unspecified cirrhosis of liver
>
>   K74.69 Other cirrhosis of liver
>
> You can see that *Portal cirrhosis of the liver* is not specified in codes K74.3 or K74.4. You cannot honestly report K74.60 because the physician DID specify the type of cirrhosis. Therefore, to be accurate, you must report **K74.69 Other cirrhosis of liver.**

> **GUIDANCE CONNECTION**
>
> Read the ICD-10-CM Official Guidelines for Coding and Reporting, section **I. Conventions, General Coding Guidelines and Chapter Specific Guidelines**, subsection **A. Conventions for the ICD-10-CM**, paragraph **14. "And."**

> **GUIDANCE CONNECTION**
>
> Read the ICD-10-CM Official Guidelines for Coding and Reporting, section **I. Conventions, General Coding Guidelines and Chapter Specific Guidelines**, subsection **A. Conventions for the ICD-10-CM**, paragraph **15. "With."**

Confirmed
Found to be true or definite.

Other Specified
Additional information the physician specified that isn't included in any other code description.

Unspecified
The absence of additional specifics in the physician's documentation.

Unspecified

Unspecified has the same meaning as NOS, explaining that the physician did not provide more details in his or her notes. Query the physician for specifics so you can avoid using an unspecified code. Using these codes should always be a last resort.

> ### EXAMPLES
> K64.9 Unspecified hemorrhoids
> Tumor, yolk sac, unspecified site, male C62.90

CODING BITES

Before choosing any code with NOS or *unspecified* in the description, double-check the notes and patient record to be certain you cannot find specific details to support a specific code. If not, then query the provider and ask for the additional details you need to determine a more accurate code. An unspecified or NOS code should always be a last resort.

See

In the Alphabetic Index of ICD-10-CM, you may look up a term and notice that the book instructs you to *see* another term. This is an instruction in the index that the information you are looking for is listed under a different term.

> ### EXAMPLES
> **Entamoeba, entamebic**—*see* Dysentery, amebic
> **Dysentery, dysenteric**
>   amebic (see also Amebiasis) A06.0
>   acute A06.0
>   chronic A06.1
>
> *-*-*
>
> **Glue**
>   sniffing (airplane)—*see* Abuse, drug, inhalant
> **Abuse**
>   drug
>   inhalant F18.10

GUIDANCE CONNECTION

Read the ICD-10-CM Official Guidelines for Coding and Reporting, section **I. Conventions, General Coding Guidelines and Chapter Specific Guidelines**, subsection **A. Conventions for the ICD-10-CM**, paragraph **16. "See" and "See Also."**

See Also

In other places in the Alphabetic Index, you may see that the instruction *see also* is next to the term you are investigating. *See also* explains that additional details may be found under a different term. The index is providing you with an alternate main term that may show descriptions more accurate to the physician's documentation.

> ### EXAMPLE
> **Angiofibroma** (*see also* Neoplasm, benign, by site)
>   juvenile
>   specified site—*see* Neoplasm, benign, by site
>   unspecified site D10.6
>
> You can see that the *See Also* notation provides you with an additional path to get to the correct code.

Anatomical Site
A specific location within the anatomy (body).

See Condition

The Alphabetic Index may also point you in a less concrete way, such as when you look up a term and the notation tells you to *see condition*. This can be confusing. The index is not telling you to look up the term *condition*. What it is instructing you to do is to find the term that describes the health-related situation involved with this diagnosis and look up that term. You will see this most often next to the listing for an **anatomical site**.

> **EXAMPLE**
>
> Heart—*see* condition
> Leg—*see* condition
> Patellar—*see* condition

This instruction comes back to the reason you are looking for a code in the first place. Remember, you are looking for a code to explain *why* the physician cared for the patient during the encounter. Using our example, having a heart is not a reason for a physician to meet with a patient. Everyone has a heart. Therefore, the index is telling you to look, instead, for the term that describes the condition of this patient's heart—the problem or concern about his or her heart that brought the patient together with the physician at this time. So, as an example, instead of *heart, cervix,* or *lung,* you need to look up *atrophy, fracture,* or *deformity* . . . whatever the reason *why* the patient would need the care of a health care professional.

Additional Characters Required

Box with a Checkmark and Number ☑4

A *box with a checkmark and number* located to the left of a code in the Tabular List is a symbol that notifies you that an additional character is required. The number tells you which character—fourth, fifth, sixth, or seventh—is needed. Some publishers of ICD-10-CM code books use a bullet • rather than a box. In addition, some versions of the ICD-10-CM book will use a ☑xx7, alerting you to the need for a placeholder—the letter *x*—to be used prior to the 7th character.

> **EXAMPLE**
>
> ☑4 H20 Iridocyclitis
>   ☑5 H20.0 Acute and subacute iridocyclitis
>   ☑6 H20.01 Primary iridocyclitis
>   H20.013 Primary iridocyclitis, bilateral
>
> You can see that, as each additional character is added to the code, more specific details are included in the code description. As a professional coding specialist, it is your obligation to always report the most detail possible. This is referred to as the *"highest level of specificity."* Therefore, when the ICD-10-CM code book directs you to keep reading to find an additional character, you are required to do this.

Hyphen -

A *hyphen* is used in the Alphabetic Index to indicate that additional characters are required. This alerts you to an incomplete code.

> **EXAMPLES**
>
> Cogan's syndrome H16.32-
> Discontinuity, ossicles, ear H74.2-
> Fahr Volhard disease (of kidney) I12.-

4.2 ICD-10-CM Official Guidelines for Coding and Reporting

As you work your way through this content, you may be thinking, "How can I possibly remember all of this information?" Here is the good news . . . you don't have to

> **CODING BITES**
>
> If you ever forget what one of these symbols, abbreviations, or notations means, look for the pages in your ICD-10-CM book titled *ICD-10-CM Official Guidelines for Coding and Reporting, Section 1. A. Conventions for the ICD-10-CM*. On these pages, you will find the explanation for all of the footnotes, symbols, instructional notes, and conventions used.
>
> In addition, most versions of ICD-10-CM include a legend across the bottom of the pages throughout the Tabular List with the symbols used and a brief description.

memorize because your code book contains the important information you need to code accurately. All you have to do is read carefully and completely.

In the front of your code book are the rules and directions for accurate reporting of diagnosis codes. You don't have to memorize them. All you have to do is remember that they are available, right at your fingertips, so you can make certain that the codes you report (1) are presented in the legal manner and (2) support clear communications with all parties involved in the care and reimbursement of patients. (See Figure 4-2.)

---

a. Diabetes mellitus

The diabetes mellitus codes are combination codes that include the type of diabetes mellitus, the body system affected, and the complications affecting that body system. As many codes within a particular category as are necessary to describe all of the complications of the disease may be used. They should be sequenced based on the reason for a particular encounter. Assign as many codes from categories E08-E13 as needed to identify all the associated conditions that the patient has.

1) Type of diabetes

The age of a patient is not the sole determining factor, though most type 1 diabetics develop the condition before reaching puberty. For this reason type 1 diabetes is also referred to as juvenile diabetes.

2) Type of diabetes mellitus not documented

If the type of diabetes mellitus is not documented in the medical record the default is E11.–, Type 2 diabetes mellitus.

3) Diabetes mellitus and the use of insulin

If the documentation in a medical record does not indicate the type of diabetes but does indicate that the patient uses insulin, code E11, Type 2 diabetes mellitus, should be assigned. Code Z79.4, Long-term (current) use of insulin, or Z79.84, Long-term (current) use of oral hypoglycemic drugs, should also be assigned to indicate that the patient uses insulin or oral hypoglycemic drugs. Code Z79.4 should not be assigned if insulin is given temporarily to bring a type 2 patient's blood sugar under control during an encounter.

FIGURE 4-2 An excerpt from the Official Guidelines for Coding and Reporting, section 1.C. Chapter-Specific Coding Guidelines, chapter 4. Endocrine, Nutritional, and Metabolic Diseases (E00-E89), subsection a. Diabetes Mellitus, parts 1 through 3   Source: *ICD-10-CM Official Guidelines for Coding and Reporting* The Centers for Medicare and Medicaid Services (CMS) and the National Center for Health Statistics (NCHS)

Section I. Conventions, General Coding Guidelines and Chapter-Specific Guidelines

As you can tell from this header, Section 1 has three parts:

A. Conventions for the ICD-10-CM
B. General Coding Guidelines
C. Chapter-Specific Coding Guidelines

This section contains the rules and guidelines for determining and reporting accurate, valid diagnosis codes. Take a moment and review the information in A and B. You will discover that most of these reiterate what you read in the *Introduction and Official Conventions* section. These may describe each of the items differently, so be certain to read both to ensure that you understand the guidelines.

There are a few additional elements that are important and, therefore, emphasized here.

Section I.A. Conventions for the ICD-10-CM and Section I.B. General Coding Guidelines

Multiple and Additional Codes

If the patient has several conditions or concerns, the physician might possibly indicate more than one diagnosis. Sometimes, the doctor will list the diagnoses, making it easier for you to know which additional codes are needed.

HOW MANY CODES DO YOU NEED?

A professional coding specialist's job is to tell the *whole story* about the encounter between the health care provider and the patient. With diagnosis codes, you relate the whole story about *why* the physician provided the services, treatments, and procedures to the patient at this time. You must support *medical necessity* for all of these procedures.

Let's use a scenario as an example:

> *Jenna Wilson, a 29-year-old female, came to a walk-in clinic complaining of a terrible headache in her forehead and pain in her cheeks. She stated that this is the third time over the last few months she has had this pain. Dr. Jackson evaluated her, did a physical exam, and took a culture from her nasal cavity. The in-house lab identified the cause of her sinusitis as* Streptococcus pneumoniae. *Dr. Jackson diagnosed Jenna with acute recurrent frontal sinusitis due to* Streptococcus pneumoniae *and gave her a prescription for Amoxicillin.*

So, how many codes do you need?

You need as many codes as necessary to tell the *whole story* about *why* Jenna required Dr. Jackson's care at this visit. Why did Dr. Jackson examine Jenna, take the culture, perform the lab test, and then write a prescription? Because Jenna has acute frontal sinusitis caused by *Streptococcus pneumoniae*. When you look for **Sinusitis, Acute**, in the Alphabetic Index, it leads you to the Tabular List at code category

✓4	**J01**	**Acute Sinusitis**
	J01.10	Acute frontal sinusitis, unspecified
	J01.11	Acute recurrent frontal sinusitis

Dr. Jackson noted that Jenna's sinusitis was recurrent, leading you to J01.11 as the correct code. However, this does not tell the WHOLE story, does it? You need to also explain the cause of the sinusitis.

Take a look at the notations beneath J01:

> **Use additional code** *(B95–B97) to identify infectious agent*

This tells you that the second code to report will explain the cause of the sinusitis. You are already using what you have learned in just this short amount of time. You can find the correct second code by turning in your Tabular List to B95 and read all of the code descriptions in these code categories carefully. Did you find:

B95.3	Streptococcus pneumoniae as the cause of diseases classified elsewhere

So, you will report:

J01.11	Acute recurrent frontal sinusitis
B95.3	Streptococcus pneumoniae as the cause of diseases classified elsewhere

Now you can see that, with these two codes, you and anyone reading these codes clearly can understand that Dr. Jackson cared for Jenna because she had a recurring acute frontal sinus infection caused by *Streptococcus pneumoniae*. Without BOTH

GUIDANCE CONNECTION

Read the ICD-10-CM Official Guidelines for Coding and Reporting, section **I. Conventions, General Coding Guidelines and Chapter Specific Guidelines**, subsection **B. General coding guidelines**, paragraph **7. Multiple coding for a single condition.**

CODING BITES

The sinusitis is considered a *"disease classified elsewhere"* because it is a condition that is reported with a code from elsewhere in this code set. The word "classified" is used to mean assigned a code in this code set.

codes, you don't have the *whole story*. So, for every case, every encounter, every scenario, you are responsible for telling *the WHOLE STORY about the encounter.*

CODE SEQUENCING

When more than one diagnosis code is required to tell the whole story of the encounter accurately, you then must determine in which order the codes should be listed. [Yes, it does matter!] The code reporting the most important reason for the encounter is called the **principal diagnosis**.

Sometimes the ICD-10-CM book will tell you which code should come first and which should come second with the *Code first* and *Use additional code* notations. Section II and Section III of the Official Guidelines will help you with those instances when there are no notations to guide you with sequencing.

Principal Diagnosis
The condition, after study, that is the primary, or main, reason for the admission of a patient to the hospital for care; the condition that requires the largest amount of hospital resources for care.

EXAMPLE

Carl Rossen was diagnosed with myocarditis due to *E. coli*. You will find notations directing you on how to sequence these two codes.

I40.0 Infective myocarditis

Use additional code (B95–B97) to identify infectious agent

I41 Myocarditis in diseases classified elsewhere

Code first underlying disease, such as: typhus (A75.0–A75.9)

In cases when there are multiple confirmed diagnoses identified, the guidelines instruct you to list the codes in order of severity from the most severe to the least severe. Take a look at the encounter Dr. Jackson documented with Jenna Wilson. You knew to report B95.3 AFTER J01.11 because the notation beneath J01 directed you to *Use additional code*, providing you with the detail that you (1) needed a second code to complete your explanation of why Jenna required treatment and that (2) clarified the order in which to place the codes.

CODING BITES
If two (or more) diagnoses are of equal severity, then report them in order of anatomical site—head to toe.

Acute and Chronic Conditions

If a patient has a health concern diagnosed by a physician as being both acute (severe) and chronic (ongoing) and the condition offers you separate codes for the two descriptors, you should report the code for the acute condition first, as directed by the guidelines. Remember, from your medical terminology lessons—acute is more serious than chronic.

YOU CODE IT! CASE STUDY

Lorraine Pankow has acute lymphoblastic leukemia and chronic lymphocytic leukemia of B-cell type, now in remission. She is seeing Dr. Huang today for a checkup of this condition.

You Code It!

Can you determine the correct codes for Lorraine's visit with Dr. Huang?

Step #1: Read the case carefully and completely.

Step #2: Abstract the scenario. Which main words or terms describe why the physician cared for the patient during this encounter?

Step #3: Are there any details missing or incomplete for which you would need to query the physician? [If so, ask your instructor.]

Step #4: Check for any relevant guidance, including reading all of the symbols and notations in the Tabular List and the appropriate sections of the Official Guidelines.

Step #5: Determine the correct diagnosis code or codes to explain why this encounter was medically necessary.

Step #6: Double-check your work.

Answer:

Did you determine the correct codes?

> C91.01   Acute lymphoblastic leukemia, in remission
>
> C91.11   Chronic lymphocytic leukemia of B-cell type in remission

Great job!

Combination Codes

If one code exists with a description that includes two or more diagnoses identified in one patient at the same time, you must choose the code that includes as many conditions as available. You may not code each separately.

When the physician's notes indicate that the patient suffered with both **acute** respiratory failure and **chronic** respiratory failure, you must use the code J96.2-. You are not allowed to use J96.0- and J96.1-, even though, technically, you are reporting the patient's conditions accurately. It is required that you use the combination code, as discussed in the Official Guidelines.

Acute
Severe; serious.

Chronic
Long duration; continuing over an extended period of time.

EXAMPLES

J96.0- Acute respiratory failure

J96.1- Chronic respiratory failure

J96.2- Acute and chronic respiratory failure

Also, there are combination codes throughout ICD-10-CM that enable you to report an underlying condition along with a manifestation.

EXAMPLES

E10.21 Type 1 diabetes mellitus with diabetic nephropathy

... This one code reports two diagnoses: type 1 DM + diabetic nephropathy.

I73.01 Raynaud's syndrome with gangrene

... This one code reports two diagnoses: Reynaud's syndrome + gangrene.

K55.21 Angiodysplasia of colon with hemorrhage

... This one code reports two diagnoses: Angiodysplasia of colon + hemorrhage.

> **GUIDANCE CONNECTION**
>
> Read the ICD-10-CM Official Guidelines for Coding and Reporting, section **I. Conventions, General Coding Guidelines and Chapter Specific Guidelines**, subsection **B. General Coding Guidelines**, paragraphs **8. Acute and Chronic Conditions** and **9. Combination Code.**

Two or More Conditions—Only One Confirmed Diagnosis

There may be cases where the physician documents treatment of two (or more) complaints and only one is identified by a confirmed diagnosis.

> **LET'S CODE IT! SCENARIO**
>
> Cahlen Achmed, a 61-year-old male, came to see Dr. Miller. Earlier in the day, he was lightheaded and a little dizzy. In addition, he complained that his heart was beating so wildly that he thought he was having a heart attack.
>
> *(continued)*

Due to his previous diagnosis of type 1 diabetes, Dr. Miller ordered a blood glucose test. He also performed an EKG to check Cahlen's heart. After getting the results of the tests, Dr. Miller determined that Cahlen's lightheadedness and dizziness were a result of his glucose being too high and administered a shot of insulin subq, 5U. He spoke with Cahlen about how to bring his diabetes under control. He also told him that the EKG was negative and that there were no signs of a heart attack.

Let's Code It!

Dr. Miller confirmed that Cahlen's *type 1 diabetes mellitus* was the cause of his lightheadedness and dizziness. Turn to the Alphabetic Index and find:

> **Diabetes**

Turn to the Tabular List and see:

> ☑4 **E10 Type 1 diabetes mellitus**
>
> **E10.9 Type 1 diabetes mellitus without complications**

CODING BITES

Cahlen Achmed's case illustrates that sometimes asking yourself, *"Why did the physician provide a specific test, treatment, or service?"* can help you find the necessary diagnostic key words for an encounter.

Type 1 diabetes mellitus seems to be the only confirmed diagnosis in Dr. Miller's notes. However, the doctor performed an EKG. A diagnosis for diabetes does not provide any medical necessity for doing an EKG. In addition, the test was negative and, therefore, provided no diagnosis. So you still need a diagnosis code to report the medical necessity for running the EKG. Why did Dr. Miller perform the EKG? Because Cahlen complained of a *rapid heartbeat*. The Alphabetic Index suggests:

> **Rapid, heart (beat) R00.0**

The Tabular List confirms

> ☑4 **R00 Abnormalities of heart beat**
>
> **R00.0 Tachycardia, unspecified**

CODING BITES

An electrocardiogram may be referred to as either an ECG or an EKG. *Tachycardia* is the medical term for rapid heartbeat.

For the encounter, you have one confirmed diagnosis (the diabetes) and one symptom (rapid heartbeat).

Check the top of this subsection and the head of this chapter in ICD-10-CM. There is a **NOTE**, an **EXCLUDES1** notation, and an **EXCLUDES2** notation. Read carefully. Do any relate to Dr. Miller's diagnosis of Cahlen? No. Turn to the Official Guidelines and read Section 1.c.4, particularly a. Diabetes mellitus. There is nothing specifically applicable here either.

The guidelines state that a confirmed diagnosis should precede a sign or symptom, so you will list the diabetes code first and then the tachycardia.

E10.9 Type 1 diabetes mellitus without complications

R00.0 Tachycardia, unspecified

Differential Diagnosis
When the physician indicates that the patient's signs and symptoms may closely lead to two different diagnoses; usually written as "diagnosis A vs. diagnosis B."

Differential Diagnosis

In the case where a provider indicates a **differential diagnosis** by using the word *versus* or *or* between two diagnostic statements, you need to code both as if they were confirmed, and either may be listed first. This means that the physician has determined that the patient's signs and symptoms lead equally to two different diagnoses.

YOU CODE IT! CASE STUDY

Gilbert Albun, a 57-year-old male complaining of chest pain and shortness of breath, was seen by his family physician. Dr. Pressman admitted him into the hospital with a differential diagnosis of congestive heart failure versus pleural effusion with respiratory distress.

You Code It!

Review the notes of the encounter between Dr. Pressman and Gilbert Albun, and determine the applicable diagnosis code(s).

Step #1: Read the case carefully and completely.

Step #2: Abstract the scenario. Which main words or terms describe why the physician cared for the patient during this encounter?

Step #3: Are there any details missing or incomplete for which you would need to query the physician? [If so, ask your instructor.]

Step #4: Check for any relevant guidance, including reading all of the symbols and notations in the Tabular List and the appropriate sections of the Official Guidelines.

Step #5: Determine the correct diagnosis code or codes to explain why this encounter was medically necessary.

Step #6: Double-check your work.

Answer:

Did you determine the correct codes?

I50.9	**Congestive heart failure, unspecified**
J90	**Pleural effusion, not elsewhere classified**
R06.00	**Dyspnea, unspecified**

Other Current Conditions

Another important issue that needs to be coded is a current condition that might be subtly addressed by the physician. It might be the writing of a prescription refill or a short discussion on the state of the patient's well-being as the result of ongoing therapy for a matter other than that which brought the patient to see the physician today.

YOU CODE IT! CASE STUDY

Deanna Franklin, a 45-year-old female, came to see Dr. Carter for a follow-up on a previous diagnosis of paroxysmal atrial fibrillation. Dr. Carter examined Deanna and did a blood test to monitor the effectiveness of the prescription medication Coumadin, a blood thinner. Dr. Carter told Deanna he was very pleased with her progress and that she was doing well. Before leaving, Deanna asked Dr. Carter for a refill of trinalin, her allergy medication. This time of year typically provoked her allergy to pollen, which caused a lot of inflammation and irritation in her nose (rhinitis). Dr. Carter wrote the refill prescription.

You Code It!

Read Dr. Carter's notes regarding this encounter with Deanna, and determine the correct diagnostic code or codes.

Step #1: Read the case carefully and completely.

Step #2: Abstract the scenario. Which main words or terms describe why the physician cared for the patient during this encounter?

(continued)

Step #3: Are there any details missing or incomplete for which you would need to query the physician? [If so, ask your instructor.]

Step #4: Check for any relevant guidance, including reading all of the symbols and notations in the Tabular List and the appropriate sections of the Official Guidelines.

Step #5: Determine the correct diagnosis code or codes to explain why this encounter was medically necessary.

Step #6: Double-check your work.

Answer:

Did you determine the correct codes?

I48.0	Paroxysmal atrial fibrillation
J30.1	Allergic rhinitis, due to pollen (hayfever)
Z79.01	Long-term (current) use of anticoagulants

The code for the atrial fibrillation supports the office visit and exam, the code for long-term use of the Coumadin (an anticoagulant) justifies the blood test, and the code for the allergic rhinitis supports the medical necessity for the trinalin prescription.

Placeholder Character

There are times when a fifth, sixth, or seventh character is required, yet there are no fourth, fifth, or sixth characters. In these cases, ICD-10-CM uses a placeholder character, the letter "**x**," so the following characters will fall into their correct locations. The symbols in the Tabular List will lead you to filling out your code accurately. Just pay attention to each character as well as in what position each character belongs. Let's look at ✓xx7 as an example. This symbol tells you that you will need to add a placeholder **x** in the fifth position and a placeholder **x** in the sixth position before determining which of the seventh character options to place at the end of the code.

> **GUIDANCE CONNECTION**
>
> Read the ICD-10-CM Official Guidelines for Coding and Reporting, section **I. Conventions, General Coding Guidelines and Chapter Specific Guidelines**, subsection **A. Conventions for the ICD-10-CM**, paragraph **4. Placeholder character**.

EXAMPLES

S02.611A	Fracture of condylar process of right mandible, initial encounter
T47.2x2D	Poisoning by stimulant laxatives, intentional self-harm, subsequent encounter
W89.1xxS	Exposure to tanning bed, sequela
W85.xxxA	Exposure to electric transmission lines, initial encounter

As you can see, all of these codes require a seventh character, yet the initial codes were shorter. These codes are examples of how the placeholder character "**x**" is used so that all of the characters fall into their proper placement.

Seventh Character

Some ICD-10-CM codes require a seventh character. Different subsections of the code book use this position—the seventh character—to add varying types of information. Most often, the character choices are listed at the top of the code category to be used for all codes within that category. With this in mind, you must always begin reading at the top of the code category or subsection for this information.

The Tabular List contains all the details you need. All you have to do is read the options and determine which is the most accurate, as per the physician's documentation.

> **GUIDANCE CONNECTION**
>
> Read the ICD-10-CM Official Guidelines for Coding and Reporting, section **I. Conventions, General Coding Guidelines and Chapter Specific Guidelines**, subsection **A. Conventions for the ICD-10-CM**, paragraph **5. 7th Characters**.

Section I.C. Chapter-Specific Coding Guidelines

This subsection of the Official Guidelines is further divided and sorted by the chapters in the Tabular List. The process of determining the code or codes for a specific encounter will lead you to various places throughout the ICD-10-CM code set. It is important to always reference these chapter-specific official guidelines to ensure you are considering all of the facets of this complex job before you report a code on an assessment in class or on a claim form or report when you are on the job.

Section II. Selection of Principal Diagnosis and Section III. Reporting Additional Diagnoses

Earlier in this chapter, you learned about reporting multiple diagnosis codes and about the basics of sequencing codes. It might seem straightforward right now, but there are times when sequencing and reporting multiple codes become more complicated. Determining the sequencing of the diagnosis codes reported is very important, so you want to get it right every time. With the Official Guidelines readily available for you to reference while you are coding, you can report codes with confidence.

Section IV. Diagnostic Coding and Reporting Guidelines for Outpatient Services

This section of the Official Guidelines covers specific differences when reporting for an **outpatient** service, including a hospital emergency department, same-day surgical center, walk-in clinic, or physician's office.

Essentially, the guidelines for inpatient and outpatient coding are the same or similar when it comes to reporting the reasons *why* a patient needs care except for one main difference—unconfirmed diagnoses.

Unconfirmed Diagnoses

The Official Guidelines are different for reporting unconfirmed diagnoses for patients who are treated as outpatient versus inpatient.

Outpatient Services

The guideline *Section IV.H, Uncertain diagnosis* states that you are to use the code or codes that identify the condition to its highest level of certainty. This means that you code only what you know for a fact. You are *not permitted* to assign an ICD-10-CM diagnosis code for a condition that is described by the provider as *probable, suspected, possible, questionable,* or *to be ruled out*. If the health care professional has not been able to confirm a diagnosis, then you must code the signs, symptoms, abnormal test results, or other element stated as the reason for the visit or service.

> **EXAMPLE**
>
> Ellyn Cragen, a 27-year-old female, came to see Dr. Jenisha in his office because of nausea and absence of her period for 2 months. After doing a thorough examination, Dr. Jenisha suspects that Ellyn may be pregnant, so he orders a blood test. If the blood test comes back *positive* to confirm her pregnancy (after the physician documents it in the file), you would use the following code:
>
> **Z32.01 Encounter for pregnancy test, result positive**
>
> If the blood test comes back *negative*, this confirms that Ellyn is not pregnant. Therefore, you would need to report what you know to be true:
>
> **N91.2 Amenorrhea, unspecified**
> **R11.0 Nausea**
> **Z32.02 Encounter for pregnancy test, results negative**

Inpatient Services

The rules for coding uncertain diagnoses for patients of an **inpatient facility** are different from those for outpatients. As directed by the guideline *Section II.H, Uncertain*

CODING BITES

Inpatient coding calls the most serious diagnosis code, the code that is reported first, as the **principal diagnosis** code.

Outpatient coding calls the most serious diagnosis code the **first-listed** diagnosis code.

Principal Diagnosis
The condition, after study, that is the primary, or main, reason for the admission of a patient to the hospital for care; the condition that requires the largest amount of hospital resources for care.

First-Listed
"First-listed diagnosis" is used, when reporting outpatient encounters, instead of the term "principal diagnosis."

Outpatient
An **outpatient** is a patient who receives services for a short amount of time (less than 24 hours) in a physician's office or clinic, without being kept overnight. An **outpatient facility** includes a hospital emergency room, ambulatory care center, same-day surgery center, or walk-in clinic.

GUIDANCE CONNECTION

Read the ICD-10-CM Official Guidelines for Coding and Reporting, section **IV. Diagnostic Coding and Reporting Guidelines for Outpatient Services**, paragraph **H. Uncertain Diagnosis.**

Inpatient Facility
An establishment that provides health care services to individuals who stay overnight on the premises.

diagnosis, if the diagnosis is described as probable, possible, suspected, likely, or still to be ruled out at the time of discharge, you must code that condition as if it existed. This directive applies only when you are coding services provided in a short-term, acute, long-term care, or psychiatric hospital or facility. It is one of the few circumstances in which you will find the guidelines differ between coding for outpatient and inpatient services.

YOU CODE IT! CASE STUDY

Howard Tamar, a 61-year-old male, was admitted to the hospital for observation after he complained of having severe chest pain radiating to his left shoulder and down his left arm. After 24 hours in the telemetry unit, Dr. Norwalk discharged him with a diagnosis of suspected variant angina pectoris.

You Code It!

As the hospital's coder, go through the steps of coding and determine the diagnosis code or codes that should be reported for this encounter between Dr. Norwalk and Howard Tamar.

Step #1: Read the case carefully and completely.

Step #2: Abstract the scenario. Which main words or terms describe why the physician cared for the patient during this encounter?

Step #3: Are there any details missing or incomplete for which you would need to query the physician? [If so, ask your instructor.]

Step #4: Check for any relevant guidance, including reading all of the symbols and notations in the Tabular List and the appropriate sections of the Official Guidelines.

Step #5: Determine the correct diagnosis code or codes to explain why this encounter was medically necessary.

Step #6: Double-check your work.

Answer:

Did you determine this to be the code?

    I20.1   Angina pectoris with documented spasm (variant angina)

Good job!

Appendix I. Present-On-Admission Reporting Guidelines

You will learn more about Present-On-Admission (POA) indicators in the chapter *Inpatient (Hospital) Diagnosis Coding*. These indicators are only used for reporting diagnoses for patients treated in a hospital as an inpatient. The Appendix I rules about how to use POA indicators will come in very handy later in your learning.

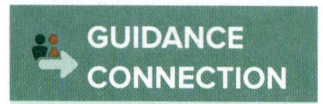

4.3 The Alphabetic Index and Ancillaries

GUIDANCE CONNECTION

Read the ICD-10-CM Official Guidelines for Coding and Reporting, section **II. Selection of Principal Diagnosis**, paragraph **H. Uncertain Diagnosis.**

In the *Abstracting Clinical Documentation* chapter, you learned how to identify the diagnosis-related main words abstracted from the physician's notes (the terms that explain *why* the physician needed to care for the patient during the encounter). Let's practice looking for the main term or terms in the Alphabetic Index of your ICD-10-CM code book [also titled ICD-10-CM Index to Diseases and Injuries] (see Figure 4-3), as well as the ancillary sections of the code set.

A

Aarskog's syndrome Q87.1

Abandonment—*see* Maltreatment

Abasia (-astasia) (hysterical) F44.4

Abderhalden-Kaufmann-Lignac syndrome (cystinosis) E72.04

Abdomen, abdominal—*see also* condition
- acute R10.0
- angina K55.1
- muscle deficiency syndrome Q79.4

Abdominalgia—*see* Pain, abdominal

Abduction contracture, hip or other joint—*see* Contraction, joint

FIGURE 4-3 Example from ICD-10-CM Alphabetic Index: Main terms Aarskog's syndrome through Abduction contracture, hip or other joint Source: *ICD-10-CM Official Guidelines for Coding and Reporting* The Centers for Medicare and Medicaid Services (CMS) and the National Center for Health Statistics (NCHS)

Index to Diseases and Injuries (aka Alphabetic Index)

Index to Diseases and Injuries, most often referred to as the **Alphabetic Index**, is the part of the code book that lists all of the diagnoses and other reasons to provide health care by their main word or term, alphabetically from A to Z.

You will use the Alphabetic Index to guide you to the correct page or area in the Tabular List. Codes in the Alphabetic Index are only suggested codes. Often, the code shown in the Index will require additional characters, will need to be coupled with another code, or will be the wrong interpretation altogether.

Conditions are shown in the Alphabetic Index by:

- **Condition** (e.g., infections, fractures, and wounds)
- **Eponyms** (e.g., Epstein-Barr syndrome and Cushing's disease)
- Other descriptors (e.g., history, family history)

After you abstract the documentation and open the Alphabetic Index, you will realize that looking for a main word of a diagnosis in the Alphabetic Index may, sometimes, be easy and direct, and you will be able to determine the code right away!

For example, suppose you read that *"Dr. Gaseor diagnosed Belinda Alfonzo with Tourette's disorder."*

Turning in the Alphabetic Index in your codebook, you will find (Figure 4-4):

The Alphabetic Index's suggestion is clear:

> **Tourette's syndrome F95.2**

There are times, however, when finding the suggested code requires a bit more work. Consider this diagnostic statement, *"Dr. Mulford noted that Charlie has suffered an abrasion on his chin."* Did you determine the main term to be "abrasion"? Good job! Let's find this term in the Alphabetic Index (Figure 4-5).

This is not as straightforward, is it? Notice that the long list indented below the main term Abrasion (and you can see in your ICD-10-CM book that it is much longer than what is shown here) is a list, in alphabetical order, of anatomical sites: abdomen, alveolar, ankle, etc. Go back to the diagnostic statement: *"Dr. Mulford noted that Charlie has suffered an abrasion on his chin."* On what anatomical site was Charlie's abrasion? His chin. Now read down the long list and find the suggested code:

> **Abrasion, chin S00.81**

Good work! You are really learning.

Alphabetic Index
The section of a code book showing all codes, from A to Z, by the short code descriptions.

Condition
The state of abnormality or dysfunction.

Eponym
A disease or condition named for a person.

CODING BITES

Find the condition or issue ("main term") in the ICD-10-CM Alphabetic Index.

If you cannot identify a "main term" from all the words in the diagnostic statement, just look up all the words, one at a time, in the ICD-10-CM Alphabetic Index. You will get to the correct "main term" and find the suggested code. Write the suggested code down on a piece of scratch paper and move to the next step.

Torture, victim of Z65.4
Torula, torular (histolytica) (infection)—see Cryptococcosis
Torulosis—see Cryptococcosis
Torus—see (mandibularis) (palatinus) M27.0
- fracture—see Fracture, by site, torus
Touraine's syndrome Q79.8
Tourette's syndrome F95.2
Tourniquet syndrome—see Constriction, external, by site
Tower skull Q75.0
- with exophthalmos Q87.0
Toxemia R68.89
- bacterial—see Sepsis
- burn—see Burn

FIGURE 4-4 ICD-10-CM, Alphabetic Index, partial, from Torture to Toxemia Source: *ICD-10-CM Official Guidelines for Coding and Reporting* The Centers for Medicare and Medicaid Services (CMS) and the National Center for Health Statistics (NCHS)

Abrasion T14.8
- abdomen, abdominal (wall) S30.811
- alveolar process S00.512
- ankle S90.51-
- antecubital space—see Abrasion, elbow
- anus S30.817
- arm (upper) S40.81-
- auditory canal—see Abrasion, ear
- auricle—see Abrasion, ear
- axilla—see Abrasion, arm
- back, lower S30.810
- breast S20.11-
- brow S00.81
- buttock S30.810
- calf—see Abrasion, leg
- canthus—see Abrasion, eyelid
- cheek S00.81
-- internal S00.512
- chest wall—see Abrasion, thorax
- chin S00.81
- clitoris S30.814
- cornea S05.0-
- costal region—see Abrasion, thorax
- dental K03.1
- digit(s)
-- foot—see Abrasion, toe
-- hand—see Abrasion, finger
- ear S00.41-
- elbow S50.31-
- epididymis S30.813
- epigastric region S30.811
- epiglottis S10.11
- esophagus (thoracic) S27.818
-- cervical S10.11
- eyebrow—see Abrasion, eyelid

(continued)

> - eyelid S00.21-
> - face S00.81
> - finger(s) S60.41-
> -- index S60.41-
> -- little S60.41-
> -- middle S60.41-
> -- ring S60.41-
> - flank S30.811
> - foot (except toe(s) alone) S90.81-
> -- toe—see Abrasion, toe
> - forearm S50.81-
> -- elbow only—see Abrasion, elbow
> - forehead S00.81

FIGURE 4-5 ICD-10-CM Alphabetic Index, partial, from Abrasion to Abrasion, forehead   Source: *ICD-10-CM Official Guidelines for Coding and Reporting* The Centers for Medicare and Medicaid Services (CMS) and the National Center for Health Statistics (NCHS)

It is important for you to remember that the ICD-10-CM code book has information that can really help you do your job well. Consider Dr. Johnson, a pediatrician, caring for Melinda, who has a problem with her right eye. Dr. Johnson documents that Melinda has "*pink eye.*" Pink eye is not actually a medical term. It is a common term. But this is all you have to go on, so let's take a chance with this in the Alphabetic Index. Eye is an anatomical site, so you know that having an eye is not a reason to see the physician. Look for the term "**pink**" and find, not a suggested code, but a reference (see Figure 4-6).

The ICD-10-CM Alphabetic Index actually tells you the medical term for "pink eye" and that you need to look this up using this term. Turn in the Alphabetic Index to find the main term, **Conjunctivitis** (see Figure 4-7).

Similar to the situation with Abrasion, you see a long list indented beneath this main term, meanin, you need more details from the documentation, or in this case, the previous Alphabetic Index notation. Check back to what you read when you looked at **Pink**, eye—*see* Conjunctivitis, acute, mucopurulent. Now, read the indented list beneath **Conjunctivitis** carefully and find acute. Then, indented beneath that, find:

Conjunctivitis, acute, mucopurulent H10.02-

You may find that a medical dictionary can also help you find synonyms for terms used in the physician documentation that does not match an item in the Alphabetic Index. Build the habit to use all of your resources to help you determine the accurate code.

> **Pinhole meatus** (*see also* Stricture, urethra) N35.9
> **Pink**
> - disease—see subcategory T56.1
> - eye—*see* Conjunctivitis, acute, mucopurulent
> **Pinkus' disease** (lichen nitidus) L44.1

FIGURE 4-6 ICD-10-CM Alphabetic Index, partial, from Pinhole meatus through Pinkus' disease   Source: *ICD-10-CM Official Guidelines for Coding and Reporting* The Centers for Medicare and Medicaid Services (CMS) and the National Center for Health Statistics (NCHS)

> **CODING BITES**
>
> **Never, never, never** code *only* from the Alphabetic Index. *You are required to check* every code in the Tabular List. Only then can you read the entire code description and all notations to determine the most accurate code.

> **CODING BITES**
>
> **Neoplasm Table:** A table that lists the suggested codes for benign and malignant neoplasms (tumors). The list is organized in alphabetic order by the anatomical location of the neoplasm.

Neoplasm Table
The Neoplasm Table lists all possible codes for benign and malignant neoplasms, in alphabetic order by anatomical location of the tumor.

> **Conjunctiva**—*see* condition
>
> **Conjunctivitis** (staphylococcal) (streptococcal) **NOS** H10.9
> - Acanthamoeba B60.12
> - acute H10.3-
> -- atopic H10.1-
> -- chemical (see also Corrosion, cornea) H10.21-
> -- mucopurulent H10.02-
> --- follicular H10.01-
> -- pseudomembranous H10.22-
> -- serous except viral H10.23-
> --- viral—*see* Conjunctivitis, viral
> -- toxic H10.21-
> - adenoviral (acute) (follicular) B30.1
> - allergic (acute)—*see* Conjunctivitis, acute, atopic
> -- chronic H10.45
> --- vernal H10.44
> - anaphalactic—*see* Conjunctivitis, acute, atopic
> - Apollo B30.3
> - atopic (acute)—*see* Conjunctivitis, acute, atopic
> - Béal's B30.2
> - blennorrhagic (gonococcal) (neonatorum) A54.31
> - chemical (acute) (*see also* Corrosion, cornea) H10.21-

FIGURE 4-7 ICD-10-CM Alphabetic Index, partial, Conjuctiva to Conjunctivitis, chemical Source: *ICD-10-CM Official Guidelines for Coding and Reporting* The Centers for Medicare and Medicaid Services (CMS) and the National Center for Health Statistics (NCHS)

Neoplasm Table

The **Neoplasm Table** is a breakout section of the Alphabetic Index, listing the suggested codes for benign and malignant neoplasms. These pages are set up as a seven (7) column table (Figure 4-8) organized by the information in column 1—the anatomical location of the tumor, in alphabetic order. Moving to the right, the following six columns show the suggested code in the following order:

Malignant, Primary

Malignant, Secondary

	Malignant Primary	Malignant Secondary	Ca in situ	Benign	Uncertain Behavior	Unspecified Behavior
Neoplasm, neoplastic	C80.1	C79.9	D09.9	D36.9	D48.9	D49.9
- abdomen, abdominal	C76.2	C79.8-	D09.8	D36.7	D48.7	D49.89
-- cavity	C76.2	C79.8-	D09.8	D36.7	D48.7	D49.89
-- organ	C76.2	C79.8-	D09.8	D36.7	D48.7	D49.89
-- viscera	C76.2	C79.8-	D09.8	D36.7	D48.7	D49.89
-- wall—*see also* Neoplasm, abdomen, wall, skin	C44.509	C79.2-	D04.5	D23.5	D48.5	D49.2

FIGURE 4-8 Excerpt from the Neoplasm Table, partial listing for Abdominal neoplasm Source: *ICD-10-CM Official Guidelines for Coding and Reporting* The Centers for Medicare and Medicaid Services (CMS) and the National Center for Health Statistics (NCHS)

Ca in situ

Benign

Uncertain Behavior

Unspecified Behavior

As you have learned, there are many different variations of diseases, especially neoplasms. When the documentation uses one of these alternate terms, you can still look up the main term used by the physician, and, again, the ICD-10-CM Alphabetic Index will help you find your way in the code book.

Adenosarcoma—*see* Neoplasm, malignant, by site

You will learn more about this Table in the chapter on *Coding Neoplasms*.

Table of Drugs and Chemicals

Similar to the Neoplasm Table, the seven (7) columns in the **Table of Drugs and Chemicals** section (see Figure 4-9) provide suggested codes related to the cause of a patient being poisoned or of having an adverse reaction to a medication. This table's first column shows a list of most drugs and chemicals with which a patient might interact, listed in alphabetic order. The six columns that follow, to the right, are:

Poisoning, Accidental (unintentional)

Poisoning, Intentional Self-Harm

Poisoning, Assault

Poisoning, Undetermined

Adverse Effect

Underdosing

Later in this book, the chapter titled *Coding Injury, Poisoning, and External Causes* will provide you with full explanations for using this table.

Index to External Causes

To make it easier to determine the correct code or codes to report *how* the patient became injured or poisoned, and *where* the patient was (Place of Occurrence) when

Table of Drugs and Chemicals
The section of the ICD-10-CM code book listing drugs, chemicals, and other biologicals that may poison a patient or result in an adverse reaction.

CODING BITES

Table of Drugs and Chemicals: A table that lists pharmaceuticals and chemicals that may cause poisoning or **adverse effects** in the human body.

Adverse Effect
An unexpected bad reaction to a drug or other treatment.

Substance	Poisoning, Accidental (unintentional)	Poisoning, Intentional Self-Harm	Poisoning, Assault	Poisoning, Undetermined	Adverse Effect	Underdosing
Acetomorphine	T40.1X1	T40.1X2	T40.1X3	T40.1X4	—	—
Acetone (oils)	T52.4X1	T52.4X2	T52.4X3	T52.4X4	—	—
- chlorinated	T52.4X1	T52.4X2	T52.4X3	T52.4X4	—	—
- vapor	T52.4X1	T52.4X2	T52.4X3	T52.4X4	—	—
Acetonitrile	T52.8X1	T52.8X2	T52.8X3	T52.4X4	—	—
Acetophenazine	T43.3X1	T43.3X2	T43.3X3	T43.3X4	T43.3X5	T43.3X6
Acetophenetedin	T39.1X1	T39.1X2	T39.1X3	T39.1X4	T39.1X5	T39.1X6
Acetophenone	T52.4X1	T52.4X2	T52.4X3	T52.4X4	—	—
Acetorphine	T40.2X1	T40.2X2	T40.2X3	T40.2X4	—	—
Acetosulfone (sodium)	T37.1X1	T37.1X2	T37.1X3	T37.1X4	T37.1X5	T37.1X6

FIGURE 4-9 Excerpt from Table of Drugs and Chemicals, Acetomorphine through Acetosulfone (sodium). Source: *ICD-10-CM Official Guidelines for Coding and Reporting* The Centers for Medicare and Medicaid Services (CMS) and the National Center for Health Statistics (NCHS)

> **Fall, falling (accidental)** W19
> - building W20.1
> -- burning (uncontrolled fire) X00.3
> - down
> -- embankment W17.81
> -- escalator W10.0
> -- hill W17.81
> -- ladder W11
> -- ramp W10.2
> -- stairs, steps W10.9
> - due to
> – bumping against
> --- object W18.00
> — sharp glass W18.02
> — specified NEC W18.09
> — sports equipment W18.01

FIGURE 4-10 An excerpt from the Index to External Causes, main term Fall Source: *ICD-10-CM Official Guidelines for Coding and Reporting* The Centers for Medicare and Medicaid Services (CMS) and the National Center for Health Statistics (NCHS)

> **CODING BITES**
>
> **Index to External Causes** : The alphabetic list with short descriptions of the **external causes** of injury and poisoning.

Index to External Causes
The alphabetic listing of the external causes that might cause a patient's injury, poisoning, or adverse reaction.

External Cause
An event, outside the body, that causes injury, poisoning, or an adverse reaction.

Tabular List of Diseases and Injuries
The section of the ICD-10-CM code book listing all of the codes in alphanumeric order.

the injury or poisoning occurred, you can use the **Index to External Causes** (see Figure 4-10) to find a suggested code for the main terms you abstract from the physician's documentation.

Later in this book, the chapter titled *Coding Injury, Poisoning, and External Causes* will provide you with full explanations for using this index.

4.4 The Tabular List

Once you have a suggested code from the *Alphabetic Index, Neoplasm Table, Table of Drugs and Chemicals,* and/or the *Index to External Cause Codes,* you will need to find that code in the **Tabular List of Diseases and Injuries**. Remember, you may never report a code directly from the Alphabetic Index without checking it in the *Tabular List*.

This suggested code will point you to a section or subsection inside a chapter of the Tabular List (see Table 4-1 for a list of the Tabular List chapters).

Beginning at the top of each chapter and subchapter, you will need to carefully read *all* associated code descriptions. This part of the process helps you ensure that you determine the most accurate code to the highest level of specificity:

- Matching the details in the physician's documentation
- Regarding only one particular encounter
- In compliance with the rules and guidelines

The **Tabular List** section of the ICD-10-CM book lists every code and its complete description in alphanumeric order by code. Starting at A00, the codes go all the way through to Z99.89 (see Figure 4-11). Let's investigate the various components of this section.

Tabular List Chapter Heads

Many of the 21 chapters within the Tabular List start out with valuable information that will support your determination of the accurate code to report. For example, Chapter 1 (Figure 4-12) begins with several instructions that will affect your code decisions. As you practice your coding process, be certain to include checking the very beginning of the chapter so you can benefit from these important notations.

TABLE 4-1 Chapters in ICD-10-CM Tabular List

Chapter	Code Range	Title
1	A00–B99	Certain Infectious and Parasitic Diseases
2	C00–D49	Neoplasms
3	D50–D89	Diseases of the Blood and Blood-forming Organs and Certain Disorders Involving the Immune Mechanism
4	E00–E89	Endocrine, Nutritional, and Metabolic Diseases
5	F01–F99	Mental, Behavioral, and Neurodevelopmental Disorders
6	G00–G99	Diseases of the Nervous System
7	H00–H59	Diseases of the Eye and Adnexa
8	H60–H95	Diseases of the Ear and Mastoid Process
9	I00–I99	Diseases of the Circulatory System
10	J00–J99	Diseases of the Respiratory System
11	K00–K95	Diseases of the Digestive System
12	L00–L99	Diseases of the Skin and Subcutaneous Tissue
13	M00–M99	Diseases of the Musculoskeletal System and Connective Tissue
14	N00–N99	Diseases of the Genitourinary System
15	O00–O9A	Pregnancy, Childbirth, and the Puerperium
16	P00–P96	Certain Conditions Originating in the Perinatal Period
17	Q00–Q99	Congenital Malformations, Deformations, and Chromosomal Abnormalities
18	R00–R99	Symptoms, Signs, and Abnormal Clinical and Laboratory Findings, Not Elsewhere Classified
19	S00–T88	Injury, Poisoning, and Certain Other Consequences of External Causes
20	V00–Y99	External Causes of Morbidity
21	Z00–Z99	Factors Influencing Health Status and Contact with Health Services

Source: *ICD-10-CM Official Guidelines for Coding and Reporting* The Centers for Medicare and Medicaid Services (CMS) and the National Center for Health Statistics (NCHS)

CODING BITES

The Alphabetic Index will suggest a possible diagnosis code. Then you must find the code suggested by the Alphabetic Index in the Tabular List. This step is not a suggestion—it is mandatory. The Tabular List provides more detail in the code description as well as additional notations such as *includes* and *excludes* notes and directives for the requirement of additional characters and codes. *NEVER, NEVER, NEVER code from the Alphabetic Index.*

CODING BITES

Different publishers do things differently. So, your specific version of the ICD-10-CM code book may provide you with the meanings of the symbols in other ways, and other places. Be certain to spend a few minutes becoming familiar with YOUR code book and where things are placed. Inserting tabs on specific pages may help you find quick access to the details you need when you need them.

> **B68 Taeniasis**
> **EXCLUDES1** cysticercosis (B69.-)
> **B68.0 Taenia solium taeniasis**
> Pork tapeworm (infection)
> **B68.1 Taenia saginata taeniasis**
> Beef tapework (infection)
> Infection due to adult tapeworm Taenia saginata
> **B68.9 Taeniasis, unspecified**
> **B69 Cysticercosis**
> **INCLUDES** cysticerciasis infection due to larval form of Taenia solium
> **B69.0 Cysticercosis of central nervous system**
> **B69.1 Cysticercosis of eye**
> **B69.8 Cysticercosis of other sites**
> **B69.81 Myositis in cysticercosis**
> **B69.89 Cysticercosis of other sites**
> **B69.9 Cysticercosis, unspecified**
> **B70 Diphyllobithriasis and sparganosis**
> **B70.0 Diphyllobothriasis**
> Diphyllobothrium (adult) (latum) (pacificum) infection
> Fish tapeworm (infection)
> **EXCLUDES2** larval diphyllobothriasis (B70.1)
> **B70.1 Sparganosis**

FIGURE 4-11 Example of a page from ICD-10-CM Tabular List: code categories B67 through B70 Source: *ICD-10-CM Official Guidelines for Coding and Reporting* The Centers for Medicare and Medicaid Services (CMS) and the National Center for Health Statistics (NCHS)

> **Chapter 1**
>
> **Certain infectious and parasitic diseases (A00-B99)**
> **INCLUDES** diseases generally recognized as communicable or transmissible
> *Use additional code* to identify resistance to antimicrobial drugs (Z16.-)
> **EXCLUDES1** certain localized infections—see body system-related chapters
> **EXCLUDES2** carrier or suspected carrier of infectious disease (Z22.-)
> infectious and parasitic diseases complicating pregnancy, childbirth, and the puerperium (O98.-)
> infectious and parasitic diseases specific to the perinatal period (P35-P39)
> influenza and other acute respiratory infections (J00-J22)

FIGURE 4-12 ICD-10-CM Tabular List, chapter 1 opening notations Source: *ICD-10-CM Official Guidelines for Coding and Reporting* The Centers for Medicare and Medicaid Services (CMS) and the National Center for Health Statistics (NCHS)

The Legends

Across the bottom of every page throughout the Tabular List you will find short explanations for many of the symbols you will see among the codes and their descriptions. These legends are an abbreviation of the more complete explanations of each symbol in the front of your code book, found on the pages titled ***Overview of ICD-10-CM Official Conventions*** and ***Additional Conventions***. Once you become familiar with each symbol and notation, the legends will provide you with a quick reference to confirm you are making the correct interpretation.

Using the Tabular List

Earlier in this chapter, in 4.3 *The Alphabetic Index and Ancillaries*, you learned to use the Alphabetic Index to find suggested codes that matched diagnostic statements. Let's take each of these to the next step . . . confirming the code in the Tabular List.

Case #1 Tourette's Disorder

The first scenario you worked with in the previous section *The Alphabetic Index and Ancillaries* was "Dr. Gaseor diagnosed Belinda Alfonzo with Tourette's disorder." And you found code F95.2 suggested by the Alphabetic Index. In your ICD-10-CM code book, turn to code category F95 in the Tabular List.

☑4 F95 Tic disorder

    F95.0 Transient tic disorder
        Provisional tic disorder

    F95.1 Chronic motor or vocal tic disorder

    F95.2 Tourette's disorder
        Combined vocal and multiple motor tic disorder [de la Tourette]
        Tourette's syndrome

    F95.8 Other tic disorders

    F95.9 Tic disorder, unspecified
        Tic NOS

It appears that, at this point, F95.2 is the correct code to report this diagnosis. You are not done yet. Now, backtrack to the subchapter header to see if there are any notations that may apply to this case. [HINT: It is directly above code F90. See Figure 4-13.]

This is good information but has no impact to this specific encounter. Next, backtrack to the very beginning of this ICD-10-CM chapter 5 (see Figure 4-14) to check for any notations that you need to apply in reporting Belinda's diagnosis.

Behavioral and emotional disorders with onset usually occurring in childhood and adolescence (F90-F98)

Note: Codes within categories F90-F98 may be used regardless of the age of a patient. These disorders generally have onset within the childhood and adolescent years, but may continue throughout life or not be diagnosed until adulthood.

FIGURE 4-13 Example of a subchapter section note, from above code F90 Source: *ICD-10-CM Official Guidelines for Coding and Reporting* The Centers for Medicare and Medicaid Services (CMS) and the National Center for Health Statistics (NCHS)

Chapter 5. Mental, Behavioral, and Neurodevelopmental Disorders (F01-F99)

INCLUDES disorders of psychological development

EXCLUDES2 symptoms, signs, and abnormal clinical laboratory findings, not classified elsewhere (R00-R99)

FIGURE 4-14 Chapter opening notations, example from chapter 5 Source: *ICD-10-CM Official Guidelines for Coding and Reporting* The Centers for Medicare and Medicaid Services (CMS) and the National Center for Health Statistics (NCHS)

Again, good information, but none of these notations related to reporting Belinda's diagnosis. One more step to take—check the **ICD-10-CM Official Guidelines for Coding and Reporting, Section 1.c.5. Mental, Behavioral, and Neurodevelopmental Disorders (F01-F99).** Read all of the guidelines in this section to see if there is any guidance you need to properly report code F95.2. No? Great.

Now . . . you can report code F95.2 with confidence that it is accurate and correct to report *why* Dr. Gaseor cared for Belinda during this encounter. Good work!

Case #2 Abrasion

Let's look at the second case we covered in the section *The Alphabetic Index and Ancillaries*, "*Dr. Mulford noted that Charlie has suffered an abrasion on his chin.*" And you found code Abrasion, chin S00.81. Turn in your ICD-10-CM Tabular List to the code category:

☑4 **S00   Superficial injury of head**

> **EXCLUDES1** diffuse cerebral contusion (S06.2-)
> focal cerebral contusion (S06.3-)
> injury of eye and orbit (S05.-)
> open wound of head (S01.-)

The appropriate 7th is to be added to each code from category S00.
A Initial encounter
D Subsequent encounter
S Sequela

None of these diagnoses in the **EXCLUDES1** notation relate to Charlie's case; however, it is a good thing you started reading here because there is a box containing the available seventh characters for you to use in this code category.

Read down through all of the available fourth characters in this code category to ensure you don't find something more accurate than that suggested by the Alphabetic Index:

☑5 S00.0 Superficial injury of scalp
☑5 S00.1 Contusion of eyelid and periocular area
☑5 S00.2 Other and unspecified superficial injuries of eyelid and periocular area
☑5 S00.3 Superficial injury of nose
☑5 S00.4 Superficial injury of ear
☑5 S00.5 Superficial injury of lip and oral cavity
☑5 S00.8 Superficial injury of other parts of the head
☑5 S00.9 Superficial injury of unspecified part of head

It looks like the Alphabetic Index was sending us in the right direction. S00.8 is the best option. A fifth character is needed. Read all of the options carefully. Did you determine this?

☑7 **S00.81   Abrasion of other part of head**

You see how different this code description is from what you read in the Alphabetic Index? This is one reason why it is important to use both the Alphabetic Index and the Tabular List. Each has its own details to share. Good. However, one thing the Alphabetic Index didn't let you know is that this code must have a seventh character. Turn back to that box at the beginning of this subsection. Which is the correct character to report for Charlie's encounter with Dr. Mulford for care related to his abrasion?

The appropriate 7th is to be added to each code from category S00.
A Initial encounter
D Subsequent encounter
S Sequela

> **Chapter 19. Injury, Poisoning and Certain Other Consequences of External Causes (S00-T88)**
>
> **Note:** Use secondary code(s) from Chapter 20, External causes of morbidity, to indicate cause of injury. Codes within the T section that include the external cause do not require an additional external cause code.
>
> *Use additional code* to identify any retained foreign body, if applicable (Z18.-)
>
> **EXCLUDES1** birth trauma (P10-P15)
>
> obstetric trauma (O70-O71)
>
> **Note:** The chapter uses the S-section for coding different types of injuries related to single body regions and the T-section to cover injuries to unspecified body regions as well as poisoning and certain other consequences of external causes.

FIGURE 4-15 ICD-10-Tabular List, chapter 19 opening notations Source: *ICD-10-CM Official Guidelines for Coding and Reporting* The Centers for Medicare and Medicaid Services (CMS) and the National Center for Health Statistics (NCHS)

Did you abstract from the scenario that this was the first encounter? And you noticed that you will need to insert a placeholder letter **x** after the fifth character, so that the seventh character **A** lands in the correct spot.

S00.81xA Abrasion of other part of head, initial encounter

Look back to the beginning of this ICD-10-CM chapter to check for any notations that you might need to consider before you report this code (see Figure 4-15).

This is important information, but none of it relates to Charlie's abrasion.

One more step, check the **ICD-10-CM Official Guidelines for Coding and Reporting, Section 1.c.19. Injury, Poisoning, and Certain Other Consequences of External Causes (S00-T88).** Read all of the guidelines in this section to see if there is any guidance you need to properly report code S00.81xA. No? Great. Good work!

Case #3 Pink Eye (Conjunctivitis)

Our third scenario in the section *The Alphabetic Index and Ancillaries* was from Dr. Johnson's care for Melinda's pink eye. You used the Alphabetic Index properly to lead you to the suggested code:

Conjunctivitis, acute, mucopurulent H10.02-

In this case, the Alphabetic Index did notify you that an additional character is required by including the hyphen after the first five characters. In your ICD-10-CM's Tabular List, find the code category

✓4 **H10 Conjunctivitis**

EXCLUDES1 keratoconjunctivitis (H16.2-)

This is a match for the alternate term provided by the **EXCLUDES1** Alphabetic Index, and the notation is not related to Melinda's case, so continue reading down to investigate the fourth character options. Did you determine which one matches best?

✓5 **H10.0 Mucopurulent conjunctivitis**

You are making good progress! A fifth character is required, so read carefully and determine which you should use:

✓5 **H10.02 Other mucopurulent conjunctivitis**

This is the best because there was nothing about the pink eye diagnosis that stated it could be acute follicular conjunctivitis.

As you read the options for the sixth character, you should notice that you need a new piece of information . . . which eye was diagnosed? Right? Left? Or both (bilateral)?

> **Chapter 7. Diseases of the Eye and Adnexa (H00-H59)**
>
> **Note:** Use an external cause code following the code for the eye condition, if applicable, to identify the cause of the eye condition
>
> **EXCLUDES2** certain conditions originating in the perinatal period (P04-P96)
> certain infectious and parasitic diseases (A00-B99)
> complications of pregnancy, childbirth, and puerperium (O00-O9A)
> congenital malformations, deformations, and chromosomal abnormalities (Q00-Q99)
> diabetes mellitus related eye conditions (E09.3-, E10.3-, E11.3-, E13.3-)
> endocrine, nutritional and metabolic diseases (E00-E88)
> injury (trauma) of eye and orbit (S05.-)
> injury, poisoning, and certain consequences of external causes (S00-T88)
> neoplasms (C00-D49)
> symptoms, signs and abnormal clinical and laboratory findings, not elsewhere classified (R00-R94)
> syphilis related eye disorders (A50.01, A50.3-, A51.43, A53.71)

FIGURE 4-16 Tabular List, chapter 7, Diseases of the Eye and Adnexa, opening notations Source: *ICD-10-CM Official Guidelines for Coding and Reporting* The Centers for Medicare and Medicaid Services (CMS) and the National Center for Health Statistics (NCHS)

Go back to the documentation and read: "*Dr. Johnson . . . caring for Melinda, who has a problem with her right eye.*"

H10.021 Other mucopurulent conjunctivitis, right eye

Good work! Check the beginning of the subsection. There are no notations at all. Now, check the very beginning of this ICD-10-CM chapter (see Figure 4-16).

A lot of good information here, yet it is not related to Melinda's diagnosis, so you have only one more place to check: the **ICD-10-CM Official Guidelines for Coding and Reporting, Section 1.c.7. Diseases of the Eye and Adnexa (H00-H59).** Read all of the guidelines in this section to see if there is any guidance you need to properly report code H10.021. No? Great. You can now report H10.021 Other mucopurulent conjunctivitis, right eye with confidence.

4.5 Which Conditions to Code

As you abstract the provider's notes, you are looking for the information that will direct you to those codes that explain or describe the answer to the question, "*Why did this health care provider care for and treat this individual during this encounter?*" That is it. The codes do not report the individual's complete medical history.

Unrelated Conditions

The attending physician may include information in his or her documentation that reports a condition or diagnosis that is unrelated to this encounter. Remember that the physician does not write the notes just for you to code from. The notes have other, important purposes, such as documenting past history. You must learn to distinguish among notations. You will code only those diagnoses, signs, and/or symptoms related to procedures, services, treatments, and/or medical decision making occurring during this visit. ICD-10-CM guidelines specifically direct you to omit (do not code) any

> **GUIDANCE CONNECTION**
>
> Read the ICD-10-CM Official Guidelines for Coding and Reporting, section **I. Conventions, General Coding Guidelines and Chapter Specific Guidelines,** subsection **B. General coding guidelines,** specifically subsections **4. Signs and symptoms, 5. Conditions that are an integral part of a disease process,** and **6. Conditions that are not an integral part of a disease process.**

diagnoses or conditions from a patient's history that have no impact on the current treatment or service. So, you will have to read carefully.

Keep in mind, in some situations, the attention to a condition may be subtle. For example, the physician may renew a previous prescription for a chronic condition. You will need to report that condition to support the writing of the prescription, even if it is not the principal reason the patient is being cared for at this encounter.

Systemic Conditions

If a patient has a **systemic condition**, this means that this condition affects the entire body, for example, diabetes mellitus, hypertension, or pregnancy. The physician, therefore, must take this into consideration in the medical decision making for virtually any other condition.

> **Systemic Condition**
> A condition that affects the entire body and virtually all body systems, therefore requiring the physician to consider this in his or her medical decision making for any other condition.

LET'S CODE IT! SCENARIO

MaeBelle Abernathy, a 29-year-old female, came to see Dr. Cypher complaining of severe pain in her shoulder. She stated that she was working in the garden and a loose branch fell out of her magnolia tree onto her left shoulder. MaeBelle is 15 weeks pregnant. Normally, Dr. Cypher would have sent MaeBelle for an x-ray. However, because she is pregnant, he decided to examine her, diagnosed her with a sprained corahumeral shoulder, and strapped her shoulder and arm. He also double-checked the pain medication he prescribed to ensure that it was safe for pregnant women.

Let's Code It!

Dr. Cypher diagnosed MaeBelle with a *sprained shoulder*. Turn to the Alphabetic Index and look up *sprain, shoulder*.

Sprain, shoulder joint S43.40-

In the Tabular List, begin reading at code category S43 and read the INCLUDES and EXCLUDES2 notes carefully. There is nothing here that relates to this patient, so continue reading.

✓4 S43   Dislocation and sprain of joints and ligaments of shoulder girdle

You can see that you need additional characters, so continue reading down the column. Match the terms to the physician's notes. The fact is that Dr. Cypher did not provide any further specifics, so the most accurate code is:

S43.412A   Sprain of left corahumeral (ligament), initial encounter

This is the only diagnosis confirmed by Dr. Cypher at this encounter. However, the notes clearly indicate that MaeBelle's pregnancy influenced the way the doctor treated her. Therefore, the codes need to tell that part of the story. The code for the pregnancy must be included to accurately report this visit. The Alphabetic Index suggests

Pregnancy incidental finding Z33.1

In the Tabular List you will find:

✓4 Z33 Pregnant state

Keep reading to review the fourth-character choices. The most accurate is

Z33.1 Pregnant state, incidental

This code explains the situation perfectly. MaeBelle is pregnant and that pregnancy was involved in the treatment of her shoulder injury, but it was not the principal reason she came to see Dr. Cypher. This code means

(continued)

that her pregnancy was a factor included in the patient's treatment plan but not a part of the principal diagnosis. Perfect!

Do you remember when you read the chapter *Abstracting Clinical Documentation* that you will need external cause codes for this encounter between MaeBelle and Dr. Cypher because she was injured? Therefore, you would also include three other codes:

> **W20.8xxA Other cause of strike by thrown, projected or falling object**
>
> **Y93.H2 Activity, gardening and landscaping**
>
> **Y99.8 Other external cause status (leisure activity)**

[Don't worry . . . more details about determining external cause codes are in the upcoming chapter titled *Coding Injury, Poisoning, and External Causes*.]

Check the top of each subsection and the head of each chapter in ICD-10-CM. There are notations at the beginning of this chapter: an INCLUDES notation, a *Use Additional Code* note, an EXCLUDES1 notation, and an EXCLUDES2 notation. Read carefully. Do any relate to Dr. Cypher's diagnosis of MaeBelle? No. Turn to the **Official Guidelines** and read **Section 1.c.19, 1.c.20, and 1.c.21**. There is nothing here that will change what you have already determined, this time.

The bottom line . . . there will be five codes to report the reasons why Dr. Cypher needed to care for MaeBelle at this encounter:

S43.412A	Sprain of left corahumeral (ligament), initial encounter
Z33.1	Pregnant state, incidental
W20.8xxA	Other cause of strike by thrown, projected or falling object
Y93.H2	Activity, gardening and landscaping
Y99.8	Other external cause status (leisure activity)

In some encounters you will not report a condition, just because there was a mention of it in the documentation.

LET'S CODE IT! SCENARIO

Arthur Fleurs, a 47-year-old male, came to Dr. Davenport at the clinic because he was having a nosebleed that wouldn't stop. Arthur was in a single-car accident and his airbag expanded, hitting him in the nose, causing it to bleed. He is otherwise healthy with a history of allergic asthma. Dr. Davenport examined Arthur's nasal passages and packed the nostrils. The doctor then told Arthur to go home and rest and return the next day for a follow-up.

Let's Code It!

Arthur came to see Dr. Davenport because he had a *nosebleed*. Turn to the Alphabetic Index and look up the diagnosis.

> **Nosebleed R04.0**

Surprised it was that easy? Well, sometimes it is. Check the code in the Tabular List, and you will see

> ✓4 **R04** Hemorrhage from respiratory passages

The nose is on the head, so you are in the correct category. Continue reading down the column to review your choices for the fourth-digit:

> **R04.0 Epistaxis**
>
> **Hemorrhage from nose; nosebleed**

(continued)

> Yes. I guess it was easy. Is that all you need to code? The notes state that Arthur has a history of asthma. However, it has nothing to do with the reason he came to the doctor, and it did not affect the way Dr. Davenport treated Arthur. Therefore, you will not code it for this encounter because it had nothing to do with this visit.
>
> Check the top of this subsection and the head of this chapter in ICD-10-CM. There is a **NOTE** and an **EXCLUDES2** notation. Read carefully. Do any relate to Dr. Davenport's diagnosis of Arthur? No. Turn to the **Official Guidelines** and read **Section 1.c.18.** There is nothing specifically applicable here either.
>
> Now you can report **R04.0** with confidence.

Screenings and Other Preventive Services

When a screening test is performed (patient has no signs, symptoms, or diagnosis of a condition), you will still need to report a code to explain the reason why Fiona had her annual mammogram or Roger, after his 50th birthday, had a colonoscopy. Many times, you can identify such instances because they are usually determined not by the patient's feelings, signs, symptoms, or other active health issue, but by the calendar.

> ### EXAMPLES
>
> **Z00.00 Encounter for general adult medical examination without abnormal findings**
> . . . this code reports what is commonly known as an annual physical, which is an encounter prompted by the calendar to ensure preventive measures and early detection testing are employed to support good health.
>
> **Z02.1 Encounter for pre-employment examination**
> . . . some employers require a candidate to have a physical prior to being officially hired. This code is used to report this reason *why* the individual would see the physician.
>
> **Z12.31 Encounter for screening mammogram for malignant neoplasm of breast**
> . . . every woman over the age of 40 should be doing this annually, or every other year, to identify the presence of a malignancy at the earliest possible time, when treatment is less invasive, less intensive, and less costly. This code explains that this woman has no signs or symptoms; she and her physician just want to be smart about her health.

Test Results

Even though you didn't go to medical school, you still need to know the difference between a positive test result and a negative test result. However, you are not permitted to affirm a diagnosis from a test result without the physician's documentation. This rule applies to laboratory tests, x-rays and other imaging, pathology, and any other screening or diagnostic testing done for a patient. In such cases, especially when the health care professional has ordered additional tests based on an abnormal finding, you should query, or ask, the physician whether or not you should document the results. Be certain to get your answer in writing in the patient's record. *If it's not in writing, you can't code it!*

> ### EXAMPLE
> Laboratory report in patient's file shows:
>
> Glucose   155   Norm Range: 65–105 mg/dL
>
> You can see that the patient's glucose is abnormally high. However, you cannot code *hyperglycemia* without a physician's written interpretation and diagnostic statement.

If a physician or other health care professional has already interpreted the test results and the final report has been placed in the patient's file with a diagnostic statement, you should include the code.

> **EXAMPLE**
>
> Report from radiology states: "X-ray shows an open fracture of the anatomical neck of the humerus, right arm. Signed: Flor Rodriquez, MD, Chief of Radiology."
>
> The report, signed by a physician, includes a specific diagnostic statement that should be coded. However, you should always check with the attending physician and permit him or her the opportunity to update the patient's chart with the confirmed diagnosis. You should do this as a sign of respect.

Preoperative Evaluations

Whenever a patient is scheduled for a surgical procedure (on a nonemergency basis), there are typical tests that must be done to ensure that the patient is healthy enough to have the operation. Cardiovascular, respiratory, and other examinations are often done a couple of days prior to the date of surgery. Often these tests do not necessarily relate directly to the diagnostic reason the surgery will be performed. Therefore, they will need a different diagnosis code to report medical necessity.

Coding those encounters carries a specific guideline. In such cases, the principal, or first-listed, diagnosis code will be from the following category:

Z01.8   Encounter for other specified special examinations

Follow that code with the code or codes that identify the condition(s) documented as the reason for the upcoming surgical procedure.

> **EXAMPLE**
>
> *Kenzie Hannon was diagnosed with carpal tunnel syndrome in her right wrist. Dr. Isaacs recommended a surgical solution. Because of her history of atrial fibrillation, Kenzie was required to get approval from her cardiologist before she could have the procedure.*
>
> **G56.01, Carpal tunnel syndrome, right upper limb**, is the code that will be used to report the medical necessity for the surgery on Kenzie's wrist. However, it will not support the examination performed by her cardiologist. Think about it . . . who would agree to pay for a cardiologist to examine a patient with a diagnosis of carpal tunnel syndrome? The cardiologist is not qualified to do the job; that is better suited for an orthopedist.
>
> **Z01.810, Encounter for preprocedural cardiovascular examination** will support the cardiologist's time and expertise to clear Kenzie for the procedure on her wrist.

> **GUIDANCE CONNECTION**
>
> Read the ICD-10-CM Official Guidelines for Coding and Reporting, section **II. Selection of Principal Diagnosis** and section **III. Reporting Additional Diagnoses**.

Preoperative/Postoperative Diagnoses

You may have already noticed that procedure and operative reporting usually include both a preoperative diagnosis and a postoperative diagnosis. For cases where the two statements differ, the guidelines state that you should code the postoperative diagnosis because it is expected that it is the more accurate of the two.

4.6 Putting It All Together: ICD-10-CM Basics

Now that you have learned about how to use all of the parts of the ICD-10-CM code book, let's put all your new knowledge to the test.

LET'S CODE IT! SCENARIO

Michael Smithstone, a 45-year-old male, came in to see Dr. Opell, his internist. He complains of a fever, sweating, headaches, and pain in his muscles, joints, and back. He stated that he has also felt fatigued. Dr. Opell documents that Michael has just returned from working for a week at a goat farm in an impoverished area. He said that he was supposed to stay longer but came home early because of his illness, "whatever it is."

Dr. Opell ordered a CBC and other blood tests, which revealed that Michael was suffering from Cypress Fever, a bacterial infection caused by Brucella abortus. Dr. Opell gave Michael a prescription for Doxycycline, 100mg PO q 12 hr on the first day, then once daily for 6 weeks; and another for Rifampin, 600mg BID for 6 weeks.

Let's Code It!

First, let's identify the confirmed diagnosis of the bacterial infection:

Cypress Fever, caused by Brucella abortus

Next, which word is the main term . . . the reason why Michael needed Dr. Opell's care. You can always look up all of the words; however, as you gain more experience in identifying the main term, it will save you time. For this case, the main term is *Fever*.

Open your ICD-10-CM code book to the Index to Diseases and Injuries—more commonly referred to as the Alphabetic Index—and find the main term in bold: FEVER.

> **Fever** (inanition) (of unknown origin) (persistent) (with chills) (with rigor) R50.9
> - abortus A23.1
> - Aden (dengue) A90
> - African tick-borne A68.1
> - American
> -- mountain (tick) A93.2
> -- spotted A77.0
> - aphthous B08.8
> - arbovirus, arboviral A94
> -- hemorrhagic A94
> -- specified NEC A93.8
> - Argentinian hemorrhagic A96.0
> - Assam B55.0
> - Australian Q A78
> - Bangkok hemorrhagic A91
> - Barmah forest A92.8
> - Bartonella A44.0
> - bilious, hemoglobinuric B50.8
> - blackwater B50.8
> - blister B00.1
> - Bolivian hemorrhagic A96.1
> - Bonvale dam T73.3
> - boutonneuse A77.1
> - brain—*see* Encephalitis
> - Brazilian purpiric A48.4
> - breakbone A90
> - Bullis A77.0
> - Bunyamwera A92.8
> - Burdwan B55.0
> - Bwamba A92.8

(continued)

> - Cameroon—*see* Malaria
> - Canton A75.9
> - catarrhal (acute) J00
> -- chronic J31.0
> - cat-scratch A28.1
> - Central Asian hemorrhagic A98.0
> - cerebral—*see* Encephalitis
> - cerebrospinal meningococcal A39.0
> - Chagres B50.9
> - Chandipura A92.8
> - Changuinola A93.1
> - Charcot's (biliary) (hepatic) (intermittent)—*see* Calculus, bile duct
> - Chikungunya (viral) (hemorrhagic) A92.0
> - Chitral A93.1
> - Colombo—*see* Fever, paratyphoid
> - Colorado tick (virus) A93.2
> - congestive (remittent)—*see* Malaria
> - Congo virus A98.0
> - continued malarial B50.9
> - Corsican—*see* Malaria
> - Crimean-Congo hemorrhagic A98.0
> - Cyprus—*see* Brucellosis
> - dandy A90
> - deer fly—*see* Tularemia
> - dengue (virus) A90
> -- hemorrhagic A91

You can see the long, long list of types of fevers that a person can have. Notice these additional terms are shown in alphabetic order, so . . . what kind of fever did Michael have? Cypress Fever. Read carefully down the long list and see if you can find Cypress.

Fever

- Cyprus—*see* Brucellosis

Still in the Alphabetic Index, turn to find the main term, Brucellosis.

> **Bruce sepsis** A23.0
> **Brucellosis** (infection) A23.9
> - abortus A23.1
> - canis A23.3
> - dermatitis A23.9
> - melitensis A23.0
> - mixed A23.8
> - sepsis A23.9
> -- melitensis A23.0
> -- specified NEC A23.8
> - suis A23.2
> **Bruck-de Lange disease** Q87.1

There are several choices here as well. Go back to Dr. Opell's notes. Are there any terms that will help with this decision?

(continued)

. . . a bacterial infection caused by Brucella abortus

Therefore, *Brucellosis abortus* leads you to a suggested code **A23.1**—good. Now you have a suggested code to work with.

Turn in the Tabular List of your ICD-10-CM code book and find the code category **A23**. Remember, you must always begin reading in the Tabular List at the three-character code category.

> **A23 Brucellosis**
> INCLUDES Malta fever
> Mediterranean fever
> undulant fever
> **A23.0 Brucellosis due to Brucella melitensis**
> **A23.1 Brucellosis due to Brucella abortus**
> **A23.2 Brucellosis due to Brucella suis**
> **A23.3 Brucellosis due to Brucella canis**
> **A23.8 Other brucellosis**
> **A23.9 Brucellosis, unspecified**

Check the INCLUDES notation. This does not relate to this case. Check for any other notations. There are none. Do you need a second code to identify the specific bacteria that caused Michael's infection? No, because this is a combination code and it already includes that detail.

One final step . . . turn to the **ICD-10-CM Official Guidelines for Coding and Reporting, Section 1.c.1. Certain Infectious and Parasitic Diseases (A00-B99).** Read through the subsections. Are there any related to Cypress Fever or Brucellosis? No.

Terrific! Now you can feel confident that reporting **A23.1 Brucellosis due to Brucella abortus** will justify Dr. Opell's care for Michael.

Good job! You are really learning.

Chapter Summary

As you look back over this chapter, you should notice one very important thing: The ICD-10-CM book will almost always guide you to the correct code. The Alphabetic Index will guide you to the correct chapter and subsection in the Tabular List, so you can read all of the notations and symbols, evaluate all the options, and determine the best, most accurate code. If no codes seem to match the attending physician's notes, just go back and keep looking.

Two principles important to becoming a good ICD-10-CM coder:

1. Abstract the main term(s) from the physician's documentation so that you can determine the best, most accurate code or codes.
2. In case of an injury, poisoning, or adverse effect, you will need to add an external cause code.

The Official Coding Guidelines are always there, at your fingertips in the book for you to reference—no memorization! All the information can point you in the right direction toward the best, most accurate code. Just look and read. And when the time comes, you will have no problem transitioning from student to professional coding specialist.

The ICD-10-CM code book will lead you, step-by-step, to the correct, complete code to report medical necessity—*why* the health care provider cared for the patient—for this encounter with the highest level of specificity. However, not all diagnostic

> **CODING BITES**
> ICD-10-CM CODE BOOK CONTENTS
> Introduction
> Official Conventions
> Official Guidelines for Coding and Reporting
> The Alphabetic Index
> The Neoplasm Table
> The Table of Drugs and Chemicals
> The Index to External Causes
> The Tabular List

statements follow a straight line. Sometimes, you have to really read carefully and use your critical thinking skills to interpret accurately. Other times, you may have to use alternate terms from those used in the notes to determine the correct code description. A medical dictionary will help you, so it is recommended that you keep one by your side (especially now, while you are early in your learning). Familiarize yourself with the terms used as well as the critical thinking and interpretation skills that are part of the coding process.

CHAPTER 4 REVIEW
Introduction to ICD-10-CM

Let's Check It! Terminology

Match each key term to the appropriate definition.

Part I

E 1. LO 4.4 The section of the ICD-10-CM code book listing all of the codes in alphanumeric order.

A 2. LO 4.3 The section of a code book showing all codes, from A to Z, by the short code descriptions.

D 3. LO 4.3 The section of the ICD-10-CM code book listing drugs, chemicals, and other biologicals that may poison a patient or result in an adverse reaction.

C 4. LO 4.3 A list of all possible codes for benign and malignant neoplasms, in alphabetic order by anatomical location of the tumor.

B 5. LO 4.3 The alphabetic listing of the multitude of external causes that might result in a patient's injury.

A. Alphabetic Index
B. Index to External Causes
C. Neoplasm Table
D. Table of Drugs and Chemicals
E. Tabular List of Diseases and Injuries

Part II

B 1. LO 4.1 A specific location or part of the human body.

D 2. LO 4.1 Found to be true or definite.

E 3. LO 4.3 A condition named after a person.

J 4. LO 4.5 A condition that affects the entire body and virtually all body systems, therefore requiring the physician to consider this in his or her medical decision making for any other condition.

G 5. LO 4.2 An establishment that provides acute care services to individuals who stay overnight on the premises.

I 6. LO 4.1 Cause-and-effect relationship between an original condition, illness, or injury and an additional problem caused by the existence of that original condition.

H 7. LO 4.2 Health care services provided to individuals without an overnight stay in the facility.

C 8. LO 4.3 The state of abnormality or dysfunction.

A 9. LO 4.3 An unexpected, bad result.

F 10. LO 4.3 An event, outside the body, that causes injury, poisoning, or an adverse reaction.

A. Adverse Effect
B. Anatomical Site
C. Condition
D. Confirmed
E. Eponym
F. External Cause
G. Inpatient Facility
H. Outpatient Services
I. Sequela (Late Effect)
J. Systemic Condition

Part III

E 1. LO 4.1 Descriptors that are not absolutely necessary to have been included in the physician's notes and are provided simply to further clarify a code description; optional terms.

F 2. LO 4.1 Specifics that are not described in any other code in the ICD-10-CM book.

B 3. LO 4.2 Long duration; continuing over a long period of time.

D 4. LO 4.1 A condition caused or developed from the existence of another condition.

J 5. LO 4.1 One disease that affects or encourages another condition.

K 6. LO 4.1 The absence of additional specifics in the physician's documentation.

H 7. LO 4.1 Additional information that the physician specified and isn't included in any other code description.

I 8. LO 4.2 The condition that is the primary, or main, reason for the encounter.

G 9. LO 4.1 An indication that more detailed information is not available from the physician's notes.

A 10. LO 4.2 Severe; serious.

C 11. LO 4.2 When the physician indicates that the patient's signs and symptoms may closely lead to two different diagnoses.

A. Acute
B. Chronic
C. Differential Diagnosis
D. Manifestation
E. Nonessential Modifier
F. Not Elsewhere Classifiable (NEC)
G. Not Otherwise Specified (NOS)
H. Other Specified
I. Principal Diagnosis
J. Underlying Condition
K. Unspecified

Let's Check It! Concepts

Choose the most appropriate answer for each of the following questions.

1. LO 4.4 Which code range identifies the diseases of the digestive system?
   a. E00-E89
   b. G00-G99
   c. K00-K95
   d. R00-R99

2. LO 4.1 Turn to Hypertension in the ICD-10-CM Alphabetic Index. All of the following are listed as nonessential modifiers *except*
   a. accelerated.
   b. benign.
   c. idiopathic.
   d. organic.

3. LO 4.2 Refer to the ICD-10-CM Official Guidelines Section II. What is section II's title?
   a. Conventions, General Coding Guidelines and Chapter Specific Guidelines
   b. Selection of Principal Diagnosis
   c. Reporting Additional Diagnoses
   d. Diagnostic Coding and Reporting Guidelines for Outpatient Services

4. LO 4.2 The ICD-10-CM Official Guidelines I.A.16 are guidelines with instructions concerning which word(s)?
   a. "And"
   b. "With"
   c. "See" and "See Also"
   d. "Code Also" note

5. LO 4.1 A code surrounded within *italicized*, or *slanted*, brackets
   a. is optional.
   b. must be included.
   c. is a previously deleted code.
   d. is a manifestation.

6. LO 4.1 NEC means
   a. the hospital didn't provide more details.
   b. the physician didn't provide more details.

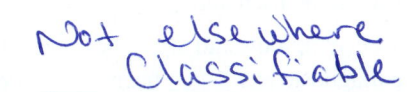

Not elsewhere Classifiable

CHAPTER 4 REVIEW

    c. the ICD-10-CM book didn't provide a code with more details.
    d. the patient didn't provide more details.

7. LO 4.3 An example of a condition is
    a. Cushing's disease.
    b. Danlos syndrome.
    c. Beck's.
    d. a wound.

8. LO 4.6 The correct code for acute and chronic respiratory failure with hypoxia is
    a. J96.01
    b. J96.12
    c. J96.21
    d. J96.92

9. LO 4.5 Which of the following would not be considered a systemic condition?
    a. diabetes mellitus
    b. sprain of left corahumeral
    c. pregnancy
    d. hypertension

10. LO 4.6 Steve is starting a new job and is required to complete a preemployment examination. Dr. Rogers completed the exam and signs the paperwork. How is this encounter coded?
    a. Z02.1
    b. Z00.00
    c. Z12.31
    d. Z02.2

Let's Check It! Guidelines

Refer to the Official Guidelines and fill in the blanks according to the Conventions and General Coding Guidelines Section I, subsections A and B.

Tabular	3	Neoplasms	separate
reported	Diseases	Excludes2	right
first	highest	placeholder	Drugs
acute	discharge	Alphabetic	same
related	External Causes	both	not
verify	once	expansion	confirmed
left	invalid	Excludes1	established
unspecified	insufficient		

1. The ICD-10-CM is divided into the _Alphabetic_ Index, an alphabetic list of terms and their corresponding code, and the _____ List, a structured list of codes divided into chapters based on body system or condition.
2. The Alphabetic Index consists of the following parts: the Index of _____ and Injury, the Index of _____ of Injury, the Table of _____, and the Table of _____ and Chemicals.
3. All categories are _____ characters.
4. A code that has an applicable seventh character is considered _____ without the seventh character.
5. The "x" is used as a _____ at certain codes to allow for future _____.
6. Codes titled _____ are for use when the information in the medical record is _____ to assign a more specific code.
7. A type _____ note is a pure excludes note. It means "NOT CODED HERE!"
8. A type _____ note represents "Not included here."
9. To select a code in the classification that corresponds to a diagnosis or reason for a visit documented in a medical record, _____ locate the term in the Alphabetic Index, and then _____ the code in the Tabular List.
10. Diagnosis codes are to be used and _____ at their _____ number of characters available.
11. Codes that describe symptoms and signs, as opposed to diagnoses, are acceptable for reporting purposes when a _____ definitive diagnosis has _____ been _____ (confirmed) by the provider.

94   PART II | REPORTING DIAGNOSES

12. If the same condition is described as both acute (subacute) and chronic, and _____ subentries exist in the Alphabetic Index at the _____ indentation level, code _____ and sequence the _____ code first.
13. Each unique ICD-10-CM diagnosis code may be reported only _____ for an encounter.
14. If no bilateral code is provided and the condition is bilateral, assign separate codes for both the _____ and _____ side.
15. If the provider documents a "borderline" diagnosis at the time of _____, the diagnosis is coded as _____, unless the classification provides a specific entry (e.g., borderline diabetes).

Let's Check It! Rules and Regulations

Please answer the following questions from the knowledge you have gained after reading this chapter.

1. LO 4.2 Explain the difference in the guidelines between coding for outpatient services and coding for inpatient services.
2. LO 4.3 When is it appropriate to code from the Alphabetic Index?
3. LO 4.1 Explain a *code first* notation.
4. LO 4.4 Explain the importance of the Tabular List.
5. LO 4.5 When the preoperative and the postoperative diagnoses differ, which diagnosis is coded and why?

YOU CODE IT! Basics

First, identify the main term in the following diagnoses; then code the diagnosis.

Example: Factitial dermatosis:
a. main term: *dermatosis* b. diagnosis: *L98.1*

1. Acute cystitis without hematuria:
   a. main term: _____ b. diagnosis: _____
2. Pulmonary necrosis:
   a. main term: _____ b. diagnosis: _____
3. Fibrocystic disease of the pancreas:
   a. main term: _____ b. diagnosis: _____
4. Chronic daily headache:
   a. main term: _____ b. diagnosis: _____
5. Inflammation of the jaw:
   a. main term: _____ b. diagnosis: _____
6. Mobile kidney:
   a. main term: _____ b. diagnosis: _____
7. Lymphoid interstitial pneumonia:
   a. main term: _____ b. diagnosis: _____
8. Adrenal fibrosis:
   a. main term: _____ b. diagnosis: _____
9. Upper respiratory infection, chronic:
   a. main term: _____ b. diagnosis: _____
10. Acute conjunctivitis, right:
    a. main term: _____ b. diagnosis: _____
11. Ulcer of lower limb, left calf with muscle necrosis:
    a. main term: _____ b. diagnosis: _____
12. Aortic endocarditis:
    a. main term: _____ b. diagnosis: _____
13. Tuberculous cystitis:
    a. main term: _____ b. diagnosis: _____
14. Acute appendicitis:
    a. main term: _____ b. diagnosis: _____
15. Systemic lupus erythematosus with lung involvement:
    a. main term: _____ b. diagnosis: _____

CHAPTER 4 REVIEW

YOU CODE IT! Practice

Using the techniques described in this chapter, carefully read through the case studies and determine the most accurate ICD-10-CM code(s) and external cause code(s), if appropriate, for each case.

1. Ralph Flower, a 27-year-old male, presents today for his annual flu vaccination.

2. Erina Castles, a 43-year-old female, presents today with a few pimples on her chest. Dr. Moss noted some slight redness and swelling in the area and orders blood tests. The results of the blood tests confirm the diagnosis that Erina is a carrier of staphylococcal, methicillin resistant (MRSA).

3. Herman Carson, a 32-year-old male, presents with a severe headache and occasional nosebleeds. Dr. Wells completed an examination recording a blood pressure reading of 180/110. Herman is hospitalized, where an ECG and echocardiogram confirm the diagnosis of malignant hypertension.

4. Anna Blanks, a 68-year-old female, presents with a cyst on the anterior wall of her vagina. After an examination, Dr. Hervey takes a tissue biopsy and orders a CT scan. Anna is diagnosed with a primary malignant neoplasm of the Skene's gland.

5. Jan McKenzie, a 68-year-old female, presents today to see Dr. McLeod due to restlessness and being anxious. Jan retired 3 months ago. Dr. McLeod notes Jan is having difficulty adjusting to retirement.

6. Margaret Carll, a 28-year-old female, presents today with the complaint of feeling dizzy and has some headaches. Dr. Dithomas notes a fever and completes an ECG, which shows an ST depression. PMH and PFH are noncontributory. Margaret is admitted to the hospital, where further blood tests, a chest CT scan, and a ventilation scan confirm the diagnosis of hyperventilation (tetany).

7. Elizabeth Hagun, a 35-year-old female, spent yesterday afternoon outside in the full sun; now she is experiencing severe itching. She comes to see Dr. Jerod, who completes an examination and notes skin redness and blistering. Elizabeth is diagnosed with acute dermatitis due to solar radiation. Code the dermatitis.

8. Audrey Harkey, a 33-year-old female, comes to see Dr. Blankenship. Audrey is accompanied by her husband, Henry. Audrey complaints of fever, a stiff neck, and headaches. Henry states he is concerned because he has noticed some confusion. Audrey is admitted to the hospital, where a lumbar puncture is performed; 5 ml of cerebrospinal fluid is drawn. Test results confirm Dr. Blankenship's diagnosis of tuberculous meningitis.

9. Gloria Leugers, a 37-year-old female, comes to see Dr. Lewis with a fever, weakness, and abdominal pain. Blood tests reveal a hemoglobin of 8.6 and UA is positive for blood. Gloria is admitted to Weston Hospital and diagnosed with schistosomiasis disorder in the kidney.

10. Lauren Wheatle, a 68-year-old female, presents today with chest discomfort when resting. Dr. Billings completes an examination with ECG. The ECG reveals an elevated ST segment. Lauren is admitted to the hospital, where blood tests show elevated cardiac enzymes and a cardiac echo confirms the diagnosis of variant angina.

11. Carolyn Mann, a 34-year-old female, presents today with intense itching and a burning sensation of her anus. Dr. Neal completes an examination and diagnoses her with pruritus ani, stage 2.

12. Sylvia McCray, a 17-year-old female, presents today with a headache and dull facial pain between and behind her eyes. Dr. Clayton orders a CT scan, which confirms the diagnosis of acute ethmoidal sinusitis, infection due to staphylococcus.

13. Shawn Phillips, a 6-year-old male, is brought in by his parents to see Dr. Smoak, his pediatrician. Shawn was eating his lunch and swallowed a piece of chicken bone, which is stuck in his throat. Shawn is having difficulty breathing. Dr. Smoak notes that the bone is causing tracheal compression. Dr. Smoak was able to remove the bone and Shawn's breathing returned to normal.

14. Christopher Crawford, a 47-year-old male, presents today with swollen, red gums that are painful to touch, but are not bleeding. Dr. Hubert diagnosed Christopher with acute gingivitis, non-plaque induced.

15. Paul Plum, an 8-month-old male, is brought in by his mother to see Dr. Wallace, Paul's pediatrician. Paul's stomach feels hard and he is also having some diarrhea and vomiting. Dr. Wallace notes Paul is failing to thrive and hospitalizes him. After blood tests and a hydrogen breath test are completed, Paul is diagnosed with congenital lactase deficiency.

YOU CODE IT! Application

The following exercises provide practice in abstracting physician documentation from our health care facility, Prader, Bracker, & Associates. These case studies are modeled on real patient encounters. Using the techniques described in this chapter, carefully read through the case studies and determine the most accurate ICD-10-CM code(s) for each case study. Remember to include external cause codes, if appropriate.

PRADER, BRACKER, & ASSOCIATES

A Complete Health Care Facility

159 Healthcare Way • SOMEWHERE, FL 32811 • 407-555-6789

PATIENT: Kassandra, Kelly

ACCOUNT/EHR #: KASSKE001

DATE: 09/16/18

Attending Physician: Oscar R. Prader, MD

S: Pt is a 19-year-old female who has had a sore throat and cough for the past week. She states that she had a temperature of 101.5 F last night. She also admits that it is painful to swallow. No OTC medication has provided any significant relief.

O: Ht 5'5" Wt. 148 lb. R 20. T 101 F. BP 125/82. Pharynx is inspected, tonsils enlarged. There is pus noted in the posterior pharynx. Neck: supple, no nodes. Chest: clear. Heart: regular rate and rhythm without murmur.

A: Acute pharyngitis

P: 1. Send pt for Strep test

    2. Recommend patient gargle with warm salt water and use OTC lozenges to keep throat moist

    3. Rx if needed once results of Strep test come back

    4. Return in 2 weeks for follow-up

ORP/pw   D: 9/16/18 09:50:16   T: 9/18/18 12:55:01

Determine the most accurate ICD-10-CM code(s).

WESTON HOSPITAL

629 Healthcare Way • SOMEWHERE, FL 32811 • 407-555-6541

PATIENT: DAVIS, HELEN

ACCOUNT/EHR #: DAVIHE001

DATE: 10/21/18

Attending Physician: Renee O. Bracker, MD

CHAPTER 4 REVIEW

Patient, an 82-year-old that presents today to see Dr. Newson. Dr. Newson saw this patient 10 days ago in office, where she was diagnosed with a UTI and prescribed nitrofurantoin po. Today she presents with the complaints of dysuria, low back pain, abdominal pain, nausea, and diarrhea. After a positive UA she was admitted to Weston Hospital.

PE: Ht: 5′3″, Wt: 112 lb., T: 97.3, P: 70, R: 19, BP: 133/62, O2 sat 97%. Dr. Newson notes LLQ tenderness and poor nutritional intake. Blood work results: WBC-16.5, RBC-5.70, HCT-50.5 indicating infection. Urine culture showed Staphylococcus. CT scan of abdomen and pelvis reveals mild diverticulitis. Chest clear, lungs clear—sounds bilaterally S1 & S2 heard. Active bowel sound. Strong muscle strength in all extremities. Pulse is regular. Skin is intact, noted redness in coccyx area. Mucous membrane is moist and pink. Functioning independently.

Laboratory results:

Sodium—133 (L); Potassium—4.7

Chloride—95 (L); CO_2—23

Glucose-Serum—122 (H); BUN—16

Creatinine—0.8; Protein—8.2

Albumin—4.7; Total Bilirubin—1.3

WBC—15.5 (H); RBC—5.70 (H)

HGB—15.9; HCT—50.5 (H)

Platelet—326; Neutrophils—65.4

Lymphocytes—27.0; Monocytes—6.3

Eosinophils—0.4; Basophils—0.9

ALT—13; AST—31; Alkaline Phosphatase—106

Patient was started on Vancomycin 200mg/IV q 6 hr, Docusate sodium 100mg/hr, and Zofran 24mg po. Patient responded to treatment and is alert & oriented x 3. If she continues to improve, she will be discharged home tomorrow.

Dx: Staphylococcal UTI, Large intestine diverticulitis

ROB/pw   D: 10/21/18 09:50:16   T: 10/25/18 12:55:01

Determine the most accurate ICD-10-CM code(s).

PRADER, BRACKER, & ASSOCIATES

A Complete Health Care Facility

159 Healthcare Way • SOMEWHERE, FL 32811 • 407-555-6789

PATIENT: HOBARTH, CHANTEL

ACCOUNT/EHR #: HOBACH001

DATE: 08/11/18

Attending Physician: Oscar R. Prader, MD

S: Pt is a 45-year-old female diagnosed with bladder cancer 4 years ago. She underwent chemotherapy and radiation treatments and is now malignant-free for 18 months. Since being malignant-free she comes in for an abdominal scan every 6 months. Pt has no signs or symptoms indicating a return of the malignancy.

O: Ht 5'5". Wt. 137 lb. R 18. T 99. BP 128/81. Abdomen appears to be normal upon manual examination. Results of CT scan indicated no abnormalities.

A: Personal history of bladder cancer

P: Pt to return PRN

ORP/pw   D: 08/11/18 09:50:16   T: 08/13/18 12:55:01

Determine the most accurate ICD-10-CM code(s).

PRADER, BRACKER, & ASSOCIATES

A Complete Health Care Facility

159 Healthcare Way • SOMEWHERE, FL 32811 • 407-555-6789

PATIENT: ROMANO, JOSEPH

ACCOUNT/EHR #: ROMAJO001

DATE: 07/11/18

Attending Physician: Renee O. Bracker, MD

S: Pt is a 32-year-old male who works at local restaurant. While at work he was preparing a chicken and cut the back of his right index finger. He states he stopped the bleed with pressure, but now he can't extend his finger. Pt. had last tetanus toxoid administered last year. He has no past history of serious illnesses, operations, or allergies. Social history and family history are noncontributory.

O: Examination reveals a 3.6-cm laceration, dorsum of right index finger, with laceration of extensor tendon, proximal to the interphalangeal joint. The patient cannot extend the finger. Pt was prepped, and a digital nerve block using 1% Carbocaine was administered. When the block was totally effective, the wound was irrigated with normal saline. The joint capsule was repaired with two sutures of 5-0 Dexon. The tendon repair was then carried out using 4-0 nylon. Dressings were applied, and a splint was applied holding the interphalangeal joint in neutral position, in full extension. The Pt tolerated the procedure well.

A: 3.6-cm laceration, dorsum of right index finger

P: 1. Rx Percocet, q4h prn for pain

2. Rx Augmentin, 250mg tid

3. Follow-up in 3 days

ROB/pw   D: 07/11/18 09:50:16   T: 07/13/18 12:55:01

Determine the most accurate ICD-10-CM code(s) for the laceration.

CHAPTER 4 REVIEW

WESTON HOSPITAL

629 Healthcare Way • SOMEWHERE, FL 32811 • 407-555-6541

PATIENT: FLORA, VINCENT

ACCOUNT/EHR #: FLORVI001

DATE: 11/19/18

Attending Physician: Oscar R. Prader, MD

S: Pt is a 37-year-old female who was on vacation with friends. On a wager she parachuted from a plane and landed in a tree. She hit her head against a rock when she fell from the tree and lost consciousness for approximately 5 minutes. She says she has a headache and is a bit nauseated.

O: Ht 5′6″ Wt. 130 lb. R 18. T 98.1. BP 122/83. HEENT unremarkable. PERRLA. Dr. Prader notes slight slurred speech. EEG shows indication of a head trauma. CT scan confirmed the brain concussion. Patient was admitted to the hospital for observation.

A: Concussion with brief loss of consciousness

P: 1. Watch for 24 hours

   2. Discharge home if no further complications.

ORP/pw D: 11/19/18 09:50:16 T: 11/23/18 12:55:01

Determine the most accurate ICD-10-CM code(s) for the concussion.

Coding Infectious Diseases

5

Learning Outcomes

After completing this chapter, the student should be able to:

LO 5.1 Interpret the details required to report an accurate code for an infection.
LO 5.2 Clarify the details about bacterial infections.
LO 5.3 Determine the specifics needed to report viral infections.
LO 5.4 Translate information about parasitic and fungal infections into diagnosis codes.
LO 5.5 Abstract documentation to identify important details about the specific pathogen causing a diagnosis.
LO 5.6 Ascertain the correct code or codes to report immunodeficiency conditions.
LO 5.7 Apply the guidelines for reporting blood infections.
LO 5.8 Analyze the documentation to identify the code or codes required to report antimicrobial resistance.

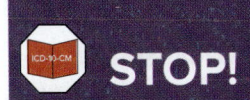

Key Terms

Acute
Asymptomatic
Bacteria
Chronic
Fungi
Human Immunodeficiency Virus (HIV)
Infection
Infectious
Inflammation
Nosocomial
Parasites
Pathogen
Sepsis
Septic Shock
Septicemia
Severe Sepsis
Systemic
Systemic Inflammatory Response Syndrome (SIRS)
Tuberculosis
Viruses

STOP! Remember, you need to follow along in your ICD-10-CM code book for an optimal learning experience.

5.1 Infectious and Communicable Diseases

Many conditions and illnesses can be disseminated from one individual to another. **Infectious** diseases are spread by personal contact, such as a handshake or the exchange of bodily fluids, while other diseases can be spread by the touch of a doorknob that has been handled by someone else. Some of these conditions, such as meningitis, hepatitis, **tuberculosis**, and **human immunodeficiency virus (HIV)**, have been in the media, and others you may never have heard of before. This chapter will help you understand how to report all of these diseases using ICD-10-CM codes.

Infections and Inflammation

There are wars going on constantly throughout your body as **pathogens** (vehicles of disease) insert themselves into your cells and multiply. There are many types of pathogens and each carries its own threat to your health. **Infection** happens once a pathogen successfully invades the body and begins to replicate. This multiplication of the organism, known as *colonization*, causes damage to cell structures and can remain localized in one area (such as an infected toe), spread to a larger area (such as infection of the foot and leg), or become **systemic** (spreading throughout the entire body). The human body is designed to alert the individual and the doctor to the existence of infection by exhibiting specific signs and symptoms:

Infectious
A condition that can be transmitted from one person to another.

Tuberculosis
An infectious condition that causes small rounded swellings on mucous membranes throughout the body.

Human Immunodeficiency Virus (HIV)
A condition affecting the immune system.

Pathogen
Any agent that causes disease; a microorganism such as a bacterium or virus.

Infection
The invasion of pathogens into tissue cells.

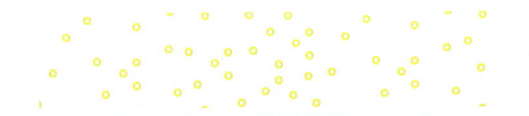

101

Systemic
Spread throughout the entire body.

Asymptomatic
No symptoms or manifestations.

Acute
Severe; serious.

Inflammation
The reaction of tissues to infection or injury; characterized by pain, swelling, and erythema.

Chronic
Long duration; continuing over an extended period of time.

- Increased body temperature (commonly known as a *fever*)
- Increased white blood cell count
- Increase (tachycardia) or decrease (bradycardia) in heart rate
- Increase (hyperventilation) or decrease (dyspnea) in respiratory rate

In some cases, a patient might not be aware that there is an infection in his or her body. This is known as a *subclinical* or **asymptomatic** infection. In other cases, the condition can become **acute** (severe) and a specific area may show signs of **inflammation**. When located in the epidermis, inflammation can be visible; it causes signs and symptoms, such as erythema (reddening), swelling, warmth to the touch, and often pain. When located internally, the inflammation can cause lack of function, especially when found within a joint. When inflammation is left untreated, or if treatment is ineffective, the condition can become **chronic** (ongoing). Any of these details may be required to determine an accurate code. You will know by reading the complete code descriptions in the Tabular List.

> **EXAMPLE**
> A39.2   Acute meningococcemia
> B39.1   Chronic pulmonary histoplasmosis capsulati
> Z21   Asymptomatic human immunodeficiency virus [HIV] infection status

Communicable Diseases

People interact in society, and, therefore, the transmission of pathogens cannot be avoided. The level of interaction and the severity of the pathogen (how aggressive it may be) will impact how many individuals are infected. There are many ways that patients can be exposed to an infection and become ill.

Health care–acquired infections (HAIs), also known as **nosocomial** infections, are those conditions that are contracted solely due to interactions with a health care facility, during which exposure to various types of pathogens occurs. Take note that HAIs are infections that occur in hospitals, nursing homes, and other health care provider locations. HAIs are not just the concern of inpatient acute care facilities.

A cough or a sneeze may send pathogens into the air, and a doorknob or a telephone receiver easily transfers pathogens to the skin that touches it next—these are methods of transportation for bacteria or viruses to travel from an infected person to another soon-to-be-infected person. Some diseases require more intimate contact, such as the exchange of bodily fluids (during sex, exposure to blood, or contact with mucus).

- *Touch exposure:* Physical interaction with blood, bodily fluids, nonintact skin, and mucous membranes can enable a long list of bloodborne pathogens to make their way from one person to another.
- *Airborne exposure:* Some pathogens travel in small particles that remain contagious in the air, such as chickenpox. Measles can live in the air of a room for 2 hours after the infected person leaves. Breathing in contaminated air by merely entering an examination room or patient area can expose someone to the disease.
- *Droplet exposure:* Some diseases, such as influenza, can be dispersed in large droplets, such as those transmitted by coughing, spitting, talking, and sneezing.
- *Contact exposure:* As with touch exposure, some infections, such as herpes simplex virus, are communicated by skin-to-skin contact or skin to other surfaces (e.g., countertops, paper).

CODING BITES

Keep references close at hand. Bookmark or mark as a favorite reliable sources such as the MedlinePlus online medical encyclopedia. This will help you increase your understanding of any infectious disease, and its inclusive signs and symptoms, that you encounter in physician documentation.

Nosocomial
A hospital-acquired condition; a condition that develops as a result of being in a health care facility.

CODING BITES

Later on, in the chapter titled *Inpatient (Hospital) Diagnosis Coding*, you will learn how to use Present-On-Admission indicators to report nosocomial conditions.

- *Needlestick/sharps injury exposure:* Bloodborne pathogens, including HIV, hepatitis B, and hepatitis C, can be highly contagious when contaminated needles or other sharp objects (e.g., scalpels, dental wire) penetrate the protective outer layer of the skin.
- *Insect bites:* Mosquitoes, deer ticks, fleas, and other insects/parasites spread disease as well. Zika is transmitted by mosquitoes, deer ticks transmit Lyme disease, and fleas spread the plague.
- *Food and water:* There are many diseases, such as *E. coli* or cholera, that are spread by ingestion of substances.

Reporting the Infectious Agent

In some cases, the code you determine to report an infection may be complete with the specific type of pathogen, such as tuberculosis, which is only caused by *Mycobacterum tuberculosis* or *Mycobacterium bovis*. This means that the specific pathogen is included in the diagnostic statement and therefore the code.

> **CODING BITES**
>
> Remember, inclusive signs and symptoms are not coded separately. This is why you need to learn what they are for each illness or disease so you know what should not and what should be coded.

> **EXAMPLE**
>
> **Tuberculosis (A15-A19)**
>
> INCLUDES infections due to Mycobacterium tuberculosis and Mycobacterium bovis

Sometimes, you will find a combination code that includes the name of the pathogen in the code description.

> **EXAMPLE**
>
> J02.0 Streptococcal pharyngitis
> J09.x3 Influenza due to identified novel influenza A virus with gastrointestinal manifestations
>
> These code descriptions are known as combination codes because they include both the condition and the specific pathogen.

Other times, an infection might be caused by any one of several different pathogens. In these cases, you will need to report a second code to specify the bacterial or viral infectious agent.

> **EXAMPLES**
>
> B95.2 Enterococcus as the cause of diseases classified elsewhere
> B96.3 Hemophilus influenzae [H. influenzae] as the cause of diseases classified elsewhere
> B97.11 Coxsackievirus as the cause of diseases classified elsewhere
>
> These code descriptions identify the specific pathogen to be reported along with the code describing the condition caused.

The part of the code description that states *"diseases classified elsewhere"* means that the condition has its own code within this code set. This underscores the fact that this is not a combination code and you will need two codes to report the condition.

> **EXAMPLE**
>
> ☑4 N30 Cystitis
>
> *Use additional code* **to identify infectious agent (B95-B97)**
>
> Very often, the ICD-10-CM will tell you that you will need this second code to identify the specific pathogen.

YOU INTERPRET IT!

What is the mode of transmission for each condition?
1. Hepatitis B _____
2. Measles _____
3. Cholera _____
4. Insect bites _____
5. Influenza _____

5.2 Bacterial Infections

Types of Bacteria

Bacteria
Single-celled microorganisms that cause disease.

Bacteria are single-celled organisms named by their shape (see Figure 5-1). Rod-shaped bacteria, called *bacilli*, are responsible for the development of diphtheria, tetanus, and tuberculosis, among others. *Spirilla*, bacterial organisms shaped like a

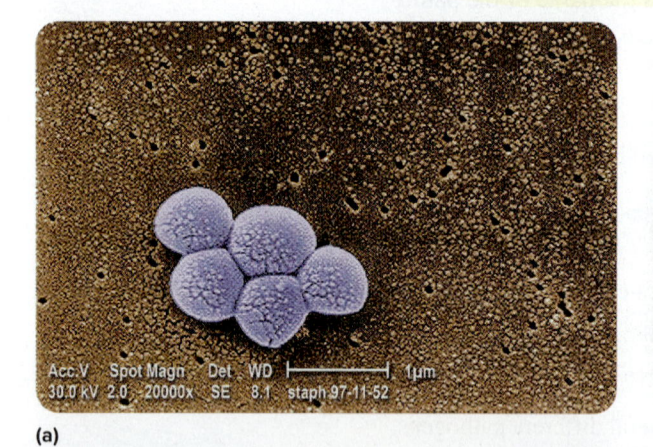

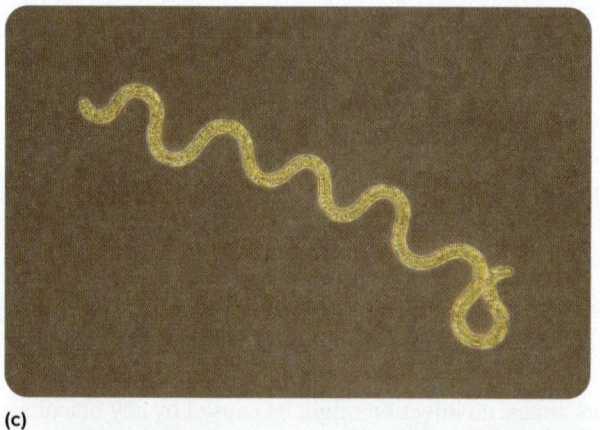

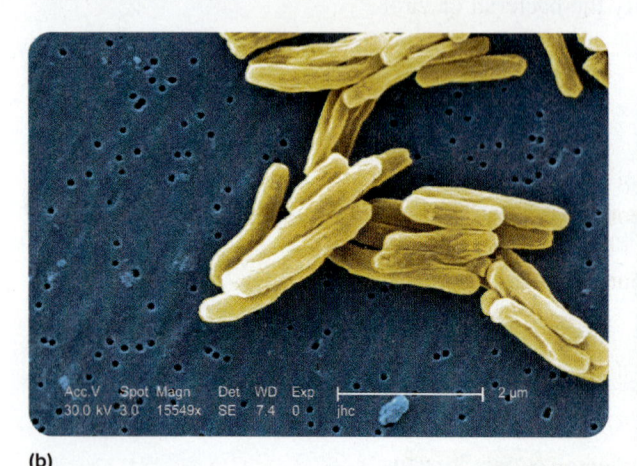

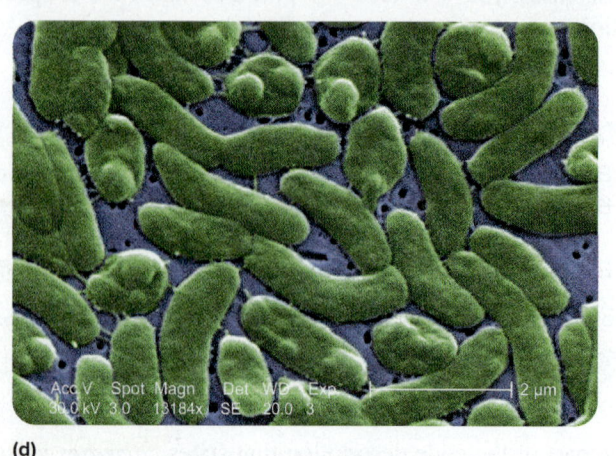

FIGURE 5-1 Types of bacteria: (a) coccus, (b) bacillus, (c) spirillum, and (d) vibrio (a) Source: CDC/Janice Carr; (b) Source: CDC/Janice Carr; (c) ©MELBA PHOTO AGENCY/Alamy Stock Photo RF; (d) Source: CDC/Janice Carr

spiral, may cause cholera or syphilis, while dot-shaped bacteria known as *cocci* cause gonorrhea, tonsillitis, scarlet fever, and bacterial meningitis.

> **EXAMPLE**
>
> A05.4   Foodborne Bacillus cereus intoxication
> A27.9   Leptospirosis, unspecified
> A49.1   Streptococcal infection, unspecified site
>
> This is a great example of why professional coders-to-be need to know these details . . . so you can recognize the name of a bacterium in diagnostic terms and phrases. Until you learn them, use your medical dictionary to confirm.

Conditions Caused by Bacteria

Impetigo

Impetigo is a common illness affecting children, caused by either a streptococcal or a staphylococcal pathogen. This means that MRSA (methicillin-resistant *Staphylococcus aureus*) is a real concern. This disease spreads through contact with fluid oozing from a bullous—or blister. Visually, impetigo is evidenced by the appearance of rings that can range from pea-size to large rings. They may itch. These blisters may ooze yellow or honey-colored fluid and then crust. Of course, the itching may result in the patient scratching, which then spreads the rash. The physician may also document swollen lymph nodes, particularly in the body areas close to the infection site. Impetigo is often reported with a code from code category L01 with additional required characters to provide additional specificity.

> **EXAMPLE**
>
> A specific, complete diagnostic statement is required to determine an accurate code for a case of impetigo:
>
> L01.01   Non-bullous impetigo
> L01.02   Brockhart's impetigo
> L01.03   Bullous impetigo
> L01.09   Other impetigo [ulcerative impetigo]
>
> Yet, notice . . . not all impetigo diagnoses are reported from this one code category . . .
>
> L40.1   Generalized pustular psoriasis [impetigo herpetiformis]

Foodborne Illness

Some bacterial infections that you will encounter in a typical health care facility are those that are foodborne, commonly called *food poisoning*. Do not let the word "poisoning" fool you. These diagnoses are not poisonings; they are actually infections. Some of the most frequently seen bacterial infections, and their sources, are shown in Table 5-1.

> **EXAMPLES**
>
> *Clostridium botulinium* is the bacterium that causes A05.1 Botulism food poisoning
>
> Foodborne *Clostridium perfringens*, the bacterium that causes enteritis necroticans, is reported with code A05.2
>
> *(continued)*

> Foodborne staphylococcal intoxication is reported with A05.0
>
> *Salmonella* foodborne intoxication and infection are reported from code category A02, which requires additional information related to the infection resulting from this bacterium.
>
> Listeriosis [listerial foodborne infection] is reported from code category A32 and requires additional detail about the patient's condition.

TABLE 5-1 Common Bacterial Infections, Their Sources, and Their Codes

Name	Source	Code
Campylobacter	From foods including raw poultry, raw meat, untreated milk	A04.5
Listeria	Untreated milk, dairy products, raw salads and vegetables	A32.-
Salmonella	Raw poultry, eggs, raw meat, untreated milk and dairy products	A02.9
Shigella	Untreated water, milk and dairy products, raw vegetables and salads, shellfish, turkey, apple cider	A03.-
Vibrio	Raw and lightly cooked shellfish	A00.-
Clostridium perfringens	Animal and human excreta, soil, dust, insects, raw meat	B96.7
Escherichia coli (E. coli 0157)	Human and animal gut, sewage, water, raw meat	A49.8

Almost all infections shown in Table 5-1 induce symptoms of diarrhea, abdominal pain, nausea, fever, and vomiting. Other serious effects include dehydration, headache, and kidney damage or failure. Therefore, you must be careful not to report unnecessary codes for signs and symptoms that are actually included in a definitive diagnosis that has been made.

LET'S CODE IT! SCENARIO

Francie Holland, a 23-year-old female, came to see Dr. Kensington due to severe abdominal pain. She had a fever and stated that she has had bloody diarrhea for the past 2 days. Dr. Kensington's examination revealed that she was dehydrated as well. Francie stated she ate at a new restaurant at the beach where she had a salad and a vegetable plate. After taking some tests, he diagnosed Francie with Shigella dysenteriae *(bacillary dysentery)*.

Let's Code It!

Dr. Kensington found Francie to be suffering from Shigella dysenteriae. Turn to the Alphabetic Index and find

Shigella (dysentery) (*see* Dysentery, bacillary)

Dysentery, bacillary A03.9

Turn to the Tabular List, and check the code's complete description:

✓4 **A03 Shigellosis**

There are no notations or directives, so read down the column to review all of the choices for the required fourth character. The code suggested by the Alphabetic Index:

A03.9 Shigellosis, unspecified

Is this the most accurate code? You will note that the other fourth-character code choices want specifics on which group (A, B, C, or D) of the Shigella infection is present. Do you know? Dr. Kensington did specify in the notes—Shigella dysenteriae, which matches the description for

> **A03.0 Shigellosis due to Shigella dysenteriae**
>
> Check the top of this subsection and the head of this chapter in ICD-10-CM. There are notations at the beginning of this chapter: an INCLUDES notation, a *Use Additional Code* note, an EXCLUDES1 notation, and an EXCLUDES2 notation. Read carefully. Do any relate to Dr. Kensington's diagnosis of Francie? No. Turn to the Official Guidelines and read Section 1.c.1. There is nothing specifically applicable here either.
> Therefore, A03.0 is the most accurate code available. Excellent!!

Cellulitis

Cellulitis is a serious infection of the skin that may be either a staph infection (the staphylococcal bacteria) or a strep infection (the streptococcal bacteria). These pathogens typically enter the body through an abnormal opening in the epidermal layer of the skin—for example, a burn, puncture wound, abrasion (also known as a scrape), or even a bite—either animal or human.

Cellulitis begins with the typical signs of inflammation: erythema (redness), heat arising from the area of infection, pain, and edema (swelling). Vesicles or bullae may appear in the infected area. In addition, the patient may develop a fever with chills, experience tachycardia (a rapid heartbeat), suffer a headache, have hypotension (low blood pressure), and, at times, become mentally confused.

Report a diagnosis of cellulitis with a code—in many cases—from code category L03. You will need specific information on the precise anatomical site affected by the condition.

> **EXAMPLES**
>
> L03.012   Cellulitis of left finger
> L03.113   Cellulitis of right upper limb
> L03.314   Cellulitis of groin
>
> These are examples of the need to identify the specific anatomical site of the cellulitis to determine an accurate code.

There is an EXCLUDES2 notation beneath L03.211, the code used to report cellulitis of the face. This long list of specific anatomical sites that might normally be included within the face are actually reported with different codes from different areas of the ICD-10-CM code book . . . such as cellulitis of the ear, reported with code H60.1, or cellulitis of the mouth, which is reported with code K12.2. As always, you must read all of the notations, carefully and completely.

L03.31—the code used to report cellulitis of the trunk—also has a list of specific anatomical sites located on the torso that are reported with codes from other chapters, such as cellulitis of anal and rectal regions, which is reported with a code from the K61 Abscess of anal and rectal regions code category, or cellulitis of the breast, which is reported from code category N61 Inflammatory disorders of the breast.

Tetanus (Lockjaw)

You are probably more familiar with the tetanus vaccine than you are with the disease. Tetanus is an infection of the nervous system and is caused by the entry of bacteria into the body through a break in the skin. It causes death in about 11% of all cases. The illness can be prevented by the administration of the tetanus toxoid, included in the DTaP, DT, and Td vaccines.

When a patient has come for inoculation with the tetanus toxoid only, you will use Z23. However, read the notes carefully. If the development of tetanus is a complication arising from the vaccination, use code T88.1. If tetanus is a result of an incident, such

> **CODING BITES**
>
> When the documentation states that an external cause, such as an animal bite, provided entry for the pathogen, external cause codes may be required. More about these in the chapter *Coding Injury, Poisoning, and External Causes.*

as stepping on a rusty nail, report it with code A35 plus an external cause code. Should this disease occur with or following an abortion or ectopic pregnancy, then you will report it as a complication of pregnancy, using A34 or O08.89. And in cases where the tetanus is affecting a neonate, it will be reported with code A33.

Tuberculosis

Mycobacterium tuberculosis, the causative agent of tuberculosis (TB), is a bacterial infection that is transmitted through the air. One version of TB is called *latent tuberculosis infection (LTBI)* because it is dormant and may not show symptoms right away. Not everyone who has been infected is symptomatic, so a test is required to confirm the diagnosis. Most types of TB and LTBI are successfully treated with medication.

There is a specific cultural group of people who will get a positive result to the skin test but not actually have the disease. A simple chest x-ray confirms that situation. Should you have a patient in such a circumstance, you will use this code:

R76.11   Nonspecific reaction to tuberculin skin test without active tuberculosis

When the documentation confirms a diagnosis of TB, you will choose the best, most appropriate code from the range A15–A19 Tuberculosis based on the specific anatomical site affected.

> ### EXAMPLE
> A15.0   Tuberculosis of lung
> A17.1   Meningeal tuberculoma
> A18.81 Tuberculosis of thyroid gland
> A19.1   Acute miliary tuberculosis of multiple sites
>
> The codes in these four code categories illustrate the extensive list of anatomical sites that may be affected with TB. Read the documentation and diagnosis carefully (as always).

As you look through the section, you will notice that TB is a disseminated disease. While most people think of TB as a pulmonary infection, infiltrating only the lungs, it can actually leach throughout the body and be identified in many different anatomical sites. You have to abstract which anatomical site is infected with the TB bacterium so that you can find the most accurate code.

YOU CODE IT! CASE STUDY

Audra Swenson was brought into the emergency department (ED) by ambulance because she was having suprapubic pain, pain in her lower back, and nocturia. Dr. Balthazar diagnosed Audra with renal tuberculosis, also known as urogential TB, confirmed histologically, with pyelonephritis.

You Code It!

Go through the steps of coding, and determine the diagnosis code or codes that should be reported for this encounter between Dr. Balthazar and Audra Swenson.

Step #1: Read the case carefully and completely.

Step #2: Abstract the scenario. Which main words or terms describe why the physician cared for the patient during this encounter?

Step #3: Are there any details missing or incomplete for which you would need to query the physician? [If so, ask your instructor.]

Step #4: Check for any relevant guidance, including reading all of the symbols and notations in the Tabular List and the appropriate sections of the Official Guidelines.

Step #5: Determine the correct diagnosis code or codes to explain why this encounter was medically necessary..

Step #6: Double-check your work.

Answer:

Did you determine the correct code?

    A18.11   **Tuberculosis of kidney and ureter (Pyelitis tuberculous)**

Terrific!

5.3 Viral Infections

Types of Viruses

There are a large number of viral **infectious** diseases that you may have to code, depending upon the type of facility that employs you, combined with geographic and other factors.

    Viruses are tiny microorganisms that are not easily treated with medication because they embed themselves within their host's cells and are, therefore, difficult to isolate (see Figure 5-2). These invaders can remain dormant (latent) for long periods of time.

Infectious
A condition that can be transmitted from one person to another.

Viruses
Microscopic particles that initiate disease, mimicking the characteristics of a particular cell; viruses can reproduce only within the body of the cell that they have invaded.

> **EXAMPLE**
>
>   A85.0   Enteroviral encephalitis
>   B18.0   Chronic viral hepatitis B with delta-agent
>   B33.21   Viral endocarditis
>
> Sometimes, the code description identifies the viral pathogen involved in a diagnosis. When a combination code is available, you will need to report it, as long as it matches the physician's documentation.

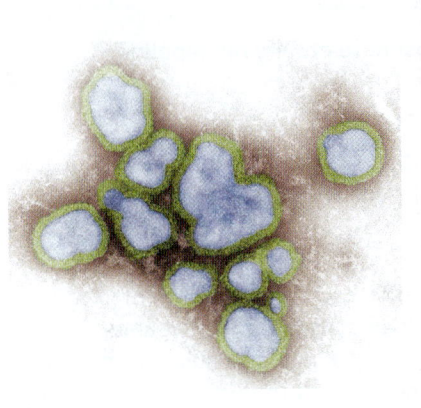

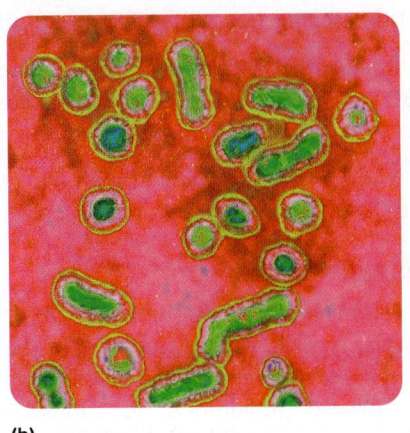

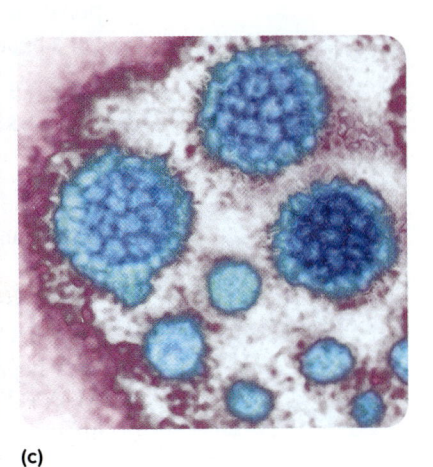

FIGURE 5-2 Types of viruses: (a) influenza, (b) hepatitis, and (c) warts (a) Source: CDC/F.A. Murphy; (b) ©BSIP/UIG/Universal Images Group/Getty Images; (c) ©James Cavallini/Science Source

> **Wart** (due to HPV) (filiform) (infectious) (viral) B07.9
> - anogenital region (venereal) A63.0
> - common B07.8
> - external genital organs (venereal) A63.0
> - flat B07.8
> - Hassal-Henle's (of cornea) H18.49
> - Peruvian A44.1
> - plantar B07.0
> - prosector (tuberculosis) A18.4
> - seborrheic L82.1
> -- inflamed L82.0
> - senile (seborrheic) L82.1
> -- inflamed L82.0
> - tuberculosis A18.4
> - venereal A63.0

FIGURE 5-3 ICD-10-CM Alphabetic Index, partial listing under the main term Wart Source: *ICD-10-CM Official Guidelines for Coding and Reporting* The Centers for Medicare and Medicaid Services (CMS) and the National Center for Health Statistics (NCHS)

Conditions Caused by Viruses

Viral Warts

Viral warts are most common in children and are rarely seen in the elderly. This virus can be spread from person to person during sexual contact or an individual with a viral wart can see it spread from one anatomical site to another.

There are several different types of warts, as you can see in Figure 5-3, so it is important that the specifics are documented. Take a look at the suggested codes, here in the Alphabetic Index: A63.0, B07.9, H18.49, L82.0 . . . located in several different chapters throughout the Tabular List. You must read the documentation carefully, including the pathology report, to point you toward the correct codes from which to choose.

Viral Hepatitis

Hepatitis (*hepat* = liver; *-itis* = inflammation) actually refers to several different viral infections. According to the Centers for Disease Control and Prevention (CDC), viral hepatitis is the most prevalent cause of malignant neoplasms of the liver. As you know, prevention is a much better path than treatment. For those coming to your facility to get a hepatitis vaccine, you will report one of these codes:

Z20.5	Contact with or (suspected) exposure to other viral hepatitis
Z22.330	Carrier of Group B Streptococcus
Z23	Encounter for immunization

For those who are already infected with one of the strains of hepatitis, it's critical to understand the different types in order to code the encounter(s) correctly.

Viral Hepatitis, Type A

The CDC estimates that an additional 25,000 people each year become infected with viral hepatitis, type A, a viral infection of the liver caused by the hepatitis A virus (HAV). The virus can travel from person to person by personal contact, as with other infections. However, in addition, one can become infected through exposure to contaminated water or ice. Shellfish harvested from sewage-contaminated water as well as fruits, vegetables, and other foods that have been contaminated and eaten uncooked may also carry the hepatitis A virus.

In some cases, a patient may develop hepatic encephalopathy (hepatic coma). This occurs when, because of the infection, the liver is unable to remove toxins from the blood, resulting in a loss of brain function.

Viral hepatitis A is reported with either:

B15.0   **Hepatitis A with hepatic coma**

or

B15.9   **Hepatitis A without hepatic coma**

Viral Hepatitis, Type B

Caused by the hepatitis B virus (HBV), viral hepatitis, type B is transmitted through contact with infected bodily fluids, such as blood or semen. The infection can also be spread by the use of equipment that has been contaminated with the virus, which is why when getting a tattoo, body piercing, or even a fingernail application one must be careful that the needles and files have been sterilized properly. The CDC estimates 43,000 new cases of hepatitis B are diagnosed each year.

To determine the most accurate code, you have to abstract these details from the documentation:

- Is the patient documented as in a hepatic coma?
- Is the condition identified as acute (code category B16) or chronic (code category B18)?
- Is hepatitis D (also known as hepatitis delta, or delta-agent) involved?

B16.0   **Acute hepatitis B with delta-agent with hepatic coma**
B16.1   **Acute hepatitis B with delta-agent without hepatic coma**
B16.2   **Acute hepatitis B without delta-agent with hepatic coma**
B16.9   **Acute hepatitis B without delta-agent and without hepatic coma**

Viral Hepatitis, Type C

The hepatitis C virus (HCV) infection is estimated by the CDC to chronically affect 3.2 million people in the United States. It is considered to be the most widespread chronic bloodborne infection. Those individuals at the highest risk for infection are those using injected drugs. Each year, it is believed that an additional 17,000 individuals become hepatitis C positive. Report this diagnosis with one of these codes:

B17.11   **Acute hepatitis C with hepatic coma**
B18.2   **Chronic hepatitis C**
B17.10   **Acute hepatitis C without hepatic coma**
B19.20   **Unspecified viral hepatitis C without hepatic coma**

Viral Hepatitis, Type D

Also known as *hepatitis delta*, this is a serious liver disease that requires the HBV (hepatitis B virus) to replicate itself. This condition is not seen often in the United States. Hepatitis D is transmitted through direct contact with infected blood, similar to how hepatitis B is passed from one person to another. Currently, there is no vaccine for hepatitis D. Hepatitis D is referred to as *hepatitis delta* in the code descriptions, and reported with this code:

B17.0   **Acute delta-(super) infection of hepatitis B carrier**

Viral Hepatitis, Type E

Occurrences of hepatitis E in the United States are rare; it is known to be common in countries with poor sanitation and contaminated water supplies. This liver disease, caused by the hepatitis E virus (HEV), does not lead to chronic infection. There is no vaccine currently approved by the FDA for hepatitis E. Report this diagnosis with

B17.2   **Acute hepatitis E**

> ### LET'S CODE IT! SCENARIO
>
> David Tranccione, a 55-year-old white male, came into our office. He complains that he feels tired all the time, no matter how much he sleeps. His muscles are sore, his stomach is upset, and he has experienced frequent bouts of diarrhea. He made an appointment with his regular physician, Dr. Cameron, when he noticed his urine was dark. Dr. Cameron ordered blood tests, and the pathology report confirmed the diagnosis of acute hepatitis B virus.
>
> #### Let's Code It!
>
> Dr. Cameron confirmed that David has acute hepatitis B virus. Open your ICD-10-CM code book to the Alphabetic Index to:
>
> **Hepatitis** K75.9
>
> Before you turn to this code category in the Tabular List, read down the long list indented beneath, just to see if you can find a listing that is more specific and in agreement with Dr. Cameron's documentation.
>
> **Hepatitis** K75.9
>   B B19.10
>   with hepatic coma B19.11
>   acute B16.9
>
> Four different listings and three very different codes. It is a good thing you keep reading. Turn to code category B16 in the Tabular List:
>
> ☑4 B16 Acute hepatitis B
>
> Read the four options for the required fourth character. What details do you need from the documentation to choose: with or without delta-agent and with or without hepatic coma. Go back to the scenario. There is no mention of either delta-agent or hepatic coma, so you can report:
>
> **B16.9** Acute hepatitis B without delta-agent and without hepatic coma
>
> Check the top of this subsection, which has an **EXCLUDES1** and an **EXCLUDES2** notation. Neither relates to David's case this time, so next, check the head of this chapter in ICD-10-CM. Above code A00, you will find an **INCLUDES** notation, a *Use additional code* note, an **EXCLUDES1** notation, and an **EXCLUDES2** notation. Read carefully. Do any relate to Dr. Cameron's diagnosis of David? No. Turn to the Official Guidelines and read Section 1.c.1. There is nothing specifically applicable here either.
> Now you can report B16.9 for David's diagnosis with confidence.
> **Good coding!**

Influenza

There is a reason why so much commotion is made annually about individuals getting their flu shots. A seemingly ordinary infection, influenza (commonly called the *flu*) can be deadly. It is caused by the influenza A or B virus and can be transmitted by casual contact, such as a handshake or touching a contaminated doorknob. It is estimated that as many as 36,000 people die in the United States each year from influenza.

The most common symptoms of the flu are

- Body or muscle aches
- Chills
- Cough
- Fever
- Headache
- Sore throat

The diagnosis of influenza will be reported with a code from these categories:

- ☑4 J09 Influenza due to certain identified influenza viruses
- ☑4 J10 Influenza due to other identified influenza viruses
- ☑4 J11 Influenza due to unidentified influenza viruses

The required additional characters will enable you to report the specific virus, such as novel influenza A, as well as manifestations of this virus.

> **EXAMPLE**
>
> J09.X1 Influenza due to identified novel influenza A virus with pneumonia
> J10.2   Influenza due to other identified influenza virus with gastrointestinal manifestations
> J11.1   Influenza due to unidentified influenza virus with other respiratory manifestations
>
> The physician's documentation, along with the pathology report, should provide you with the details you need.

Varicella

Varicella, commonly known as *chickenpox,* is generally not perceived to be serious, most particularly for children. Complications from varicella, however, may include pneumonia in adults and bacterial infections of the skin and soft tissue in affected children. The infections can be severe and can lead to septicemia, toxic shock syndrome, necrotizing fasciitis, osteomyelitis, bacterial pneumonia, and septic arthritis. There may also be a connection between varicella and development of herpes zoster, also known as *shingles,* later in life. The availability of the varicella vaccine has made the risk of contracting the infection almost nil.

Code varicella from B01.- if the patient has been diagnosed. If the patient has come to receive a varicella vaccine, then use code Z23. However, if the patient has been exposed to varicella, the code will change to Z20.820.

> **CODING BITES**
>
> Varicella is commonly called *chickenpox*.

Rubeola

The risk of catching the childhood illness of rubeola, commonly referred to as measles, is very low because of the success of the measles vaccine. Your coding experience relating to measles should be limited to office visits for administering the vaccine.

When an individual has come to get vaccinated against rubeola only, code the encounter using Z23. However, a patient who is seeing a health care professional because of having been exposed to rubeola will be reported with Z20.828. A diagnosis of rubeola (measles) should be reported with code B05.-.

> **YOU CODE IT! CASE STUDY**
>
> Gregg Espinoza brought his 3-year-old son, Raymond, to his pediatrician, Dr. Nunez, with complaints of a 102 degree F fever for 3 days' duration. The boy was coughing, had signs of a runny nose, and had conjunctivitis in both eyes. Upon examination, Dr. Nunez notes Koplik's spots inside his checks and lips. Also noted are small, generalized, maculopapular erythematous rashes on his scalp. When asked, the father agreed that the boy had been scratching his head and he had been tugging at his ears.
>
> Dr. Nunez confirmed that Raymond had measles keratoconjunctivitis.
>
> *(continued)*

CHAPTER 5 | CODING INFECTIOUS DISEASES

> **You Code It!**
>
> Read the scenario carefully and determine the diagnosis code or codes to report for this encounter with Dr. Nunez.
>
> Step #1: Read the case carefully and completely.
>
> Step #2: Abstract the scenario. Which main words or terms describe why the physician cared for the patient during this encounter?
>
> Step #3: Are there any details missing or incomplete for which you would need to query the physician? [If so, ask your instructor.]
>
> Step #4: Check for any relevant guidance, including reading all of the symbols and notations in the Tabular List and the appropriate sections of the Official Guidelines.
>
> Step #5: Determine the correct diagnosis code or codes to explain why this encounter was medically necessary.
>
> Step #6: Double-check your work.
>
> **Answer:**
>
> Did you determine this to be the code?
>
> > **B05.81**   Measles keratitis and keratoconjunctivitis
>
> Good job!

Rubella

Rubella, an acute viral disease that can affect anyone of any age, is thought of by many to be a children's disease known as the *German measles*. While the symptoms are most often not more than a mild rash, the health danger of rubella can be serious to a pregnant woman in her first trimester. When contracted during the early months of pregnancy, rubella can be associated with a condition known as *congenital rubella syndrome (CRS)*. CRS may cause any of a large number of birth defects, including deafness and possibly fetal death. The rubella vaccine has almost eliminated CRS.

Rubella is coded with B06.- when it has been diagnosed. For those cases in which a patient is being vaccinated against rubella alone, you will use Z23, and if the patient has been exposed to rubella, report this with code Z20.4.

Herpes Simplex Virus

The *herpes simplex virus*, often referred to by the abbreviation HSV, is transmitted by direct contact between individuals. Small vesicles (fluid-filled lesions) appear on reddened skin in clusters or groups, particularly in the mucous membranes. HSV type 1 may be associated with orofacial disease and type 2 is associated with infections in the genitalia.

B00 is the code category dedicated to reporting herpes simplex infections—with the exception of congenital herpesviral infection—reported with code P35.2.

> **EXAMPLE**
>
> ☑4 B00 Herpesviral [herpes simplex] infections
>
> > **EXCLUDES1** congenital herpesviral infections (P35.2)
> >
> > **EXCLUDES2** anogenital herpesviral infection (A60.-)
> >
> > gamaherpesviral mononucleosis (B27.0-)
> >
> > herpangina (B08.5)

Specific documentation is critical to determine an accurate code. You want to avoid reporting B00.9 Herpesviral infection NOS, so be certain to query your physician if you need more details to determine which of these codes to report.

Herpes Zoster

Herpes zoster or *postherpetic neuralgia* is commonly known as shingles. Herpes zoster is an infection of the varicella zoster virus—the same pathogen that causes chickenpox. Those patients who actually had chickenpox previously are at the greatest risk for developing this painful disease. Patients will feel a burning sensation or shooting pain, accompanied often by tingling or itching on only one side of the body.

Finding shingles in the ICD-10-CM Alphabetic Index will require you to search for *Herpes, zoster* . . . reported with a code from code category B02. The required additional characters will identify specific details about the anatomical location and activity of the virus.

> **EXAMPLE**
> ☑4 B02 Zoster [herpes zoster]
> INCLUDES shingles
> zona
> B02.0 Zoster encephalitis
> B02.24 Postherpetic myelitis

You may be aware of the shingles vaccine, made recently available. For those patients coming to your health care facility to take advantage of this preventive medicine, the likely ICD-10-CM diagnosis code to provide medical necessity will be Z86.19 Personal history of other infectious and parasitic diseases.

Of course, the specific disease would be varicella—commonly known as chickenpox. The documentation will need to specify this personal history to support the provision of this vaccine. Also, make note of any other qualifiers set forth by third-party payers. Some require the patient to be aged 65 or over.

Zika Virus Infections

When a physician documents a confirmed diagnosis of the Zika virus, you are going to report code A92.5 Zika virus disease. However, if the physician includes any terms of doubt, such as describing this diagnosis as "suspected" or "possible," do not report the A92.5 code. Instead, you must report either:

- the codes for the specific symptoms that are included in the documentation, such as joint pain, fever, etc.

or

- Z20.828 Contact with and (suspected) exposure to other viral communicable diseases

> **GUIDANCE CONNECTION**
>
> Read the ICD-10-CM Official Guidelines for Coding and Reporting, section **I. Conventions, General Coding Guidelines and Chapter Specific Guidelines,** subsection **C. Chapter-Specific Coding Guidelines,** chapter **1. Certain Infectious and Parasitic Diseases,** subsection **f. Zika virus infections.**

YOU INTERPRET IT!

Is the infection bacterial or viral?
6. Strep throat (a) Bacteria (b) Virus 9. Measles (a) Bacteria (b) Virus
7. The Flu (a) Bacteria (b) Virus 10. Staph infection (a) Bacteria (b) Virus
8. Plantar wart (a) Bacteria (b) Virus

5.4 Parasitic and Fungal Infections

Parasitic Infestations

Parasites are tiny living things that can invade and feed off other living things—like humans. They are one-celled organisms (protozoa), insects (lice and mites), and worms (helminths) among others (see Figure 5-4) that can interfere with a healthy body. Tapeworms, hookworms, and pinworms are internal parasites. Parasites can be transmitted in food (e.g., protozoa like *Giardia intestinalis* and *Cyclospora cayetanensis*); spread by mosquitoes and other insects through the bloodstream (as in malaria and leishmaniasis); or ingested in contaminated water (as in amebiasis and schistosomiasis).

Parasites
Tiny living things that can invade and feed off other living things.

> **EXAMPLE**
>
> B86   Scabies
> B71.9   Cestode infection, unspecified
> B87.2   Ocular myiasis
>
> Diagnoses with a pathogen that is parasitic may not always be clearly defined. Keep that medical dictionary close at hand.

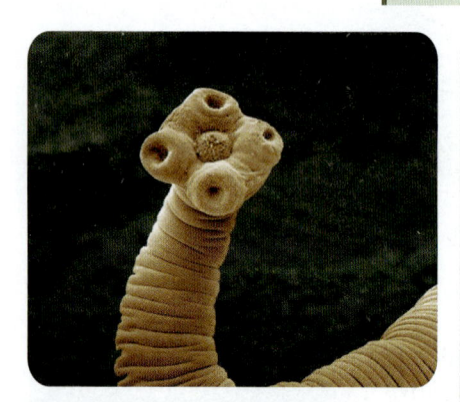

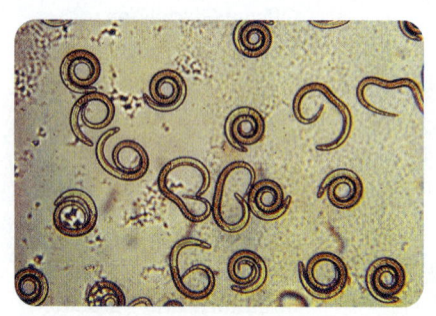

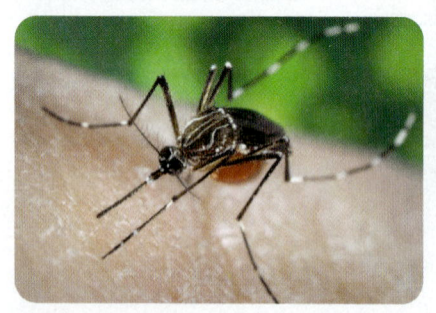

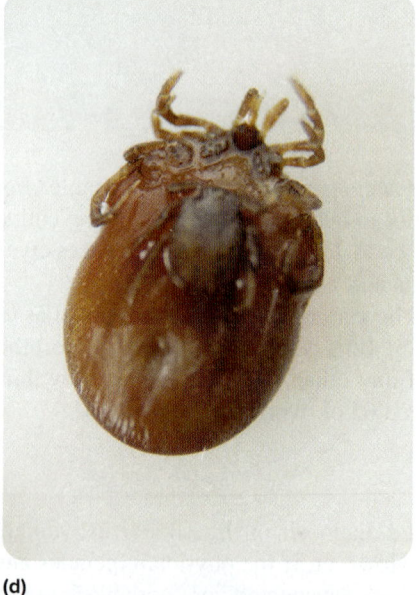

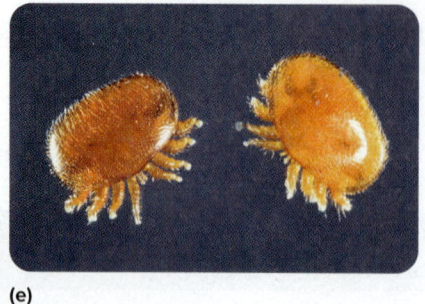

FIGURE 5-4 Parasitic worms: (a) tapeworms and (b) *Trichinella*. Parasitic insects: (c) mosquitoes, (d) deer ticks, and (e) mites (a) ©Mediscan/Alamy Stock Photo; (b) ©Dickson Despommier/Science Source; (c) Source: CDC/James Gathany; (d) ©Svetoslav Radkov/Shutterstock.com RF; (e) Source: USDA/Scott Bauer

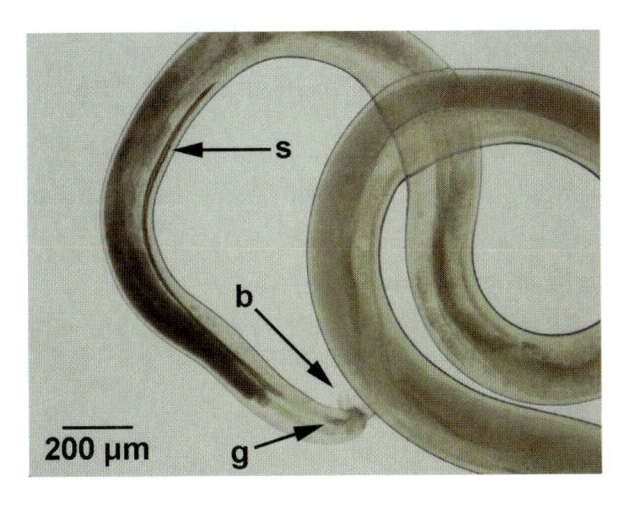

FIGURE 5-5 Angiostrongyliasis due to *Parastrongylus cantonensis,* reported with code B83.2 ©Michael S. Duffy

Protozoal diseases are caused by a single-celled, microscopic organism. There are several types of diagnoses that fall into this category:

- ☑ **B50-B54 Malaria**
- ☑ **B57 Chagas' disease (infection due to Trypanosoma cruzi)**
- ☑ **B58 Toxoplasmosis (infection due to Toxoplasma gondii)**

Helminths (from the Greek word for worms) are large organisms that grow to be visible with the naked eye. (See Figure 5-5.) Platyhelminths (flatworms) are commonly called tape worms, like acanthocephalins, which seek out the gastrointestinal tract. Ascariasis is the medical term used to describe a case of roundworm infection.

	B68.1	Taenia saginata taeniasis (infection due to adult tapeworm Taenia saginata)
☑	B76	Hookworm diseases
☑	B77	Ascariasis (roundworm infection)
	B85.3	Phthiriasis (infestation by crab-louse)

CODING BITES
These terms from Greek and Latin can be complex. However, physicians are more likely to use these terms in documentation. Therefore, keep that medical dictionary close at hand. You will need the support and accuracy of the definitions to help you determine the correct code.

YOU CODE IT! CASE STUDY

Michael McCarthey brought his 6-year-old daughter, Johannah, to see Dr. Benzzoni, complaining that his daughter keeps scratching her head. After a thorough exam, Dr. Benzzoni explains that Johannah has a case of head lice. He instructs Michael to buy Nix, an over-the-counter permethrin, and provides an instruction sheet on how to rid his child and their household of the parasites.

You Code It!

Step #1: Read the case carefully and completely.

Step #2: Abstract the scenario. Which main words or terms describe why the physician cared for the patient during this encounter?

Step #3: Are there any details missing or incomplete for which you would need to query the physician? [If so, ask your instructor.]

Step #4: Check for any relevant guidance, including reading all of the symbols and notations in the Tabular List and the appropriate sections of the Official Guidelines.

(continued)

> Step #5: Determine the correct diagnosis code or codes to explain why this encounter was medically necessary.
>
> Step #6: Double-check your work.
>
> **Answer:**
>
> Did you determine the correct code?
>
> > B85.0　　Pediculosis due to Pediculus humanus capitis [head louse infestation]
>
> Great work!

Fungal Infections

Fungi
Group of organisms, including mold, yeast, and mildew, that cause infection; fungus (singular).

There are many versions of **fungi** (the plural form of *fungus*) in our lives. Mushrooms on your pizza or in your salad and yeast in your bread or beer are tasty. Mold, a form of fungus, can be delicious when it is called blue cheese or feta cheese, and it can be helpful when developed in a pill containing penicillin. Then there are fungi that cause illness, such as *Aspergillus,* which may cause lower respiratory tract dysfunction, or *Candida albicans,* which causes infection in the oral mucosa and the walls of the vagina. *Onychomycosis* is the most common nail fungal infection.

> ### EXAMPLE
> P37.5　　Neonatal candidiasis
> B44.81　 Allergic bronchopulmonary aspergillosis
> B40.3　　Cutaneous blastomycosis
>
> With fungal infections, it may not be easy or straightforward from reading the diagnostic statement. You may need to do some research, or check in your medical dictionary.

Except in patients with compromised immune systems, fungal infections are not life-threatening.

☑ **B35 Dermatophytosis**

Ectoparasites are organisms that attach, or burrow, into the epidermis and dermis and remain there, such as ticks, fleas, lice, and mites. Often, the medical term "tinea" is used in the diagnostic statement, such as tinea pedis (commonly known as athlete's foot) or tinea cruris (also known as jock itch).

☑ **B44 Aspergillosis**

There can be serious concerns with a fungal infection when it affects the pulmonary organs, skin, or adrenal glands, known as histoplasmosis.

☑ **B38.0 Acute pulmonary coccidioidomycosis** *(also known as Valley Fever, this is an infection of the lungs)*

☑ **B39.3 Disseminate histoplasmosis capsulati**

YOU INTERPRET IT!

How are these diseases transmitted?

11. Lyme disease	(a) Parasite	(b) Fungus	14. *Aspergillus*	(a) Parasite	(b) Fungus
12. *Candida albicans*	(a) Parasite	(b) Fungus	15. Blastomycosis	(a) Parasite	(b) Fungus
13. Zika	(a) Parasite	(b) Fungus	16. Ring worm	(a) Parasite	(b) Fungus

5.5 Infections Caused by Several Pathogens

Up to this point, you have been reading about infectious and communicable diseases that are known to be caused by either a bacterium, virus, or other specific pathogen. However, there are some diagnoses that can be caused by a virus, a bacterium, or even a fungus. This means that you must abstract not only the name of the condition but also the specific type of underlying pathogen to determine an accurate code. Lab tests are required to confirm a diagnosis. Therefore, reading the pathology reports in the patient's chart can provide these details.

Pneumonia

Pneumonia is not an uncommon infection of the lungs. Actually, it is estimated that more than 3 million diagnoses of pneumonia are made each year in the U.S. Yet, as a professional coder, you need to know the specific type of pathogen that caused this infection before you can accurately determine the code.

Types of Pneumonia

Several different types of pathogens can result in fluid and pus filling the air sacs (alveoli)—the underlying cause of pneumonia. Integral signs and symptoms include cough with phlegm or pus, fever, chills, and difficulty breathing. When you look under the main term **PNEUMONIA** in the ICD-10-CM Alphabetic Index, you can see the very long list of additional descriptors needed to get to a specific code recommendation.

Bacterial Pneumonia

The *Streptococcus pneumoniae* bacterium, also known as pneumococcus, causes the most common type of pneumonia. Atypical pneumonia, commonly referred to as walking pneumonia, is also caused by bacteria, but different bacteria, including *Legionella pneumophila, Mycoplasma pneumoniae (M. pneumoniae),* and *Chlamydophila pneumoniae.*

Aspiration pneumonia is a bacterial infection that develops after the patient has inhaled food, a liquid, or vomit. The particles deteriorate and bacteria grow, causing the infection and inflammation.

> **CODING BITES**
>
> The incidence of pneumonia is also categorized by the environment in which the patient may have contracted this condition.
>
> *Community-acquired pneumonia (CAP)* identifies that pneumonia has developed in a patient who has not recently been in the hospital or another health care facility such as a nursing home or rehab facility.
>
> *Hospital-acquired pneumonia* identifies those patients who contract pneumonia while in a residential health care facility.

LET'S CODE IT! SCENARIO

Anna Carland, an 81-year-old female, was admitted to the hospital with pneumonia. She was placed on oxygen to help her breathe while labs were done to determine the type of pneumonia. Dr. Premin diagnosed her with streptococcal pneumonia. The pathology report specifies Streptococcus pneumoniae group B.

Let's Code It!

Anna was diagnosed with streptococcal pneumonia by Dr. Premin. Turn to the Alphabetic Index in your ICD-10-CM code book and find the main term:

Pneumonia (acute) (double) (migratory) (purulent) (septic) (unresolved) J18.9

Read carefully down the long, indented list beneath and find

(continued)

Pneumonia

in (due to)

all the way down this list to . . .

> Streptococcus J15.4
> > group B J15.3
> >
> > pneumoniae J13
> >
> > specified NEC J15.4

Knowing that Anna has "*Streptococcus pneumoniae*" is not enough. Remember that we are required to always code to the greatest specificity, and the code book is reminding you that you need additional details. Go back to the documentation, not only the physician's notes but the pathology report, too. Aha! The pathology report specifies "*Streptococcus* group B." Now, turn to the Tabular List to the code category J15.

☑4 **J15 Bacterial pneumonia, not elsewhere classified**

Code First associated influenza, if applicable (J09.X1, J10.0-, J11.0-)

Code Also associated lung abscess, if applicable (J85.1)

EXCLUDES1   chlamydial pneumonia (J16.0)

congenital pneumonia (P23.-)

Legionnaires' disease (A48.1)

spirochetal pneumonia (A69.8)

Read these notations carefully and determine if any of them relate to Anna's case. Not this time. Good! So, read down all of the fourth-character options and determine which matches Dr. Premin's documentation.

J15.3   Pneumonia due to streptococcus, group B

Check the head of this chapter in ICD-10-CM. There are notations at the beginning of this chapter: a **NOTE**, a *Use Additional Code* notation, and an EXCLUDES2 notation. Read carefully. Do any relate to Dr. Premin's diagnosis of Anna? No. Turn to the Official Guidelines and read Section 1.c.1. There is nothing specifically applicable here either.

Now you can report J15.3 for Anna's diagnosis with confidence.

Good coding!

Viral Pneumonia

There are some viruses that are known to cause inflammation and swelling in the lungs. The influenza A and B viruses, as well as *Hemophilus influenzae* (*H. influenzae*), can develop into viral pneumonia if not treated quickly. *Cytomegalovirus* (CMV) is most often seen in patients with a suppressed immune system, such as one going through chemotherapy or one suffering with an immunodeficiency condition.

> **EXAMPLES**
>
> ☑5 J11.0 Influenza due to unidentified influenza virus with pneumonia
> ☑4 J12 Viral pneumonia not elsewhere classified
> J14 Pneumonia due to Hemophilus influenzae

Fungal Pneumonia

The fungus *Pneumocystis jiroveci* is the cause of a fungal pneumonia, previously known as *Pneumocystis carini* or PCP pneumonia, in patients whose immune system is diminished. This is a known manifestation in those diagnosed with advanced HIV infection.

Pneumonia due to *Aspergillus* is the result of inhaling this form of mold.

Secondary Pneumonia

There are some diseases that can manifest a case of pneumonia. These conditions include rheumatic fever, schistosomiasis, and Q fever. There is a difference between this type of pneumonia and those we have just been discussing, so read carefully and possibly query the physician. This diagnosis is reported with the following code:

J17 Pneumonia in diseases classified elsewhere

Meningitis

Meningitis is the inflammation of the meningeal membranes of the brain and/or the spinal cord. Meningitis can be caused by a bacterial pathogen, such as *Meningococcus*; however, it is more often the result of a viral infection. When meningitis is caught early, the prognosis is good and complications are rare.

In order to code a diagnosis of meningitis, you have to know the specific virus or bacterium at the core of the inflammation. This will typically be found in the pathologist's report as well as the physician's documentation.

> **EXAMPLES**
>
> Some bacterial causes of meningitis would be reported with
>
> | | |
> |---|---|
> | A39.0 | Meningococcal meningitis |
> | A54.81 | Gonococcal meningitis |
> | G00.2 | Streptococcal meningitis |
>
> *Use additional code* to further identify organism (B95.0-B95.5)

> **EXAMPLES**
>
> Some viral causes of meningitis would be reported with
>
> | | |
> |---|---|
> | A87.1 | Adenoviral meningitis |
> | A87.0 | Echoviral meningitis |
> | B26.1 | Mumps (virus) meningitis |

In some cases, ICD-10-CM will identify the requirement of a second code.

> **EXAMPLES**
>
> Meningitis due to poliovirus A80.9 *[G02]*
>
> | | |
> |---|---|
> | A80.9 | Acute poliomyelitis, unspecified |
> | G02 | Meningitis in other infectious and parasitic diseases classified elsewhere |
> | G00.2 | Streptococcal meningitis |
>
> *Use additional code* to further identify organism (B95.0-B95.5)

CODING BITES

In some states, information in the patient's record relating to HIV testing (positive or negative result), HIV AIDS status, sexually transmitted diseases, genetic information (such as the results of any genetic testing), mental health conditions, and substance abuse is categorized as *superconfidential* information. This information has additional legal protection, above the requirements of HIPAA, with regard to disclosure and use. Be certain to find out if your state has this additional protection for patients as well as the requirements for compliance.

GUIDANCE CONNECTION

Read the ICD-10-CM Official Guidelines for Coding and Reporting, section **I. Conventions, General Coding Guidelines and Chapter Specific Guidelines,** subsection **C. Chapter-Specific Coding Guidelines,** chapter **1. Certain Infectious and Parasitic Diseases,** subsections **a. Human immunodeficiency virus (HIV) infections** and **a.2)(h) Encounters for testing for HIV.**

5.6 Immunodeficiency Conditions

Some conditions cause the body's immune system to stop working, meaning that infection and pathogens cannot be fought off effectively. You may remember learning about T cells, B cells, and lymphoid tissues from your physiology class. A defect involving any of these is known as a *primary (congenital) immunodeficiency* condition. A *secondary (acquired) immunodeficiency* is a manifestation caused by something that is blocking the proper immune response or depressing the response to an ineffective level. There are some viruses that trigger secondary immunodeficiency, such as with acquired immunodeficiency syndrome (AIDS). However, there are a number of potential external causes of secondary immunodeficiency, ranging from exposure to an infection, a toxic chemical, or radiation to suffering severe burns.

Primary immunodeficiency disorders include

- X-linked agammaglobulinemia (XLA)
- Common variable immunodeficiency (CVID)
- Severe combined immunodeficiency (SCID), also known as "boy in a bubble" disease
- Alymphocytosis (deficiency of lymphocytes in the blood)

Secondary immunodeficiency conditions include

- AIDS
- Leukemia and other cancers of the immune system
- Viral hepatitis and other immune-complex diseases
- Multiple myeloma (a cancer of the plasma cells)

Human Immunodeficiency Virus

Human immunodeficiency virus (HIV) infection is a serious illness. Sadly, as if this illness were not enough for a patient to deal with, it also carries a huge societal stigma. Therefore, whether you are coding for an inpatient facility (an exception to the guideline discussed earlier) or an outpatient facility, you will code this illness *only* when it has been *clearly specified in the physician's notes* that the patient is HIV-positive.

Anyone possibly exposed to HIV should be tested. Similar to so many other conditions, like malignancies, the earlier a diagnosis is made, the sooner treatment can begin. Early treatment translates into a longer, better-quality life for the patient.

Coding HIV Testing, Test Results, and Symptoms

Documenting Medical Necessity of HIV Testing

When an individual with no symptoms comes to a health care facility to be tested for a condition, you will need a diagnosis code to provide medical necessity for the test. As with other preventive health care encounters, you will use a Z code to document the need for HIV testing. For a first office visit to discuss possible exposure to HIV, you will use this code:

Z20.6   Contact with and (suspected) exposure to human immunodeficiency virus [HIV]

For the diagnosis code used to support the actual test, generally, you will use this code:

Z11.4   Encounter for screening for human immunodeficiency virus [HIV]

However, if the patient is documented by the physician as a member of a known high-risk group, you may use one of these codes:

Z72.5- High-risk sexual behavior
Z72.8- Other problems related to lifestyle

Remember, until there is a specific diagnostic statement in the physician's notes, you are not to report anything connected to HIV. If the patient is tested because of specific signs and/or symptoms, you will code those signs and symptoms, rather than any of the above.

> **CODING BITES**
>
> NEVER report a code for HIV infection or illness without a specific physician diagnostic statement—a confirmed diagnosis.

LET'S CODE IT! SCENARIO

Michael Callahan got drunk and had unprotected intercourse last night. He comes to Dr. Ansara's office to discuss his concerns about possible exposure to HIV.

Let's Code It!

Michael went to see Dr. Ansara because he was concerned that he had been *exposed to HIV.* Let's turn to the Alphabetic Index and look up *exposure:*

Exposure (to)
  human immunodeficiency virus (HIV) Z20.6

Confirm the complete code description in the Tabular List; start reading at the top of the chapter subsection titled

Persons with potential health hazards related to communicable diseases (Z20-Z29)

Be certain to read the **EXCLUDES1** and **EXCLUDES2** notes. While these excluded diagnoses do not relate to our current case of Michael's visit to Dr. Ansara, always reading up and down and around the code that was suggested by the Alphabetic Index is a critical habit that you need to build. This time, the notes do not apply, but next time, they might. Continue reading down the column.

☑4 Z20 Contact with or (suspected) exposure to communicable diseases

This fits the documentation, which notes that Michael is concerned that he has been "exposed." Keep reading down the column to find that required fourth digit. You will see this code:

Z20.6 Contact with and (suspected) exposure to human immunodeficiency virus [HIV]

Directly beneath this code is another **EXCLUDES1** notation:

Asymptomatic human immunodeficiency virus [HIV] infection status (Z21)

This reminds you that contact or exposure is not the same as a positive status asymptomatic HIV diagnosis.

Check the top of this subsection and the head of this chapter in ICD-10-CM. There is a **NOTE** at the beginning of this chapter. Read carefully. Does it relate to Dr. Ansara's diagnosis of Michael? No. Turn to the Official Guidelines and read Section 1.c.1. There is nothing specifically applicable here, either.

Now you can report code Z20.6 with confidence!

Test Negative

There are rapid HIV tests using oral swabs or finger sticks that can provide results in minutes. Other HIV tests may take several days to provide an answer. Therefore, a return visit to the health care provider will sometimes be required.

The entire experience of being tested and then having to wait for the results can be psychologically difficult, even when the news is good and the test is negative. It is the health care professional's responsibility to counsel the patient on how to prevent future risk. Therefore, when an individual returns to get the results of an HIV test, even when the results are negative, counseling should be provided. For that reason, when documented, report:

Z71.7   Human immunodeficiency virus [HIV] counseling

Test Inconclusive

It can happen that the serology (pathology testing) comes back inconclusive for HIV. There can be no specific diagnosis for HIV or any direct manifestations of the illness because there is nothing to confirm or deny HIV-positive status. In such cases, you have to use this code:

R75   Inconclusive laboratory evidence of human immunodeficiency virus [HIV]

Test Positive but Asymptomatic

Thanks to research and the development of new drug therapies, patients who have HIV are living longer and with a better quality of life. Therefore, testing positive for HIV is not quite as devastating as it was years ago. When a patient comes to receive the HIV test results that are positive but the patient has no signs, symptoms, or manifestations, the patient is **asymptomatic.** You will assign this code:

Z21   Asymptomatic human immunodeficiency virus [HIV] infection status

When the physician provides counseling for the patient, discusses therapeutic treatments, and/or any other elements of dealing with the disease, you should report the counseling code as well.

Test Positive with Symptoms or Manifestations

Once the individual has been diagnosed and exhibits any manifestations associated with HIV, the code to report the condition will change from Z21 to

B20   Human immunodeficiency virus [HIV] disease

Code B20 includes a diagnosis of acquired immune deficiency syndrome (AIDS), which is essentially HIV with manifestations. When you use code B20, you have to follow it with a code or codes to identify the specific manifestations, such as pneumonia or HIV-2 infection. There is a notation in the ICD-10-CM book, below code B20's description in the Tabular List, reminding you to do this. If the patient is seen for a condition or illness directly related to his or her HIV-positive status, list code B20 first, followed by the code or codes for the conditions.

> **CODING BITES**
> Once a patient has been diagnosed with manifestations of HIV-positive status, you are no longer permitted to use code Z21, even when the manifestations are no longer present.

Asymptomatic
No symptoms or manifestations.

> **CODING BITES**
> *Positive status* means that laboratory tests have confirmed that the patient does have the virus in his or her system (positive status).
>
> *Asymptomatic* means that the patient is currently not exhibiting any signs or symptoms of the disease.

LET'S CODE IT! SCENARIO

Alfredo Zimoso has been HIV-positive for 10 years. He comes to see Dr. Chang because of severe headaches and vision problems. After a complete physical examination (PE) and appropriate tests, Dr. Chang diagnoses Alfredo with noninfectious acute disseminated encephalomyelitis, secondary to HIV.

Let's Code It!

Alfredo has been diagnosed with *noninfectious acute disseminated encephalomyelitis, secondary to HIV.* Do you know whether the noninfectious acute disseminated encephalomyelitis is an HIV-related manifestation? There are two ways to tell. First, the physician's notes state that the condition is *secondary to HIV.* This means that not only are the two conditions related to each other but that the HIV is also the underlying condition (it came first). The second way to tell is shown in the Tabular List. Let's first go to the Alphabetic Index to find encephalomyelitis. The indented descriptions of encephalomyelitis include terms used by the physician in her notes.

> **Encephalomyelitis**
>> **acute disseminated (ADEM) (postinfectious) G04.01**

Notice that this description also includes the term *postinfectious*. Alfredo was diagnosed with noninfectious encephalomyelitis. Keep reading down and find:

> **Encephalomyelitis, acute disseminated, noninfectious G04.81**

That seems to match the doctor's notes, so now, let's turn to the Tabular List and read the complete descriptions. Start reading at

> ✓4 **G04**   **Encephalitis, myelitis, and encephalomyelitis**

This code category contains INCLUDES, EXCLUDES1, and EXCLUDES2 notes, which you need to read carefully. Is there anything that leads you away from this code category? No, there isn't, so you need to read down the column to find the most accurate, required fourth digit:

> ✓5 **G04.8 Other causes of encephalitis, myelitis, and encephalomyelitis**

None of the other descriptions match Dr. Chang's notes, so this looks like the best option. Take a look at your choices for the required fifth digit:

> **G04.81 Other encephalitis and encephalomyelitis**
> **G04.89 Other myelitis**

Check the notes and you will see that Alfredo was diagnosed with encephalomyelitis, leading you directly to code:

> **G04.81 Other encephalitis and encephalomyelitis; noninfectious acute disseminated encephalomyelitis (noninfectious ADEM)**

That matches Dr. Chang's notes exactly.

Now you need the code for Michael's HIV-positive status. You know that the encephalomyelitis is a manifestation of that status and you should be clear as to what the code should be. In the Alphabetic Index, find:

> **Human immunodeficiency virus (disease) (infection) B20**
>> **asymptomatic status Z21**

Which one should you follow? You know from the notes that Alfredo does have symptoms and has manifested a secondary illness. Therefore, turn to the Tabular List to confirm:

> **B20   Human immunodeficiency virus [HIV] disease**

You now have two codes to report the reasons Dr. Chang cared for Alfredo at this encounter. Which gets listed first? The notation below the description reminds you to "*use additional code(s)* to identify all manifestations of HIV." This tells you that B20 is listed first.

Check the top of this subsection and the head of this chapter in ICD-10-CM. There are notations at the beginning of this chapter: an INCLUDES notation, a *Use additional code* note, an EXCLUDES1 notation, and an EXCLUDES2 notation. Read carefully. Do any relate to Dr. Chang's diagnosis of Alfredo? No. Turn to the Official Guidelines and read Section 1.c.1. Read subsection (a) Human Immunodeficiency virus (HIV) infections, particularly (2) Selection and sequencing of HIV codes, (a) Patient admitted for HIV-related condition.

So your report for Dr. Chang's encounter with Alfredo will show:

> **B20   Human immunodeficiency virus [HIV] disease**
> **G04.81   Other causes of encephalitis, noninfectious acute disseminated encephalomyelitis**

Good job!

> **GUIDANCE CONNECTION**
>
> Read the ICD-10-CM Official Guidelines for Coding and Reporting, section **I. Conventions, General Coding Guidelines and Chapter Specific Guidelines,** subsection **C. Chapter-Specific Coding Guidelines,** chapter **1. Certain Infectious and Parasitic Diseases,** subsection **a. 2)(f) Previously diagnosed HIV-related illness.**

HIV Status with Unrelated Conditions

An individual who is HIV-positive can still be affected by conditions, illnesses, or injuries that have nothing to do with his or her HIV status. As you have learned, the first-listed code should answer the question, "Why did the health care provider care for the patient at this encounter?" Therefore, the code for the condition that caused the patient to visit the physician should come first. Because HIV is a systemic disease, affecting the entire body, you have to include a code for that condition as well. Even if it has nothing to do with the services or treatment provided by the physician, it will have an impact on the physician's decision making and therefore must be included.

> **GUIDANCE CONNECTION**
>
> Read the ICD-10-CM Official Guidelines for Coding and Reporting, section **I. Conventions, General Coding Guidelines and Chapter Specific Guidelines,** subsection **C. Chapter-Specific Coding Guidelines,** chapter **1. Certain Infectious and Parasitic Diseases,** subsection **a.2)(b):** "If a patient with HIV disease is admitted for an unrelated condition (such as a traumatic injury), the code for the unrelated condition (e.g., the nature of injury code) should be the principal diagnosis. Other diagnoses would be B20 followed by additional diagnosis codes for all reported HIV-related conditions."

EXAMPLE

Gayle Robbins came to see Dr. Tigliano because she slipped on the ice this morning and hurt her ankle. Dr. Tigliano examined her and took x-rays that confirmed a sprain of the deltoid ligament of the left ankle. Gayle was diagnosed with HIV 2 years ago and is asymptomatic.

S93.422A Sprain, of deltoid ligament of left ankle, initial encounter
Z21   Asymptomatic human immunodeficiency virus [HIV]

EXAMPLE

Yuri Kastachen fell off a ladder and hurt his lower back. Dr. Lang determined that Yuri had a fractured coccyx. Last year, Yuri was hospitalized with HIV-related pneumonia.

S32.2xxA Fracture of coccyx, initial encounter
B20   Human immunodeficiency virus [HIV] disease

HIV Status in Obstetrics

When a woman with HIV-positive status is pregnant, giving birth, or in the postpartum period, the systemic disease must be a consideration in determining her care. Therefore, whether or not she has symptoms or manifestations of the HIV condition, the first-listed code must be

O98.7- Human immunodeficiency virus [HIV] disease complicating pregnancy, childbirth, or the puerperium

This should be followed by the appropriate HIV-positive status code: Z21 or B20.

YOU CODE IT! CASE STUDY

Maureen Dunbar, a 27-year-old female, 23 weeks pregnant, was playing tennis when she felt a pain in her right knee. She went to see her physician, Dr. Rummur, who diagnosed her problem as a derangement of the anterior horn of the lateral cystic meniscus. Maureen has been HIV-positive and asymptomatic for 5 years.

> **You Code It!**
>
> Go through the steps of coding, and determine the diagnosis code(s) to be reported for this encounter between Dr. Rummur and Maureen Dunbar.
>
> Step #1: Read the case carefully and completely.
>
> Step #2: Abstract the scenario. Which main words or terms describe why the physician cared for the patient during this encounter?
>
> Step #3: Are there any details missing or incomplete for which you would need to query the physician? [If so, ask your instructor.]
>
> Step #4: Check for any relevant guidance, including reading all of the symbols and notations in the Tabular List and the appropriate sections of the Official Guidelines.
>
> Step #5: Determine the correct diagnosis code or codes to explain why this encounter was medically necessary.
>
> Step #6: Double-check your work.
>
> **Answer:**
>
> Did you determine the correct codes?
>
> | | |
> |---|---|
> | M23.041 | Cystic meniscus, anterior horn of lateral meniscus, right knee |
> | O98.712 | Human immunodeficiency virus [HIV] disease complicating pregnancy, childbirth, or the puerperium, antepartum condition, second trimester |
> | Z21 | Asymptomatic human immunodeficiency virus [HIV] infection status |
>
> Good job!

Are you wondering why the knee condition is listed first when the guideline for HIV infection in pregnancy states the O98.7- code category should be listed first? In this case, you have two guidelines that need to be followed:

> Section I.C.1.a.2)(b) Patient with HIV disease admitted for unrelated condition
> Section I.C.1.a.2)(g) HIV infection in pregnancy, childbirth, and the puerperium

To break the tie, let's look at one more guideline, either

> Section II. Selection of Principal Diagnosis (for inpatient encounters)

or

> Section IV. Diagnostic Coding and Reporting Guidelines for Outpatient Services, Subsection H (for outpatient encounters)

Whether you are coding for outpatient or inpatient services, the guidelines agree that the principal, or first-listed, diagnosis code should be the condition "chiefly responsible" for the encounter. In Maureen's case, the reason she went to the doctor for care was the pain in her knee—not the pregnancy and not the HIV. Then why code them at all? Because Dr. Rummur must take Maureen's pregnant status and her HIV status into consideration in his medical decision-making process to determine the best way to treat her knee.

YOU INTERPRET IT!

Which condition code is sequenced first [principal diagnosis]?
17. HIV-positive patient admitted with fractured leg _____
18. Patient admitted with pneumocystis carinii, HIV-positive since 2015 _____
19. Patient, 38 weeks pregnant, HIV-positive, delivers _____
20. Patient seen for type 1 diabetes, HIV-positive _____

5.7 Septicemia and Other Blood Infections

Blood infections are very dangerous, as you might imagine, because of their potential effect on the entire body. Blood circulates through the body and touches all the cells and organs in some fashion. So you can understand that if the blood circulating through the body is carrying a disease, it can have the potential to cause serious problems. There are several types of blood infections, and each needs to be coded differently.

Septicemia

Essentially, **septicemia** is identified as the presence of a microorganism or toxin in the bloodstream. The organism might be a virus, a fungus, a bacterium, or another pathologic substance. Septicemia is very serious. A physician may refer to this condition as *bacteremia;* however, they are really not the same. Bacteremia may not be clinically significant, but septicemia is always significant.

The code used for a diagnosis of septicemia may be taken from category

> **A41.9**   Sepsis, unspecified sepsis (Septicemia NOS)

You will need to determine a more accurate code by the pathogen or toxin found in the blood, such as streptococcus or staphylococcus.

A diagnosis of **systemic inflammatory response syndrome (SIRS)** is used when the basic cause, or *pathogen,* is unknown. The human body is amazing and is designed to fight any and all intruders (disease or infection). The system's response to infection may be

- Increased body temperature.
- Change in heart rate.
- Change in respiratory rate.
- Increased white blood cell count.

> **Systemic inflammatory response syndrome (SIRS) of non-infectious origin R65.10**
> **Systemic inflammatory response syndrome (SIRS) of non-infectious origin with acute organ dysfunction R65.11**

Septicemia
Generalized infection spread through the body via the bloodstream; blood infection.

Systemic Inflammatory Response Syndrome (SIRS)
A definite physical reaction, such as fever, chills, etc., to an unspecified pathogen.

GUIDANCE CONNECTION

Read the ICD-10-CM Official Guidelines for Coding and Reporting, section **I. Conventions, General Coding Guidelines and Chapter Specific Guidelines,** subsection **C. Chapter-Specific Coding Guidelines,** chapter **1. Certain Infectious and Parasitic Diseases,** subsection **d. Sepsis, severe sepsis, and septic shock.**

YOU CODE IT! CASE STUDY

Priscilla Christopher, a 17-year-old female, was brought by her mother to see Dr. Fasold. Priscilla claimed that her muscles ache, she has been sweating, and she has chills at the same time. She stated that she has been coughing and short of breath for several days. After running some tests, Dr. Fasold diagnosed Priscilla with sepsis due to Hemophilus influenzae.

You Code It!

Go through the steps of coding, and determine the diagnosis code or codes that should be reported for this encounter between Dr. Fasold and Priscilla.

Step #1: Read the case carefully and completely.

Step #2: Abstract the scenario. Which main words or terms describe why the physician cared for the patient during this encounter?

Step #3: Are there any details missing or incomplete for which you would need to query the physician? [If so, ask your instructor.]

Step #4: Check for any relevant guidance, including reading all of the symbols and notations in the Tabular List and the appropriate sections of the Official Guidelines.

Step #5: Determine the correct diagnosis code or codes to explain why this encounter was medically necessary.

Step #6: Double-check your work.

Answer:

Did you determine the correct code?

    A41.3   Sepsis due to Hemophilus influenzae

Terrific!

Sepsis

When an individual exhibits two or more systemic responses or when the presence of a specific pathogen has been identified in the bloodstream, the diagnosis is typically **sepsis**.

Reporting a diagnosis of sepsis will begin with the identification of the underlying systemic infection—the pathogen that initiated the septic condition. This code will come from category A40.- or A41.-. You may find this detail in the physician's documentation or the pathology report.

On occasion, a physician might diagnose a patient with *urosepsis*. This is not a synonym for sepsis and cannot be coded as sepsis. Should you find this term used in the documentation, you will need to query the physician for clarification.

A patient may be diagnosed with sepsis and acute organ failure during the same encounter, without a relationship (or cause and effect) between the two. In these situations, the organ failure is a co-morbidity and is reported separately from the sepsis.

> **EXAMPLE**
> Bernard Madison was in the hospital and diagnosed with group A streptococcus sepsis.
>
>   A40.0   Sepsis due to streptococcus, group A

Severe Sepsis

When left untreated, sepsis may become severe and cause an organ to fail—a life-threatening condition. In some cases, this can occur when treatment is provided but is ineffective. A diagnosis of sepsis in combination with acute organ failure due to the septic condition is reported as **severe sepsis**. The physician's notes that contain a diagnosis of severe sepsis will be reported with

- *First:* the code for the underlying systemic infection, such as streptococcus or other bacteria (e.g., a code from A40.- or A41.-). If the organism is not known, you may report A41.9 Sepsis, unspecified organism.
- *Followed by:* a code from subcategory R65.2 Severe sepsis. An additional character is required to report whether or not the physician has documented that the patient is in "septic shock."
- *Followed by:* a code to report the specific organ failure caused by the septic condition. To remind you, code subcategory R65 has a *Use additional code* notation.

Sepsis
Condition typified by two or more systemic responses to infection; a specified pathogen.

GUIDANCE CONNECTION

Read the ICD-10-CM Official Guidelines for Coding and Reporting, section **I. Conventions, General Coding Guidelines and Chapter Specific Guidelines,** subsection **C. Chapter-Specific Coding Guidelines,** chapter **1. Certain Infections and Parasitic Diseases,** subsection **d.3) Sequencing of severe sepsis,** which warns you that a code from subcategory **R65.2 Severe sepsis** is *never* permitted to be the first-listed or principal diagnosis code reported.

Severe Sepsis
Sepsis with signs of acute organ dysfunction.

CHAPTER 5 | CODING INFECTIOUS DISEASES

> ### LET'S CODE IT! SCENARIO
>
> *Dr. Kahanni admitted Burton Chapel with acute renal failure due to severe sepsis resulting from pneumonia.*
>
> #### Let's Code It!
>
> Dr. Kahanni diagnosed Burton with "acute renal failure due to severe sepsis resulting from pneumonia." Remember the Official Guideline at Section l.c.1.d(1)(b): The coding of severe sepsis requires first a code for the underlying systemic infection, followed by a code from R65.2-, and then the code for the acute organ dysfunction. Turn to the Alphabetic Index and find
>
> > **Sepsis**
> >> **Pneumococcal A40.3**
>
> Turn to the Tabular List to confirm this code:
>
> > ☑4 **A40**   **Steptococcal sepsis**
>
> Read the fourth-character choices and find
>
> > **A40.3**   **Sepsis due to Streptococcus pneumoniae (Pneumococcal sepsis)**
>
> Next, let's turn to R65.2- and see what will accurately report Dr. Kahanni's diagnosis for Burton.
>
> > ☑5 **R65.2**   **Severe sepsis**
>
> Read the fifth-character descriptions, and determine which one matches:
>
> > **R65.20**   **Severe sepsis without septic shock**
>
> The notations above this code help you further. They remind you to "*Code first underlying infection*," which you have done already with the pneumococcal sepsis code. The second notation directs you to
>
> > *Use additional code* to specify acute organ dysfunction, such as: acute kidney failure (N17.-)
>
> Next, confirm the code for the acute renal (kidney) failure:
>
> > ☑4 **N17**   **Acute kidney failure**
>
> Carefully read the *Code also* and **EXCLUDES1** notes. There is no relevance here to Burton's diagnosis at this encounter, so read down the column to review all of your choices for the required fourth character. With no documentation of any lesions on Burton's kidneys, the best choice is
>
> > **N17.9**   **Acute renal failure, unspecified**
>
> Check the top of this subsection and the head of this chapter in ICD-10-CM. There are notations at the beginning of this chapter: an **INCLUDES** notation, a *Use additional code* note, an **EXCLUDES1** notation, and an **EXCLUDES2** notation. Read carefully. Do any relate to Dr. Kahanni's diagnosis of Burton? No. Turn to the Official Guidelines and read Section 1.c.1, particularly d. Sepsis, severe sepsis, and septic shock.
>
> Now you can report, with confidence, these codes in the order specified by the guidelines: A40.3, R65.20, N17.9 . . .
> Good job!

Septic Shock
Severe sepsis with hypotension; unresponsive to fluid resuscitation.

Septic Shock

Should a patient also develop hypotension (low blood pressure) in addition to having severe sepsis, the diagnosis becomes **septic shock**. Septic shock cannot be present without the existence of severe sepsis—and it all must be documented. When coding septic shock, report the codes in the following order:

1. The code for the systemic infection (e.g., A40.-).
2. The code for the severe sepsis with septic shock (e.g., R65.21).
3. The code for the organ dysfunction.

> **CODING BITES**
> The code for septic shock may not be the principal or first-listed diagnosis.

Sepsis and Septic Shock Relating to Pregnancy or Newborns

Sepsis during Labor

During the process of giving birth, a woman might develop a septic infection. In this case, code O75.3 Other infection during labor (Sepsis during labor) is reported. A code from B95–B97 Bacterial and viral infectious agents should follow to specify the pathogen causing the infection.

Puerperal Sepsis

Puerperal sepsis, also known as *postpartum sepsis, puerperal peritonitis,* or *puerperal pyemia*, results from an infection that develops in a woman's reproductive organs and that was initiated during or following miscarriage or childbirth. This diagnosis is reported with code O85 Puerperal sepsis.

In addition, a code from B95-B97 Bacterial and viral infectious agents is required to specify the pathogen causing the infection. If severe sepsis is documented, a code from R65.2- should also be reported.

Neonatal Sepsis

A fetus may contract an infection in utero, during the birth process (delivery), or during the first 28 days after birth. In these cases, when a neonate is diagnosed with sepsis, the code will be reported from category P36 Bacterial sepsis of newborn. An additional character is required to identify the pathogen that caused the infection. If severe sepsis is documented, a code from R65.2- should also be reported.

> **GUIDANCE CONNECTION**
> Read the ICD-10-CM Official Guidelines for Coding and Reporting, section **I. Conventions, General Coding Guidelines and Chapter Specific Guidelines,** subsection **C. Chapter-Specific Coding Guidelines,** chapter **1. Certain Infectious and Parasitic Diseases,** subsection **d. 2) Septic shock.**

Septic Condition Resulting from Surgery

Should a patient develop sepsis from an infection as a complication of a surgical procedure, you will list a code for that situation first. In the Alphabetic Index, find

> **Sepsis, postprocedural T81.4**

In the Tabular List, find

> **T81.4xx- Infection following a procedure**

You can see, included with other non-essential modifiers *Sepsis following a procedure* is listed.

Read the EXCLUDES1 note. You will see that there are three diagnoses that would be easy to code incorrectly from this subcategory:

> **obstetric surgical wound infection (O86.0)**
> **postprocedural fever NOS (R50.82)**
> **postprocedural retroperitoneal abscess (K68.11)**

This is a great example of why it is so important to read carefully.

> **GUIDANCE CONNECTION**
> Read the ICD-10-CM Official Guidelines for Coding and Reporting, section **I. Conventions, General Coding Guidelines and Chapter Specific Guidelines,** subsection **C. Chapter-Specific Coding Guidelines,** chapter **1. Certain Infectious and Parasitic Diseases,** subsection **d. 5) Sepsis due to a postprocedural infection.**

Next, carefully read the three diagnoses listed in the EXCLUDES2 note.

> bleb associated endophthalmitis (H59.4-)
>
> infection due to infusion, transfusion and therapeutic injection (T80.2-)
>
> infection due to prosthetic devices, implants and grafts (T82.6-T82.7, T83.5-T83.6, T84.5-T84.7, T85.7)

Don't forget the *Use Additional Code* notations, also:

> *Use additional code* to identify infection
>
> *Use additional code* (R65.2-) to identify severe sepsis, if applicable

Then, continue with the usual coding sequence for sepsis, as reviewed earlier in this section. Remember to refer to the physician's documentation and the pathology report to gather all of the details you need to code accurately.

YOU CODE IT! CASE STUDY

Gregory Parrale, a 31-year-old male, had his appendix taken out last week. He comes to Dr. Gorman's office for his postsurgical follow-up visit. Dr. Gorman finds the surgical wound is erythematous, swollen, and painful to the touch. He takes a swab of the fluid oozing from the site. The lab confirms a postoperative staph infection.

You Code It!

Go through the steps of coding, and determine the diagnosis code(s) to be reported for this encounter between Dr. Gorman and Gregory Parrale.

Step #1: Read the case carefully and completely.

Step #2: Abstract the scenario. Which main words or terms describe why the physician cared for the patient during this encounter?

Step #3: Are there any details missing or incomplete for which you would need to query the physician? [If so, ask your instructor.]

Step #4: Check for any relevant guidance, including reading all of the symbols and notations in the Tabular List and the appropriate sections of the Official Guidelines.

Step #5: Determine the correct diagnosis code or codes to explain why this encounter was medically necessary.

Step #6: Double-check your work.

Answer:

Did you determine the correct codes?

T81.4xxA	Infection following a procedure, initial encounter
B95.8	Unspecified staphylococcus as the cause of diseases classified elsewhere

Good job!

Systemic Inflammatory Response Syndrome (SIRS) without Infection

Systemic inflammatory response syndrome (SIRS) can develop in patients who have not developed an infection. Instead the reaction may occur due to the presence of a burn or other trauma, a malignant neoplasm, or the presence of pancreatitis. In such cases, coding the condition will change slightly. You will code the following sequence:

1. The code for the underlying condition (e.g., T22.311- Third-degree burn of right forearm).
2. The code for SIRS from the subcategory R65.1- Systemic inflammatory response syndrome (SIRS) of non-infectious origin.
3. The code for the acute organ dysfunction, when applicable.

If the documentation indicates that the patient later developed an infection, you will code the diagnosis for the infection as shown earlier in this section, along with the additional code for the underlying trauma or condition.

> **GUIDANCE CONNECTION**
>
> Read the ICD-10-CM Official Guidelines for Coding and Reporting, section **I.Conventions, General Coding Guidelines and Chapter Specific Guidelines,** subsection **C. Chapter-Specific Coding Guidelines,** chapter **18. Symptoms, signs, and abnormal clinical laboratory findings, not elsewhere classified,** subsection**g. SIRS due to non-infectious process.**

5.8 Antimicrobial Resistance

There are individuals who go to the doctor or clinic demanding a prescription for an antibiotic for the slightest sniffle. Touch a cart at the supermarket? Wipe antimicrobial gel on your hands. Unfortunately, there is an ongoing war on germs and, it turns out, the pathogens are winning. A natural phenomenon of adaptation to survive is one of the reasons why antimicrobial drugs are no longer working. Biologists call this "adaptive immunity" . . . a concept similar to the process of vaccinations affording a patient ultimate resistance to the effects of a specific pathogen. Only, in this case, it is the pathogen building its own immunity.

In 1928, bacteriologist Alexander Fleming realized that a mold growing on a culture plate actually had antibacterial benefit. The mold became known as "penicillin" and it was found to be very effective against *staphylococci* bacteria—a serious and life-threatening human infection. This discovery saved millions of lives as penicillins and other antibiotics were able to kill infection and prevent patients from dying. More than eight decades later, antibiotics are no longer halting the spread of infectious disease. And, in one perspective, they may actually be contributing to the spread.

The World Health Organization (WHO) defines "antimicrobial resistance (AMR)" as the ". . . *resistance of a micro-organism to an antimicrobial medicine to which it was originally sensitive.*" In addition to adaptive immunity, AMR is caused by the overuse of antibiotics. In the United States, antibiotics are prescribed for patients who actually do not need them an estimated 50% of the time. The Centers for Disease Control and Prevention (CDC) recommends that physicians wait for the results of cultures and lab tests before writing that prescription to ensure the bacteria or virus proven to cause the patient's infection can be fought off with the most effective drug. And these tests will also identify when no prescription is in the patient's best interests, saving the money that would have been spent on medication that would not work anyway.

Both inpatient and outpatient facilities are guilty of having less than effective infection control and prevention—the third underlying cause of AMR. The invisibility of these tiny organisms makes it difficult for some individuals to believe and remember to wash up or, at least, access antibacterial gel/foam.

Several codes are available to you to report AMR.

Coding for AMR

The CDC identified three pathogens as urgent threats: *Clostridium difficile* (*C. diff*), carbapenem-resistant *Enterobacteriaceae,* and drug-resistant *Neisseria gonorrhoeae.* Let's look at some details about these three concerns.

Primarily, one code category is used to report AMR. There is a note and a notation for you:

☑4 **Z16 Resistance to antimicrobial drugs**
NOTE: The codes in this category are provided as *Use additional codes* to identify the resistance and non-responsiveness of a condition to antimicrobial drugs.
Code first **the infection.**

> **CODING BITES**
>
> A *Physician's Desk Reference* (PDR) or a Drug Guide can help you connect the name of a specific drug to a family name of drugs. For example, the quinolones are a family of synthetic broad-spectrum antibiotics. Ciprofloxacin, also known as Cipro, and levofloxavin, also known as Levaquin, are part of the quinolones family of drugs.

Clostridium difficile (C. diff)

C. diff is a spore-forming, gram-positive anaerobic bacillus that causes life-threatening diarrhea and that has been documented as causing about 250,000 infections each year, which have resulted in about 14,000 deaths. Of those patients aged 65 and older infected with *C. diff*, more than 90% died. In total, *C. diff* costs us an estimated $1 billion in excess health care costs. At greatest risk for contracting *C. diff* are hospitalized patients, those who have been recently hospitalized, and those who have recently received medical care with a course of antibiotic therapy.

The CDC is calling for more data as they track these AMRs. ICD-10-CM gives us the tools to collect and submit these details. For example, these codes may be reported for a patient with *C. diff* who is not responding to antibiotics:

| Z16.23 | Resistance to quinolones and fluoroquinolones |
| Z16.24 | Resistance to multiple antibiotics |

Carbapenem-Resistant *Enterobacteriaceae* (CRE)

CRE refers to a collection of microorganisms that have developed resistance to antibiotics. This grouping, or family, includes *Klebsiella* species and *Escherichia coli* (*E. coli*). Carbapenem antibiotics are beta-lactam antibiotics used as a last resort for many bacterial infections (brand names include Invanz®, Primaxin®, and Merrem®); however, increased resistance to these antibiotics has made them virtually ineffective.

Klebsiella pneumoniae carbapenemase (KPC) and *New Delhi Metallo-beta-lactamase* (NDM), both types of CRE, are the enzymes responsible for rendering carbapenems ineffective. CRE causes a variety of diseases, ranging from pneumonia to urinary tract infections to serious bloodstream or wound infections. Patients who are ill, exposed to hospital environments, and in long-term care facilities are most susceptible to CRE infection.

| Z16.19 | Resistance to other specified beta lactam antibiotics |

Neisseria gonorrhoeae Bacterial Infection

Gonorrhea is caused by the *Neisseria gonorrhoeae* bacterium and is most often transmitted by sexual contact. This microorganism replicates easily in the warm, moist areas of the reproductive tract, as well as in the mouth, throat, eyes, and anus. Approximately 30% of gonorrhea infections are found to be drug resistant and, often, patients infected with drug-resistant *Neisseria gonorrhoeae* do not exhibit any signs or symptoms. This disease can have long-lasting effects on the patient, including pelvic inflammatory disease that can result in infertility in women and epididymitis (an inflammation of the structure within the testis that stores sperm and transports the sperm to the vas deferens) in men. A patient who has contracted gonorrhea is more susceptible to contracting the human immunodeficiency virus (HIV).

When the physician's documentation states the patient is resistant to one of these antibiotics, normally prescribed to combat a diagnosis of *Neisseria gonorrhoeae*, report one of these codes in addition to the code for the infection (based on the anatomical site). Code Z16.19 or Z16.29 explains why the physician prescribed a different antibiotic.

Z16.19 Resistance to other specified beta lactam antibiotics (resistance to cephalosporins)

Z16.29 Resistance to other single specified antibiotic (resistance to macrolides) (resistance to tetracyclines)

Methicillin-Resistant *Staphylococcus aureus* Infection

Methicillin-resistant *Staphylococcus aureus* (MRSA) is a bacterial (staph) infection that is essentially unaffected by certain antibiotics. MRSA is spread from one person to another by direct contact with the infection, such as touching a skin bump or infection that is draining pus. MRSA can be spread directly, for example, by touching an infected person's rash, or it can be spread indirectly, such as by touching a used bandage contaminated with MRSA or by sharing a towel or razor that has come in contact with infected skin. One of the most frequent anatomical sites of MRSA colonization is the nose; bacteria can be found in nasal secretions.

To properly report these diagnoses, code the current infection due to MRSA and the MRSA infection separately with codes:

A49.02 Methicillin resistant Staphylococcus aureus infection, unspecific site

B95.62 Methicillin resistant Staphylococcus aureus infection as the cause of diseases classified elsewhere

Combination Codes

There are some infections commonly known to be caused by the patient's current MRSA status. In these cases, ICD-10-CM provides a combination code that can be used—the one code instead of two different codes. Two examples of these combination codes are

A41.02 Sepsis due to Methicillin resistant Staphylococcus aureus

J15.212 Pneumonia due to Methicillin resistant Staphylococcus aureus

Notice that the code descriptions include both the MRSA and another infection: septicemia in the first code and pneumonia in the second.

> **GUIDANCE CONNECTION**
>
> Read the ICD-10-CM Official Guidelines for Coding and Reporting, section **I. Conventions, General Coding Guidelines and Chapter Specific Guidelines,** subsection **C. Chapter-Specific Coding Guidelines,** chapter **1. Certain Infectious and Parasitic Diseases,** subchapter **e. Methicillin resistant Staphylococcus aureus (MRSA) conditions.**

> **EXAMPLE**
>
> Sally Hayes-Meyer was diagnosed with acute cystitis due to MRSA.
>
> N30.00 Acute cystitis without hematuria
>
> B95.62 Methicillin resistant Staphylococcus aureus infections as the causes of diseases classified elsewhere

Methicillin-Resistant *Staphylococcus aureus* Colonization

When a patient is documented as having a MRSA screening or nasal swab test that is positive yet there is no current illness, this is called colonization. Colonization indicates that the patient is a carrier. When this is the case, report either

Z22.321 Carrier or suspected carrier, Methicillin susceptible Staphylococcus aureus (MSSA)

or

Z22.322 Carrier or suspected carrier, Methicillin resistant Staphylococcus aureus (MRSA)

The coding guidelines state that it is possible for one patient to be a MRSA carrier *and* have a current MRSA infection at the same encounter. When this is the case, you are permitted to report code Z22.322 and a code for the MRSA infection.

YOU CODE IT! CASE STUDY

REFERRING PHYSICIAN: Audra Starch, MD

REASON FOR CONSULTATION: MRSA pneumonia, fever.

HISTORY OF PRESENT ILLNESS: This 77-year-old male has a history of recent stroke. Garden Nursing Home, where he is a resident, requested a consultation due to his increased cough, along with some pulmonary congestion. Dr. Starch prescribed an extended spectrum penicillin (Zosyn, 4.5g q 6hr via IV bedside) for the patient's low-grade fever. Sputum cultures evidenced MRSA, leading to the request for this consultation.

Patient is post-CVA aphasic. Daughter is present and serves as primary relator. Nurse's notes document that the patient has been aspirating in conjunction with the increasing frequency of cough. Overall status has decreased due to these situations. At this time, the patient appears to be resting comfortably without any complaints.

ASSESSMENT AND PLAN:

1. Pathology report shows: positive sputum cultures with methicillin-resistant *Staphylococcus aureus*.
2. Fever, most likely secondary to pneumonia.

RX: Vancomycin, 500mg q 6hr IV x 10 days to treat MRSA
   ceftriazone, 2 g q 12, IM x 7 days to treat UTI/*E. coli*

You Code It!

Read Dr. Starch's documentation about this patient's condition and determine the accurate diagnosis code or codes.

Step #1: Read the case carefully and completely.

Step #2: Abstract the scenario. Which main words or terms describe why the physician cared for the patient during this encounter?

Step #3: Are there any details missing or incomplete for which you would need to query the physician? [If so, ask your instructor.]

Step #4: Check for any relevant guidance, including reading all of the symbols and notations in the Tabular List and the appropriate sections of the Official Guidelines.

Step #5: Determine the correct diagnosis code or codes to explain why this encounter was medically necessary.

Step #6: Double-check your work.

Answer:

Did you determine this to be the correct code?

J15.212   Pneumonia due to methicillin resistant Staphylococcus aureus

Good job!

NOTE: The fever is not reported separately because it is an inclusive sign of the pneumonia.

Chapter Summary

The contagious nature of infectious diseases makes them very serious. The coding of such conditions, and their treatments, has statistical significance, in addition to the importance of reimbursement.

Ordinary day-to-day activities, such as sneezing, coughing, having sex, or playing baseball, may pass an infectious disease from one person to another. Health care advancements have enabled the use of vaccines to prevent such conditions as measles, mumps, varicella, or human papillomavirus (HPV). Other conditions require behavioral or lifestyle changes to prevent their spread.

In any case, the health care industry is charged with helping patients, and it is, or will be, your job to code all of these infectious diseases correctly.

> **CODING BITES**
>
> *Did you know . . . ?*
> - Number of visits to physician offices for infectious and parasitic diseases: 20.2 million (2012)
> - Number of new tuberculosis cases: 9,582 (2013)
> - Number of new salmonella cases: 50,634 (2013)
> - Number of new Lyme disease cases: 36,307 (2013)
> - Number of new meningococcal disease cases: 556 (2013)

You Interpret It! Answers

1. Needlestick, **2.** Airborne, **3.** Drinking water, **4.** Insect bites, **5.** Droplets, **6.** Bacteria (streptococcus bacteria), **7.** Virus (influenza virus A or B), **8.** Virus (human papillomavirus (HPV)), **9.** Virus (measles virus), **10.** Bacteria (staphylococcus bacteria), **11.** Parasite (deer tick), **12.** Fungus (bodily fluid exchange), **13.** Parasite (mosquito), **14.** Fungus (airborne, contaminated water), **15.** Parasite (lice), **16.** Fungus (microsporum), **17.** Fracture, **18.** HIV, **19.** Complication of pregnancy, **20.** Type 1 diabetes

CHAPTER 5 REVIEW
Coding Infectious Diseases

Let's Check It! Terminology

Match each key term to the appropriate definition.

Part I

1. LO 5.1 A hospital-acquired condition. **J**
2. LO 5.2 A singxle-celled microorganism that causes disease. **C**
3. LO 5.1 A condition that can be transmitted from one person to another. **H**
4. LO 5.1 Long-lasting; ongoing. **D**
5. LO 5.1 A condition affecting the immune system. **F**
6. LO 5.4 Group of organisms, including mold, yeast, and mildew, that cause infection. **E**
7. LO 5.1 Severe. **A**
8. LO 5.1 The invasion of pathogens into tissue cells. **G**
9. LO 5.1 No symptoms or manifestations. **B**
10. LO 5.1 The reaction of tissues to infection or injury; characterized by pain, swelling, and erythema. **I**

A. Acute
B. Asymptomatic
C. Bacteria
D. Chronic
E. Fungi
F. Human Immunodeficiency Virus (HIV)
G. Infection
H. Infectious
I. Inflammation
J. Nosocomial

Part II

1. LO 5.3 Microscopic particles that initiate disease, mimicking the characteristics of a particular cell, and can reproduce only within the body of the cells that they have invaded. **J**
2. LO 5.4 Tiny living things that can invade and feed off of other living things. **A**
3. LO 5.1 Any agent that causes disease; a microorganism such as a bacterium or virus. **B**
4. LO 5.7 Generalized infection spread through the body via the bloodstream; blood infection. **E**
5. LO 5.7 Sepsis with signs of acute organ dysfunction. **F**
6. LO 5.7 A definite physical reaction, such as fever, chills, etc., to an unspecified pathogen. **H**
7. LO 5.1 Spread throughout the entire body. **G**
8. LO 5.2 An infectious condition that causes small rounded swellings on mucous membranes throughout the body. **I**
9. LO 5.7 Condition typified by two or more systemic responses to infection; a specified pathogen. **C**
10. LO 5.7 Severe sepsis with hypotension; unresponsive to fluid resuscitation. **D**

A. Parasites
B. Pathogen
C. Sepsis
D. Septic Shock
E. Septicemia
F. Severe Sepsis
G. Systemic
H. Systemic Inflammatory Response Syndrome (SIRS)
I. Tuberculosis
J. Viruses

Let's Check It! Concepts

Choose the most appropriate answer for each of the following questions.

1. LO 5.1 The body's response to an infection may include the sign or symptom of
   a. rash.   b. blurred vision.   **c. increased body temperature.**   d. reduced body temperature.
2. LO 5.2 _____ is a serious infection of the skin that may be either a staph infection (staphylococcal bacteria) or a strep infection (streptococcal bacteria).
   a. Impetigo   **b. Cellulitis**   c. Hepatitis   d. Meningitis
3. LO 5.3 Grant Harris, a 19-year-old male, is diagnosed with herpes zoster keratoconjunctivitis. How is this coded?
   a. B02.30   b. B02.31   c. B02.32   **d. B02.33**
4. LO 5.4 All of the following are parasites *except*
   a. lice.   b. mites.   **c. warts.**   d. worms.
5. LO 5.5 Aspiration pneumonia is a
   a. viral infection.   **b. bacterial infection.**   c. fungal infection.   d. parasitic infection.
6. LO 5.6 A woman with HIV-positive status is pregnant and in her second trimester. What must be the first-listed code?
   a. O98.7   b. O98.71   c. O98.711   **d. O98.712**
7. LO 5.6 Exposure to HIV will be coded with which code?
   a. Z20.4   b. Z20.5   **c. Z20.6**   d. Z20.7
8. LO 5.7 When coding for SIRS in a patient who has *not* developed an infection, you would code in which sequence?
   a. the code for the acute organ dysfunction, the code for SIRS, the code for the underlying condition
   b. the code for SIRS, the code for the acute organ dysfunction, the code for the underlying condition
   c. the code for the underlying condition, the code for SIRS, the code for the acute organ dysfunction
   d. none of these

9. LO 5.7 The code for septic shock may be all of the following *except*
   a. the first-listed diagnosis code.
   b. an additional code.
   c. used to identify the inclusion of hypotension.
   d. added to the codes required for severe sepsis.
10. LO 5.8 Methicillin-resistant *Staphylococcus aureus* (MRSA) is spread from one person to another by
    a. direct contact.
    b. indirect contact.
    c. both direct and indirect contact.
    d. none of these.

Let's Check It! Guidelines

Refer to the Official Guidelines and fill in the blanks according to the Chapter 1, Certain Infectious and Parasitic Diseases, Chapter-Specific Coding Guidelines.

I.C.16.f	R65.2	infection	synonymous
informed	confirmed	diagnosis	underlying
Septic	B95.62	2	inconclusive
unrelated	documentation	sepsis	organ
R75	severe	urosepsis	Z71.1
postprocedural	queried	principal	

1. Code only _____ cases of HIV infection/illness. This is an exception to the hospital inpatient guideline _____.
2. If a patient with HIV disease is admitted for an _____ condition, the code for the unrelated condition should be the _____ diagnosis.
3. Patients with _____ HIV serology, but no definitive _____ or manifestations of the illness, may be assigned code _____.
4. When a patient returns to be _____ of his/her HIV test results and the test is negative, use code _____.
5. The term _____ is a nonspecific term. It is not to be considered _____ with sepsis. Should a provider use this term, he/she must be _____ for clarification.
6. The coding of severe sepsis requires a minimum of _____ codes: first code for the _____ systemic infection, followed by a code from subcategory _____, Severe sepsis.
7. _____ shock generally refers to circulatory failure associated with _____ sepsis, and therefore, it represents a type of acute _____ dysfunction.
8. As with all _____ complications, code assignment is based on the provider's _____ of the relationship between the _____ and the procedure.
9. Newborn _____ See Section _____. Bacterial sepsis of Newborn.
10. When there is documentation of a current infection due to MRSA, and that infection does not have a combination code that includes the causal organism, assign the appropriate code to identify the condition along with code _____.

Let's Check It! Rules and Regulations

Please answer the following questions from the knowledge you have gained after reading this chapter.

1. LO 5.2/5.3 Explain the difference between a bacterial infection and a viral infection, and give examples of each.
2. LO 5.4 What is the difference between a parasitic and a fungal infection? Include an example of each in your answer.

3. **LO 5.1** What is a nosocomial infection, and where do such infections occur?
4. **LO 5.7** Discuss the difference between septicemia and SIRS.
5. **LO 5.8** What is MRSA and how is it spread?

YOU CODE IT! Basics

First, identify the main term in the following diagnoses; then code the diagnosis.

Example: Neonatal candidiasis:

   a. main term: <u>candidiasis</u>   b. diagnosis: <u>P37.5</u>

1. Allergic bronchopulmonary aspergillosis:
   a. main term: _____   b. diagnosis: _____
2. Chronic active hepatitis:
   a. main term: _____   b. diagnosis: _____
3. Sepsis, streptococcal, group B:
   a. main term: _____   b. diagnosis: _____
4. Pulmonary cryptococcosis:
   a. main term: _____   b. diagnosis: _____
5. Herpes zoster meningitis:
   a. main term: _____   b. diagnosis: _____
6. Chronic otitis media, right ear:
   a. main term: _____   b. diagnosis: _____
7. Jungle yellow fever:
   a. main term: _____   b. diagnosis: _____
8. Kaposi's sarcoma of the lymph nodes:
   a. main term: _____   b. diagnosis: _____
9. Cellulitis of upper right limb:
   a. main term: _____   b. diagnosis: _____
10. Generalized blastomycosis:
    a. main term: _____   b. diagnosis: _____
11. Acute disseminated, noninfectious, encephalomyelitis:
    a. main term: _____   b. diagnosis: _____
12. Laryngeal diphtheria:
    a. main term: _____   b. diagnosis: _____
13. Retroperitoneal tuberculosis:
    a. main term: _____   b. diagnosis: _____
14. Shigellosis, group C:
    a. main term: _____   b. diagnosis: _____
15. Ringworm honeycomb:
    a. main term: _____   b. diagnosis: _____

YOU CODE IT! Practice

Using the techniques described in this chapter, carefully read through the case studies and determine the most accurate ICD-10-CM code(s) and external cause code(s), if appropriate, for each case.

1. Ben Kenton, a 49-year-old male, presents today with a high fever, chills, nausea, and diarrhea. After an examination and reviewing the results of the blood tests, Dr. Daniels diagnoses Ben with West Nile fever.
2. Robin Pullen, a 36-year-old female, comes to see Dr. Ditolla because she is running a fever and has a sore throat and overall body aches. Test results are positive for H1N1. Robin is diagnosed with swine influenza.
3. Joan Kenney, a 27-year-old female, is having difficulty breathing. Dr. Aung documents a fever of 101 F and facial edema. Joan recently returned home from a trip to Asia. Joan said they were contending with some sort of larval infestation in Asia. Joan is diagnosed with nasopharyngeal myiasis.

4. Babbs Fisher, a 48-year-old female, just returned from an African vacation. Babbs is brought in by her husband, George, who noticed she was acting confused. Dr. Carla notes a low fever. Babbs states she feels tired and has a sore throat. She started vomiting this morning and admits to abdominal pain. Dr. Carla examines Babbs and orders an enzyme-linked immunosorbent assay (ELISA) test, which confirms the diagnosis of Ebola virus. Babbs is admitted to Weston Hospital for treatment.

5. Steven Jordan, a 51-year-old male, comes to see Dr. Kolb because he is experiencing nausea and vomiting and his stool is unusually light in color. Steven is accompanied by his wife, Sally. Sally says her husband seems confused and less alert lately. Upon examination, Dr. Kolb notes hepatosplenomegaly, jaundice, and RUQ tenderness. Steven is admitted to the hospital, where blood test results confirm the presence of IgG anti-HAV antibodies. Steven is diagnosed with acute hepatitis A.

6. John Brennen, a 7-year-old male, is brought in by his parents. Johnny has developed a hard cough and says his sides hurt. Dr. Travis, Johnny's pediatrician, completes blood work and takes a CXR and nasopharyngeal specimen. A subconjunctival hemorrhage is noted in the left eye. Test results confirm a diagnosis of whooping cough due to *Bordetella pertussis* with pneumonia. Johnny is admitted to Weston Hospital.

7. Frances Lowder is having difficulty breathing. She also admits to a bad headache, sore throat, and no appetite. She is 28 weeks pregnant and was diagnosed with HIV 3 years ago. Dr. Mabry notes a temperature of 102 F and papules over her upper body. Blood tests confirm the diagnosis of varicella with pneumonia. Frances is admitted to Weston Hospital.

8. Jenny Cassidy, a 4-year-old female, is brought in by her parents to see her pediatrician, Dr. Harmon. Jenny has a fever and a rash on her back. Dr. Harmon notes a "strawberry tongue." The completed CBC test confirms a diagnosis of scarlet fever.

9. Lee Greenwalt, a 9-year-old male, is brought in by his parents. Lee is not feeling well and is losing weight. Mrs. Greenwalt states Lee seems to be sweating at night. Dr. Moon documents a bitonal cough, a temperature of 100 F, and a general weakening. Lee is admitted to Weston Hospital. Test results confirm a diagnosis of tuberculosis of tracheobronchial lymph nodes.

10. Donald Rampey, a 72-year-old male, was admitted to the hospital with severe sepsis due to streptococcus, group B. Donald developed acute hepatic failure.

11. Mendenhall Aguirre, a 37-year-old male, presents today with a burning sensation during urination. Dr. Boykin collects a penile swab specimen for a microscopic examination, which confirms trichomonal prostatitis.

12. Gayle Cassels, a 12-year-old female, is brought in by her mother to see Dr. Kellum. Gayle has had a fever for 3 days with a head cold. Dr. Kellum notes conjunctivitis, an erythematous rash on the head and neck, as well as Koplik's spots on the inside of Gayle's mouth. The salivary measles-specific IgA test confirmed the diagnosis of measles.

13. Steven Crooks, a 16-year-old male, presents today with a sore throat. Dr. Hoffman notes acute pharyngitis with a low-grade fever, as well as petechiae on the roof of the mouth. A serological test confirms the diagnosis of Epstein–Barr infectious mononucleosis.

14. Donna Burgess, a 33-year-old female, comes to see Dr. Freeman today with a headache, fever, and chest pain. The ELISA serological test confirms a diagnosis of Coxsackie B virus infection with pericarditis.

15. Victor Lockhart, a 29-year-old male, presents today with a fever of 100.6 F. He says 1 minute he is sweating and the next he is shivering and his stomach hurts. Dr. Osterlund documents paleness and tenderness in the right hypochondria region. Victor is admitted to Weston Hospital, where blood tests, a liver function test, and a CT scan confirm the diagnosis of amebic liver abscess due to *Entamoeba histolytica*.

YOU CODE IT! Application

The following exercises provide practice in abstracting physicians' documentation from our textbook's health care facility, Prader, Bracker, & Associates. These case studies are modeled on real patient encounters. Using the techniques described in this chapter, carefully read through the case studies and determine the most accurate ICD-10-CM code(s) for each case study.

WESTON HOSPITAL

629 Healthcare Way • SOMEWHERE, FL 32811 • 407-555-6541

PATIENT: GALEANA, ROBERT

ACCOUNT/EHR #: GALERO001

DATE: 09/16/18

Attending Physician: Oscar R. Prader, MD

This 33-year-old male was admitted for a high fever, abdominal pain, and a noted moderate decrease in alertness. Robert has been on oral antibiotics for a left ear infection for approximately 7 days. I last saw the patient in the office four days ago when his left ear spontaneously drained.

PE: Ht: 5' 11", Wt: 194, T: 101.2, R: 19, BP: 134/86. Pt seems confused. Left ear drainage continues.

CSF analysis reveals normal pressure, a slightly thicker viscosity with a cloudy appearance. Results of CSF exam showed 6875 WBC, 35 g/L protein, and 23 mg/dL glucose.

Arbovirus is identified in two blood cultures. Pt responds positively to antimicrobial therapy.

DX: Meningitis due to arbovirus, urban yellow fever, acute suppurative otitis media.

ORP/pw   D: 09/16/18 09:50:16   T: 09/18/18 12:55:01

Determine the most accurate ICD-10-CM code(s).

WESTON HOSPITAL

629 Healthcare Way • SOMEWHERE, FL 32811 • 407-555-6541

PATIENT: MURPHY, ADRIENNE

ACCOUNT/EHR #: MURPAD001

DATE: 08/11/18

Attending Physician: Renee O. Bracker, MD

Pt is admitted with a chief complaint of shortness of breath of approximately 7 to 10 days duration and a feeling of uneasiness and discomfort. Pt was found to be HIV-positive in May 2014, and diagnosed with AIDS in February 2016. Patient also complains of vision loss. She states she can't see and it hurts when you touch her eyes and face.

PE: Ht: 5'4", Wt: 126, T: 101.6. The physician notes pustules on forehead, right eye, and bridge of nose. A Tzanck smear with methylene blue stain was performed; results positive.

DX: Herpesviral keratoconjunctivitis (simplex), secondary to AIDS

Plan: Acyclovir, IV: 10mg/kg q 8 hr

ROB/pw   D: 08/11/18 09:50:16   T: 08/13/18 12:55:01

Determine the most accurate ICD-10-CM code(s).

PRADER, BRACKER, & ASSOCIATES
A Complete Health Care Facility
159 Healthcare Way • SOMEWHERE, FL 32811 • 407-555-6789

PATIENT: LUPO, THERESA

ACCOUNT/EHR #: LUPOTH001

DATE: 09/16/18

Attending Physician: Renee O. Bracker, MD

Pt presented to office with a laceration to the left knee that occurred approximately 10 days ago. Theresa states that she fell as she was getting up from a chair in her backyard. She cleaned the area and put an OTC antibiotic ointment on the bandage before applying it to the wound. She has changed the bandage daily.

PE: Ht: 5"2", Wt: 120, T: 99.6, R: 18, BP: 128/78. After removing the bandage, a widely infected wound was found with small pieces of gravel, with resulting cellulitis to the knee. Extensive irrigation and debridement using sterile water were performed, but closure was not attempted pending resolution of the infection. Culture of the wound revealed streptococcus D.

1,200 units of Bicillin CR IM was given.

Rx for oral antibiotics was given to Pt.

Pt to return in 3 days for follow-up.

ROB/pw   D: 09/16/18 09:50:16   T: 09/18/18 12:55:01

Determine the most accurate ICD-10-CM code(s).

PRADER, BRACKER, & ASSOCIATES
A Complete Health Care Facility
159 Healthcare Way • SOMEWHERE, FL 32811 • 407-555-6789

PATIENT: PLATTENBAUM, BENJAMIN

ACCOUNT/EHR #: PLATBE001

DATE: 08/11/18

Attending Physician: Oscar R. Prader, MD

Pt, a 32-year-old male, presents with continued complaints of nasal drainage, pressure behind his eyes, and a sore throat. I last saw Ben two weeks ago when he was diagnosed with acute frontal sinusitis due to *Staphylococcus aureus*. Prescription for amoxicillin 250mg q 8 hr. was given.

PE: Ht: 6' 2", Wt: 210, T 100.1, R 20, BP: 134/86. Nasal endoscopy confirms the diagnosis that acute sinusitis is still present. MRSA, specifically to penicillins, is apparent. IV injection levofloxacin, 500 mg.

Rx: Levofloxacin, 250 mg q 24 hr x 10 days

Recommendation for bed rest, lots of fluids. Pt to return prn.

ORP/pw   D: 08/11/18 09:50:16   T: 08/13/18 12:55:01

Determine the most accurate ICD-10-CM code(s).

CHAPTER 5 REVIEW

WESTON HOSPITAL

629 Healthcare Way • SOMEWHERE, FL 32811 • 407-555-6541

PATIENT: SAMUELS, BERNARD

ACCOUNT/EHR #: SAMUBE001

DATE: 09/16/18

Attending Physician: Oscar R. Prader, MD

This 82-year-old male was admitted to the hospital with high fever, myalgia, headache, rhinitis, and a nonproductive cough. He also shows signs of confusion.

PE: Ht: 5'9", Wt: 173, T: 103.2, R: 22, BP: 90/59. Pt's condition deteriorated with definite signs of septic shock, pneumonia, and hypotension. He is now in acute renal failure.

DX: Influenza with pneumonia due to *E. coli*; septic shock, acute renal failure.

ORP/pw   D: 09/16/18 09:50:16   T: 09/18/18 12:55:01

Determine the most accurate ICD-10-CM code(s).

Coding Neoplasms

6

Learning Outcomes

After completing this chapter, the student should be able to:

LO 6.1 Identify the medical necessity for screenings and diagnostic testing for malignancies.

LO 6.2 Discern the various types of neoplasms.

LO 6.3 Interpret the Table of Neoplasms accurately.

LO 6.4 Employ the directions provided in the Chapter Notes at the head of the Neoplasms section of the Tabular List.

LO 6.5 Apply the guidelines for sequencing admissions due to complications of neoplasms and/or their treatments.

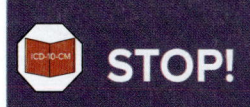

Key Terms

Benign
Carcinoma
Ectopic
Functional Activity
Malignant
Mass
Metastasize
Morphology
Neoplasm
Overlapping Boundaries
Topography

STOP! Remember, you need to follow along in your ICD-10-CM code book for an optimal learning experience.

6.1 Screening and Diagnosis

Screenings

You may already know about screenings. Screenings are provided with the intention of identifying a disease or abnormality as early as possible. When a neoplasm is detected and treated early in its formation, the treatment is less intense, making the process easier on the patient and less costly. Also important is the proven fact that the earlier a malignancy is dealt with, the better the chances of recovery and survival. Patients with *no* signs or symptoms are typically scheduled for various screenings based on guidelines related to age, family history, or personal history.

When you are coding for a patient encounter for a screening for a possible malignant neoplasm, such as a mammogram or a colonoscopy, you will report a code from this category:

Z12 Encounter for screening for malignant neoplasms

> **GUIDANCE CONNECTION**
>
> Read the ICD-10-CM Official Guidelines for Coding and Reporting, section **I. Conventions, General Coding Guidelines and Chapter Specific Guidelines,** subsection **C. Chapter-Specific Coding Guidelines,** chapter **21. Factors influencing health status and contact with health services (Z00-Z99),** subsection **c.5) Screening**

EXAMPLE

You would report code:

Z12.5 Encounter for screening for malignant neoplasm of prostate

for an encounter when a 59-year-old man goes in for a screening prostate exam, as per recommendations for men aged 55 to 69 years of age.

Read the notation directly below the Z12 code category:

> **Screening is the testing for disease or disease precursors in asymptomatic individuals so that early detection and treatment can be provided for those who test positive for the disease.**

Also, read the next notation carefully:

Use additional code to identify any family history of malignant neoplasm (Z80.-)

ICD-10-CM reminds you that an additional code should be reported when the prompting factor for the screening is not age but family history. Family history means that someone in the patient's past bloodline had been diagnosed with the condition being screened for, and it is known that this places the patient at a higher risk for developing the condition.

> ### EXAMPLE
> You would report code:
>
> Z80.42 Family history of malignant neoplasm of prostate
>
> *in addition to* code Z12.5 for an encounter when a 44-year-old man goes in for a screening prostate exam because his father and brother were both diagnosed with prostate cancer, dramatically increasing his risk.

A personal history code (Z85.-) should be reported for those patients who may receive screening tests more frequently than others. For example, a woman with a history of breast cancer may get mammograms every 6 months rather than annually. The personal history of breast cancer code will support medical necessity for this increase in the frequency of testing.

> ### EXAMPLE
> You would report code:
>
> Z85.3 Personal history of malignant neoplasm of breast
>
> *in addition to* code **Z12.31 Encounter for screening mammogram for malignant neoplasm of breast** for an encounter when a 57-year-old female goes in for a screening mammogram every 6 months, instead of the usual (once a year), because the fact that she had a malignant neoplasm of her breast a few years ago dramatically increases her risk for a recurrence.

> **GUIDANCE CONNECTION**
>
> Read the ICD-10-CM Official Guidelines for Coding and Reporting, section **I. Conventions, General Coding Guidelines and Chapter Specific Guidelines,** subsection **C. Chapter-Specific Coding Guidelines,** chapter **21. Factors influencing health status and contact with health services (Z00-Z99),** subsection **c.4) History (of).**

The Z12 code category also carries an **EXCLUDES1** notation to remind you of the difference between a diagnostic test, which is performed when a patient <u>does</u> exhibit signs or symptoms, and a screening test, which is performed with the intention of early detection of disease without signs or symptoms.

EXCLUDES1 encounter for diagnostic examination—code to sign or symptom

> ### EXAMPLE
> You would report code:
>
> N63.- Unspecified lump in breast
>
> for an encounter when a 62-year-old female goes in for a mammogram because she felt a lump in her breast during her monthly self-check and her gynecologist confirmed it was suspicious.

Confirming a Diagnosis

Once the patient exhibits signs, such as a lump found during a physical examination or an abnormality identified during a screening test, a pathologist must determine the essence of the neoplasm. This is the only way to factually distinguish between benign cells and malignant cells.

Generally, specimens may be provided to the laboratory in various forms: blood (capillary or vein), urine, semen, sputum, swabs (that carry tissue cells, pus, or other excretion), or tissue specimens (surgical samples taken during a biopsy). Most often with neoplasms, a biopsy is necessary. You will need to ensure that an accurate ICD-10-CM diagnosis code is presented with the specimen to confirm medical necessity for the diagnostic testing, such as signs and symptoms.

> **EXAMPLES**
>
> R91.8 Other nonspecific abnormal finding of lung field (mass on lung)
> R93.1 Abnormal findings on diagnostic imaging of heart and coronary circulation
>
> Abnormal findings of diagnostic tests justify the need for additional tests and procedures.

CODING BITES

The only way to confirm a diagnosis of a malignancy is for the physician to perform a biopsy (surgical removal of all or part of the tumor tissue) and submit that tissue for pathological examination. Therefore, you can understand why reporting a malignancy and not specifying the anatomical location of the tumor would be unlikely.

Blood tests can also provide important information with regard to malignancies in the body. For example, an increased white blood cell (WBC) count, also known as *leukocytosis*, may be a sign that neoplastic cells have been produced in the bone marrow and released into the bloodstream—common in conditions such as leukemic neoplasia and other myeloproliferative disorders. Many types of pathological and imaging tests can provide critical information to the physician seeking to confirm, or deny, a diagnosis of a malignancy. Tests available depend upon the anatomical site and the type of malignancy (see Table 6-1).

Test Results

You will see pathology reports in the patient's chart, whether you work in a hospital or a physician's office. Some examples of reports include

- Histopathology: A punch biopsy of the overlying skin reveals an adenocarcinoma with diffuse involvement of the dermis and extensive invasion of the dermal lymphatics. The adenocarcinoma is composed of irregular nests with some areas forming tubercles. Mitotic figures, including atypical forms, are seen. The tumor was ER −, PR −, Her2 +, CK7 +, and CK 20 −.
- Tissue biopsy culture: Negative for any growth
- Lumbar puncture: negative for organisms
- Blood culture: 2/2 positive for *Neisseria meningitidis*
- Labs: WBC: 8.6, Hgb/Hct: 9.4/26.3, Platelets: 222, BUN: 71, Creatinine: 6.8, U/A: 2+ protein, 3+ blood, ANA: negative, Hepatitis B surface antigen: negative, Hepatitis C antibody: negative, Serum cryoglobulins: negative, HIV: negative, cANCA: positive (1:1280), Tissue culture: negative, Initial blood cultures: negative, CXR: bilateral opacities.

Pathology reports may also provide information on the grading and/or staging of the tumor. Grading a tumor is the microscopic analysis of the tumor cells and tissue to describe how abnormal they appear. Staging, however, evaluates the size and location of the tumor, as well as determination of any signs or evidence of metastasis. In some cases, you will need to know the grade of a patient's tumor so you can determine the correct code.

> **EXAMPLES**
>
> C82.07 Follicular lymphoma grade 1, spleen
> C82.16 Follicular lymphoma grade II, intrapelvic lymph nodes
>
> These two codes are examples of those with code descriptions that require you to check the physician's documentation and pathology reports to identify the grade of the tumor.

CHAPTER 6 | CODING NEOPLASMS 147

TABLE 6-1 Some Common Tests Performed When Various Types of Malignancies Are Suspected

Malignant Neoplasm of the Cervix
- Abdominal ultrasound
- Cervical biopsy
- Colposcopy
- CT scan of the abdomen and pelvis

Malignant Neoplasm of the Colon and Rectum
- Barium enema
- Carcinoembryonic antigen (CEA)
- Colonoscopy
- Stool for occult blood

Leukemia/Lymphoma
- Blood smear
- Bone marrow biopsy
- Cell surface immunophenotyping
- Cryoglobulins

Malignant Neoplasm of the Lung
- Alpha-1 antitrypsin
- Bone scan
- Bronchoscopy
- Chest x-ray
- Lung biopsy

Malignant Neoplasm of the Ovary
- CA-125
- Laparoscopy
- Paracentesis
- Pyelography

Malignant Neoplasm of the Prostate
- Acid phosphatase
- CT scan of the pelvis
- Cystoscopy
- MRI of the prostate
- Prostate specific antigen (PSA)

TABLE 6-2 Cancer Stages

Tumor Stage	What the Stage Describes
Stage 0	Abnormal cells are present but have not spread to nearby tissue. Also known as carcinoma in situ, or CIS. CIS is not malignant, but it may evolve into malignancy.
Stage I, Stage II, Stage III	Malignant cells are present. The higher the number, the larger the malignant tumor and the more it has metastasized to nearby tissues.
Stage IV	Malignant cells have metastasized to distant parts of the body.

Source: cancer.gov

The pathologist will also stage the tumor tissue specimen (see Table 6-2 for more details on the stages of cancer).

Physicians, most often oncologists, use tumor grading in addition to staging, a patient's age, and overall health to determine a prognosis and create a treatment plan.

CODING BITES

Find out more about Cancer Registries at https://www.cdc.gov/cancer/npcr/value/index.htm

Cancer registries collect population-based cancer incidence data, as required under federal law, to support research and government funding to support the impact of cancer on a community.

> ### YOU INTERPRET IT!
>
> Is this order for a screening or a diagnostic test?
> 1. Susie's annual mammogram — (a) Screening (b) Diagnostic
> 2. Dr. McFadden felt a lump in Arthur's arm. Dr. McFadden did a biopsy. — (a) Screening (b) Diagnostic
> 3. Edith told her doctor she is coughing, is wheezing, and suffers from unexplained weight loss. Her doctor ordered a lung CT. — (a) Screening (b) Diagnostic
> 4. At Roger's annual checkup, Dr. Concord ordered a PSA test to be completed. — (a) Screening (b) Diagnostic

6.2 Abstracting the Details About Neoplasms

When normal cells mutate, they may create a **neoplasm**, also known as a *tumor*. A tumor is an overgrowth or abnormal mass of tissue, and it may be either benign or malignant (cancerous). In all cases, a physician should check the abnormality and determine a course of action.

Once a diagnosis is confirmed, you will need to accurately report it with the specific code or codes. Begin by ensuring you understand the details.

In some cases, you will see the term **mass** used to describe a patient's condition. Mass is *not* the same as a neoplasm. More often, mass is used to identify a cyst or other thickening of tissue.

While many people think that *neoplasm* and *cancer* are synonymous, they are not. Cancer is the common term for **carcinoma** (see Figure 6-1).

Terms Used to Identify Neoplasms

Neoplasms might be **malignant** or **benign** or have aspects of both characteristics. In diagnoses, neoplasms may also be defined by an individual name. The physician's notes may state a different term. Some examples of these terms are

- Adenoma
- Melanoma
- Leukemia
- Papilloma

Neoplasm
Abnormal tissue growth; tumor.

Mass
Abnormal collection of tissue.

Carcinoma
A malignant neoplasm or cancerous tumor.

Malignant
Invasive and destructive characteristic of a neoplasm; possibly causing damage or death.

Benign
Nonmalignant characteristic of a neoplasm; not infectious or spreading.

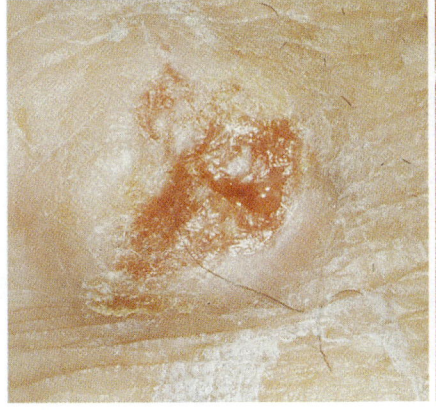

(a) © Biophoto Associates/Science Source
(b) © Biophoto Associates/Science Source
(c) © James Stevenson/Science Source

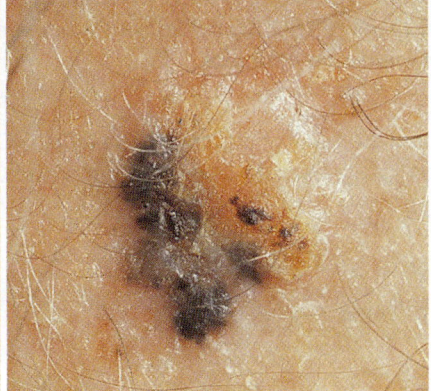

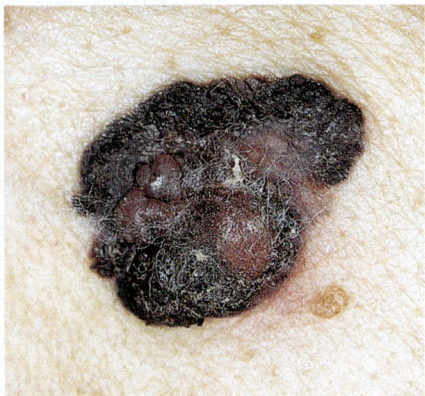

FIGURE 6-1 Types of skin cancer: (a) squamous cell carcinoma, (b) basal cell carcinoma, and (c) malignant melanoma

> **CODING BITES**
>
> In medical terminology, the suffix *-oma* means tumor.

When the physician uses a term such as adenoma, melanoma, or other specific name rather than the more generic term of neoplasm, it is more efficient for you to look for that specific term in the Alphabetic Index first, before looking under the term *neoplasm.* At the very least, the Alphabetic Index can tell you if that type of tumor is known to be malignant or benign.

Often, when you look up one of these specific neoplasm terms in the Alphabetic Index, it will provide you with some specific information about the tumor. Let's take a look in the ICD-10-CM Alphabetic Index under the term written by the physician . . .

> **Fibroxanthoma** (see also Neoplasm, connective tissue, benign)
> atypical — *see* Neoplasm, connective tissue, uncertain behavior
> malignant — *see* Neoplasm, connective tissue, malignant
> **Fibroxanthosarcoma** — *see* Neoplasm, connective tissue malignant

You can see that while you might not know if a fibroxanthoma is malignant or benign, the Alphabetic Index will tell you.

LET'S CODE IT! SCENARIO

Abby Shantner, a 41-year-old female, comes to see Dr. Branson to get the results of her biopsy. Dr. Branson explains that Abby has an alpha cell adenoma of the pancreas. Dr. Branson spends 30 minutes discussing treatment options.

Let's Code It!

Dr. Branson has diagnosed Abby with an *alpha cell adenoma of the pancreas.* You have been working with Dr. Branson as his coder for a while, so you know that an adenoma is a neoplasm, but what kind of neoplasm is it—benign or malignant? To help you determine this, instead of going to *neoplasm,* let's see if there is a listing in the Alphabetic Index under *adenoma.* When you find *adenoma,* the book refers you to

> **Adenoma** (*see also* Neoplasm, benign, by site)

This tells you an adenoma is a benign tumor. Or you can continue down this list to the indented term, and find

> **Adenoma**
> alpha-cell,
> pancreas **D13.7**

Turn to the Tabular List and read the complete description of code category D13:

> ☑4 **D13** **Benign neoplasm of other and ill-defined parts of digestive system**
> The **EXCLUDES1** note does not relate to this patient's diagnosis for this encounter, so continue reading down the column to review all of the choices for the required fourth character.
> **D13.7** **Benign neoplasm of endocrine pancreas**

That matches Dr. Branson's diagnosis.

Check the top of this subsection and the head of this chapter in ICD-10-CM. There are several **NOTES.** Read carefully. Do any relate to Dr. Branson's diagnosis of Abby? No. Turn to the Official Guidelines and read Section 1.c.2. There is nothing specifically applicable here, either.

Good job!

Malignant Primary

The term *primary* indicates the anatomical site (the place in the body) where the malignant neoplasm was first seen and identified. If the physician's notes do not specify primary or secondary, then the site mentioned is primary.

Malignant Secondary

The term *secondary* identifies the anatomical site to which the malignancy **metastasized**. One very strange thing about cancerous cells is that they travel through the body and do not necessarily spread to adjoining body parts. Cancer can be identified in the breast as the primary site and metastasize to the liver without actually affecting anything in between. Notes will state that a site is "secondary to" *(primary site)*, "metastasized from" *(primary site)*, or *(primary site)* "metastasized to" *(secondary site)*.

The terms *disseminated cancer, generalized cancer,* or *widely metastatic* would indicate that the malignancy has infiltrated the body throughout and affects all or most of the patient's anatomy. This would be coded as a malignant neoplasm without specification of site (code C80.0). In such cases, it is not that the physician forgot to specify the site. It is that there are too many sites to list.

Ca in Situ

The term *Ca in situ* indicates that the tumor has undergone malignant changes but is still limited to the site where it originated (i.e., it has not spread). *Ca* is short for carcinoma, and you can remember *situ* as in the word *situated*. So think of it as a cancerous tumor that is staying in place.

Benign

The term *benign* means there is no indication of invasion of adjacent cells. Essentially, benign means not cancerous.

Uncertain

The classification *uncertain* indicates that the pathologist is not able to specifically determine whether a tumor is benign or malignant because indicators of both are present.

Unspecified Behavior

Choose codes that describe *"Unspecified Behavior"* when the physician's notes do not include any specific information regarding the nature of the tumor. Before choosing one of these codes, please query the physician and make certain that a laboratory report is not available or on its way with the information you need.

YOU INTERPRET IT!

What type of neoplasm is this: benign or malignant; primary or secondary?
5. Metastatic lung cancer   _____
6. Melanoma   _____
7. Squamous cell carcinoma   _____
8. Pancreatic lymph gland neoplasm   _____
9. Adenoma   _____

6.3 Reporting the Neoplastic Diagnosis

Once you have determined the anatomical location and type of tumor that has been documented, you will need to find a suggested code in the ICD-10-CM Neoplasm Table, found directly after the Alphabetic Index.

The Neoplasm Table is a seven-column table set in alphabetic order by the anatomical site (the part of the body where the tumor is located), shown in the first column. To the right of the first column, there are six columns across: Malignant

---

CODING BITES

Always begin with the terms the physician writes in his or her notes. Then, only when that does not bring you to a suggested code, you can look up alternate terms. This rule of thumb will save you a lot of time.

Metastasize
To proliferate, reproduce, or spread.

CODING BITES

To determine the code to report a neoplasm, you need to know
1. Where in the body (specifically, which anatomical site) is the neoplasm located?
2. Is the neoplasm benign, malignant, in situ, or uncertain? Uncertain is a pathologic determination and is *not* the same as unspecified.
3. If the neoplasm is malignant, is this the first diagnosis of malignancy for this patient? If so, this is the primary site. If not, this is a secondary malignancy because it metastasized from the primary.

CODING BITES

If you turn to the term *Neoplasm* in the Alphabetic Index in the regular alphabetic order, you will see the notation *(see also Table of Neoplasms)*.

	Malignant Primary	Malignant Secondary	Ca in situ	Benign	Uncertain Behavior	Unspecified Behavior
Neoplasm, neoplastic	C80.1	C79.9	D09.9	D36.9	D48.9	D49.9
- abdomen, abdominal	C76.2	C79.8-	D09.8	D36.7	D48.7	D49.89
-- cavity	C76.2	C79.8-	D09.8	D36.7	D48.7	D49.89
-- organ	C76.2	C79.8-	D09.8	D36.7	D48.7	D49.89
-- viscera	C76.2	C79.8-	D09.8	D36.7	D48.7	D49.89
-- wall — *see also Neoplasm, abdomen, wall, skin*	C44.509	C79.2-	D09.5	D23.5	D48.5	D49.2
--- connective tissue	C49.4	C79.8-	—	D21.4	D48.1	D49.2
--- skin	C44.509					
---- basal cell carcinoma	C44.519	—	—	—	—	—
---- specified type NEC	C44.599	—	—	—	—	—
---- squamous cell carcinoma	C44.529	—	—	—	—	—
- abdominopelvic	C76.8	C79.8-	—	D36.7	D48.7	D49.89

FIGURE 6-2 The Neoplasm Table, in part, showing codes for various abdominal neoplasms and abdominopelvic neoplasms

Primary, Malignant Secondary, Ca in situ, Benign, Uncertain Behavior, and Unspecified Behavior (see Figure 6-2) . . . the types of neoplasms you read about previously in this chapter. It is here, in this Table, that you can find the suggested code to report the specific type and location of the tumor documented by the physician.

After abstracting the physician's documentation to identify the anatomical site of the tumor, turn to the Neoplasm Table and find that anatomical site in the first column in the Table. Remember to carefully review indented lists below the main term of the anatomical site so you can determine the code for the greatest specificity.

> **EXAMPLE**
>
> Epiglottis
>   anterior aspect or surface
>   cartilage
>   free border (margin)
>   junctional region
>   posterior (laryngeal) surface
>
> You can see in this one example that knowing the anatomical site of the tumor—the *epiglottis*—is not enough information. You need to identify, from the documentation, where the tumor is located on the epiglottis.

Once you have found the most specific match for the anatomical site identified as the location of the tumor in the documentation, go back to the physician's notes. This time, look for the type of neoplasm in the diagnosis: Malignant Primary, Malignant Secondary, Ca in situ, Benign, Uncertain, or Unspecified Behavior. Now, back in the Neoplasm Table, read straight across to the right of the anatomical site line. At the top of the page, each of these six columns has a title. Find which column has the title that matches the diagnosis, and then go down until you hit the conjunction of the anatomical site line and the type of neoplasm in question. This is your suggested code.

EXAMPLE

Dr. Tomlinsonn diagnosed Elsa with a malignant neoplasm of the abdominal viscera, noted as Ca in situ.

	Malignant Primary	Malignant Secondary	Ca in situ	Benign	Uncertain Behavior	Unspecified Behavior
Neoplasm, neoplastic	C80.1	C79.9	D09.9	D36.9	D48.9	D49.9
- abdomen, abdominal	C76.2	C79.8-	D09.8	D36.7	D48.7	D49.89
-- cavity	C76.2	C79.8-	D09.8	D36.7	D48.7	D49.89
-- organ	C76.2	C79.8-	D09.8	D36.7	D48.7	D49.89
-- viscera	C76.2	C79.8-	D09.8	D36.7	D48.7	D49.89
-- wall — *see also* Neoplasm, abdomen, wall skin	C44.509	C79.2-	D04.5	D23.5	D48.5	D49.2

In the Neoplasm Table, in the first column, find **Abdomen,** then indented below that the specific site **-- viscera.**

Then, across to the right you can see suggested codes for each type of tumor. For Elsa's diagnosis, code D09.8 is *suggested*.

Next, turn in the Tabular List to check this code, and all of the notations. Because the Neoplasm Table is a part of the Alphabetic Index, the rule still applies . . . never, never report a code directly from here. You must check the suggested code in the Tabular List, read the symbols and notations, read the complete code description and all of the options, and check the Official Guidelines before you can confirm and report a code.

LET'S CODE IT! SCENARIO

Aaron Docker, a 65-year-old male, returns to see Dr. Cabrera. The results of his colonoscopy and laboratory tests on the biopsy have come back. Dr. Cabrera confirms Aaron has a benign neoplasm of the ascending colon.

Let's Code It!

Dr. Cabrera confirmed Aaron has *a benign neoplasm of the ascending colon.* Turn to the Neoplasm Table in your ICD-10-CM code book. Go down the list of anatomical sites until you reach *colon*. There is a notation that directs you to *"see also* Neoplasm, intestine, large." The ascending colon is actually the portion of the large intestine that goes from the cecum to the transverse colon. Indented under *colon* are the words *and rectum*. Go back to Dr. Cabrera's notes. His diagnosis does not include the rectum, so follow the book's advice and turn to the listing for *intestine, large,* and read what is shown there.

Continue through the list until you get to *intestine, intestinal.* Beneath the term *intestine,* you will find the word *large* indented. Indented under *large* is *colon.* Indented under *colon,* you see *ascending.* This matches Dr. Cabrera's diagnosis of Aaron's neoplasm exactly! Now, read across the table to the right to the "Benign" column. Here, the code D12.2 is suggested. Remember the rule: Never, never code from the Alphabetic Index, and that includes the Neoplasm Table, so turn to the Tabular List to confirm this suggested code. Start reading at the three-character code category:

✓4 **D12** Benign neoplasm of colon, rectum, anus, and anal canal

The EXCLUDES1 note does not relate to this patient's diagnosis for this encounter, so continue reading down the column to review all of the choices for the required fourth character.

D12.2 Benign neoplasm of ascending colon

(continued)

Check the top of this subsection and the head of this chapter in ICD-10-CM. There are several **NOTES** at the beginning of this chapter. Read carefully. Do any relate to Dr. Cabrera's diagnosis of Aaron? No. Turn to the Official Guidelines and read Section 1.c.2. There is nothing specifically applicable here, either.

Now you can report D12.2 for Aaron's diagnosis with confidence.

Good coding!

A Pregnant Patient with a Malignancy

Conditions that may complicate a pregnancy have their very own chapter in ICD-10-CM. You will learn about this in depth in the chapter *Coding Genitourinary, Gynecology, Obstetrics, Congenital, and Pediatrics*. However, when a pregnant woman is diagnosed with a malignancy, a code from code subcategory O9A.1- Malignant neoplasm complicating pregnancy, childbirth, and the puerperium will be reported as the principal diagnosis, followed by the code for the primary malignancy. To reinforce this, you can see the notation beneath this code subcategory that reminds you to *Use additional code* to identify neoplasm.

> **EXAMPLE**
>
> Fran has been diagnosed with malignant melanoma on her right shoulder. She is 21 weeks pregnant.
>
> O9A.112   Malignant neoplasm complicating pregnancy, second trimester
>
> C43.61   Malignant melanoma of right upper limb, including shoulder
>
> Z3A.21   21 weeks gestation of pregnancy

Malignancies in Remission or Relapse

There are certain types of malignancies, such as multiple myeloma (malignancy of the plasma cells in the bone marrow) or leukemia (malignancy of the bone marrow and bone-forming tissues), that may be described differently. For example:

> C90.00   Multiple myeloma not having achieved remission
> C90.01   Multiple myeloma in remission
> C90.02   Multiple myeloma in relapse

These categorizations are not available for all malignancies; however, when they are, you already know to match the code description to the documentation.

CODING BITES

Professional coding specialists must be cautious when determining the difference between a patient *in remission* and a patient with a *personal history of a condition*. If the documentation is not absolutely clear on this, you must query the physician for clarification. There is a big difference between these two diagnostic identifications.

LET'S CODE IT! SCENARIO

PATIENT: Roberta Wolfe
DATE OF CONSULTATION: 05/25/2018
CONSULTING PHYSICIAN: Oliver Cannon, MD
REQUESTING PHYSICIAN: Theresa Calabressi, MD

Thank you for referring the patient for medical oncology consultation.

HISTORY OF PRESENT ILLNESS: The patient is a 29-year-old female with noninvasive left breast cancer. The patient had a screening mammogram 4 months ago, which revealed a left upper outer breast abnormality. Stereotactic biopsy previously confirmed ductal carcinoma in situ. The patient underwent needle localization excision with pathology confirming ductal carcinoma in situ grade 2, ER positive, PR positive. She received ipsilateral breast radiation. Her course has been complicated by apparent incision site infection, which has resulted in persistent low-grade oozing of blood and occasional extrusion of pus. She has been treated with several courses of antibiotics. However, the scant bloody discharge continued. Over the past 1 week, she has noted increasing tenderness at the site of bleeding and apparent infection. She otherwise offers no complaints.

PAST MEDICAL HISTORY: Remarkable for anemia attributed to iron deficiency for which she takes iron supplements. Unremarkable for hypertension, diabetes, hypercholesterolemia, or prior cardiac, pulmonary, or hepatic dysfunction. Normal monthly cycles; however, the last cycle has been particularly prolonged at 9 days.

MEDICATIONS: She takes no regular prescription medications.

ALLERGIES: NO KNOWN ALLERGIES.

FAMILY HISTORY: Remarkable for sister with diagnosis of breast cancer at age 43, presently 51, in remission. No other known family history of breast or ovary cancer. Father died at age 82 of cardiac disease, mother aged 79 with history of heart disease; 2 brothers, 3 sons, and 2 daughters are healthy.

SOCIAL HISTORY: Married. Denies cigarettes, alcohol, drugs.

REVIEW OF SYSTEMS: Denies fever, chills, sweats, headaches, seizures, syncope, blurred vision, dysphagia, cough, chest pain, shortness of breath, abdominal pain, nausea, vomiting, diarrhea, constipation, melena, hematochezia, dysuria, hematuria, flank pain, back pain, abnormal bleeding, bruising, lymph node swelling, or focal paresthesias or weakness.

PHYSICAL EXAMINATION

GENERAL: The patient is well developed, well nourished, in no acute distress.

VITAL SIGNS: Temperature 98.8, heart rate 63, blood pressure 110/81, weight 135.4 pounds, and height 57 inches.

SKIN: Skin clear. No visible rash, ecchymosis or petechia.

HEENT: Normocephalic. No scleral icterus. No mucosal lesions.

NECK: Supple without thyromegaly.

LYMPH NODES: No secondary neck, axillary, or inguinal nodes.

BREASTS: Without dominant mass bilaterally. There is moderate induration of approximately 2.8 cm across, underlying the left upper outer quadrant incision. There is no fluctuance or erythema and patient denies significant tenderness to the area.

CHEST: Clear to auscultation and percussion.

CARDIAC: Regular rate and rhythm. No murmur, rub, or gallop.

ABDOMEN: Soft and nontender. No masses or hepatosplenomegaly.

RECTAL AND GENITAL: Deferred.

EXTREMITIES: No clubbing, cyanosis, or edema.

MUSCULOSKELETAL: No back tenderness. No bony or joint deformity.

NEUROLOGIC: Alert and oriented. Cranial nerves, sensory and motor system, and gait are normal.

IMPRESSION: Ductal carcinoma in situ, left breast, stage 0 (Tis N0 M0), ER positive, PR positive, status post lumpectomy to negative surgical margins and has set up breast radiation. Overall prognosis is excellent with estimated risk of local recurrence in the 5% range. Risk of systemic metastasis is negligible. Thus, adjuvant systemic therapy is not warranted. She is, of course, at increased risk for second malignancy; thus tamoxifen chemoprevention would be a reasonable option.

RECOMMENDATIONS AND PLAN: Diagnosis, prognosis, and management options were discussed in detail with the patient and questions were answered. Tamoxifen chemoprevention was discussed in detail and she, at this time, appears agreeable to initiation of therapy. I provided a prescription for tamoxifen 20 mg daily. On the assumption that

(continued)

she desires continuing oncologic follow-up, any follow-up appointment will be made in 6 months. Alternatively, if she should decline tamoxifen chemoprevention or if her gynecologic physician, Dr. Calabressi, would be willing to prescribe tamoxifen and provide continuing oncologic follow-up, then medical oncology follow-up will be on an as-needed basis.

Let's Code It!

Dr. Cannon examined and evaluated Roberta Wolfe with regard to her post-procedural condition for breast cancer. Read the entire documentation. Can you find his conclusion or impression of her condition? In the section marked IMPRESSIONS, he documents, *"Ductal carcinoma in situ, left breast."*

Turn in your ICD-10-CM Alphabetic Index, Table of Neoplasms. What is the anatomical site of this neoplasm? "breast, duct." Find this in the first column:

breast (connective tissue) (glandular tissue) (soft parts)

Read all of the specific components of the breast shown in the indented list below this. Can you find "duct"? Neither can I. However, you know that this is the location within the breast that has the neoplasm. Hmm. Read across to the third column to the right, titled Ca in situ. Notice that the majority of these have the same code category suggested: D05. Perhaps we can find a more specific description for the duct in the Tabular List. Turn to find D05 in the Tabular List.

☑4 **D05** Carcinoma in situ of breast

Check the **EXCLUDES1** notation. None of these diagnoses relate to Roberta's diagnosis, so read down and review the four options you have for a fourth character. One seems to be what you are looking for:

☑5 **D05.1** Intraductal carcinoma in situ of breast

Read the three options for the required fifth character. Which one matches Dr. Cannon's documentation?

D05.12 Intraductal carcinoma in situ of left breast

However, before you can report this code, you must check the top of this subsection and the **INCLUDES** note above code D00. Next, check the notations at the head of this chapter in ICD-10-CM. There are notations at the beginning of this chapter; you will learn more about these specific notations in the next part of this chapter. Read carefully. Do any relate to Dr. Cannon's diagnosis of Roberta? No. Turn to the Official Guidelines and read Section 1.c.2. There is nothing specifically applicable here either.

Now you can report D05.12 for Roberta's diagnosis with confidence.

D05.12 Intraductal carcinoma in situ of left breast

Good work!

6.4 Neoplasm Chapter Notes

In the ICD-10-CM Tabular List, take a look at the beginning of Chapter 2: Neoplasms (directly above code C00). There are four notes here to help you determine the most accurate neoplasm code.

Functional Activity

The functional activity of a neoplasm notes whether or not the tumor is causing the secretion of hormones. This would be documented in the pathology report and may need to be reported.

The first note in the Neoplasms chapter of ICD-10-CM helps you when certain neoplasms require an additional code to report **functional activity**. This note states:

Functional Activity
Glandular secretion in abnormal quantity.

"All neoplasms are classified in this chapter, whether they are functionally active or not. An additional code from chapter 4 may be used to identify such functional activity associated with any neoplasm."

Chapter 4 of the ICD-10-CM Tabular List is titled: Endocrine, nutritional, and metabolic diseases (E00–E89). The note beneath the heading for Chapter 4 (directly above code E00) reminds you of this detail:

Note: All neoplasms, whether functionally active or not, are classified in Chapter 2. Appropriate codes in this chapter (i.e. E05.8, E07.0, E16–E31, E34.-) may be used as additional codes to indicate either functional activity by neoplasms and ectopic endocrine tissue or hyperfunction and hypofunction of endocrine glands associated with neoplasms and other conditions classified elsewhere.

What this note means is that if a patient has been diagnosed with a neoplasm affecting the individual's glandular function, you have to identify the functional activity (of the gland) with an additional code.

For example, take a look beneath code category C56 Malignant neoplasm of ovary. There is a notation that says:

Use additional code to identify any functional activity

This note regarding functional activity also appears under the following terms:

- Benign neoplasm of ovary
- Malignant neoplasm of endocrine glands
- Benign neoplasm of endocrine glands
- Malignant neoplasm of islets of Langerhans
- Benign neoplasm of islets of Langerhans
- Malignant neoplasm of the testis
- Benign neoplasm of the testis
- Malignant neoplasm of thyroid glands
- Benign neoplasm of thyroid glands

EXAMPLES

Catecholamine-producing malignant pheochromocytoma of thyroid

| C73 | Malignant neoplasm of thyroid gland |
| E27.5 | Adrenomedullary hyperfunction |

Ovarian carcinoma, right side, with hyperestrogenism

| C56.1 | Malignant neoplasm of right ovary |
| E28.0 | Estrogen excess |

Basophil adenoma of pituitary with Cushing's disease

| C75.1 | Malignant neoplasm of pituitary gland |
| E24.0 | Pituitary-dependent Cushing's disease |

LET'S CODE IT! SCENARIO

Daniel Coleman, a 41-year-old male, came to see Dr. Lucano for a checkup. He was diagnosed with functioning thyroid carcinoma. Dr. Lucano reviews with Daniel the results of his latest thyroid scan, TSH and TRH stimulation tests, and an ultrasonogram. Dr. Lucano informs Daniel that he has developed hyperthyroidism.

(continued)

> ### Let's Code It!
>
> Dr. Lucano has diagnosed Daniel with *functioning thyroid carcinoma* and *hyperthyroidism*. The hyperthyroidism is the functional activity of the thyroid carcinoma. Turn to the Alphabetic Index and look for
>
> **Carcinoma —** *see also* **Neoplasm, by site, malignant**
>
> Look down the list. Neither the term *functioning* nor the term *thyroid* is shown here, so you will need to turn to the Neoplasm Table and find
>
> **Neoplasm, thyroid, malignant, primary C73**
>
> Let's go to the Tabular List, to confirm:
>
> **C73   Malignant neoplasm of thyroid gland**
>
> *Use additional code* to identify any functional activity
>
> This code is correct, and the ICD-10-CM book is telling you that you need an additional code to report the functional activity. The only other detail Dr. Lucano included in her diagnostic statement is hyperthyroidism. Turn back to the Alphabetic Index and look up hyperthyroidism:
>
> **Hyperthyroidism (latent) (preadult) (recurrent) E05.90**
>
> Turn to the Tabular List to confirm this suggested code.
>
> ☑4 **E05   Thyrotoxicosis [hyperthyroidism]**
>
> The **EXCLUDES1** note mentions nothing that relates to this encounter for our patient, so read down the column to review the choices for the required fourth character.
>
> ☑5 **E05.9   Thyrotoxicosis unspecified**
>
> This matches the notes, so you are in the correct place. The symbol to the left of the code tells you that an additional character is required.
>
> **E05.90   Thyrotoxicosis unspecified without mention of thyrotoxic crisis or storm**
>
> Did you notice that this code is located in Chapter 4 and is describing the functional activity of the neoplasm? Great!
>
> Check the top of this subsection and the head of this chapter in ICD-10-CM. A **NOTE** and an **EXCLUDES1** notation are shown at the beginning of this chapter. Read carefully. Do any relate to Dr. Lucano's diagnosis of Daniel? Yes. Both chapters have **NOTES** regarding the coding of neoplasms and functional activity. Double-check to make certain you are complying with these directions. Next, turn to the Official Guidelines and read both Sections 1.c.2 and 1.c.4. There is nothing specifically applicable here either.
>
> Now, you can report C73 and E05.90 for this encounter with Daniel with confidence.
> Good coding!

Morphology (Histology)

The second note at the top of Chapter 2 relates to the classifications of neoplasms.

Topography
The classification of neoplasms primarily by anatomical site.

Morphology
The study of the configuration or structure of living organisms.

Chapter 2 classifies neoplasms primarily by site (topography) with broad groupings for behavior, malignant, in situ, benign, etc. The Table of Neoplasms should be used to identify the correct topography code. In a few cases, such as for malignant melanoma and certain neuroendocrine tumors, the morphology (histologic type) is included in the category and codes.

In addition to the code for a neoplasm, you may be required to include a separate code with additional information about the tumor's morphology. "Morphology of Neoplasms" is available as a separate book, the *International Classification of Diseases for Oncology* (ICD-O). Morphology codes are not structured like the other diagnosis codes. The codes always begin with the letter "M," which is followed by four characters, a slash (/), and a single character. A neoplasm's histology is described by the first four characters of the M code.

M codes are used for providing specific data about the site (topography) and the histology (morphology) of the affected tissue to tumor and cancer registries. Pathologists may also use the codes to provide more detail about a particular tissue sample. Normally, M codes are not used for reimbursement and are not placed on insurance claim forms. Cancer registries use them in their cataloging of data.

Primary Malignant Neoplasms Overlapping Site Boundaries

The third note here, at the head of Chapter 2, Neoplasms, in ICD-10-CM, is concerned with primary malignant tumors that overlap anatomical sites.

> **A primary malignant neoplasm that overlaps two or more contiguous (next to each other) sites should be classified to the subcategory/code 8 ("overlapping lesion"), unless the combination is specifically indexed elsewhere. For multiple neoplasms of the same site that are not contiguous, such as tumors in different quadrants of the same breast, codes for each site should be assigned.**

The nature of a malignant neoplasm includes its potential to spread to adjoining tissue. As you learned earlier in this chapter, you code malignancies by their anatomical site in the order in which the malignancy developed: primary and secondary. However, there are cases where the condition of the patient involves more than one code subcategory. Neoplasms with **overlapping boundaries**, also known as *contiguous,* may blur anatomical descriptors.

> **CODING BITES**
> The phrase "**subcategory/code .8**" refers to the fourth character of 8.

Overlapping Boundaries
Multiple sites of carcinoma without identifiable borders.

EXAMPLE
C05.8   Malignant neoplasm of overlapping sites of palate
C17.8   Malignant neoplasm of overlapping sites of small intestine
C57.8   Malignant neoplasm of overlapping sites of female genital organs

For cases in which the physician cannot identify a specific site, usually because the malignancy has metastasized so dramatically, the code category C76 enables you to report the malignancy by identifying only the section of the patient's body, such as head, abdomen, or lower limb.

EXAMPLE
C76.0   Malignant neoplasm of head, face, and neck
C76.51   Malignant neoplasm of right lower limb

Malignant Neoplasms of Ectopic Tissue

The last note at the head of Chapter 2 in the Tabular List states:

> **Malignant neoplasms of ectopic tissue are to be coded to the site mentioned, e.g., ectopic pancreatic malignant neoplasms are coded to pancreas, unspecified (C25.9)**

This notation provides you with direction on how to determine the code for a case when the neoplasm is located in an unusual and hard-to-determine location in the body. The term *ectopic* means outside of an organ. Therefore, if the diagnostic statement describes the tumor as being ectopic, report the condition to the nearest, identified organ.

Ectopic
Out of place, such as an organ or body part.

> **EXAMPLE**
> Dr. Laveign documented that Evan's biopsy confirmed that he has an ectopic malignant neoplasm of the prostate.
> Report this with the following code:
>
> C61   Malignant neoplasm of prostate

6.5 Admissions Related to Neoplastic Treatments

When you are coding encounters with a patient who has been diagnosed with a neoplasm, whether benign or malignant, the same rule for identifying the principal diagnosis still applies.

Why did the health care professional care for this patient today?

Admission for Treatment of Malignancy

If a patient's encounter is only for therapeutic treatment of a malignancy, such as the administration of chemotherapy, immunotherapy, or radiation therapy, then the principal (first-listed) code will report this fact, followed by a code or codes to report details about the malignancy being treated.

One of these codes would be reported as the principal diagnosis code:

- Z51.0   Encounter for antineoplastic radiation therapy
- Z51.11 Encounter for antineoplastic chemotherapy
- Z51.12 Encounter for antineoplastic immunotherapy

Note that there is a notation for the Z51 code category that reminds you to

Code also condition requiring care

This would be the code or codes with the details about the malignancy, the reason *why* the patient would need this radiation, chemotherapy, or immunotherapy treatment.

> **EXAMPLE**
> *Warren Spencer was admitted to McGraw Hospital for his third chemotherapy infusion . . . treatment for the malignant neoplasm on the tail of his pancreas.*
>
> Z51.11   Encounter for antineoplastic chemotherapy
> C25.2   Malignant neoplasm of tail of pancreas
>
> Because Warren was admitted for the purpose of receiving his chemotherapy treatment, his chemotherapy is reported first (the principal diagnosis code), followed by the reason Warren needs this chemotherapy—pancreatic cancer.

Excised Malignancies/Personal History

Thanks to modern medical science and technology, health care professionals are more successful than ever at getting rid of certain neoplasms (tumors), often by excising them (surgically cutting them out). Postoperatively, the patient no longer has the anatomical site where the malignancy was located. Therefore, the patient can no longer have that condition. At that time, the code will change from a malignancy code (C00–C96) to a personal history of a malignancy code (category Z85).

EXAMPLE

Martha Peterson was diagnosed with a malignant neoplasm of the upper-inner quadrant of the right breast. The diagnosis code was

    C50.211   Malignant neoplasm of upper-inner quadrant of right female breast

She underwent a mastectomy, a surgical procedure to remove her breast. Once the anatomical site (her breast) that contained the malignant neoplasm was removed, she no longer had the disease, and no additional treatment was needed. From this point on, the diagnosis code is

    Z85.3   Personal history of malignant neoplasm, breast

> **GUIDANCE CONNECTION**
>
> Read the ICD-10-CM Official Guidelines for Coding and Reporting, section **I. Conventions, General Coding Guidelines and Chapter Specific Guidelines,** subsection **C. Chapter-Specific Coding Guidelines,** chapter **2. Neoplasms,** subsection **d. Primary malignancy previously excised.**

Suppose a patient has a primary site of malignancy and the disease has already metastasized to a second location. If the primary site is removed, the secondary malignancy is still coded as secondary but listed first. Confusing? Let's look at an example.

EXAMPLE

Ronald Albertson was diagnosed with prostate cancer. It spread to his liver before he was able to have surgery. The diagnosis codes, in this sequence, are

    C61   Malignant neoplasm of the prostate
    C78.7   Secondary malignant neoplasm of liver, and intrahepatic bile duct

Dr. Isaacson removes Ronald's prostate successfully. He no longer required any treatment. The new codes are

    C78.7   Secondary malignant neoplasm of liver, and intrahepatic bile duct
    Z85.46   Personal history of malignant neoplasm, prostate

Once Ronald has the site of his primary malignancy removed, his prostate condition becomes "history." The code for his secondary malignancy in the liver moves up in order, but it will always be the *secondary* site at which Ronald developed a malignancy.

> **GUIDANCE CONNECTION**
>
> Read the ICD-10-CM Official Guidelines for Coding and Reporting, section **I. Conventions, General Coding Guidelines and Chapter Specific Guidelines,** subsection **C. Chapter-Specific Coding Guidelines,** chapter **2. Neoplasms,** subsection **b. Treatment of secondary site.**

YOU CODE IT! CASE STUDY

Frederick Westchester, a 53-year-old male, came to see Dr. Henner, his dermatologist, for an annual checkup. Two years ago, Dr. Henner removed a malignant melanoma from Frederick's left forearm. The malignancy was totally removed, but he comes to see his physician for a checkup once a year.

You Code It!

Go through the steps of coding, and determine the diagnosis code or codes that should be reported for this encounter between Dr. Henner and Frederick.

Step #1: Read the case carefully and completely.

Step #2: Abstract the scenario. Which main words or terms describe why the physician cared for the patient during this encounter?

Step #3: Are there any details missing or incomplete for which you would need to query the physician? [If so, ask your instructor.]

Step #4: Check for any relevant guidance, including reading all of the symbols and notations in the Tabular List and the appropriate sections of the Official Guidelines.

(continued)

Step #5: Determine the correct diagnosis code or codes to explain why this encounter was medically necessary.

Step #6: Double-check your work.

Answer:

Did you determine the following diagnosis code?

Z85.820   Personal history of malignant melanoma of skin

Good job!

Complications and Complications of Treatment

You probably are aware that some of the most frequently used treatments to eradicate malignant cells, such as chemotherapy and radiation, manifest other conditions.

In those cases where the patient is admitted for therapy (radiation, chemotherapy, or immunotherapy) and develops complications during the encounter, report the Z51.0, Z51.11, or Z51.12 as the principal diagnosis code, *followed* by the code or codes to report the specific complications, such as uncontrolled nausea and vomiting or dehydration.

When the patient is admitted for treatment of anemia that is a manifestation of the malignancy, and only the anemia is treated during this stay, report the code for the neoplasm as the principal diagnosis *followed* by code D63.0 Anemia in neoplastic disease.

However, if the patient is admitted for treatment of anemia that is the result of the neoplastic treatment (chemotherapy or immunotherapy), you will report a code for the anemia first, *followed* by code T45.1x5- Adverse effect of antineoplastic and immunosuppressive drugs [seventh character is required to identify the encounter].

Anemia that is manifested as an effect from radiation treatments is reported a bit differently. For this patient, the code to report the anemia is reported as the principal diagnosis, *followed* by the code explaining the neoplasm for which the radiation was administered, *followed* by code Y84.2 Radiological procedure and radiotherapy as the cause of abnormal reaction of the patient, or of later complication, without mention of misadventure at the time of the procedure.

When the patient is admitted for treatment of dehydration, manifestation from the malignancy, and only the dehydration is treated during this stay, report the code for the dehydration as the principal diagnosis *followed* by the code for the neoplasm that was the reason the treatment was needed.

Treatment of Secondary Site Only

There are instances where a physician may treat only the secondary site of malignancy for a patient in a given encounter. In this case, you would report the secondary site as the principal diagnosis and the primary site malignancy after this.

> **GUIDANCE CONNECTION**
>
> Read the ICD-10-CM Official Guidelines for Coding and Reporting, section **I. Conventions, General Coding Guidelines and Chapter Specific Guidelines,** subsection **C. Chapter-Specific Coding Guidelines,** chapter **2. Neoplasms,** subsection **c. Coding and sequencing of complications.**

> **GUIDANCE CONNECTION**
>
> Read the ICD-10-CM Official Guidelines for Coding and Reporting, section **I. Conventions, General Coding Guidelines and Chapter Specific Guidelines,** subsection **C. Chapter-Specific Coding Guidelines,** chapter **2. Neoplasms,** subsection **l. Sequencing of neoplasm codes.**

> **EXAMPLE**
>
> Marvin's prostate cancer has spread to his lungs. Today, he has come to see Dr. Dunbar, a pulmonologist specializing in lung cancer, for evaluation and treatment.
>
> Report the codes in this order:
>
> 1. Secondary lung cancer
> 2. Primary prostate cancer
>
> Note that the primary cancer site is still identified and coded as "primary" even though it is the second code reported.

> **YOU CODE IT! CASE STUDY**
>
> Eric Swanson is a 43-year-old male with a malignant neoplasm of the laryngeal cartilage. He has become dehydrated due to the course of radiation therapy treatments. Dr. Leistner admitted Eric today to receive rehydration therapy.
>
> ### You Code It!
>
> Abstract the details related to the reasons why Dr. Leistner met with Eric.
>
> Step #1: Read the case carefully and completely.
>
> Step #2: Abstract the scenario. Which key words or terms describe why the physician cared for the patient during this encounter?
>
> Step #3: Are there any details missing or incomplete for which you would need to query the physician? [If so, ask your instructor.]
>
> Step #4: Check for any relevant guidance, including reading all of the symbols and notations in the Tabular List and the appropriate sections of the Official Guidelines.
>
> Step #5: Determine the correct diagnosis code or codes to explain why this encounter was medically necessary.
>
> Step #6: Double-check your work.
>
> **Answer:**
>
> Did you determine these to be the correct codes?
>
> | | |
> |---|---|
> | E86.0 | Dehydration |
> | C32.3 | Malignant neoplasm of laryngeal cartilage |

Prophylactic Organ Removal

Advances in science have given us genetic predisposition testing and other identification exams. The information these tests provide, along with personal and family histories, enables patients and health care professionals to predict an individual's risk for cancer and other diseases more accurately. Studies show, for example, that a woman who has inherited a mutation in the BRCA1 or BRCA2 gene faces a dramatically higher risk for developing breast cancer by age 65. A strong family history of colon cancer may lead an individual to be tested for a variant in the APC gene. There are many genes that can now be tested for various hereditary or familial conditions.

Prophylactic, or preventive, surgery can reduce risk of cancer in these situations by as much as 90%. In the case of breast cancer, preventive action would mean having a double mastectomy (the surgical removal of both breasts) while a patient is still healthy and without any signs or symptoms of carcinoma.

As a coder, the question becomes: How do you code a diagnosis for a surgical procedure on a healthy anatomical site? You will use a code from this sub-category:

> **Z40.0-** Encounter for prophylactic surgery for risk factors related to malignant neoplasms (Admission for prophylactic organ removal)
> *Use additional code* to identify risk factor

For those patients who have had genetic testing with a confirmed abnormal gene, you will also use a second code from category Z15 Genetic susceptibility to disease.

If the reason for the preventive surgery is due to a family history of cancer, you will add another code from the Z80 Family history of primary malignant neoplasm category.

YOU CODE IT! CASE STUDY

Angelina Constantine, a 27-year-old female, was admitted today for the prophylactic removal of her breasts. Her grandmother, mother, and sister have all had breast cancer, so she had genetic testing performed. It indicated that she did have a genetic susceptibility to breast cancer. She elected to have the surgery instead of taking chances with her health.

You Code It!

Go through the steps of coding, and determine the diagnosis code or codes that should be reported for Angelina's surgery.

Step #1: Read the case carefully and completely.

Step #2: Abstract the scenario. Which main words or terms describe why the physician cared for the patient during this encounter?

Step #3: Are there any details missing or incomplete for which you would need to query the physician? [If so, ask your instructor.]

Step #4: Check for any relevant guidance, including reading all of the symbols and notations in the Tabular List and the appropriate sections of the Official Guidelines.

Step #5: Determine the correct diagnosis code or codes to explain why this encounter was medically necessary.

Step #6: Double-check your work.

Answer:

Did you determine the following diagnosis codes?

Z40.01	Prophylactic removal of breast
Z15.01	Genetic susceptibility to malignant neoplasm of breast
Z80.3	Family history of malignant neoplasm, breast

Good job!

Chapter Summary

In this chapter, you learned how to identify the key words in physicians' documentation and test results reports that can guide you toward the most accurate code or codes. You learned the differences in the types of neoplasms and the proper sequencing of codes. In addition, you reviewed the correct way to sequence the codes when a patient has had a malignant site excised or been admitted for treatment or a complication.

There have been, and continue to be, incredible advancements made in the treatments of all types of neoplasms, as well as modifications to sociological behaviors to help prevent the development of those insidious health concerns. As a professional coding specialist, your ability to properly code the medical necessity for diagnostic tests and therapeutic procedures used in the care of individuals can open many job opportunities for you.

You Interpret It! Answers

1. (a) Screening, **2.** (b) Diagnostic, **3.** (b) Diagnostic, **4.** (a) Screening, **5.** Malignant, secondary, **6.** Malignant, primary, **7.** Malignant, primary, **8.** Malignant, secondary, **9.** Benign

CODING BITES

Did you know that medical coders have foundational knowledge to become **Cancer Registrars**?

Run by the CDC, the National Program of Cancer Registries (NPCR) collates data amassed by local cancer registries. This important health information provides public health professionals with the ability to assess and make plans for ways to alleviate the cancer burden on patients, families, and the community more effectively.

According to the National Cancer Registrars Association (NCRA), "*cancer registrars capture a complete summary of the history, diagnosis, treatment, and disease status for every cancer patient. Registrars' work leads to better information that is used in the management of cancer, and ultimately, cures.*"

Cancer registrars work in hospitals, state and regional cancer registries, federal government agencies, pharmaceutical companies, and other locations working with these data.

CHAPTER 6 REVIEW
Coding Neoplasms

Let's Check It! Terminology

Match each key term to the appropriate definition.

1. LO 6.2 Invasive and destructive characteristic of a neoplasm; possibly causing damage or death. **E**
2. LO 6.4 Glandular secretion in abnormal quantity. **D**
3. LO 6.2 Nonmalignant characteristic of a neoplasm; not infectious or spreading. **A**
4. LO 6.2 A malignant neoplasm or cancerous tumor. **B**
5. LO 6.2 Abnormal tissue growth; tumor. **I**
6. LO 6.2 To proliferate, reproduce, or spread. **G**
7. LO 6.4 Out of place, such as an organ or body part. **C**
8. LO 6.4 The classification of neoplasms primarily by anatomical site. **K**
9. LO 6.4 Multiple sites of carcinoma without identifiable borders. **J**
10. LO 6.2 Abnormal collection of tissue. **F**
11. LO 6.4 The study of the configuration or structure of living organisms. **H**

A. Benign
B. Carcinoma
C. Ectopic
D. Functional Activity
E. Malignant
F. Mass
G. Metastasize
H. Morphology
I. Neoplasm
J. Overlapping Boundaries
K. Topography

Let's Check It! Concepts

Choose the most appropriate answer for each of the following questions.

1. LO 6.2 A neoplasm is the same as a
   a. tumor.   b. cancer.   c. malignancy.   d. metastasis.
2. LO 6.2 Different types of neoplasms include all of the following *except*
   a. adenoma.   b. melanoma.   c. papilloma.   **d. chemotherapy.**

CHAPTER 6 REVIEW

3. **LO 6.2** The term _____ indicates that the tumor has undergone malignant changes but is still limited to the site where it originated.
   a. uncertain   **b. Ca in situ**   c. benign   d. secondary

4. **LO 6.4** Morphology codes are used
   a. for reimbursement.
   b. to describe treatment.
   c. to describe the topography and histology of the neoplasm.
   d. for identification of manifestations.

5. **LO 6.5** At subsequent encounters after the surgical removal of a neoplasm and no additional treatment, the diagnosis code changes to a
   a. personal history of malignancy code.   b. malignancy code.
   c. late effects code.   d. co-morbidity code.

6. **LO 6.5** When a patient is admitted for chemotherapy to treat a malignant neoplasm and that is the extent of treatment, the first code listed is the code for
   a. the primary malignancy.   b. the secondary malignancy.
   c. the chemotherapy.   d. observation in a hospital.

7. **LO 6.5** When a patient is admitted for treatment for a complication, such as anemia or dehydration, as the result of a neoplastic treatment, the code for this complication should be listed
   a. after the primary malignancy.   **b. first.**
   c. after the chemotherapy or radiation code.   d. as a Z code.

8. **LO 6.3** The correct code for a solitary plasmacytoma in remission is
   a. C90.3   b. C90.30   **c. C90.31**   d. C90.32

9. **LO 6.1** All of the following are common diagnostic tests for a suspected malignancy of the lung *except*
   a. alpha-1 antitrypsin.   **b. CA-125**   c. bronchoscopy.   d. bone scan.

10. **LO 6.2** When coding a neoplasm, you must know
    a. the anatomical site.   b. whether it is primary or secondary.
    c. whether it is benign or malignant.   **d. all of these.**

Let's Check It! Guidelines

Refer to the Official Guidelines and fill in the blanks according to the Chapter 2, Neoplasms, Chapter-Specific Coding Guidelines.

benign	Z85	anemia	primary
Z51.11	principal	extent	Z51.12
first-listed	malignancy	properly	M84.5
pathological	metastasis	dehydration	first
excised	principal/first-listed	Z51.0	

1. To _____ code a neoplasm it is necessary to determine from the record if the neoplasm is _____, in-situ, malignant, or of uncertain histologic behavior.

2. If the treatment is directed at the malignancy, designate the malignancy as the _____ diagnosis.

3. When a patient is admitted because of a _____ neoplasm with _____ and treatment is directed toward the secondary site only, the secondary neoplasm is designated as the principal diagnosis even though the primary malignancy is still present.

4. When admission/encounter is for management of an _____ associated with the malignancy, and the treatment is only for anemia, the appropriate code for the malignancy is sequenced as the principal or _____ diagnosis followed by the appropriate code for the anemia.

5. When the admission/encounter is for management of _____ due to the malignancy and only the dehydration is being treated (intravenous rehydration), the dehydration is sequenced first, followed by the code(s) for the _____.

6. When a primary malignancy has been previously _____ or eradicated from its site and there is no further treatment directed to that site and there is no evidence of any existing primary malignancy, a code from category _____, Personal history of malignant neoplasm, should be used to indicate the former site of the malignancy.

7. If a patient admission/encounter is solely for the administration of chemotherapy, immunotherapy, or radiation therapy assign code _____, Encounter for antineoplastic radiation therapy, or _____, Encounter for antineoplastic chemotherapy, or _____, Encounter for antineoplastic immunotherapy as the first-listed or principal diagnosis.

8. When the reason for admission/encounter is to determine the _____ of the malignancy or for a procedure such as paracentesis or thoracentesis, the primary malignancy or appropriate metastatic site is designated as the principal or first-listed diagnosis, even though chemotherapy or radiotherapy is administered.

9. If the reason for the encounter is for treatment of a primary malignancy, assign the malignancy as the _____ diagnosis.

10. When an encounter is for a _____ fracture due to a neoplasm, and the focus of treatment is the fracture, a code from subcategory _____, Pathological fracture in neoplastic disease, should be sequenced _____, followed by the code for the neoplasm.

Let's Check It! Rules and Regulations

Please answer the following questions from the knowledge you have gained after reading this chapter.

1. LO 6.2 Explain the difference between benign and malignant.
2. LO 6.2 What is the difference between primary, secondary, Ca in situ, uncertain, and unspecified behavior?
3. LO 6.4 Explain what overlapping boundaries are, and give another term for overlapping boundaries.
4. LO 6.4 What is morphology, and why is it important?
5. LO 6.5 Discuss prophylactic organ removal, its advantage, and how this should be coded.

YOU CODE IT! Basics

First, identify the main term in the following diagnoses; then code the diagnosis.

Example: Malignant primary neoplasm of lung, right upper lobe:

a. main term: *neoplasm*   **b.** diagnosis *C34.11*

1. Acute megakaryocytic leukemia in relapse:
   a. main term: _____   **b.** diagnosis: _____
2. Benign neoplasm of uterine ligament, broad:
   a. main term: _____   **b.** diagnosis: _____
3. Papillary adenocarcinoma, intraductal, left breast:
   a. main term: _____   **b.** diagnosis: _____
4. Malignant carcinoid tumor of the colon:
   a. main term: _____   **b.** diagnosis: _____
5. Hemangioma of intra-abdominal structures:
   a. main term: _____   **b.** diagnosis: _____
6. Adenoma of the liver cell:
   a. main term: _____   **b.** diagnosis: _____

7. Follicular grade III lymphoma lymph nodes of inguinal region and lower limbs:

   a. main term: _____   b. diagnosis: _____

8. Acral lentiginous, right heel melanoma:

   a. main term: _____   b. diagnosis: _____

9. Lipoma of the kidney:

   a. main term: _____   b. diagnosis: _____

10. Primary malignant neoplasm of right male breast, upper-outer quadrant:

    a. main term: _____   b. diagnosis: _____

11. Malignant odontogenic tumor, upper jaw bone:

    a. main term: _____   b. diagnosis: _____

12. Secondary malignant neoplasm of vallecula:

    a. main term: _____   b. diagnosis: _____

13. Carcinoma in situ neoplasm of left eyeball:

    a. main term: _____   b. diagnosis: _____

14. Benign neoplasm of cerebrum peduncle:

    a. main term: _____   b. diagnosis: _____

15. Myelofibrosis with myeloid metaplasia:

    a. main term: _____   b. diagnosis: _____

YOU CODE IT! Practice

Using the techniques described in this chapter, carefully read through the case studies and determine the most accurate ICD-10-CM code(s) and external cause code(s), if appropriate, for each case study.

1. George Donmoyer, a 58-year-old male, presents today with a sore throat, persistent cough, and earache. Dr. Selph completes an examination and appropriate tests. The blood-clotting parameters, the thyroid function studies, as well as the tissue biopsy confirm a diagnosis of malignant neoplasm of the extrinsic larynx.

2. Monica Pressley, a 37-year-old female, comes to see Dr. Wheaten today because she has been having diarrhea and abdominal cramping and states her heart feels like its quavering. The MRI scan confirms a diagnosis of benign pancreatic islet cell adenoma.

3. Suber Wilson, a 57-year-old male, was diagnosed with a malignant neoplasm of the liver metastasized from the prostate; both sites are being addressed in today's encounter.

4. William Amerson, a 41-year-old male, comes in for his annual eye examination. Dr. Leviner notes a benign right conjunctiva nevus.

5. Edward Bakersfield, a 43-year-old male, presents with shortness of breath, chest pain, and coughing up blood. After a thorough examination, Dr. Benson notes stridor and orders an MRI scan. The results of the MRI confirm the diagnosis of bronchial adenoma.

6. Elizabeth Conyers, a 56-year-old female, presents with unexplained weakness, weight loss, and dizziness. Dr. Amos completes a thorough examination and does a work-up. The protein electrophoresis (SPEP) and quantitative immunoglobulin results confirm the diagnosis of Waldenström's macroglobulinemia.

7. James Buckholtz, a 3-year-old male, is brought in by his parents. Jimmy has lost his appetite and is losing weight. Mrs. Buckholtz tells Dr. Ferguson that Jimmy's gums bleed and he seems short of breath. Dr. Ferguson notes splenomegaly and admits Jimmy to Weston Hospital. After reviewing the blood tests, MRI scan, and bone marrow aspiration results, Jimmy is diagnosed with acute lymphoblastic leukemia.

8. Kelley Young, a 39-year-old female, presents to Dr. Clerk with the complaints of sudden blurred vision, dizziness, and numbness in her face. Kelley states she feels very weak and has headaches. Dr. Clerk admits Kelley to the hospital. After reviewing the MRI scan, her hormone levels from the blood workup, and urine tests, Kelley is diagnosed with a primary malignant neoplasm of the pituitary gland.

9. Ralph Bradley, a 36-year-old male, comes to see Dr. Harper because he is weak, losing weight, and vomiting and has diarrhea with some blood showing. Ralph was diagnosed with HIV 3 years ago. Dr. Harper completes an examination noting paleness, tachycardia, and tachypnea. Ralph is admitted to the hospital. The biopsied tissue from an endoscopy confirms a diagnosis of Kaposi's sarcoma of gastrointestinal organ.

10. Ben Jameson, a 31-year-old male, was admitted today for the prophylactic removal of his prostate. Both Ben's father and brother have prostate cancer that has spread to the lungs and liver. Ben decides to have a laparoscopic radical prostatectomy while he is still healthy.

11. Phillip DeLorne, a 21-year-old male, presents with a sore on his left ear of approximately 5-weeks duration. Philip says it just won't get well. Dr. Duruy notes a pink lump on Philip's pinna and a biopsy is taken, which confirms a diagnosis of melanoma in situ of the left external ear.

12. Mitchell Lane, a 48-year-old male, presents with the complaints of night sweats and weight loss. Dr. Clark completes an examination noting hemoptysis and takes a chest x-ray, which reveals a mass. Mitchell is admitted to Weston Hospital where a CT-guided needle biopsy is then performed. Mitchell is diagnosed with a malignant primary neoplasm of the posterior mediastinum.

13. Raykeem McFadden, a 63-year-old female, was last seen in this office 6 months ago for her annual checkup; no concerns were noted at that time. She presents today because of excessive itching after a warm bath. She also complains of a burning sensation in her arms, especially her left arm. Dr. Dingle completes a physical exam and notes aphasia, hepatosplenomegaly, and some loss of physical coordination. Raykeem is admitted to the hospital. The laboratory tests and bone marrow aspiration confirm a diagnosis of polycythemia vera.

14. Terry Shelton, a 33-year-old female, had chemotherapy 3 days ago, for gallbladder cancer. She presents today to see Dr. China due to extreme weakness and chest pain. Dr. China notes an irregular heartbeat and a CBC reveals a hemoglobin of 8.3 g/dL. Terry is diagnosed with anemia due to antineoplastic chemotherapy and admitted to Weston Hospital for treatment of her anemia.

15. Kewane Childs, a 44-year-old female, has a history of smoking cigarettes for 15 years; she quit last year. Kewane sees Dr. Cope for a dry cough, hoarse voice, and coughing up blood. Dr. Cope notes crepitation and dyspnea. Kewane is admitted to the hospital. The MRI scan and lung function tests confirm a diagnosis of neoplasm of the trachea, malignant primary.

YOU CODE IT! Application

The following exercises provide practice in abstracting physicians' documentation from our health care facility, Prader, Bracker, & Associates. These case studies are modeled on real patient encounters. Using the techniques described in this chapter, carefully read through the case studies and determine the most accurate ICD-10-CM code(s) and external cause code(s), if appropriate, for each case study.

WESTON HOSPITAL

629 Healthcare Way • SOMEWHERE, FL 32811 • 407-555-6541

PATIENT: KAHN, SERENA

ACCOUNT/EHR #: KAHNSE001

DATE: 09/16/18

Attending Physician: Oscar R. Prader, MD

HPI: This patient is being admitted to Weston Hospital for wide excision of a level 2 melanoma, right side of the face. She was referred from Dr. Robinson. Patient states she has had the lesion forever. Dr. Robinson found it disturbing and decided to take a biopsy; results, melanoma, level 2.

This lesion is located just anterior to the ear on the right zygomatic region; we should get a reasonably good margin.

PAST MEDICAL HISTORY: Hypothyroidism and takes thyroid replacement medication.

PAST SURGICAL HISTORY: The patient had carcinoma of the breast and underwent a left mastectomy in 2012. She had a hysterectomy for benign ovarian tumors in 2015.

ALLERGIES: NKA

SOCIAL HISTORY: Nonsmoker. Drinks alcohol socially.

FAMILY HISTORY: The patient's sister is diabetic.

ROS: Negative.

PHYSICAL EXAMINATION: Ht: 5'6", Wt: 142, T: 98.6, R: 18, BP 170/70. HEENT: Head is atraumatic, normocephalic; there is a pigmented lesion just anterior to the right ear over the zygomatic region, which is slightly irregular in shape and different shades of brown. Biopsied site is noted and healing within normal limits.

NECK: Negative.

CHEST: Clear and symmetrical

HEART: Regular rhythm, no murmurs

ABDOMEN: Soft, nontender, no masses or organomegaly

EXTREMITIES: No cyanosis, clubbing, or edema

NEUROLOGIC: Grossly intact

IMPRESSION: Melanoma of the right cheek, level 2

PLAN: Wide excision with flap advancement closure

ORP/pw   D: 9/16/18 09:50:16   T: 9/18/18 12:55:01

Determine the most accurate ICD-10-CM codes.

WESTON HOSPITAL

629 Healthcare Way • SOMEWHERE, FL 32811 • 407-555-6541

PATIENT: DAWSON, WILSON

ACCOUNT/EHR #: DAWSWI001

DATE: 08/11/18

Attending Physician: Renee O. Bracker, MD

Pt is a 47-year-old male with left breast carcinoma, terminal stage, metastatic to the brain and liver. Wilson is undergoing chemotherapy and has become dehydrated, showing signs of confusion and disorientation. He is admitted to Weston Hospital for rehydration. Procalamine 3%, IV, 50mL/hr was given for 12 hours. Patient stabilized and was discharged home with no other treatment.

ROB/pw   D: 08/11/18 09:50:16   T: 08/13/18 12:55:01

Determine the most accurate ICD-10-CM codes.

WESTON HOSPITAL
629 Healthcare Way • SOMEWHERE, FL 32811 • 407-555-6541

PATIENT: OAKWOOD, QUENTIN

ACCOUNT/EHR #: OAKWQU001

DATE: 09/16/18

Attending Physician: Oscar R. Prader, MD

Pt is a 63-year-old male who was diagnosed with prostate cancer 3 years ago. 18 months ago he had a radical prostatectomy. 1 year ago he was diagnosed with bone and liver metastasis. Patient has a high level of pain associated with his liver cancer and is being admitted for an insertion of a tunneled centrally inserted port-a-cath VAD (venous access device) with a sub q port for delivery of pain control medication.

ORP/pw   D: 9/16/18 09:50:16   T: 9/18/18 12:55:01

Determine the most accurate ICD-10-CM codes.

PRADER, BRACKER, & ASSOCIATES
A Complete Health Care Facility
159 Healthcare Way • SOMEWHERE, FL 32811 • 407-555-6789

PATIENT: CHARLES, KAREN

ACCOUNT/EHR #: CHARKA001

DATE: 08/11/18

Attending Physician: Renee O. Bracker, MD

Patient, a 43-year-old female, presents today to discuss pathological findings of recent exploratory laparotomy. Patient is 4 days' status post lysis of adhesions; total abdominal hysterectomy; bilateral salpingo-oophorectomy; partial omentectomy; excision of small and large bowel implants; pelvic-abdominal peritoneal stripping; placement of intraperitoneal port-a-cath; and enterolyses.

The ovaries were found to be poorly differentiated; serous carcinoma extended to the left fallopian tube. The right fallopian tube was found to have serosal fibrosis consistent with tubo-ovarian adhesion. A broad-based endometrial polyp was found in the endometrium while the myometrium showed leiomyomata, adenomyosis, and multifocal serosal implants of poorly differentiated ovarian serous carcinoma.

The specimen from the omentum was found to be metastatic adenocarcinoma consistent with ovarian origin.

Lastly, the specimens from both the small and large bowel were positive for metastatic, poorly differentiated ovarian serous carcinoma.

The histomorphologic features of poorly differentiated ovarian serous carcinoma closely resemble that of a poorly differentiated fallopian tube primary adenocarcinoma. The bilateral ovarian involvement supports the primary ovarian origin of the neoplasm.

ASSESSMENT: Metastatic adenocarcinoma of the omentum; metastatic carcinoma of the small and large intestines.

ROB/pw   D: 08/11/18 09:50:16   T: 08/13/18 12:55:01

Determine the most accurate ICD-10-CM codes.

WESTON HOSPITAL
629 Healthcare Way • SOMEWHERE, FL 32811 • 407-555-6541

PATIENT: BENTONN, VERNON

ACCOUNT/EHR #: BENTVE001

DATE: 09/16/18

Attending Physician: Oscar R. Prader, MD

PREOP DIAGNOSIS: Lower extremity ischemia with rest pain and gangrene of the right third toe, probable atheroembolic disease to the right lower extremity.

POSTOP DIAGNOSIS: Atheroembolic disease to the right lower extremity.

PROCEDURE: Right, axillary femoral-femoral bypass utilizing an 8.0-mm ringed Gore-Tex axillary-to-femoral graft and a 6.0-mm ringed Gore-Tex femoral cross-over graft, right third toe amputation.

OPERATIVE INDICATIONS: This is a 69-year-old male, presenting with local rectal carcinoma, recurrent, with miliary metastases to the liver.

PATHOLOGICAL FINDINGS: Specimen: Third right toe consistent with ischemic necrosis.

PLAN/RECOMMENDATIONS: At this time, given known early liver metastases and extensive local regional recurrence in the pelvis, I do not feel that further antineoplastic therapy will be of great benefit.

Specifically, patient has had chemotherapy up until September of this year and this disease has recurred. In addition, he has a history of full radiotherapy to the pelvis.

Secondly, evidence-based medicine for recurrent colorectal cancer has shown that secondline chemotherapy has been of little to no value.

Pain management: I would recommend continuing his Duragesic patch, advise the addition of a low dose of Elavil to help reduce neurogenic pain. Efforts will be made to improve mobility.

ORP/pw   D: 9/16/18 09:50:16   T: 9/18/18 12:55:01

Determine the most accurate ICD-10-CM codes.

Coding Conditions of the Blood and Immunological Systems

7

Learning Outcomes

After completing this chapter, the student should be able to:

LO 7.1 Differentiate between various blood conditions and how this affects the determination of the code.

LO 7.2 Determine the codes to report coagulation defects and hemorrhagic conditions accurately.

LO 7.3 Identify the different types of blood and the importance of Rh factoring involved in malfunction.

LO 7.4 Interpret the details of white blood cell disorders and diseases of the spleen.

LO 7.5 Evaluate the factors involved in immunodeficiency disorders.

Key Terms

- Agglutination
- Antibodies
- Antigen
- Blood
- Blood Type
- Coagulation
- Hematopoiesis
- Hemoglobin (hgb or Hgb)
- Hemolysis
- Hemostasis
- Plasma
- Platelets (PLTs)
- Red Blood Cells (RBCs)
- Rh (Rhesus) Factor
- Transfusion
- White Blood Cells (WBCs)

STOP! Remember, you need to follow along in your ICD-10-CM code book for an optimal learning experience.

7.1 Reporting Blood Conditions

As with any other part of the body, malfunction of the blood-forming organs, the blood itself, or one of its components can result in problems affecting the entire body.

Blood is actually a type of connective tissue consisting of **red blood cells (RBCs)**, **white blood cells (WBCs)**, and **platelets (PLTs)**—all contained within liquid **plasma**. It is the transportation system used to deliver oxygen (nourishment) for cells throughout the body and to carry carbon dioxide (cell waste products) so it can be expelled from the body. The average adult has between 5 and 6 liters of blood constantly circulating throughout.

The Formation of Blood

Blood is created in the red bone marrow (see Figure 7-1) during a series of steps called **hematopoiesis**. During gestation, blood cells originate in the yolk sac from the mesenchyme (the section of the embryo in which blood, lymphatic vessels, bones, cartilage, and connective tissues form). As the fetus continues to develop, the liver, spleen, and thymus begin to produce blood cells. Then, at about the 20th week of gestation, the red bone marrow also begins to contribute to production. Once the baby is born, blood cell formation becomes the responsibility of the red bone marrow only, specifically in the sternum, ribs, and vertebrae. Red bone marrow produces red blood cells (erythrocytes) through a process called *erythropoiesis* and white blood cells (leukocytes) through a process called *leukopoiesis*.

Blood
Fluid pumped throughout the body, carrying oxygen and nutrients to the cells and wastes away from the cells.

Red Blood Cells (RBCs)
Cells within the blood that contain hemoglobin responsible for carrying oxygen to tissues; also known as *erythrocytes*.

White Blood Cells (WBCs)
Cells within the blood that help to protect the body from pathogens; also known as *leukocytes*.

Platelets (PLTs)
Large cell fragments in the bone marrow that function in clotting; also known as *thrombocytes*.

Plasma
The fluid part of the blood.

Hematopoiesis
The formation of blood cells.

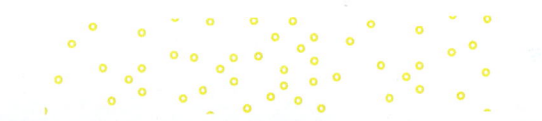

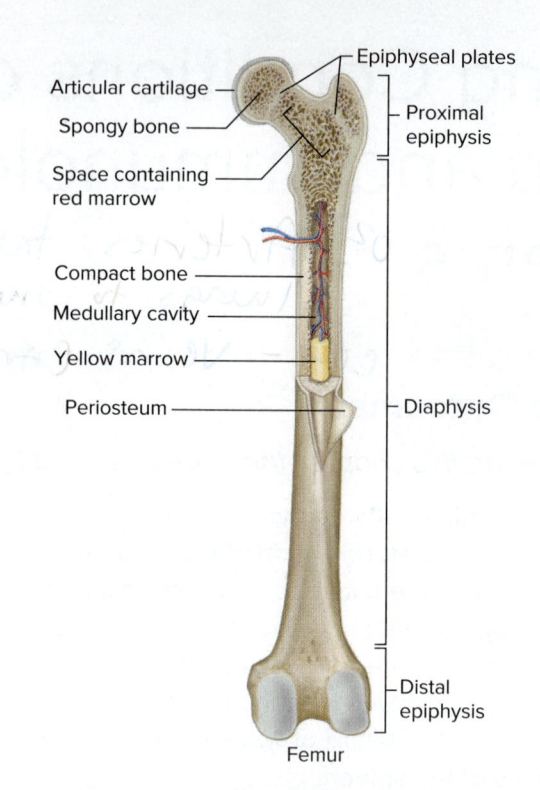

FIGURE 7-1 Bone marrow Source: David Shier et al., *Hole's Human Anatomy & Physiology*, 12/e. ©2010 McGraw-Hill Education. Figure 7.2, p. 194. Used with permission.

How many blood cells does a healthy body need? Normal counts (per microliter of blood) are

- *Red blood cell count:* 4 to 6 million cells.
- *White blood cell count:* 4,000 to 11,000 cells.
- *Platelet count:* 150,000 to 400,000 platelets.

Too many cells or too few cells may indicate a problem. This is why one of the first diagnostic tests run when a physician is trying to figure out what is wrong with the patient is a complete blood count (CBC).

Blood Roles

Blood's primary job is transporting oxygen from the lungs and delivering it to tissue cells throughout the body. As the oxygen passes from the lungs to the blood, it binds to the red blood cells and the **hemoglobin (hgb or Hgb)** inside those RBCs (see Figure 7-2), so it can travel through the heart and out through the body via the arteries. After delivering the oxygen (O_2) to the cells, the blood picks up carbon dioxide (CO_2) and carries it back to the lungs for expulsion from the body.

Anemias

While many believe anemia is the result of an iron deficiency, this is only one cause of an abnormally low count of hemoglobin, hematocrit, and/or RBCs. The low volume of RBCs reduces the amount of oxygen being transported, causing tissue hypoxia (low levels of oxygen). Blood loss, lack of red blood cell production, and high rates of red blood cell destruction are the three most common causes of anemia. Classic signs and symptoms include tachycardia, dyspnea, and sometimes fatigue.

Hemoglobin (hgb or Hgb)
The part of the red blood cell that carries oxygen.

CODING BITES

While professional coding specialists are not permitted to diagnose a patient, understanding these details from a pathology or lab report can support your understanding of the documentation or explain medical necessity—or it may alert you, as the coder, to query the physician about missing or ambiguous notes.

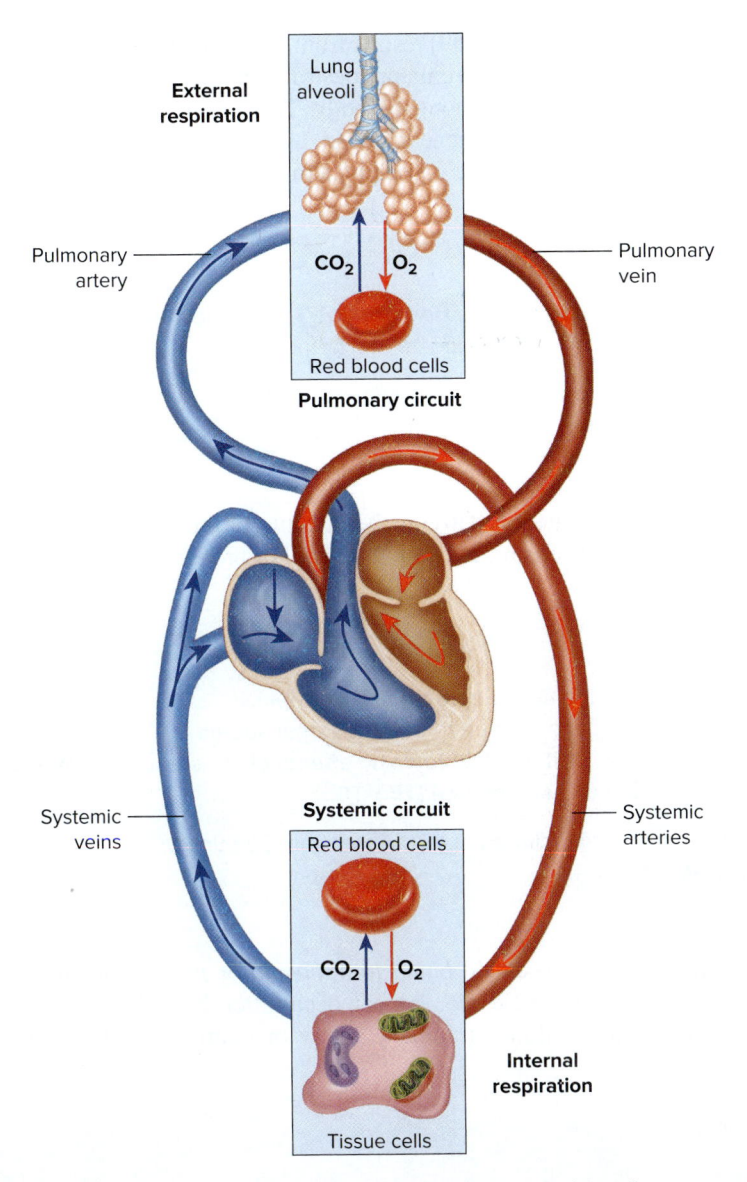

FIGURE 7-2 Oxygen and carbon dioxide exchanging in blood

Nutritional anemia, reported with a code from the D50–D53 range, is caused by an insufficient intake or absorption into the body of certain key nutrients. For example, pernicious anemia is a genetic condition that causes dysfunction of the ileum so it cannot properly absorb vitamin B_{12}; iron deficiency anemia may be caused by a diet lacking iron-rich foods.

> **EXAMPLES**
>
> D50.0 Iron deficiency anemia secondary to blood loss (chronic)
> D51.0 Vitamin B12 deficiency anemia due to intrinsic factor deficiency (pernicious (congenital) anemia)
> D52.0 Dietary folate deficiency anemia
> D53.2 Scorbutic anemia
>
> Specific details about the underlying cause of the anemia are required to report an accurate code.

Hemolytic anemia (codes D55–D59) results from an insufficient number of healthy red blood cells due to abnormal or premature destruction, thereby retarding the delivery of oxygen to the tissues throughout the body. This premature destruction of the red blood cells may be caused by a genetic defect, an infection, or exposure to certain toxins. Hemolytic anemia can also be caused by a mismatched blood transfusion.

EXAMPLES

D55.1   Anemia due to other disorders of glutathione metabolism
D56.4   Hereditary persistence of fetal hemoglobin

Sickle-cell disorders are included in this subsection. See upcoming section for more on these diagnoses.

Aplastic anemia (code category D61) is the inability of the bone marrow to manufacture enough new blood cells required by the body for proper function.

EXAMPLES

D61.01   Constitutional (pure) red blood cell aplasia
D61.2   Aplastic anemia due to other external agents
              Code first, if applicable, toxic effects of substances chiefly non-medicinal as to source (T51-T65)

Sickle-cell disorders are included in this subsection. See upcoming section for more on these diagnoses.

Hemorrhagic anemia, also called *blood loss anemia* or *posthemorrhagic anemia* (code D62 Acute posthemorrhagic anemia), can occur after the patient has lost a great deal of blood. This can be after a traumatic injury or internal bleeding, such as an untreated gastric ulcer.

LET'S CODE IT! SCENARIO

Carter McMannus, an 18-month-old male, was brought by his mother to Dr. Hampshire, a pediatrician specializing in hematologic (blood) disorders. Dr. Hampshire noted jaundice, an enlarged spleen on palpation, and other signs of failure to thrive. Dr. Hampshire recognized these signs and symptoms and confirmed with blood tests a diagnosis of Cooley's anemia.

Let's Code It!

Dr. Hampshire diagnosed Carter with *Cooley's anemia*. Turn to the Alphabetic Index and find

Anemia

Are you surprised by the long indented list of different types of anemia? Read down the list and find

Anemia
     Cooley's (erythroblastic) D56.1

Now let's go to the Tabular List to confirm this code. Remember, always begin reading at the three-character category.

     ✓4 **D56**   Thalassemia

> Thalassemia is an inherited group of hemolytic anemias (*hemo* = blood + *-lytic* = involving lysis, the decomposition of a cell). Cooley's anemia, also known as *thalassemia major,* is one type of beta thalassemia, the most common form of this condition.
> Read down the fourth-character choices and find
>
> **D56.1   Beta thalassemia (Cooley's anemia)**
>
> Check the top of this subsection and the head of this chapter in ICD-10-CM. There is an **EXCLUDES2** notation at the beginning of this chapter. Read carefully. Does this relate to Dr. Hampshire's diagnosis of Carter? No. Turn to the Official Guidelines and read Section 1.c.3. Interesting, there are no guidelines for this chapter.
> Now you can report D56.1 for Carter's diagnosis with confidence.
> Good job!

Sickle Cell Disease and Sickle Cell Trait

Sickle cell disease (SCD) is not actually one diagnosis, but represents several genetically passed disorders of the red blood cells (RBCs). Normal RBCs are round, whereas an individual with SCD develops red blood cells that are a C-shape and are unusually firm and sticky. The shape of these abnormal cells resembles a tool known as a sickle, leading to the name for this condition. In addition to the shape and nature of these cells, they have a shorter life span, resulting in a continuing shortage of RBCs. The sticky texture of these cells also increases the opportunity for the cells to stick to the walls of the blood vessels, manifesting obstructions and an ineffective delivery of oxygen via the hemoglobin.

SCD can be diagnosed in utero or in newborn blood screenings. The earlier the diagnosis, the sooner treatments can be implemented.

As a professional coder, you will need to know more than a diagnosis of SCD; you will need to know specifics about the condition, as well as any manifestations.

Hb-SS

D57.00	Hb-SS disease with crisis, unspecified
D57.01	Hb-SS disease with acute chest syndrome
D57.02	Hb-SS disease with splenic sequestration

Hb-SS disease is a condition in which the patient has inherited two sickle cell genes ("S"), one from each parent. Commonly referred to as *sickle cell anemia,* this is typically the most acute form of this condition.

Hb-C, HB-S, or HB-SC

D57.20	Sickle-cell/Hb-C disease without crisis
D57.211	Sickle-cell/Hb-C disease with acute chest syndrome
D57.212	Sickle-cell/Hb-C disease with splenic sequestration
D57.219	Sickle-cell/Hb-C disease with crisis, unspecified

Sometimes known as Hb-SC or Hb-S disease, this patient has inherited a sickle cell gene ("S") from one parent and a gene for abnormal hemoglobin called "C" from the other parent.

HbS Beta Thalassemia

D57.40	Sickle-cell thalassemia without crisis
D57.411	Sickle-cell thalassemia with acute chest syndrome
D57.412	Sickle-cell thalassemia with splenic sequestration
D57.419	Sickle-cell thalassemia with crisis, unspecified

CODING BITES

Be certain to read the notation at the code category of ☑4 **D57 Sickle-cell disorders,** which directs you to *Use additional code* for any associated fever (R50.81)

This form of SCD manifests when the patient inherits one sickle cell gene ("S") from one parent and the gene for beta thalassemia from the other parent.

HbSD and HbSE

D57.80	Other sickle-cell disorders without crisis
D57.811	Other sickle-cell disorders with acute chest syndrome
D57.812	Other sickle-cell disorders with splenic sequestration
D57.819	Other sickle-cell disorders with crisis, unspecified

When a patient inherits one sickle cell gene ("S") and one gene with an abnormal type of hemoglobin ("D," "E," or "O") it would be documented as Hb-SD, Hb-SE, or Hb-S.

Sickle Cell Trait

D57.3	Sickle-cell trait

Sickle-cell trait (SCT) develops when the patient has inherited one sickle cell gene ("S") from one parent and a normal gene ("A") from the other parent. Individuals diagnosed with SCT do not typically exhibit any signs or symptoms of the disease. When this patient considers having children, this should be noted because this can be passed along to future children.

Hematologic Malignancies

Both lymphomas and leukemias are included in this category. Leukemia is the presence of malignant cells within the bone marrow that produces blood cells (hematopoietic tissues), causing a reduction in the production of RBCs, WBCs, and platelets. This anemic state makes the patient very susceptible to infections and hemorrhaging.

There are several types of leukemia reported from several ICD-10-CM code categories:

code category C92 Myeloid leukemia
code category C93 Monocytic leukemia
code category C94 Other leukemia of specified cell type
code category C95 Leukemia of unspecified cell type

The aspiration of bone marrow (known as a bone marrow biopsy) is typically taken from the posterior superior iliac spine. This specimen is tested to quantify the white blood cells. When a rapid reproduction of immature WBCs is evidenced, this confirms a diagnosis of acute leukemia. In addition, the results of a differential leukocyte count can specifically identify the type of cell and a lumbar puncture (aka spinal tap) can reveal whether or not there is involvement of the meninges.

7.2 Coagulation Defects and Other Hemorrhagic Conditions

Hemostasis
The interruption of bleeding.

Coagulation
Clotting; the change from a liquid into a thickened substance.

In addition to transporting oxygen, blood also controls **hemostasis** (stopping the bleeding process) via **coagulation** (clotting).

Essentially, there are two types of clotting disorders: hemostatic and thrombotic. A *hemostatic disorder* is a failure in the system to repair a damaged blood vessel. Because there is no clot to stop it, the vessel continues to bleed. These coagulation deficiencies—where clotting does not occur as it should (see Figure 7-3)—may be seen with bleeding into the muscles, joints, and viscera or with the appearance

FIGURE 7-3 The four main events in hemostasis

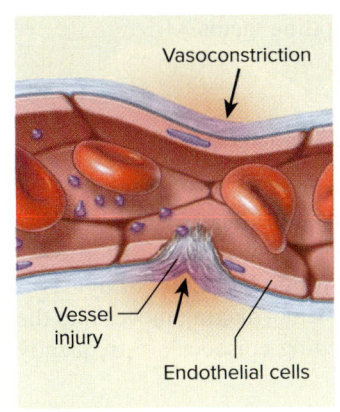

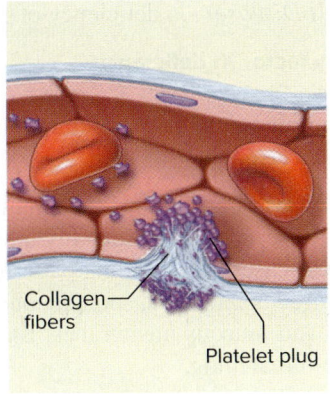

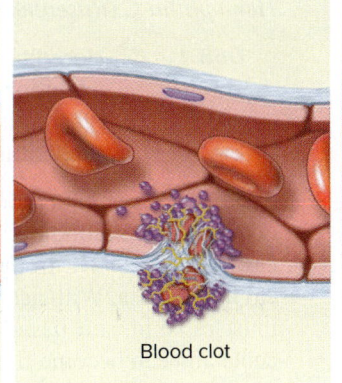

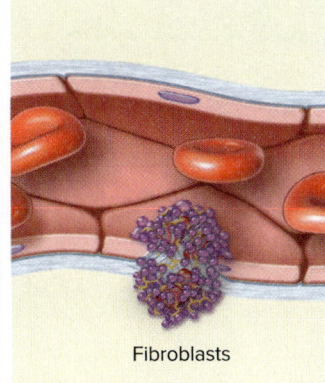

(a) Blood vessel spasm
(b) Platelet plug formation
(c) Blood clotting
(d) Fibrinolysis

of purpura (dysfunction of blood vessels). Hemophilia is a common hemostatic condition, reported with code D66 Hereditary factor VIII deficiency (Classical hemophilia).

Thrombotic disorders are the opposite: The blood clots without purpose, forming thrombi (blood clots) within the vessels, causing a blockage. Beyond the dangers from the thrombi themselves, should a clot dislodge (embolus) and travel through the blood vessels, it might get caught going through the lungs or heart, causing a blockage that could be deadly. Thrombophilia is an example of a thrombotic condition, reported with, for example, ICD-10-CM code D68.59 Other primary thrombophilia (Hypercoagulable state NOS).

Hemophilia

Hemophilia is a genetic mutation that establishes a deficiency lacking a protein (clotting factor) in the blood necessary in the clotting process. Therefore, the patient's blood will not clot when needed to prevent hemorrhaging. The lower the quantity of the clotting factor, the higher the probability that the patient might hemorrhage and have it become life-threatening.

The majority of patients diagnosed with hemophilia have a deficiency of either factor VIII or factor IX.

Types of Hemophilia

There are four types of Hemophilia: A, B, C, and Acquired.

Hemophilia A (Classic Hemophilia) . . . deficiency of clotting factor VIII. This is reported with one of two codes:

D66	Hereditary factor VIII deficiency (Hemophilia A) (Deficiency factor VIII with functional defect)
D68.0	Von Willebrand's disease (factor VIII deficiency with vascular defect)

Hemophilia B (Christmas Disease) . . . deficiency of clotting factor IX.

D67	Hereditary factor IX deficiency (Hemophilia B) (Deficiency factor IX with functional defect) (Christmas disease)

Hemophilia C (Rosenthal's Disease) . . . deficiency of clotting factor XI.

D68.1   **Hereditary factor XI deficiency (Hemophilia C)**
Plasma thromboplastin antecedent [PTA} deficiency (Rosenthal's disease)

Acquired hemophilia (secondary hemophilia) . . . actually an autoimmune disease that occurs when antibodies are created that mistakenly attack healthy tissue, specifically clotting factor VIII. In these cases, the bleeding pattern is quite different from classical hemophilia. With acquired hemophilia, spontaneous hemorrhaging moves into the muscles, skin, soft tissue, and mucous membranes. Bleeding episodes are frequently acute and can become life-threatening.

D68.311   **Acquired hemophilia (Secondary hemophilia)**

D68.4   **Acquired coagulation factor deficiency (Deficiency of coagulation factor due to liver disease) (Deficiency of coagulation factor due to vitamin K deficiency)**

LET'S CODE IT! SCENARIO

Dr. Victor ordered a coagulation profile, including a partial thromboplastin time (PTT) and prothrombin time (PT), to be done on Louis Langer prior to scheduling his surgery. The pathology report showed an abnormally prolonged PTT. The surgery will be delayed until Dr. Victor can confirm the cause.

Let's Code It!

The lab report identified an abnormal coagulation profile, and Dr. Victor did not provide any confirmed diagnosis. Therefore, this is all you know for a fact, and this is what must be reported. Turn to the Alphabetic Index and find

Abnormal

This is going to take some analysis. There is no listing under *Abnormal* for *Test* or *Coagulation*. Think about this. What is the body's reason for coagulation? To stop bleeding. Look for *Blood* or *Bleeding*. Did you find

Abnormal
    Bleeding time R79.1

Now let's go into the Tabular List to check this out. Remember, always begin reading at the three-character category.

☑4 **R79**   **Other abnormal findings of blood chemistry**

Read down the fourth-character choices and find

R79.1   **Abnormal coagulation profile (abnormal or prolonged partial thromboplastin time [PTT])**

Read the EXCLUDES1 and EXCLUDES2 notations directly below this code.

Check the top of this subsection; there is an EXCLUDES1 notation. Read it carefully to see if any of those conditions apply. At the head of this chapter in ICD-10-CM, you will find a long **NOTE** and an EXCLUDES2 notation. Read carefully. Do any relate to Dr. Victor's diagnosis of Louis? Yes, so confirm that there is no more specific diagnosis that can be reported instead. There is not. Now, turn to the Official Guidelines and read Section 1.c.18. There is nothing specifically applicable here either.

Now you can report R79.1 for Louis's diagnosis with confidence.
Good job!

Thrombocytopenia

This is a low platelet count most often due to increased platelet destruction, decreased platelet production, or malfunctioning platelets. Underlying conditions might include splenomegaly (enlarged spleen); destruction of bone marrow by medication, chemotherapy, or radiation therapy; or aplastic anemia. The condition will be reported most often with a code from ICD-10-CM code category D69 Purpura and other hemorrhagic conditions, although not exclusively. For example, postpartum puerperal thrombocytopenia is reported with code O72.3 Postpartum coagulation defects and neonatal, transitory thrombocytopenia is reported with code P61.0 Transient neonatal thrombocytopenia.

YOU CODE IT! CASE STUDY

Marissa Rubine, a 27-year-old female, came to see Dr. Post with complaints of bruising "suddenly appearing" on her arms and legs. She states she had two recent episodes of epistaxis but denies any other bleeding. She denied taking any drugs or smoking, and states she has no risk factors for HIV. Physical examination revealed the spleen was not palpable. Petechiae are noted scattered on her legs bilaterally.

Blood work results:

- hemoglobin (138 g/L)—normal
- white cell count—normal
- platelet count of 10×10^9/L—low (normal >150×10^9/L)
- erythrocyte sedimentation rate was 6 mm/h
- direct Coombs' test—negative
- antinuclear—absent
- DNA-binding antibodies—absent
- rheumatoid factor—absent

Bone marrow aspiration: high number of normal megakaryocytes but otherwise normal

Dx: Immune thrombocytopenia purpura

She is placed on a short course of prednisolone.

You Code It!

Go through the steps of coding, and determine the code or codes that should be reported for this encounter between Dr. Post and Marissa.

Step #1: Read the case carefully and completely.

Step #2: Abstract the scenario. Which main words or terms describe why the physician cared for the patient during this encounter?

Step #3: Are there any details missing or incomplete for which you would need to query the physician? [If so, ask your instructor.]

Step #4: Check for any relevant guidance, including reading all of the symbols and notations in the Tabular List and the appropriate sections of the Official Guidelines.

Step #5: Determine the correct diagnosis code or codes to explain why this encounter was medically necessary.

Step #6: Double-check your work.

(continued)

> **Answer:**
>
> Did you determine this to be the correct code?
>
> **D69.3**   Immune thrombocytopenic purpura
>
> Great work!

7.3 Conditions Related to Blood Types and the Rh Factor

Antigens on Red Blood Cells

Antigens sit on the surface of red blood cells, while **antibodies** are located within the blood plasma. Antigens are proteins that cause antibodies to form, and each antibody can connect with only one specific type of antigen. Antigens that are located on RBCs are categorized in two ways: blood type and Rh factor.

Blood Type

You may know what **blood type** you have: type A, type B, type AB, or type O. This is something that is inherited from your parents.

- An individual with type A blood has only antigen A on his or her red blood cells.
- An individual with type B blood has only antigen B on his or her red blood cells.
- An individual with type AB blood has both antigens—A and B.
- An individual with type O blood has neither antigen—neither A nor B.

Rh Factor

Another antigen that may or may not be present on the surface of a red blood cell is called **Rh (Rhesus) factor**. This is also an inherited situation.

- An individual identified as Rh-negative does *not* have the Rh antigen.
- An individual identified as Rh-positive *does* have the Rh antigen.

Because Rh factor is inherited, there is concern about additional complications if an Rh-negative woman becomes pregnant with a Rh-positive fetus (the father is Rh-positive). The good news is, often, the placenta will prevent the mother's blood from mixing with the baby's blood, keeping both mother and baby safe.

> ### EXAMPLE
>
> O36.012   Maternal care for anti-D (Rh) antibodies, second trimester
> Z31.82   Encounter for Rh incompatibility status
>
> When the mother is seen so Rh compatibility can be determined and, if necessary, dealt with, these codes are examples for reporting why the encounter was medically necessary.

When the mother is Rh-negative and her body makes antibodies to her fetus's Rh-positive blood cells, and the antibodies cross the placenta, it can result in Rh incompatibility, resulting in a large number of red blood cells in the fetus's bloodstream that may be destroyed, known as hemolytic disease of the newborn.

Antigen
A substance that promotes the production of antibodies.

Antibodies
Immune responses to antigens.

Blood Type
A system of classifying blood based on the antigens present on the surface of the individual's red blood cells; also known as *blood group*.

Rh (Rhesus) Factor
An antigen located on the red blood cell that produces immunogenic responses in those individuals without it.

> **EXAMPLES**
>
> P55.0   Rh isoimmunization of newborn [hemolytic disease (newborn)]
> P55.1   ABO isoimmunization of newborn
>
> A neonate affected by the Rh factor may be diagnosed with a hemolytic disease.

When proper precautions have not been taken while the baby is in utero, hydrops fetalis due to hemolytic disease, also known as immune hydrops fetalis, can develop. This is a known complication of Rh incompatibility and leads the neonate's entire body to swell, interfering with the proper function of body organs and systems.

P56.0   **Hydrops fetalis due to isoimmunization**

LET'S CODE IT! SCENARIO

Neonate Alvarez, male, was born vaginally yesterday, 09/05/2018, at 15:25 without incident. Apgar scores: 1 min.—10, 5 min.—10.

Four hours later, extensive purpura became visible on his abdomen, arms, and legs. No jaundice was observed. His 29-year-old mother was given a blood transfusion for a postpartum hemorrhage after her first pregnancy 3 years earlier. The mother's serum was found to contain IgG antibodies to the father's platelets and to some of a panel of platelets from normal, unrelated donors. These antibodies were typed as specific anti-HPA-1A antibodies and had been incited by the previous pregnancy and transfusion.

These antibodies crossed the placenta, manifesting as alloimmune thrombocytopenia in this neonate. Additionally, the neonate was found to have red cell incompatibility.

An exchange transfusion was performed to compensate for hemolysis. While it is unusual for an ABO incompatibility to require an exchange transfusion, it worked. The neonate's platelet count returned to normal quickly due to free reactant antibody to platelets having been removed by the exchange.

We kept the neonate for observation for another 48 hours and then discharged him to his mother. She was told to follow up in 1 week at the office or phone PRN.

Let's Code It!

The baby was born and diagnosed with *alloimmune thrombocytopenia*. In the Alphabetic Index, let's find our key term:

Thrombocytopenia

As you read down the indented list, there are two choices that may pop out at you:

Thrombocytopenia
     Congenital D69.42
     Neonatal, transitory P61.0
         Due to
             Exchange transfusion P61.0

Congenital means "present at birth," and this condition was. However, the patient is a neonate, and the documentation states that this condition is due to the exchange with his mother. One thing to always remember: You can always look up both terms in the Tabular List. So let's do just that—take a look at them both:

D69.42   **Congenital and hereditary thrombocytopenia purpura**
P61.0   **Transient neonatal thrombocytopenia**

(continued)

Let's go back to the documentation. The physician notes that the baby contracted this condition as a result of the transfusion his mother received previously. So, this is not actually inherited because it is not the result of genetics; it is the result of circumstances. In addition, the treatment worked, so the baby no longer has the blood problem, meaning the thrombocytopenia was temporary (transient). This points us toward the accurate code of

P61.0   **Transient neonatal thrombocytopenia**

Check the top of this subsection as well as the head of this chapter in ICD-10-CM. You will find a **NOTE**, an INCLUDES notation, and an EXCLUDES2 notation at the beginning of this chapter. Read carefully. Do any relate to this neonate's diagnosis? No. Turn to the Official Guidelines and read Section 1.c.16. There is nothing specifically applicable here either.

Now you can report P61.0 for baby boy Alvarez's diagnosis with confidence.

Good work!

Transfusions

Due to the existence of antigens located on the surface of the patient's red blood cells, any time a patient requires a **transfusion** of blood, it must be checked for compatibility with regard to type and Rh factor; otherwise, serious consequences could occur.

People with type O blood have neither antigen; anyone can accept this blood type. Individuals with type O blood are known as *universal donors*. So, a patient with type A blood can receive a transfusion of *only* type A or type O blood. An individual with type B blood can receive *only* type B or type O blood. Those with type AB blood have both types of antigens, so they can receive type A blood, type B blood, or type O blood. For this reason, they are known as *universal recipients*.

However, attention must still be paid to Rh factor compatibility. A patient with Rh-positive blood can receive either Rh-positive or Rh-negative blood. However, patients with Rh-negative blood should only receive Rh-negative blood. Because of these facts, in an emergency, when time cannot be taken to test the patient's blood, Rh-negative blood is used.

The concern about both blood type and Rh factor compatibility arises from the dangers that can happen when the correct antibodies and antigens are not in place. For example, if an Rh-negative patient receives Rh-positive blood, anti-Rh antibodies would be created, causing red blood cell **agglutination** and **hemolysis**. Agglutination occurs when antibodies merge with antigens, causing red blood cells to clump together. Hemolysis is the process of cells rupturing—destroying red blood cells and releasing hemoglobin into the bloodstream.

Transfusion
The provision of one person's blood or plasma to another individual.

Agglutination
The process of red blood cells combining together in a mass or lump.

Hemolysis
The destruction of red blood cells, resulting in the release of hemoglobin into the bloodstream.

EXAMPLES

Complications of incompatibility can occur when a transfusion is administered without a valid match to the patient. Because this condition is a complication of the transfusion, this diagnosis is not reported from Chapter 3 in ICD-10-CM. As the result of an External Cause, this is reported from the following code category:

☑4 T80	Complications following infusion, transfusion, and therapeutic injection
T80.411A	Rh incompatibility with delayed hemolytic transfusion reaction, initial encounter
T80.310A	ABO incompatibility with acute hemolytic transfusion reaction
T80.A10A	Non-ABO incompatibility with acute hemolytic transfusion reaction

7.4 Disorders of White Blood Cells and Blood-Forming Organs

White Blood Cell Disorders

Remember from when you took anatomy class, there are five major types of white blood cells, each of which can malfunction and be unable to perform its job keeping the body working properly.

- *Neutrophils* contain enzymes that work to destroy parts of bacterial pathogens that have been consumed by phagocytes.
- *Lymphocytes* are critical in the immune response.
- *Monocytes* are large blood cells that travel throughout the body and destroy damaged red blood cells.
- *Eosinophils* destroy some parasites in addition to controlling inflammation and allergic reactions.
- *Basophils* create heparin, a blood-thinning agent that prevents inappropriate blood clotting, and create histamines, involved in allergic reactions.

Neutropenia

Neutropenia is a condition when the patient's bone marrow produces an abnormally low number of white blood cells. This may be an ineffective number of cells being created or a loss of neutrophils at a rate faster than they can be replaced by new cells. Remember that white blood cells fight infection. Once created in the bone marrow, these cells are released into the bloodstream, so they can move about the body to wherever they are needed.

A diagnosis of neutropenia may be a congenital condition, an adverse reaction to chemotherapy or other medications, or a malfunction of the hematopoiesis process.

D70.0	**Congenital agranulocytosis**
	(congenital neutropenia)
	(Kostmann's disease)
D70.1	**Agranulocytosis secondary to cancer chemotherapy**
	Code also underlying neoplasm
	Use additional code for adverse effect, if applicable, to identify drug (T45.1X5)
D70.2	**Other drug-induced agranulocytosis**
	Use additional code for adverse effect, if applicable, to identify drug (T36-T50 with fifth or sixth character 5)
D70.3	**Neutropenia due to infection**
D70.4	**Cyclic neutropenia**

Leukopenia and Leukocytosis

In leukopenia, the body is not producing the required number of leukocytes.

D72.810	**Lymphocytopenia**
D72.819	**Decreased white blood cell count, unspecified**

Of course, while an insufficient quantity of cells is not going to accomplish what is needed by the body, too many can also cause havoc. In leukocytosis, the body creates too many leukocytes. This may be a correct action because these cells are part of the immune response to certain pathogens. In that case, the elevated white blood cell count would be a sign that an infection is present, and not reported separately. Without a reason stated, this may be a malfunction, and its own condition.

D72.820	**Lymphocytosis (symptomatic)**
D72.829	**Elevated white blood cell count, unspecified**

> **CODING BITES**
>
> Leukemia is a malignancy of the white blood cells, resulting in the bone marrow producing abnormal white blood cells that do not function as needed. This is why it is reported from the Neoplasms section of ICD-10-CM, specifically the C91–C95 code categories.

Monocytic, Eosinophilic, and Basophilic Conditions

It is logical that the malfunctions causing too few, or too many, neutrophils and leukocytes might also occur to the other types of white blood cells.

D72.818	Other decreased white blood cell count (Basophilic leukopenia) (Eosinophilic leukopenia) (Monocytopenia)
D72.821	Monocytosis (symptomatic)
D72.823	Leukemoid reaction (Basophilic leukemoid reaction) (Monocytic leukemoid reaction) (Neutrophilic leukemoid reaction)

Splenic Dysfunction

The spleen is part of the lymphatic system, but it contains white blood cells that work to fight infection. Damage to this organ can be caused by disease or trauma. Problems with the spleen caused by pathogens are reported from this section of ICD-10-CM.

> ### EXAMPLES
>
> D73.0   Hyposplenism (Atrophy of spleen)
> D73.3   Abscess of spleen
>
> A pathogen or other disease that interferes with the proper function of the spleen is reported from this chapter of ICD-10-CM.

However, an injury to the spleen caused by a traumatic event would be reported from the *Injury, Poisoning, and Certain Other Consequences of External Causes* chapter of ICD-10-CM.

> ### EXAMPLES
>
> S36.021A   Major contusion of spleen, initial encounter
> S36.030A   Superficial (capsular) laceration of spleen, initial encounter
>
> Even though the spleen is part of the immune system, traumatic injuries are still reported from the appropriate chapter in ICD-10-CM.

When the problem with the spleen is a congenital anomaly, the appropriate codes will be found in the *Congenital Malformations, Deformations, and Chromosomal Abnormalities* chapter of ICD-10-CM.

> ### EXAMPLES
>
> Q89.01   Asplenia (congenital)
> Q89.09   Congenital malformations of spleen
>
> These codes explain that the malfunction of this organ (the spleen) occurred in utero.

Manifestations of Other Diseases

When a condition causes a malfunction in the blood system and/or the blood-forming organs, it might be a manifestation. If this is the case, the underlying condition will be reported first, followed by this code:

D77   Other disorders of blood and blood-forming organs in diseases classified elsewhere

YOU CODE IT! CASE STUDY

PATIENT: Frank Copeland

DISCHARGE SUMMARY

DATE OF ADMISSION: 03/15/2018
DATE OF DISCHARGE: 03/21/2018
ADMISSION DIAGNOSIS: Neutropenic fever.
DISCHARGE DIAGNOSES:

1. Neutropenic fever.
2. Acute myelogenous leukemia, status post induction and three cycles of high-dose Ara-C.
3. Thrombocytopenia.

PROCEDURES PERFORMED:

1. Two-view chest x-ray.
2. One unit of PRBC transfusion.

HOSPITAL COURSE: The patient is a very pleasant 54-year-old male with acute myelogenous leukemia who has undergone three cycles of high-dose Ara-C. He was transferred here after he presented to an outside facility with a 1-day onset of fevers and chills. He had a measured temperature at the outside hospital at that time of 102 degrees. He was transferred to this facility and admitted to the oncology service.

He was initially placed on cefepime, and blood cultures were drawn. All cultures throughout the course of his hospitalization turned out to be negative. He, however, remained febrile for the majority of his hospitalization. Upon presentation, he did complain of 1-day onset of profuse watery diarrhea that was extremely foul smelling. Of note, he was on p.o. prophylactic Levaquin due to his neutropenia. He was also on prophylactic acyclovir. Due to his being on antibiotics and history of diarrhea, a stool PCR was collected but resulted negative. Before the stool PCR resulted, he was placed on Flagyl as empiric coverage for suspected *C. diff* colitis. After the stool PCR resulted negative, Flagyl was discontinued.

During the short 24 hours when he was on Flagyl, he seemed to have defervesced, and his fever curve trended down. However, after the Flagyl was discontinued, he started having worsened diarrhea and the fevers went back up again. For this reason, a *C. diff* PCR was ordered and the Flagyl was resumed. The *C. diff* PCR was also negative. Until that point, he remained on cefepime and the Flagyl was also decided to be continued since the patient seemed to improve with it. The thinking was that he may have had some colitis that was not related to *C. diff.*

Six days into his hospitalization, he continued to have fever. At this juncture, vancomycin was added to see if this would help. Repeat blood cultures were negative. Cultures were even drawn from the port that he had. There was some discussion as to whether his fevers may have been caused by the cefepime. The cefepime was discontinued. At this time, however, his fever curve had already started slightly trending down. Over the next 48 hours, he remained afebrile.

The vancomycin and Flagyl were discontinued the day before discharge, and he remained afebrile that night. His diarrhea had resolved over the last 4 to 5 days of his hospitalization and he received Imodium for this. The remainder of his hospitalization was unremarkable and he felt well. Of note, he did complain of poor appetite. We advised him to try to eat as much as he can and at the very least remain hydrated with Gatorade, and he understood that it may take some time for his appetite to completely return to normal.

He did frequently have hypokalemia and hypomagnesemia. This was presumed to be secondary to the diarrhea. Both of these electrolytes were replaced appropriately. However, even after the diarrhea resolved, he continued to have hypokalemia despite replacement. He later notified us that this issue is not new and that he actually takes potassium supplementation at home. He reported that he had p.o. potassium chloride at home and that he did not need medication or a refill for this. He could not, however, recall the dosage. We do not know the etiology of his

(continued)

hypokalemia as this was not worked up while he was inpatient due to again thinking that his hypokalemia was a result of his diarrhea.

On the day of discharge, he was also instructed to resume his prophylactic Levaquin and acyclovir.

DISCHARGE MEDICATIONS:

1. Acyclovir 400 mg p.o. b.i.d.
2. HCTZ 25 mg p.o. daily.
3. Lopressor 25 mg p.o. b.i.d.
4. Pravastatin 10 mg p.o. at bedtime.
5. Norethindrone 5 mg p.o. daily.
6. Levaquin 500 mg p.o. daily.
7. Zofran 4 mg sublingually q.8 hours p.r.n. nausea.
8. Norco 5/325 one tablet p.o. q.4 hours p.r.n. pain.

FOLLOWUP APPOINTMENT: Dr. Constantine Revorsky in 1 week for followup for chemotherapy.
FOLLOWUP LABS AND STUDIES: CBC, CMP before appointment with Dr. Revorsky.
DISCHARGE DIET: Regular as tolerated.
DISCHARGE ACTIVITY: As tolerated.

You Code It!

Read this Discharge Summary for Frank Copeland and determine only the principal diagnosis code.

Step #1: Read the case carefully and completely.

Step #2: Abstract the scenario. Which main words or terms describe why the physician cared for the patient during this encounter?

Step #3: Are there any details missing or incomplete for which you would need to query the physician? [If so, ask your instructor.]

Step #4: Check for any relevant guidance, including reading all of the symbols and notations in the Tabular List and the appropriate sections of the Official Guidelines.

Step #5: Determine the correct diagnosis code or codes to explain why this encounter was medically necessary.

Step #6: Double-check your work.

Answer:

Did you determine this to be the principal diagnosis code?

    D70.9   Neutropenia, unspecified

Antibodies
Immune responses to antigens.

Antigen
A substance that promotes the production of antibodies.

7.5 Disorders Involving the Immune System

The immune system is the armed forces network that develops special forces, known as **antibodies**, produced by plasma cells in the blood to protect the body from pathogens and other invaders (**antigens**) that may disrupt proper function. In the previous section, you learned about the role that the different types of white blood cells play in guarding the good health of the body . . . your immune system.

Researchers continue to study and learn more about the actual mechanisms in place, to employ in the development of more effective and efficient treatments when the body cannot fight alone. The integration of technology and the greater availability of genetic details support these efforts to eliminate past and current illness and disease, and to fight off or prevent new conditions from evolving.

Immunodeficiencies

Immunodeficiency disorders are conditions when the patient's immune response is diminished or totally ineffective. Typically, immunodeficiency disorders occur when T or B lymphocytes (special white blood cells) do not work properly. Immunodeficiency disorders may be inherited (genetically passed from parent to child) or acquired, an adverse effect to another illness, such as HIV-positive status or some malignancies; long-term use of certain medications, such as corticosteroids; chemotherapy treatments; or a manifestation of a splenectomy (the surgical removal of the spleen).

- Hereditary hypogammaglobulinemia, also known as autosomal recessive agammaglobulinemia, is an inherited immunodeficiency disorder often causing pulmonary and digestive disorders—reported with code D80.0 Hereditary hypogammaglobulinemia
- Agammaglobulinemia with immunoglobulin-bearing B-lymphocytes is a nonfamilial (acquired) defect in the body's antibodies—reported with code D80.1 Nonfamilial hypogammaglobulinemia

> **CODING BITES**
>
> Generally, allergies are reported by either the substance or object to which the patient is allergic or by the response suffered by the patient.
>
> K52.2- Allergic and dietetic gastroenteritis and colitis
>
> J30.1 Allergic rhinitis due to pollen
>
> J30.81 Allergic rhinitis due to animal (cat) (dog) hair and dander

Allergies

An allergy is actually an immune system false alarm, responding to something as if it were a pathogen able to harm the body, when, in reality, it is not. In medical terminology, this is known as a hypersensitivity reaction. These reactions are divided into four classes. Classes I, II, and III are caused by antibodies, IgE or IgG, which are produced by B cells in response to an allergen. Class IV reactions are caused by T cells. In these cases, the T cells might turn traitor and cause damage to the body, or they may ignite macrophages and eosinophils, which, in turn, may damage host cells.

Sarcoidosis

The specific etiology of sarcoidosis is still unknown; however, most researchers believe it is a combination of a genetic susceptibility with a certain exposure to something that triggers the immune system to release chemicals that are ineffective at combating inflammation. Instead, the cells clump together and become granulomas (tumors that result from an ulcerated infection) situated within certain organs throughout the body, such as the lungs, liver, or skin. This diagnosis is reported with a code from category D86 Sarcoidosis.

> **EXAMPLES**
>
> D86.0 Sarcoidosis of lung
> D86.3 Sarcoidosis of skin
> D86.84 Sarcoidosis pyelonephritis
>
> As you can see from these three examples, you will need to know the specific anatomical site of the sarcoidosis before you can determine an accurate code.

Wiskott-Aldrich Syndrome

When a patient suffers from Wiskott-Aldrich syndrome, this genetic mutation causes white blood cells to malfunction, increasing the body's susceptibility to inflammatory diseases and other immunodeficiency disorders. Eczema, thrombocytopenia, and pyogenic infections often develop and put the patient at a higher-than-normal risk of autoimmune diseases. This condition is reported with code D82.0 Wiskott-Aldrich syndrome.

YOU CODE IT! CASE STUDY

Carol-Anne Nieman, a 41-year-old female, came in complaining of discomfort and tenderness under her arms and in her neck. Dr. Rothenberg performed a physical exam, revealing swollen lymph nodes. Lab work showed she was suffering with sarcoidosis of her lymph nodes.

You Code It!

Go through the steps of coding, and determine the code or codes that should be reported for this encounter between Dr. Rothenberg and Carol-Anne.

Step #1: Read the case carefully and completely.

Step #2: Abstract the scenario. Which main words or terms describe why the physician cared for the patient during this encounter?

Step #3: Are there any details missing or incomplete for which you would need to query the physician? [If so, ask your instructor.]

Step #4: Check for any relevant guidance, including reading all of the symbols and notations in the Tabular List and the appropriate sections of the Official Guidelines.

Step #5: Determine the correct diagnosis code or codes to explain why this encounter was medically necessary.

Step #6: Double-check your work.

Answer:

Did you determine this to be the correct code?

D86.1   Sarcoidosis of lymph nodes

Great work!

CODING BITES

- One-third (about 33%) of people with DVT/PE will have a recurrence within 10 years.
- Approximately 5 to 8% of the U.S. population has one of several genetic risk factors, also known as inherited thrombophilia, in which a genetic defect can be identified that increases the risk for thrombosis.

Source: http://www.cdc.gov/ncbddd/dvt/data.html

Chapter Summary

Blood flows through your arteries and veins, transporting oxygen (O_2) to nourish tissues and carrying away the waste (CO_2) from those cells. Production of the components of the blood, including red blood cells, white blood cells, and platelets, occurs within the red bone marrow, specifically, within the sternum, ribs, and vertebrae in the adult. Since blood is systemic (traveling throughout the entire body), blood tests are an excellent diagnostic tool because the minor invasiveness of venipuncture can yield massive amounts of information about the health of the body. When the blood system malfunctions, serious health consequences result.

CHAPTER 7 REVIEW
Coding Blood Conditions

Let's Check It! Terminology

Match each key term to the appropriate definition.

1. LO 7.3 A system of classifying blood based on the antigens present on the surface of the individual's red blood cells. **E**
2. LO 7.1 Cells within the blood that help to protect the body from pathogens. **P**
3. LO 7.3 The process of red blood cells combining together in a mass or lump. **A**
4. LO 7.3 Immune responses to antigens. **B**
5. LO 7.2 Clotting; the change from a liquid into a thickened substance. **F**
6. LO 7.2 The interruption of bleeding. **J**
7. LO 7.3 An antigen located on the red blood cell that produces immunogenic responses in those individuals without it. **N**
8. LO 7.3 The provision of one person's blood or plasma to another individual. **O**
9. LO 7.1 Fluid pumped throughout the body, carrying oxygen and nutrients to the cells and wastes away from the cells. **D**
10. LO 7.1 The fluid part of the blood. **K**
11. LO 7.1 Cells within the blood that contain hemoglobin responsible for carrying oxygen to tissues. **M**
12. LO 7.1 The part of the red blood cell that carries oxygen. **H**
13. LO 7.3 The destruction of red blood cells resulting in the release of hemoglobin into the bloodstream. **I**
14. LO 7.1 Large cell fragments in the bone marrow that function in clotting. **L**
15. LO 7.1 The formation of blood. **G**
16. LO 7.3 A substance that promotes the production of antibodies. **C**

A. Agglutination
B. Antibody
C. Antigen
D. Blood
E. Blood Type
F. Coagulation
G. Hematopoiesis
H. Hemoglobin
I. Hemolysis
J. Hemostasis
K. Plasma
L. Platelets (PLTs)
M. Red Blood Cells (RBCs)
N. Rh Factor
O. Transfusion
P. White Blood Cells (WBCs)

Let's Check It! Concepts

Choose the most appropriate answer for each of the following questions.

1. LO 7.1 Blood is composed of all of the following *except*
   a. RBCs.
   b. WBCs.
   c. Plats.
   d. HCT.

2. LO 7.1 Red bone marrow produces white blood cells through which process?
   a. erythrocytes
   b. leukopoiesis
   c. lymphocytes
   d. erythropoiesis

3. LO 7.3 An individual with blood type B− can receive only which type(s) of blood in a transfusion?
   a. type B−
   b. type B+
   c. type O+
   d. type B− or type O−

4. LO 7.4 _____ create heparin, a blood thinning agent that prevents inappropriate blood clotting, and create histamines, involved in allergic reactions.
   a. Neutrophils
   b. Lymphocytes
   c. Eosinophils
   d. Basophils

CHAPTER 7 REVIEW

5. LO 7.1 Which type of anemia results from an insufficient number of healthy red blood cells due to abnormal or premature destruction?
   a. aplastic anemia
   b. hemolytic anemia
   c. nutritional anemia
   d. hemorrhagic anemia

6. LO 7.2 _____ is a low platelet count most often due to increased platelet destruction, decreased platelet production, or malfunctioning platelets.
   a. Pancytopenia
   b. Leukocytopenia
   c. Thrombocytopenia
   d. Erythrocytopenia

7. LO 7.1 Donny Cobin, a 19-year-old male, has been diagnosed with sickle-cell thalassemia with acute chest syndrome. How would you code this?
   a. D57.40
   b. D57.411
   c. D57.811
   d. D57.812

8. LO 7.3 Antigens are _____ that sit on the surface of red blood cells.
   a. proteins
   b. sugars
   c. markers
   d. chromosomes

9. LO 7.5 Typically, immunodeficiency disorders occur when _____ do not work properly.
   a. T lymphocytes
   b. B lymphocytes
   c. T or B lymphocytes
   d. None of these

10. LO 7.5 The genetic mutation causing white blood cells to malfunction, increasing the body's susceptibility to inflammatory diseases and other immunodeficiency disorders, is known as _____.
    a. Clarke-Hadfield Syndrome
    b. Heubner-Herter Syndrome
    c. Wiskott-Aldrich Syndrome
    d. Lennox-Gastaut Syndrome

Let's Check It! Rules and Regulations

Please answer the following questions from the knowledge you have gained after reading this chapter.

1. LO 7.1 Discuss what blood is, how it is created, and what it consists of; include how many blood cells are needed for a healthy body.
2. LO 7.2 Explain the two types of clotting disorders.
3. LO 7.3 When a patient requires a transfusion of blood, it must first be checked for compatibility. What does this mean?
4. LO 7.4 Discuss the difference between neutropenia, leukopenia, and leukocytosis.
5. LO 7.5 What are immunodeficiency disorders and are they inherited or acquired?

YOU CODE IT! Basics

First, identify the main term in the following diagnose; then code the diagnosis.

Example: Posthemorrhagic anemia, chronic
   a. main term: *anemia*   b. diagnosis *D50.0*

1. Hemoglobin H disease:
   a. main term: _____   b. diagnosis: _____

2. Purpura fulminans:
   a. main term: _____   b. diagnosis: _____

3. Anemia due to vitamin B12 intrinsic factor deficiency:
   a. main term: _____   b. diagnosis: _____

4. Cyclic hematopoiesis:
   a. main term: _____ b. diagnosis: _____
5. Antineoplastic chemotherapy–induced pancytopenia:
   a. main term: _____ b. diagnosis: _____
6. Minor alpha thalassemia:
   a. main term: _____ b. diagnosis: _____
7. Medullary hypoplasia:
   a. main term: _____ b. diagnosis: _____
8. Infantile pseudoleukemia:
   a. main term: _____ b. diagnosis: _____
9. Deficiency factor VIII:
   a. main term: _____ b. diagnosis: _____
10. Congenital neutropenia:
    a. main term: _____ b. diagnosis: _____
11. Sickle-cell Hb-C with crisis disease:
    a. main term: _____ b. diagnosis: _____
12. Agranulocytosis due to infection:
    a. main term: _____ b. diagnosis: _____
13. Hemolytic-uremic syndrome:
    a. main term: _____ b. diagnosis: _____
14. Polycythemia due to erythropoietin:
    a. main term: _____ b. diagnosis: _____
15. Non-Langerhans cell histiocytosis:
    a. main term: _____ b. diagnosis: _____

YOU CODE IT! Practice

Using the techniques described in this chapter, carefully read through the case studies and determine the most accurate ICD-10-CM code(s) and external cause code(s), if appropriate, for each case study.

1. James Abney, a 7-month-old male, is brought in by his parents to see Dr. Fay, his pediatrician. Dr. Fay notes a temperature of 106 F, jaundice, and generalized weakness and admits James to Weston Hospital for a full work-up. The CBC and Coombs' test results confirm the diagnosis of favism anemia.

2. Sam Goodman, a 9-year-old male, presents today for a sports physical in order to play on his school baseball team. Dr. Inabinet notes splenomegaly. The results from the CBC test and peripheral blood smear confirm a diagnosis of Hb-C disease.

3. Arthur Hylton, a 45-year-old male, presents today with the complaint of general weakness and overall tiredness. Arthur works for an industrial factory and has been exposed to a large quantity of benzene. Dr. Burger completes an examination, noting an irregular heartbeat and hand tremors. Arthur is admitted to the hospital. The results of the bone marrow biopsy confirm a diagnosis of aplastic anemia due to accidental poisoning by benzene.

4. Rosalyn Burkett, a 37-year-old female, presents today with the complaint of migraines and blurred vision. After an examination and a review of the laboratory tests, Dr. Flick diagnoses Rosalyn with Lupus anticoagulant syndrome.

5. Tilley Cabe, a 9-month-old female, is brought in to see Dr. Peterson, her pediatrician. Tilley has had a persistent low-grade fever for 4 days that has not diminished. Dr. Peterson notes a temperature of 100.2 and splenomegaly. Tilley is not thriving. Dr. Peterson admits her to the hospital. The laboratory results reveal Tilley has a low natural killer cell activity and cytopenia, which confirm the diagnosis of hemophagocytic lymphohistiocytosis (HLH).

6. Glenn Carballero, a 15-year-old male, presents today with the complaint of weakness and generalized muscular pains. Dr. Douglass notes an erythematous periorofacial macular rash. After a thorough examination and laboratory tests are completed, Glenn is diagnosed with biotinidase deficiency.

7. Sadie Thompson, an 18-month-old female, was born with TAR syndrome (thrombocytopenia with absent radius). Sadie is brought in today by her mother with the complaint of excessive bruising without significant trauma. After an examination and the laboratory tests are completed, Dr. Dotson diagnosis Sadie with congenital thrombocytopenia purpura.

8. Victor Motts, a 6-month-old male, is brought in by his mother to see his pediatrician, Dr. Stewart. Victor experienced a type of spasm. Dr. James notes skeletal abnormalities and cyanosis as well as some hearing difficulties and admits him to Weston Hospital. A fluorescence in situ hybridization (FISH) blood test confirms a diagnosis of Di George's syndrome.

9. Lindsey Williams, a 33-year-old female, has not been feeling well and is seen by Dr. Goldburg, who notes jaundice. Lindsey admits to feeling weak and being dizzy. Blood tests return a hemoglobin of 6.3 g/dL. Lindsey is admitted to the hospital for a blood transfusion; while there, a peripheral blood smear was performed that showed echinocytes, confirming a diagnosis of pyruvate kinase deficiency anemia.

10. Antonio Scott, a 47-year-old male, presents today with the complaint of a cough, runny nose, and a sore throat. Dr. Benton completes an examination and reviews the results of the CBC test and diagnoses Stanley with lymphocytopenia.

11. Ivory Presnell, a 75-year-old female, comes in today complaining of fever, chills, and night sweats. She says she feels tired and has lost 5 lbs. within a week. Dr. Shirley notes nail clubbing and completes an in-house CBC test; results: hemoglobin of 7.9 g/dL. Ivory is admitted to Weston Hospital, where a tissue biopsy is taken, returning a positive reading for extra-pulmonary tuberculosis. Ivory is diagnosed with anemia due to tuberculosis.

12. Buddy Dent, a 59-year-old male with chronic kidney disease, stage 4, comes to see Dr. Wilberly complaining of extreme weakness. Dr. Wilberly completes a full blood workup and notes the following results: hemoglobin—8.2 g/dL, creatinine—52 mg/dL, and BUN—102 mg/dL. Buddy is diagnosed with anemia due to chronic kidney disease and is scheduled for a transfusion.

13. Juanita Ilderton, a 41-year-old female, received a blood transfusion 12 hours ago; now she is experiencing fever, chills, and dizziness. A direct Coombs' test is performed, which confirms a diagnosis of acute Rh blood transfusion incompatibility after a transfusion.

14. Richard Greene, 33-year-old male, comes to see Dr. Walter with the complaints of tiredness and weakness. Dr. Walter completes bloodwork and a bone marrow biopsy. Richard is diagnosed with chronic lymphocytic, B-cell type leukemia.

15. Billy Stevenson, a 10-year-old-male, is brought in by his father to see Dr. Loveichelle. Billy has developed a cough and fever. Billy says he feels really tired. Mr. Stevenson also stated they can't get Billy to eat. Dr. Loveichelle completes an examination and an in-house CBC. Billy's hemoglobin is 7.4 g/dL. Billy is admitted to the hospital for a full workup. Once all the laboratory results have been reviewed, Billy is diagnosed with hookworm anemia.

YOU CODE IT! Application

The following exercises provide practice in abstracting physicians' documentation from our health care facility, Prader, Bracker, & Associates. These case studies are modeled on real patient encounters. Using the techniques described in this chapter, carefully read through the case studies and determine the most accurate ICD-10-CM code(s) and external cause code(s), if appropriate, for each case study.

PRADER, BRACKER, & ASSOCIATES

A Complete Health Care Facility

159 Healthcare Way · SOMEWHERE, FL 32811 · 407-555-6789

PATIENT: KRIESEL, BROOKE

ACCOUNT/EHR #: KRIEBR001

DATE: 09/23/18

Attending Physician: Oscar R. Prader, MD

Brooke Kriesel, a 41-year-old female, presents today with the complaint of fatigue—2 weeks duration. She admits to moderate shortness of breath with exertion; denies chest pain with exertion or at rest. No bright red blood per rectal exam or melena. She has had heavy menstrual periods—1 year duration.

PAST MEDICAL HISTORY: Noncontributory

FAMILY HISTORY: Noncontributory

OTC medication—aspirin, 81 mg daily—3 month duration.

PHYSICAL EXAM:

General appearance: Pale, no acute distress.

Vital signs: Ht: 5' 7', Wt: 146, T: 99.8, R: 15, HR: 81 and regular, BP: 128/81. Pale conjunctiva; mucous membranes, moist with no apparent lesions; chest, clear; heart, regular rate and rhythm, no murmurs, rubs, or gallops. The abdomen—soft, nontender, and nondistended; no hepatosplenomegaly; rectal examination—no masses and heme negative, brown stool is present.

Hemoglobin level—7.4 g/dL. There is evidence of marked microcytosis and hypochromia with a decreased hemoglobin level.

DIAGNOSIS: Anemia due to iron deficiency

ORP/pw   D: 09/25/18 09:50:16   T: 09/25/18 12:55:01

Determine the most accurate ICD-10-CM code(s).

PRADER, BRACKER, & ASSOCIATES

A Complete Health Care Facility

159 Healthcare Way • SOMEWHERE, FL 32811 • 407-555-6789

PATIENT: LAKEMONT, CALEB

ACCOUNT/EHR #: LAKECA001

DATE: 10/03/18

Attending Physician: Oscar R. Prader, MD

Calib Lakemont, a 29-year-old male, came to see me with complaints of bruising easily and prolonged nosebleeds. He also showed me a rash, nonpainful/nonitchy, on his ankles and shins. He denies making any recent changes in body soap or household detergents. Dr. Prader notes bruises on his arms and trunk; patient denies any type of trauma that would cause bruising.

PE: Ht: 5' 11", Wt: 185, T: 98.4, R: 13, HR: 57, BP: 115/79. No lymphadenopathy or hepatosplenomegaly. Stool sample testing is guaiac positive.

Lab results: CBC and peripheral smear confirm patient is thrombocytopenic. There is no evidence of a coagulation disorder.

DIAGNOSIS: Autoimmune thrombocytopenia (ITP)

ORP/pw   D: 10/05/18 09:50:16   T: 10/05/18 12:55:01

Determine the most accurate ICD-10-CM code(s).

CHAPTER 7 REVIEW

WESTON HOSPITAL

629 Healthcare Way • SOMEWHERE, FL 32811 • 407-555-6541

PATIENT: FUENTES, ERIN

ACCOUNT/EHR #: FUENER001

DATE: 09/16/18

Attending Physician: Renee O. Bracker, MD

Pt is a 9-year-old female brought in by her parents to see Dr. Bracker. I last saw Erin 6 months ago, at which time she was thriving. Erin has experienced several nosebleeds over the last week. After questioning Erin, she admits she gets tired easily and doesn't feel much like eating.

PE: Ht: 52.5", Wt: 60 lb., T: 101.2, R: 18, HR: 81, BP: 125/70. Dr. Bracker notes that Erin is having difficulty focusing and articulating. Weight loss of 3 lb. since last visit. A CBC is performed; results show a hemoglobin of 6.8 g/dL. Erin is admitted.

CV: Normal S1, S2, regular.

Pulm: Unlabored respiration, clear, bilaterally.

Abd: Soft, nontender, nondistended, without organomegaly or mass.

Extr: Warm, well perfused, no edema, notable for several 3 cm ecchymoses on the forearms and thighs bilaterally; in addition, there is a petechial rash over the ankles and feet bilaterally.

Neuro: Alert and oriented

Laboratory results:

Hemoglobin—6.7 g/dL

Platelet count—35 × 10/L

Leukocyte count—3.1 × 10/L

Neutrophil count—1.4 × 10/L

INR—1.5

PT—16.2

Bone marrow aspirate was performed—20% promyelocytes.

Dx: Acute promyelocytic leukemia (APL)

P: Chemotherapy with ATRA

ROB/pw   D: 09/16/18 09:50:16   T: 09/18/18 12:55:01

Determine the most accurate ICD-10-CM code(s).

WESTON HOSPITAL

629 Healthcare Way • SOMEWHERE, FL 32811 • 407-555-6541

PATIENT: FLOWERS, CATLYNNE

ACCOUNT/EHR #: FLOWCA001

DATE: 09/16/18

Attending Physician: Renee O. Bracker, MD

S: Catlynne Flowers, a 22-year-old female, presents to the emergency room today with dyspnea and cough.

O: Ht: 5' 3", Wt: 131 lb., R: 30, T: 101.2, BP: 110/67. Catlynne was diagnosed with sickle-cell disease 3 years ago. Patient appears to be in crisis. Chest x-ray confirms pulmonary infiltration. A broncho-alveolar lavage was performed; specimen was taken for culture, which confirmed the diagnosis.

A: Sickle-cell/Hb-C crisis with acute chest syndrome ACS

P: Admit to inpatient

ROB/pw   D: 09/16/18 09:50:16   T: 09/18/18 12:55:01

Determine the most accurate ICD-10-CM code(s).

WESTON HOSPITAL
629 Healthcare Way • SOMEWHERE, FL 32811 • 407-555-6541

PATIENT: ARNOLD, CAMERON

ACCOUNT/EHR #: ARNOCA001

DATE: 08/11/18

Attending Physician: Oscar R. Prader, MD

Cameron Arnold, a 39-year-old female, comes in to see Dr. Prader with complaints of weakness and several spontaneous nosebleeds that last approximately 10 minutes—10 days duration. She states that she bruises easily without any injury—3 times in the last month alone—and her menstrual periods have been notably heavier. Dr. White, the referring physician, asks that we rule out coagulopathy. PMH: non-contributory. PFH: no history of family bleeding.

Preliminary laboratory results reveal a hemoglobin of 6.7 g/dL. The mean corpuscular volume (MCV) is 71 fl. PT and APTT are within normal range.

A von Willebrand factor antigen assay, a von Willebrand factor activity assay, and factor VIII measurement were ordered; results confirm the diagnosis of von Willebrand disease.

ORP/pw   D: 08/11/18 09:50:16   T: 08/13/18 12:55:01

Determine the most accurate ICD-10-CM code(s).

8 Coding Endocrine Conditions

Key Terms

Cushing's Syndrome
Diabetes Mellitus (DM)
Dyslipidemia
Gestational Diabetes Mellitus (GDM)
Hyperglycemia
Hypoglycemia
Hypoglycemics
Hypothyroidism
Parathyroid Glands
Polydipsia
Polyuria
Secondary Diabetes Mellitus
Thyroid Gland
Type 1 Diabetes Mellitus
Type 2 Diabetes Mellitus

Learning Outcomes

After completing this chapter, the student should be able to:

LO 8.1 Identify the various disorders affecting the thyroid gland.
LO 8.2 Evaluate the details about a diabetes mellitus diagnosis to determine the correct code.
LO 8.3 Assess the relationship between diabetes mellitus and its manifestations.
LO 8.4 Interpret the documentation related to the reporting of other endocrinologic diseases.
LO 8.5 Identify the aspects of nutrition and weight required for accurate code determination.
LO 8.6 Analyze the details related to metabolic disorder diagnoses to determine the correct code.

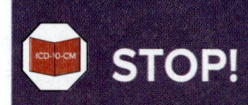

STOP! Remember, you need to follow along in your ICD-10-CM code book for an optimal learning experience.

8.1 Disorders of the Thyroid Gland

Thyroid Gland

Thyroid Gland
A two-lobed gland located in the neck that reaches around the trachea laterally and connects anteriorly by an isthmus. The thyroid gland produces hormones used for metabolic function.

The **thyroid gland** is located in the neck. Each of its two lobes reaches around the trachea laterally; they connect anteriorly by an isthmus (see Figure 8-1).

The anterior pituitary gland transmits thyroid-stimulating hormone (TSH) to the thyroid, which then extracts iodine from the blood system to create two hormones. The two hormones secreted by this gland—triiodothyronine (T_3) and thyroxine (T_4)—are collectively known as *thyroid hormone (TH)*. Thyroid hormone is responsible for stimulating the production of proteins in virtually every tissue in the body, controlling the body's metabolic rate, and increasing the quantity of oxygen used by each cell. In addition, calcitonin is produced here from the C cells located in the follicles. This hormone, secreted in response to hypercalcemia (too much calcium in the blood), promotes the deposit of calcium and works in the formation of bone.

EXAMPLES

E03.1 Congenital hypothyroidism without goiter
E07.81 Sick-euthyroid syndrome

Parathyroid Glands

Parathyroid Glands
Four small glands situated on the back of the thyroid gland that secrete parathyroid hormone.

In the posterior aspect of the thyroid gland are four partially embedded **parathyroid glands**. When stimulated by hypocalcemia (too little calcium in the blood), they

Pharynx (posterior view)

Thyroid gland

Parathyroid glands

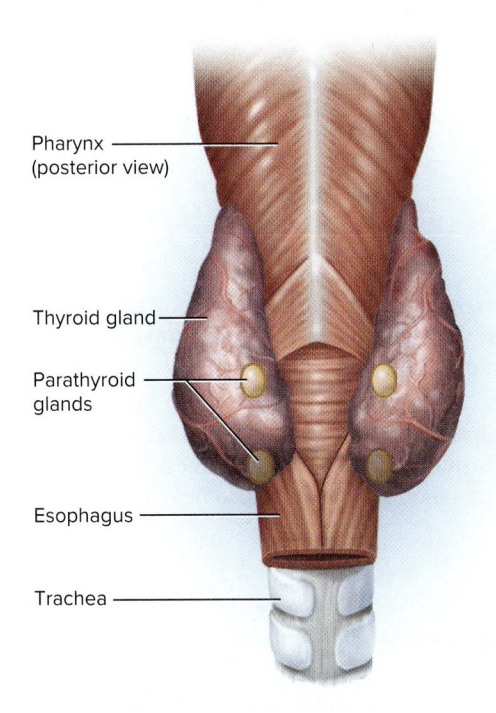

Esophagus

Trachea

FIGURE 8-1 The thyroid gland, illustrated as part of the anatomical sites within the neck
©McGraw-Hill Education

produce parathyroid hormone (PTH). PTH works in the opposite way of how calcitonin (produced by the thyroid) works.

> **EXAMPLES**
>
> E20.1   Pseudohypoparathyroidism
> E21.0   Primary hyperparathyroidism

Hypothyroidism (Adults)

Hypothyroidism is caused by an insufficient production of thyroid hormone (TH). When a patient has hypothyroidism, the thyroid converts energy more slowly than normal, resulting in an otherwise unexplained weight gain and fatigue. In addition, hypercholesterolemia, unexplained increase in weight, forgetfulness, and even unusual sensitivity to colder temperatures may be evidence of early signs of this condition.

This might be the result of irradiation therapy, infection, Hashimoto's disease (chronic autoimmune thyroiditis), or pituitary failure to produce the required amount of thyroid-stimulating hormone (TSH).

To confirm this diagnosis, radioimmunoassay and/or lab tests are performed to look at the levels of TSH. Lab tests can identify the patient's TSH levels; however, reference ranges may fluctuate depending upon the patient's age and family history. Treatment for hypothyroidism includes medication, such as levothyroxine, to replace TH.

Hypothyroidism
A condition in which the thyroid converts energy more slowly than normal, resulting in an otherwise unexplained weight gain and fatigue.

> **EXAMPLES**
>
> E03.1   Congenital hypothyroidism without goiter
> E03.2   Hypothyroidism due to medicaments and other exogenous substances
>
> *Code first* poisoning due to drug or toxin, if applicable (T36-T65 with fifth or sixth character 1-4 or 6)
> *Use additional code* for adverse effect, if applicable, to identify drug (T36-T50 with fifth or sixth character 5)
>
> *(continued)*

CHAPTER 8 | CODING ENDOCRINE CONDITIONS

> **CODING BITES**
>
> If you recognize a patient's condition from a lab report, but the physician did not document a confirmed diagnosis, you must *query* the physician. You may *not* code from the lab report.

> E03.3   Postinfectious hypothyroidism
>
> As you can see, the underlying cause of the hypothyroidism is key to determining an accurate code.

Hyperthyroidism

Hyperthyroidism, also known as *thyrotoxicosis,* is a condition in which the thyroid secretes too many hormones, more than the body needs to function properly. Interestingly, hyperthyroidism is most often a manifestation of another disease, including Graves' disease or thyroiditis.

Signs and symptoms include unexplained weight loss, rapid heart rate, and sensitivity to heat. Also, because the body systems are faster due to the excess of these hormones, irritability, trouble sleeping, hand tremors, and mood swings may also be exhibited.

> **EXAMPLES**
>
> E05.00   Thyrotoxicosis with diffuse goiter without thyrotoxic crisis or storm (Graves' disease)
> E05.11   Thyrotoxicosis with toxic single thyroid nodule with thyrotoxic crisis or storm
> E05.20   Thyrotoxicosis with toxic multinodular goiter without thyrotoxic crisis or storm
>
> As you can see from these few examples, the term *thyrotoxicosis* is used by the code descriptions, rather than the more common term *hyperthyroidism.*

Graves' Disease

Graves' disease (toxic diffuse goiter) is an autoimmune disorder. This malfunction of the immune system creates an antibody called *thyroid stimulating immunoglobulin (TSI)* that affixes itself to thyroid cells. TSI then accelerates the overproduction of the thyroid hormone.

Thyroid Nodules

Thyroid nodules are adenomas, benign neoplasms that grow in the thyroid. These nodules may stimulate the thyroid to become overactive. A toxic multinodular goiter is an accumulation of several thyroid nodules multiplying the effects, and the quantity of thyroid hormone that is overproduced.

Thyroiditis

Thyroiditis is an inflammation of the thyroid that causes thyroid hormone stored within the thyroid gland to leak out. Initially, the leakage can be identified by increased hormone levels showing in the blood. If the leak continues, this can cause hyperthyroidism.

E06.0   Acute thyroiditis
(Abscess of thyroid)
(Pyogenic thyroiditis)
Use additional code (B95–B97) to identify infectious agent

E06.1   Subacute thyroiditis
(de Quervain thyroiditis)
(Giant cell thyroiditis)
EXCLUDES1: autoimmune thyroiditis (E06.3)

E06.2   Chronic thyroiditis with transient thyrotoxicosis
EXCLUDES1: autoimmune thyroiditis (E06.3)

E06.3   Autoimmune thyroiditis
(Hashimoto's thyroiditis)
(Lymphocytic thyroiditis)

E06.4   Drug-induced thyroiditis
Use additional code for adverse effect, if applicable, to identify drug (T36-T50 with fifth or sixth character 5)

E06.5   Other chronic thyroiditis
(Chronic fibrous thyroiditis)
(Ligneous thyroiditis)
(Riedel thyroiditis)

Postpartum thyroiditis develops during the postpartum period.

O90.5   Postpartum thyroiditis

Other Disorders of the Thyroid

Additional disorders of the thyroid include

- *Nontoxic goiter,* reported from code category E04
- *Hashimoto's thyroiditis,* reported with code E06.3
- *Myxedema,* a type of hypothyroidism, is reported with code E03.9

LET'S CODE IT! SCENARIO

PATIENT: Angela Tanner

Preprocedural Diagnosis: Right thyroid tumor

Postprocedural Diagnosis: Benign tumor of right thyroid

Procedure: Isthmectomy, Right thyroidectomy

Surgeon: Samuel Rodriguez, MD

DESCRIPTION OF OPERATION: The patient was intubated with a Xomed nerve monitor endotracheal tube. The neck was extended with a shoulder roll and a transverse cervical incision was made along the skin crease, leaning to the right side. The skin incision was made and the platysma was divided. A superior flap was developed to the thyroid notch and inferior flap to the sternal notch. Crossing jugular veins were ligated with 2-0 and 3-0 silk ties. The strap muscles were separated in the midline. The right strap muscles were then lifted off of a markedly enlarged right thyroid gland. The lateral border of the gland was identified. The middle thyroid vein and its branches were doubly ligated with 3-0 silk ties and divided. The recurrent laryngeal nerve was identified at the base of the neck and we traced this superiorly. The inferior thyroid vascular bundle was noted to be quite anterior to this. We doubly ligated this with 2-0 silk ties and divided it as it entered the thyroid gland. The inferior right parathyroid gland was identified. It was noted to be adherent to the thyroid gland. We separated the two glands and placed the right inferior parathyroid gland in the base of the neck. We then identified the superior pole of the right thyroid gland. The superior thyroid vascular bundle was doubly ligated with 2-0 silk ties and divided. The right upper parathyroid gland was separated from the thyroid gland. This was also adherent to the thyroid gland. We then mobilized the gland medially. A small amount of thyroid tissue was left behind in the upper pole. The stump was doubly ligated with 2-0 silk ties and divided. This allowed us to mobilize the thyroid gland medially, and we slowly separated the nerve from the posterior surface of the thyroid gland. This nerve was adherent to the thyroid gland. The gland was left intact as we separated the thyroid gland from it, and then we lifted the thyroid gland off of the trachea. Dissection was then carried beyond the isthmus, and with the right thyroid gland in the isthmus lifted off of the trachea, we then clamped the medial

(continued)

aspect of the right thyroid lobe and we then excised the specimen. The stump was then suture ligated with running 2-0 silk stitch. Specimen was sent for pathology, and on analysis, there was no evidence of a malignancy. The thyroid stump was inspected. No bleeding was noted. No bleeding was noted from the right upper or lower parathyroid glands. The recurrent laryngeal nerve was noted to be functional throughout its course, and the inferior and superior vascular bundles were noted to be hemostatic. With assurance of hemostasis, the strap muscles were closed with running 4-0 Vicryls, platysma was closed with interrupted 4-0 Vicryls, and 5-0 Monocryls were used for subcuticular skin closure. Local anesthesia was infiltrated. The patient tolerated the procedure well. Sponge and needle counts were correct. Blood loss was minimal. The patient was extubated and taken to the recovery room in stable condition.

Let's Code It!

Dr. Rodgriquez operated on Angela to remove her right thyroid because there was a tumor on it. How do you know that the tumor was benign? The documentation states, "*Specimen was sent for pathology, and on analysis, there was no evidence of a malignancy.*"

Turn to the Neoplasm Table in your ICD-10-CM code book and find Thyroid in the first column . . .

Thyroid (gland)

Carefully read across, on that same row, to the fourth column to the right, the column titled, "Benign." Code D34 is suggested.

Now turn in the Tabular List to:

D34 Benign neoplasm of thyroid gland

This matches. But wait, there is a notation beneath this code:

Use additional code to identify any functional activity

Hmm. There is nothing in the procedure note about functional activity, and there would not be. This would be noted in the diagnostic statement. In real life, you would need to look at the other parts of the patient's record, or query the physician about this detail. For now, consider that there is documentation in the patient's medical record that the functional activity with this tumor is corticoadrenal insufficiency.

Turn back to the Alphabetic Index and find

Insufficiency, insufficient

. . . read all the way down the list to find the indented . . .

    corticoadrenal E27.40

      --primary E27.1

In the Tabular List, find

   ✓4 E27 Other disorders of adrenal gland

      E27.1 Primary adrenocortical insufficiency

   ✓5 E27.4 Other and unspecified adrenocortical insufficiency

      E27.40 Unspecified adrenocortical insufficiency

Before you report these codes, be certain to check the top of this subsection; there is an **EXCLUDES1** notation above code E20. This has no relation to this case. At the beginning of the chapter, you will find a **NOTE** and an **EXCLUDES1** notation. Read carefully. Do any relate to Dr. Rodriguez's diagnosis of Angela? No. Turn to the Official Guidelines and read Section 1.c.4. There is nothing specifically applicable here either.

Now you can report these two codes for Angela's diagnosis, evidencing the medical necessity for this procedure, with confidence.

D34   **Benign neoplasm of thyroid gland**
E27.40   **Unspecified adrenocortical insufficiency**

Good work!

YOU CODE IT! CASE STUDY

Emily Benko, a 2-month-old female, was having dyspnea and her cry sounded hoarse. In addition, Dr. Jenkins noticed her skin color was jaundiced. Her mother, Danielle, stated that she is a good baby and sleeps all the time. After running a TSH blood test and performing a thyroid scan, Dr. Jenkins diagnosed Emily with infantile cretinism, also known as congenital hypothyroidism. Dr. Jenkins also noted mild cognitive impairment, which is associated with the cretinism. He explained to Emily's mother that the mental impairment is likely to be progressive.

You Code It!

Go through the steps of coding, and determine the code or codes that should be reported for this encounter between Dr. Jenkins and Emily.

Step #1: Read the case carefully and completely.

Step #2: Abstract the scenario. Which main words or terms describe why the physician cared for the patient during this encounter?

Step #3: Are there any details missing or incomplete for which you would need to query the physician? [If so, ask your instructor.]

Step #4: Check for any relevant guidance, including reading all of the symbols and notations in the Tabular List and the appropriate sections of the Official Guidelines.

Step #5: Determine the correct diagnosis code or codes to explain why this encounter was medically necessary.

Step #6: Double-check your work.

Answer:

Did you determine these to be the correct codes?

E03.1	Congenital hypothyroidism without goiter
G31.84	Mild cognitive impairment, so stated

Good for you!

8.2 Diabetes Mellitus

Diabetes Mellitus

Diabetes mellitus (DM) is a chronic disease and a result of insulin deficiency or resistance due to a malfunction of the pancreatic beta cells. The body has a difficult time metabolizing carbohydrates, proteins, and fats. It is estimated that 16 million people have DM; however, many (possibly as many as 50%) do not know it yet.

A physician can diagnose diabetes with a glucose lab test and the presence of the following signs and symptoms:

- Excessive thirst (**polydipsia**)
- Excessive appetite
- Increased urination (**polyuria**)
- Unusual weight change (loss or gain)
- Fatigue
- Nausea, vomiting
- Blurred vision

Diabetes Mellitus (DM)
A chronic systemic disease that results from insulin deficiency or resistance and causes the body to improperly metabolize carbohydrates, proteins, and fats.

Polydipsia
Excessive thirst.

Polyuria
Excessive urination.

- Frequent vaginal infections (females)
- Yeast infections (both males and females)
- Dry mouth
- Slow-healing sores or cuts
- Itchy skin, especially in the groin or vaginal area

Measures for detecting diabetes include a glucose tolerance test (GTT) and evaluation of the results. Diabetes may be indicated by

- A casual plasma glucose value greater than or equal to 200 mg/dL
- A fasting plasma glucose level greater than or equal to 126 mg/dL
- A plasma glucose value in the 2-hour sample of the oral glucose tolerance test greater than or equal to 200 mg/dL

(*Note:* Normal blood glucose levels are less than 110 mg/dL)
There are four types of diabetes mellitus:

Type 1 Diabetes Mellitus
A sudden onset of insulin deficiency that may occur at any age but most often arises in childhood and adolescence; also known as *insulin-dependent diabetes mellitus (IDDM), juvenile diabetes,* or *type I.*

Type 2 Diabetes Mellitus
A form of diabetes mellitus with a gradual onset that may develop at any age but most often occurs in adults over the age of 40; also known as *non-insulin-dependent diabetes mellitus (NIDDM)* or *type II.*

Dyslipidemia
Abnormal lipoprotein metabolism.

Secondary Diabetes Mellitus
Diabetes caused by medication or another condition or disease.

Gestational Diabetes Mellitus (GDM)
Usually a temporary diabetes mellitus occurring during pregnancy; however, such patients have an increased risk of later developing type 2 diabetes.

- **Type 1 DM:** The malfunction of the pancreatic beta cells, resulting in no production of insulin naturally, is the underlying cause of type 1 (juvenile) diabetes mellitus, although there is no documented known etiology for idiopathic DM. Therapeutically, type 1 DM patients must administer insulin every day in addition to following specific diet and exercise programs. Implanted insulin pumps may be used for those requiring multiple dose regimens. This diagnosis will be reported from ICD-10-CM code category E10 with additional characters required to identify specific information about complications (manifestations).

- **Type 2 DM:** In type 2 patients, the pancreatic beta cells do produce insulin; however, the glucose transport is ineffective, thereby failing to deliver the required amount to the rest of the body. Type 2 diabetics often suffer pathologic effects, including increased body fat (obesity), especially when the individual does not exercise regularly. Family history of DM, co-morbidities of hypertension or **dyslipidemia**, or a personal history of gestational DM will increase the likelihood of developing this condition. In addition, patients of African-American, Latino, or Native American heritage are found to have a high risk. Diet and exercise are the first level of treatment and may resolve the condition. However, oral antidiabetic medications, such as sulfonylureas, may be prescribed to stimulate pancreatic beta cell function if diet and exercise fail to show sufficient improvement. Some type 2 DM patients require the administration of insulin. A type 2 diagnosis will be reported from ICD-10-CM code category E11 with additional characters required to identify specific information about complications (manifestations).

- **Secondary DM:** Certain drugs or chemicals can negatively affect the pancreatic beta cells and may prevent them from producing the required amount of insulin. Also, other diseases and conditions, such as Cushing's syndrome, can cause the patient to develop diabetes mellitus. This diagnosis is reported from code category E08 Diabetes mellitus due to underlying condition, E09 Drug or chemical induced diabetes mellitus, or E13 Other specified diabetes mellitus; additional characters are required to provide specific information about complications. The underlying condition, drug, or chemical causing the secondary DM will be reported first, and any codes required to identify specific manifestations will be reported following the E08, E09, or E13 code.

- **Gestational DM (GDM):** When a woman is pregnant, the weight gain, along with the higher levels of estrogen and the increase of placental hormones, may retard the production of insulin. This is considered a temporary type of DM due to the fact that, typically, the problem with the pancreatic beta cells resolves itself after the baby is delivered. Report this with a code from the ICD-10-CM code subcategory O24.4 Gestational diabetes mellitus, with an additional character to report additional details.

Diabetic Manifestations

Due to its involvement with the blood system as well as muscle and fat tissue, there can be serious manifestations—the development of other illnesses and conditions—caused by suffering with DM long term, especially when the condition goes untreated.

Ophthalmic Manifestations

The problems that diabetics frequently experience with their eyes are actually related to vascular concerns. *Diabetic retinopathy,* one of the leading causes of irreversible blindness, may be one of several types:

- *Background retinopathy:* blood vessel damage with no current vision problems.
- *Maculopathy:* damage to the macula part of the eye, resulting in a considerable loss of vision.
- *Proliferative retinopathy:* a microvascular complication of diabetes in which the small vessels of the eye become diseased as a result of diminishing oxygen.
- *Other eye problems often suffered by diabetics:* diabetic cataracts and macular edema.

Diabetic retinopathy is evidenced by microcirculatory changes in the eye that interfere with the blood supply and therefore the health of the eye. Nonproliferative diabetic retinopathy is seen in the blood vessels of the retina leaking plasma or fatty substances, resulting in diminished blood flow. Proliferative diabetic retinopathy encourages neovascularization (the growth of new blood vessels) in the vitreous of the eye; these vessels then rupture, causing a hemorrhage and sudden loss of vision. Without treatment, this can cause blindness. A diagnosis of type 1 diabetic retinopathy would be reported with a code from ICD-10-CM code subcategory E10.3 Type I diabetes mellitus with ophthalmic complications, with the required additional characters determined by the specifics (proliferative/nonproliferative, with/without macular edema, mild/moderate/severe).

> **GUIDANCE CONNECTION**
>
> Read the ICD-10-CM Official Guidelines for Coding and Reporting, section **I. Conventions, General Coding Guidelines and Chapter Specific Guidelines,** subsection **C. Chapter-Specific Coding Guidelines,** chapter **4. Endocrine, Nutritional, and Metabolic Diseases (E00-E89),** subsection **a. Diabetes mellitus,** and chapter **15. Pregnancy, childbirth, and the puerperium,** subsections **g. Diabetes mellitus in pregnancy** and **i. Gestational (pregnancy induced) diabetes.**

Neurologic Manifestations

Uncontrolled diabetes can cause damage to the patient's nerves, causing diabetic neuropathy—in particular, sensory diabetic neuropathy, or a lack of feeling. Sensory diabetic neuropathy can be dangerous because the damaged nerves do not transmit feelings of heat, cold, or pain. Such a patient might be burned or cut and not know it. The injuries might become infected, causing additional health problems. In addition, the nerve damage can retard healing, making additional complications more viable.

Renal Manifestations

Diabetic nephropathy develops due to the reduced control of blood sugar. Almost 30% of diabetics develop diabetic nephropathy (kidney disease) or other kidney-related problems, such as bladder infections and nerve damage to the bladder. The nephrons within the kidneys thicken, and the scarring that forms results in leakage of albumin (protein) into the urine. Quantitative lab tests examine the levels of albumin in the patient's urine (microalbuminuria), as well as other levels such as blood urea nitrogen (BUN) and serum creatinine. Diabetic kidney disease can cause severe illness and possibly death. Therefore, early diagnosis and treatment to prevent the progression of the condition are important. Angiotensin-converting enzyme (ACE) inhibitors as well as angiotensin receptor blockers (ARB) are considered the best medications in these cases. A diagnosis of type 2 diabetic nephropathy is reported from ICD-10-CM subcategory E11.2 Type 2 diabetes mellitus with kidney complications, with an additional character to report a chronic or other condition.

You may need a second code to identify the exact nature of the renal complication, such as the stage of the chronic kidney failure. Type 2 diabetes–related chronic kidney disease may be reported with E11.22 Type 2 diabetes mellitus with diabetic chronic kidney disease; diabetic nephropathy may be reported with E10.21 Type 1 diabetes mellitus with diabetic nephropathy.

CHAPTER 8 | CODING ENDOCRINE CONDITIONS 205

Circulatory Manifestations

Peripheral vascular disease is another likely complication because diabetes mellitus disturbs the blood flow, increasing the development of ulcers. It is estimated that as many as 10% of diabetics develop foot ulcers. Gangrene, a condition by which necrosis (tissue death) occurs as a result of lack of blood, is another relatively common manifestation. When gangrene is not caught early enough, the resulting treatment to stop the spread of the necrosis is often amputation. You might report one of these diagnoses with code E09.52 Drug or chemical induced diabetes mellitus with diabetic peripheral angiopathy with gangrene or E11.51 Type 2 diabetes mellitus with diabetic peripheral angiopathy without gangrene.

LET'S CODE IT! SCENARIO

Brittany Hatthaway, a 53-year-old female, came to see Dr. DeRupo for her annual checkup. She is a type 1 insulin-dependent diabetic and has been feeling fine. There are no diabetic-related manifestations noted.

Let's Code It!

Dr. DeRupo's notes state that Brittany has *type 1 diabetes mellitus* with *no complications*. When you turn to the Alphabetic Index, you see

Diabetes, diabetic (mellitus) (sugar) E11.9

When you turn to the Tabular List, you confirm:

☑4 **E11**   **Type 2 diabetes mellitus**

Oh, wait a minute. This code category is for type 2 diabetes. Dr. DeRupo's notes document that Brittany has type 1 diabetes. Turn the pages and review this whole section to see if you can find a more accurate code category. Did you find this code category?

☑4 **E10**   **Type 1 diabetes mellitus**

There is an INCLUDES note as well as an EXCLUDES1 notation listing several diagnoses. Take a minute to review them and determine if any apply to Brittany's condition. No, none of them do, so continue down and review all of the fourth-character choices. Which matches Dr. DeRupo's notes?

E10.9   **Type 1 diabetes mellitus without complications**

Perfect!

CODING BITES

The code for long-term insulin use is not reported for patients with type 1 diabetes mellitus. Remember, type 1 DM is known as insulin-dependent diabetes, making Z79.4 unnecessary.

Long-Term Drug Use

Long-Term Insulin Use

There are cases where a patient, who has been diagnosed with type 2 diabetes, gestational diabetes, or secondary diabetes, has been prescribed insulin on a regular basis. This is not a standard of care, so you will have to include a code stating this fact:

Z79.4   **Long-term (current) use of insulin**

You can see the notation at the beginning of the E11 Type 2 diabetes mellitus code category to remind you:

Use additional code **to identify** control using:

    insulin (Z79.4)
    oral antidiabetic drugs (Z79.84)
    oral hypoglycemic drugs (Z79.84)

Long-Term Hypoglycemic Use

There are now several new drugs, known as **hypoglycemics**. These medications are not insulin; however, they work to lower a patient's glycemic level. You may see names of drugs such as Orinase, Glucotrol, Avandia, or Glucophage in the physician's documentation. When a diabetic patient has been using one of these medications for a while, you will need to add a code:

Z79.84 Long term (current) use of oral hypoglycemic drugs

Be careful not to confuse code Z79.84 with code Z79.4. Insulin and hypoglycemic drugs are different. And remember, both of these codes report that the use of the insulin or hypoglycemic drug is not a one-time or temporary treatment.

Hypoglycemics
Prescription, non-insulin medications designed to lower a patient's glycemic level.

GUIDANCE CONNECTION

Read the ICD-10-CM Official Guidelines for Coding and Reporting, section **I. Conventions, General Coding Guidelines and Chapter Specific Guidelines**, subsection **C. Chapter-Specific Coding Guidelines**, chapter **4. Endocrine, Nutritional, and Metabolic Diseases (E00–E89)**, subsection **a.3) Diabetes mellitus and the use of insulin and oral hypoglycemics** and **a.6)(a) Secondary diabetes mellitus and the use of insulin or hypoglycemic drugs.**

YOU CODE IT! CASE STUDY

Alec Kustra, a 37-year-old male, was diagnosed with type 2 diabetes a year ago. Dr. Lockhart had prescribed tolbutamide to stimulate his pancreatic insulin release. However, 6 months ago, he became concerned that the medication was not working and started Alec on a regime of insulin injections. Alec is here today for Dr. Lockhart to check his insulin levels.

You Code It!

Go through the steps of coding, and determine the code or codes that should be reported for this encounter between Dr. Lockhart and Alec Kustra.

Step #1: Read the case carefully and completely.

Step #2: Abstract the scenario. Which main words or terms describe why the physician cared for the patient during this encounter?

Step #3: Are there any details missing or incomplete for which you would need to query the physician? [If so, ask your instructor.]

Step #4: Check for any relevant guidance, including reading all of the symbols and notations in the Tabular List and the appropriate sections of the Official Guidelines.

Step #5: Determine the correct diagnosis code or codes to explain why this encounter was medically necessary.

Step #6: Double-check your work.

Answer:

Did you determine these to be the correct codes?

E11.9	Type 2 diabetes mellitus without complications
Z79.4	Long-term (current) use of insulin

8.3 Diabetes-Related Conditions

Hyperglycemia and Hypoglycemia

Hyperglycemia
Abnormally high levels of glucose.

Hypoglycemia
Abnormally low glucose levels.

A patient with **hyperglycemia** is *not* diagnosed with diabetes. Hyperglycemia, just like **hypoglycemia**, is a separate condition.

Chronic hyperglycemia may impair one's resistance to infection, resulting in diabetic skin problems and urinary tract infections. A diabetic patient that has hypoglycemia may have administered too much insulin or antidiabetic medication.

LET'S CODE IT! SCENARIO

Jessica Gundersen, a 61-year-old female, has been feeling excessively tired and irritable. She tells Dr. Vickers that she has felt edgy and nervous while experiencing cold sweats and trembling. Dr. Vickers performs a glucose-screening test using a reagent strip, resulting in a reading of less than 45 mg/dL. He orders a lab test to confirm a diagnosis of reactive hypoglycemia and provides Jessica with a diet to follow and a referral to a nutritionist.

Let's Code It!

Jessica has been diagnosed with *reactive hypoglycemia*. Let's turn to the Alphabetic Index and look it up:

> Hypoglycemia (spontaneous) E16.2

Read all the way down the indented list to find

> Reactive (not drug-induced) E16.1

The Tabular List describes the code as

> ✓4 E16   Other disorders of pancreatic internal secretion

There are no notations or directives, so keep reading down the column.

> E16.1   Other hypoglycemia
> E16.2   Hypoglycemia, unspecified

How do you decide between these two codes? Let's think about this. Dr. Vickers *did* specify the type of hypoglycemia that Jessica has, so you cannot report that this detail was "unspecified." This eliminates E16.2 and confirms that E16.1 Other hypoglycemia is accurate.

Notice that the **EXCLUDES1** note under code E16.1 states that neither hypoglycemia in infant of diabetic mother (P70.1) nor neonatal hypoglycemia is to be reported with this code. Does it apply to Jessica's case? Dr. Vickers indicated that Jessica is an adult; therefore, it does not apply.

The correct diagnosis code for the encounter between Dr. Vickers and Jessica is this:

> E16.1   Other hypoglycemia

Excellent!

Insulin Pumps

Technology has provided patients with an easier and more controlled manner by which to get their insulin: an insulin pump. However, nothing is perfect, so there may be a concern with the patient as a result of the insulin pump not working correctly.

Underdose of Insulin

It can be very dangerous for a patient to receive less than the proper amount of insulin, as prescribed by the physician, on schedule. If that occurs and is the reason the physician is caring for the patient at the encounter, your first-listed code should be this:

T85.614A   Breakdown (mechanical) of insulin pump, initial encounter

Follow that code with the proper diabetes mellitus code and any other appropriate codes, including codes for any effects, or conditions, caused by the insulin underdose.

If the patient's ill health is caused by an underdose of insulin that the patient injects by hand (not using a pump), meaning that the patient is not taking the correct amount as often as it was prescribed, you might use the following code:

Z91.120   Patient's intentional underdosing of medication regimen due to financial hardship

Also note that beneath code Z91.12 and Z91.13 is a notation:

Code first underdosing of medication (T36-T50) with fifth or sixth character 6

This T code will enable you to report which specific medication was underdosed. So, in this example, you would also report this code:

T38.3x6D   Underdosing of insulin and oral hypoglycemic (antidiabetic) drugs, subsequent encounter

> **GUIDANCE CONNECTION**
>
> Read the ICD-10-CM Official Guidelines for Coding and Reporting, section **I. Conventions, General Coding Guidelines and Chapter Specific Guidelines,** subsection **C. Chapter-Specific Coding Guidelines,** chapter **4. Endocrine, Nutritional, and Metabolic Diseases (E00-E89),** subsection a.5) Complications due to insulin pump malfunction.

YOU CODE IT! CASE STUDY

Tori Anderson, a 19-year-old female, was diagnosed with type 1 diabetes 2 years ago. Starting college, Tori kept forgetting to take her insulin as prescribed. She comes into the University Health Center because she feels dizzy, weak, and confused. Dr. Griffith, the on-call physician, finds her to have poor skin turgor and dry mucous membranes. He diagnoses her with dehydration caused by insulin deficiency and diabetes mellitus, type 1, uncontrolled.

You Code It!

Go through the steps of coding, and determine the code or codes that should be reported for this encounter between Dr. Griffith and Tori Anderson.

Step #1: Read the case carefully and completely.

Step #2: Abstract the scenario. Which main words or terms describe why the physician cared for the patient during this encounter?

Step #3: Are there any details missing or incomplete for which you would need to query the physician? [If so, ask your instructor.]

Step #4: Check for any relevant guidance, including reading all of the symbols and notations in the Tabular List and the appropriate sections of the Official Guidelines.

Step #5: Determine the correct diagnosis code or codes to explain why this encounter was medically necessary.

Step #6: Double-check your work.

Answer:

Did you determine these to be the correct codes?

E86.0	Dehydration
E10.9	Type 1 diabetes mellitus without complications
T38.3x6A	Underdosing of insulin and oral hypoglycemic (antidiabetic) drugs, initial encounter
Z91.138	Patient's unintentional underdosing of medication regimen for other reason

Overdose of Insulin

Patients with an insulin pump that malfunctions can dose with a higher quantity of insulin than prescribed by the attending physician. For such a case, you will use the following code (which is the same as the code for an underdose):

T85.614A   Breakdown (mechanical) of insulin pump, initial encounter

Follow that code with a poisoning code, for example:

T38.3x1A   Poisoning by insulin and oral hypoglycemic (antidiabetic) drugs, accidental (unintentional), initial encounter

Follow that code with the appropriate diabetes mellitus code and any other appropriate codes, including the codes identifying the reaction or conditions caused by the overdose.

If the patient delivers a dose of insulin manually and suffers an overdose, you will code it the same way you do any other poisoning, including the determination of the cause of the overdose (such as accident, attempted suicide, or assault). Unless the health concern with the patient is an adverse reaction to the insulin and not related to the actual dosage, you will not use the code reporting therapeutic usage.

8.4 Other Endocrine Gland Disorders

Diabetes Insipidus

Another type of diabetes that few people have heard of is *diabetes insipidus (DI)*. DI is a disorder of water metabolism that is the result of an antidiuretic hormone (ADH) deficiency. Intracranial neoplastic or metastatic lesions, hypophysectomy or other neurosurgery, or skull fractures or other head trauma that damages the neurohypophyseal structures can all incite DI. The condition can also result from infection. Diabetes insipidus is also known as *pituitary diabetes insipidus* and is coded using E23.2 from the subsection for disorders of the pituitary gland.

Nephrogenic diabetes insipidus, another form of DI, is a very rare congenital disturbance of water metabolism resulting from a renal tubular resistance to vasopressin. Interestingly, it is not coded from the congenital anomalies but is reported using code N25.1 Nephrogenic diabetes insipidus.

YOU CODE IT! CASE STUDY

Roy Holvang, a 25-year-old male, comes to see Dr. Fletcher with complaints of extreme thirst and muscle weakness. During examination, Dr. Fletcher identifies that Roy has poor tissue turgor, dry mucous membranes, and hypotension. UA results show urine of low osmolality at 75 mOsm/kg. Dr. Fletcher diagnoses Roy with diabetes insipidus and prescribes vasopressin IM qid.

You Code It!

Go through the steps of coding, and determine the code or codes that should be reported for this encounter between Dr. Fletcher and Roy Holvang.

Step #1: Read the case carefully and completely.

Step #2: Abstract the scenario. Which main words or terms describe why the physician cared for the patient during this encounter?

> Step #3: Are there any details missing or incomplete for which you would need to query the physician? [If so, ask your instructor.]
>
> Step #4: Check for any relevant guidance, including reading all of the symbols and notations in the Tabular List and the appropriate sections of the Official Guidelines.
>
> Step #5: Determine the correct diagnosis code or codes to explain why this encounter was medically necessary.
>
> Step #6: Double-check your work.
>
> **Answer:**
>
> Did you determine this to be the correct code?
>
>   **E23.2**   **Diabetes insipidus**
>
> Good job!

Cushing's Syndrome

Cushing's syndrome is caused by excessive production of corticotropin (ACTH) in the hypothalamus and too much secretion from the adenohypophysis (pituitary gland). This may be caused by a tumor in another organ affecting this process—possibly a bronchogenic tumor or a malignant neoplasm of the pancreas. Approximately 30% of such cases are the result of a benign neoplasm of the adrenal gland.

Cushing's syndrome may cause diabetes mellitus, hypokalemia (low potassium in the blood), pathologic fractures, slow wound healing, hypertension, irritability, and other conditions. Lab tests for plasma steroid levels measured by 24-hour urine samples can be used to confirm a diagnosis of Cushing's syndrome. An adrenal tumor can be seen on an ultrasound, CT scan, or angiography, while MRI and CT scans can illuminate the presence of a pituitary tumor.

Administration of radiation therapy, drug therapy with a medication such as aminoglutethimide, or surgery to remove the tumor can be successful to control or reverse the effects of Cushing's syndrome. ICD-10-CM code category E24 Cushing's syndrome requires an additional character to provide more specific information about the condition.

> **Cushing's Syndrome**
> A condition resulting from the hyperproduction of corticosteroids, most often caused by an adrenal cortex tumor or a tumor of the pituitary gland.

EXAMPLES

    E24.0   Pituitary-dependent Cushing's disease
    E24.2   Drug-induced Cushing's disease
              Use additional code for adverse effect, if applicable, to identify drug (T36-T50 with fifth or sixth character 5)
    E24.4   Alcohol-induced pseudo-Cushing's disease

As you can see, you will need to abstract additional details related to the diagnosis of Cushing's disease in order to determine a specific code.

Postprocedural Endocrine System Complications

Due to the incredible connections between all aspects of the human body, there are times when a procedure employed to treat one condition results in a malfunction elsewhere in the body.

Should a malfunction in the endocrine system be a documented postprocedural complication, you must report this using a designated code category: E89 Postprocedural endocrine and metabolic complications and disorders, not elsewhere classified.

> **CODING BITES**
> The postprocedural time frame is generally considered the time from the surgical procedure's conclusion until the physician releases the patient from care. This typically aligns with the global period standard for the specific procedure provided.

> **EXAMPLES**
>
> E89.0   Postprocedural hypothyroidism
> E89.3   Postprocedural hypopituitarism
> E89.5   Postprocedural testicular hypofunction
>
> These complications may be predictable. For example, it would be expected, after the surgical removal of the patient's thyroid, that hypothyroidism would develop. However, this is not always the case.

8.5 Nutritional Deficiencies and Weight Factors

Nutritional Deficiencies

My mother said it a thousand times, as do physicians and the media . . . eat good food so you can get all your vitamins. Even with the large number of supplements available on the market, individuals still lack certain vitamins and other vital nutrients required for a healthy body.

Vitamin A deficiencies can manifest with diagnosed ophthalmological conditions. You will need to know this when reporting the vitamin A deficiency diagnosis. Two examples:

E50.0   Vitamin A deficiency with conjunctival xerosis
E50.4   Vitamin A deficiency with keratomalacia

Niacin, riboflavin, calcium, magnesium . . . and so many more deficiencies are reported from the subsection of the Endocrine, Nutritional, and Metabolic Diseases chapter in ICD-10-CM.

E52   Niacin deficiency [pellagra]
E56.0   Deficiency of vitamin E
E61.1   Iron deficiency

> **CODING BITES**
>
> Remember, in earlier chapters you learned the difference between a manifestation and a sequela. When a patient is diagnosed with a sequela of malnutrition or other nutritional deficiency, report the condition (the sequela) first, followed by a code from the E64 code category:
>
> E64.0   Sequela of protein-calorie malnutrition
> E64.1   Sequela of vitamin A deficiency
> E64.2   Sequela of vitamin C deficiency
> E64.3   Sequela of rickets
> E64.8   Sequela of other nutritional deficiencies

YOU CODE IT! CASE STUDY

Shakeia and Robert Malabwa just adopted Benjamin, a 3-year-old male, from an orphanage in Africa. They brought him in to see Dr. D'Onofrio, a pediatrician, for this first American checkup. After reviewing what was available about his history, and a complete physical examination, Dr. D'Onofrio diagnosed Ben with moderate protein-energy malnutrition. They sat together and discussed a treatment plan and diet to help him improve. Lactose intolerance can manifest, so he suggested that they avoid foods with lactose.

> **You Code It!**
>
> Go through the steps of coding, and determine the code or codes that should be reported for this encounter between Dr. D'Onofrio and Benjamin Malabwa.
>
> Step #1: Read the case carefully and completely.
>
> Step #2: Abstract the scenario. Which main words or terms describe why the physician cared for the patient during this encounter?
>
> Step #3: Are there any details missing or incomplete for which you would need to query the physician? [If so, ask your instructor.]
>
> Step #4: Check for any relevant guidance, including reading all of the symbols and notations in the Tabular List and the appropriate sections of the Official Guidelines.
>
> Step #5: Determine the correct diagnosis code or codes to explain why this encounter was medically necessary.
>
> Step #6: Double-check your work.
>
> **Answer:**
>
> Did you determine the correct diagnosis code?
>
> E44.0   Moderate protein-calorie malnutrition

Obesity

The definitions of *overweight, obese,* and *morbidly obese* can get lost in societal norms and self-perception. Of course, the health care industry has its own official determinations of these conditions, further specified by reporting the patient's body mass index (BMI).

Overweight merely means weighing too much. This can be a reference to the individual's muscles, bones, fat, or fluid retention when calculated along with the person's height. This condition is calculated as a BMI of 25 to 29.9.

Obesity is a condition calculated as a body mass index of 30 to 38.9. Typically, a person becomes obese when more calories are consumed than expended. While some critics believe extra pounds are caused only by eating too much and not exercising enough, the facts are that one's genetics and current medications (including herbal supplements) can also influence this condition.

Being diagnosed as obese is a true health condition that not only can result in self-esteem problems and social anxiety but also may increase the risk of developing diabetes, heart disease, arthritis, stroke, and even certain malignancies.

Morbid obesity is diagnosed when a patient's current overweight status increases to the extent that it actually interferes with normal, daily activities. This condition is calculated as a BMI over 39.

> **EXAMPLES**
>
> code category E66   Overweight and obesity
>
> *Use additional code* **to identify Body Mass Index (BMI) if known (Z68.-)**
>
> E66.01   Morbid (severe) obesity due to excess calories
> E66.09   Other obesity due to excess calories
> E66.1   Drug-induced obesity
> E66.2   Morbid (severe) obesity with alveolar hypoventilation
> E66.3   Overweight
> E66.8   Other obesity
> E66.9   Obesity, unspecified

CODING BITES

Several different types of health care professionals, such as a dietitian or a nutritionist, may be involved in the care of a patient determined to be overweight, obese, or morbidly obese. However, the first time this diagnosis code is reported, it may be coded only from physician documentation.

As you can see, ICD-10-CM reminds you to use an additional code to specify the patient's BMI.

Body Mass Index

It is important for health care professionals to determine specifically what is a healthy amount of body fat and what falls or rises to an unhealthy level. Body mass index (BMI) is a calculation using an individual's actual weight and current height to determine a workable measure of body fat. However, some people, such as athletes, may have a BMI that indicates he or she is overweight even though there is no excess body fat. This can occur because BMI does not actually measure body fat but instead determines a ratio with which to work. BMI is just an indicator of potential health risks related to an individual's being outside the normal weight range.

BMI ranges are listed differently for adults than they are for children and teens. The pediatric ranges, used for individuals aged 2 to 20 years, are based on the growth charts of the Centers for Disease Control and take into account the normal differences in body fat for various ages as well as differences between boys and girls.

Z68   **Body Mass Index [BMI]**

Adult BMI codes range from Z68.1–Z68.45. The pediatric BMI code is

Z68.5-   **Body Mass Index [BMI] pediatric**

Underweight

With all the discussion regarding how many people in the United States are overweight or clinically obese, the opposite—being underweight—can also cause health concerns. Unlike the codes for overweight conditions, codes for reporting an abnormal weight loss or underweight condition are listed in the *Symptoms, Signs, and Abnormal Clinical and Laboratory Findings* section of ICD-10-CM. In certain cases, the BMI will also need to be reported.

EXAMPLES

R63.4   Abnormal weight loss
R63.6   Underweight
           Use additional code to identify Body Mass Index (BMI) if known (Z68.-)

CODING BITES

While you may see issues of overweight status accompanying diagnoses such as diabetes mellitus or hypertension, in cases of underweight patients, be alert to initial or additional diagnoses of malnutrition.

When a patient is diagnosed with anorexia, you may need more information from the physician before determining the correct code.

R63.0   **Anorexia**

(This is used when the cause of the anorexia has not been determined as organic [physiological] or nonorganic [psychological].)

F50.0-   **Anorexia nervosa**
F50.2   **Bulimia nervosa**
F50.8-   **Other eating disorders**

YOU CODE IT! CASE STUDY

PATIENT: ERIC MICOH

REASON FOR CONSULTATION: Preoperative evaluation for bariatric surgery.

HISTORY OF PRESENT ILLNESS: The patient is a 47-year-old morbidly obese male with a BMI of 46.3 and multiple medical problems including hypertension, diabetes, and dyslipidemia. He has been overweight most of his life. The patient was considering bariatric surgery and he is planning to go for a lap band procedure. He says that snoring is not a very common complaint of his wife. He snores mainly when he drinks; otherwise, it could be soft snoring or sometimes no snoring at all. There was no mention of witnessed apneas. He does not wake himself up choking or gasping for air. He is a very quiet sleeper with not much tossing and turning. He wakes up feeling refreshed for the most part, unless he sleeps for 5 hours or so. He goes on with his day with no difficulty as far as excessive daytime sleepiness or fatigue. He is only tired if he had a really busy long day. His Epworth sleepiness score today was between 5 and 6. He has never fallen asleep behind the wheel or got himself in an accident. His weight has been steady. He has been overweight since he was 15 years old. He never had any symptoms suggestive of cataplexy, sleep paralysis, or hypnagogic or hypnopompic hallucinations. He denies any symptoms of restless legs. No symptoms of parasomnia. No sleep onset or sleep maintenance insomnia.

ASSESSMENT AND PLAN:

1. Even though this patient does not have any of the cardinal symptoms of obstructive sleep apnea including snoring, witnessed apneas, or excessive daytime sleepiness, he does have physical features that increase the risk for sleep apnea including obesity, large neck circumference, crowded airway with a high Mallampati class, as well as his multiple associated cardiovascular and metabolic disorders including hypertension that is not very well controlled on different blood pressure medicines, diabetes, and dyslipidemia.

2. I had a long discussion with him today about the need for a sleep study to rule out obstructive sleep apnea, even though he does not have the classic symptoms. I also explained to him the risks in the perioperative period for patients with obstructive sleep apnea that has not been treated. At this point, he wants to wait and think about it as well as talk it over with the bariatric surgery team. He does not think he has sleep apnea. He does not think he would be able to perform the sleep study, as he will have a hard time sleeping outside his house.

3. I explained to him the risks involved with untreated moderate-to-severe obstructive sleep apnea, including worsening cardiovascular disease, arrhythmias, risk of stroke, and increased overall mortality.

4. I also mentioned to him that there is a possibility of doing a portable sleep study at home if that would be something he is willing to pursue.

5. In the meantime, he should continue to lose weight, avoid alcohol and sedatives, exercise routinely, and avoid driving if drowsy.

6. We will follow up with him as needed if he is willing to pursue this further.

You Code It!

Read this evaluation of Eric Micoh and determine the diagnosis code or codes to report.

Step #1: Read the case carefully and completely.

Step #2: Abstract the scenario. Which main words or terms describe why the physician cared for the patient during this encounter?

Step #3: Are there any details missing or incomplete for which you would need to query the physician? [If so, ask your instructor.]

Step #4: Check for any relevant guidance, including reading all of the symbols and notations in the Tabular List and the appropriate sections of the Official Guidelines.

(continued)

> Step #5: Determine the correct diagnosis code or codes to explain why this encounter was medically necessary.
>
> Step #6: Double-check your work.
>
> **Answer:**
>
> Did you determine these to be the correct codes?
>
> | | |
> |---|---|
> | E66.01 | Morbid (severe) obesity due to excess calories |
> | E11.9 | Type 2 diabetes mellitus without complications |
> | I10 | Essential (primary) hypertension |
> | E78.5 | Hyperlipidemia, unspecified |
> | Z68.42 | Body mass index [BMI] 45.0-49.9, adult |

8.6 Metabolic Disorders

When you eat, it is your metabolism that processes nutrition into energy. The chemicals in the digestive system portion out glucose and acids from the carbohydrates, fats, and proteins in the food. This process is known as *metabolization*. The energy created by this process can be used right away—for example, when someone eats before taking a test or running a race. If the body doesn't need the energy at this time, the tissues in the liver and the muscular system, as well as the adipose (body fat), can store it for future use.

Dysfunction of the metabolic processes can interfere with the various systems of the body getting what they need to work properly. This may be realized as too little of a chemical needed, such as when the pancreas cannot create enough insulin (a condition known as *diabetes mellitus*). You have already learned about what havoc can be caused in the other organs and systems when this disorder continues. Metabolic disorders can also result in too much of a chemical being present in the body. For example, hyperchloremia is an excessive level of chloride anion in the blood and can cause tachycardia (rapid heartbeat), hypertension, dyspnea (shortness of breath), and agitation.

The long list of metabolic diagnoses includes:

- Acid lipase disease
- Amyloidosis
- Barth's syndrome
- Central pontine myelinolysis
- Farber's disease
- G6PD deficiency
- Gangliosidoses
- Hunter's syndrome
- Hyperoxaluria
- Lesch-Nyhan syndrome
- Lipid storage diseases
- Metabolic myopathies
- Mitochondrial myopathies
- Mucolipidoses
- Mucopolysaccharidoses (MPS)
- Oxalosis
- Pompe's disease

- Trimethylaminuria
- Type I glycogen storage disease
- Urea cycle disorder

Let's take a look at some of the more common metabolic conditions, and review the details required to accurately code them.

Cystic Fibrosis

Cystic fibrosis (CF) is a hereditary malfunction of the secretory glands. Many laypeople think of this as a malfunction of the pulmonary system. However, as you can see by the code descriptions, the effects of this genetic condition reach to other body systems as well.

A defect in the CFTR gene affects the glands that produce mucus and sweat, resulting in the creation of thick, sticky mucus and very salty sweat. There are manifestations that can develop in the respiratory, digestive, and reproductive systems, as well as other maladies.

E84.0	Cystic fibrosis with pulmonary manifestations
	Use additional code to identify any infectious organism present, such as Pseudomonas (B96.5)
E84.11	Meconium ileus in cystic fibrosis
E84.19	Cystic fibrosis with other intestinal manifestations
E84.8	Cystic fibrosis with other manifestations

Other manifestations, reported with E84.8, include male neonates born without a vas deferens or females who may have an overproduction of mucus blocking the cervix.

Dehydration may result due to the large loss of salt in the CF patient's perspiration; clubbing and low bone density may both occur later in life.

YOU CODE IT! CASE STUDY

Rachel Ward brought her 3-year-old son Ethan to his pediatrician, Dr. Inger. She was very distressed because Ethan had eruptions on his arms, legs, and face that appeared after he had spent the day at the beach. She had also noticed that his urine appeared to be reddish in color. Dr. Inger examined Ethan and discovered that he had splenomegaly (enlargement of the spleen). The blood test came back positive for hemolytic anemia. Both of these conditions are signs of erythropoietic porphyria, also known as Gunther's disease. Dr. Inger diagnosed Ethan with this condition.

You Code It!

Go through the steps of coding, and determine the code or codes that should be reported for this encounter between Dr. Inger and Ethan Ward.

Step #1: Read the case carefully and completely.

Step #2: Abstract the scenario. Which main words or terms describe why the physician cared for the patient during this encounter?

Step #3: Are there any details missing or incomplete for which you would need to query the physician? [If so, ask your instructor.]

Step #4: Check for any relevant guidance, including reading all of the symbols and notations in the Tabular List and the appropriate sections of the Official Guidelines.

Step #5: Determine the correct diagnosis code or codes to explain why this encounter was medically necessary.

(continued)

> Step #6: Double-check your work.
>
> **Answer**:
>
> Did you determine this to be the correct code?
>
> **E80.0**   **Hereditary erythropoietic porphyria**
>
> Good job!

Lactose Intolerance

If you know anyone with a lactose intolerance, you understand how challenging this can be to quality of life. While the symptoms of this condition evidence in the digestive system, this is a metabolic disorder because a lactose intolerance develops after the small intestine is unable to digest lactose due to abnormally low production of lactase (also known as lactase deficiency).

As you have learned many times, while this sounds like a complete diagnostic statement, you will need to abstract the type of lactase deficiency before you will be able to determine the accurate code.

- *Congenital lactase deficiency* is an extremely rare, genetic disorder in which there is a failure of the small intestine to produce any, or enough, of the lactase enzyme. This diagnosis is reported with code E73.0 Congenital lactase deficiency.
- *Secondary lactase deficiency* manifests when an infection or disease causes the small intestine to malfunction in this way. These cases can be reversed with successful treatment of the underlying disease. This diagnosis is reported with code E73.1 Secondary lactase deficiency.
- *Other lactose intolerance* may be prompted by *developmental lactase deficiency*, a short-term condition seen in premature neonates, or *primary lactase deficiency (lactase nonpersistence)*, the most frequently seen type of lactase deficiency. Typically, in these patients, the small intestine's production of lactase begins to decline around 2 years of age. Any of these diagnoses are reported with code E73.8 Other lactose intolerance.

Chapter Summary

The glands of the endocrine system produce and release various types of hormones that are used by numerous organs throughout the body—all a part of the function of a healthy body. When a component of this system does not function properly, the harm can cascade and reveal itself as signs and symptoms evident with other body systems, such as the urinary system or reproductive system. Diabetes mellitus is probably the most common of the conditions and diseases affecting the endocrine system. From the hypothalamus of the brain to the genitals, every part of this system, like all of the others that make up the human body, can malfunction or become diseased.

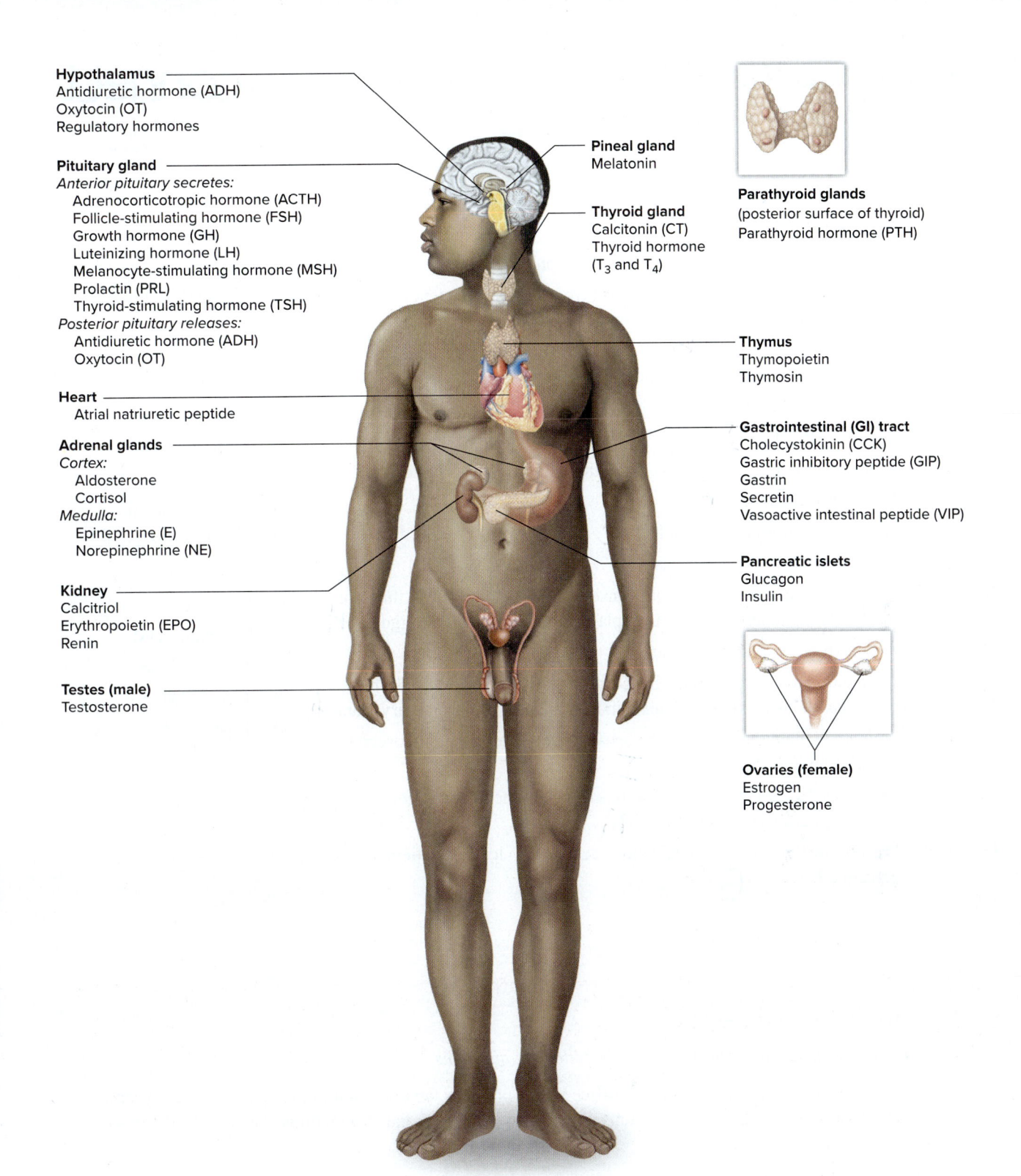

Hypothalamus
Antidiuretic hormone (ADH)
Oxytocin (OT)
Regulatory hormones

Pituitary gland
Anterior pituitary secretes:
　Adrenocorticotropic hormone (ACTH)
　Follicle-stimulating hormone (FSH)
　Growth hormone (GH)
　Luteinizing hormone (LH)
　Melanocyte-stimulating hormone (MSH)
　Prolactin (PRL)
　Thyroid-stimulating hormone (TSH)
Posterior pituitary releases:
　Antidiuretic hormone (ADH)
　Oxytocin (OT)

Heart
　Atrial natriuretic peptide

Adrenal glands
Cortex:
　Aldosterone
　Cortisol
Medulla:
　Epinephrine (E)
　Norepinephrine (NE)

Kidney
Calcitriol
Erythropoietin (EPO)
Renin

Testes (male)
Testosterone

Pineal gland
Melatonin

Thyroid gland
Calcitonin (CT)
Thyroid hormone
(T_3 and T_4)

Parathyroid glands
(posterior surface of thyroid)
Parathyroid hormone (PTH)

Thymus
Thymopoietin
Thymosin

Gastrointestinal (GI) tract
Cholecystokinin (CCK)
Gastric inhibitory peptide (GIP)
Gastrin
Secretin
Vasoactive intestinal peptide (VIP)

Pancreatic islets
Glucagon
Insulin

Ovaries (female)
Estrogen
Progesterone

CHAPTER 8 | CODING ENDOCRINE CONDITIONS　219

CHAPTER 8 REVIEW
Coding Endocrine Conditions

Let's Check It! Terminology

Match each key term to the appropriate definition.

1. LO 8.2 A form of diabetes mellitus with a gradual onset. **O**
2. LO 8.2 A chronic systemic disease that results from insulin deficiency or resistance and causes the body to improperly metabolize carbohydrates, proteins, and fats. **B**
3. LO 8.2 A temporary diabetes mellitus occurring during pregnancy. **D**
4. LO 8.3 Abnormally high levels of glucose. **E**
5. LO 8.2 Excessive thirst. **J**
6. LO 8.2 Diabetes caused by medication or another condition or disease. **L**
7. LO 8.2 Excessive urination. **K**
8. LO 8.2 Abnormal lipoprotein metabolism. **C**
9. LO 8.3 Abnormally low glucose levels. **F**
10. LO 8.1 A condition in which the thyroid converts energy more slowly than normal, resulting in an otherwise unexplained weight gain and fatigue. **H**
11. LO 8.2 A sudden onset of insulin deficiency. **N**
12. LO 8.4 A condition resulting from the hyperproduction of corticosteroids, most often caused by an adrenal cortex tumor or a tumor of the pituitary gland. **A**
13. LO 8.1 Four small glands situated on the back of the thyroid gland that secrete parathyroid hormone. **I**
14. LO 8.1 Two lobes located in the neck that reach around the trachea laterally and connect anteriorly by an isthmus. **M**
15. LO 8.3 Prescription, non-insulin medications designed to lower a patient's glycemic level. **G**

A. Cushing's Syndrome
B. Diabetes Mellitus
C. Dyslipidemia
D. Gestational Diabetes Mellitus (GDM)
E. Hyperglycemia
F. Hypoglycemia
G. Hypoglycemics
H. Hypothyroidism
I. Parathyroid Glands
J. Polydipsia
K. Polyuria
L. Secondary DM
M. Thyroid gland
N. Type 1 DM
O. Type 2 DM

Let's Check It! Concepts

Choose the most appropriate answer for each of the following questions.

1. LO 8.3 Daniel Gupta is seen at his doctor's office with a previous lab test result of positive for hyperglycemia. Dr. Ansewa writes in his chart that his diagnosis is suspected diabetes mellitus. The correct diagnosis code would report
   a. diabetes mellitus with unspecified complication.
   b. hyperglycemia.
   c. hyperglycemia; diabetes mellitus uncomplicated.
   d. diabetes mellitus with specified complication.

2. LO 8.2 Karin is diagnosed with diabetes mellitus, type 2 with Kimmelstiel-Wilson disease. What is the correct code for this diagnosis?
   a. E11.00   b. E11.01   **c. E11.21**   d. E11.29

3. LO 8.2 Diabetic retinopathy may be manifested in all of the following *except*
   a. background.   b. maculopathy.   c. proliferative.   d. neurologic.
4. LO 8.2 Gestational diabetes is a condition that can affect only an individual
   a. over the age of 65.   b. under the age of 4.   c. who is pregnant.   d. with hypertension.
5. LO 8.5 What are the correct codes for a patient with type 1 DM who is overweight and has been diagnosed with Refsum's disease?
   a. E10.51, E66.00, G60.8
   b. E11.9, E66.3, G60.2
   c. E11.49, E66.01, G60.0
   d. E10.9, E66.3, G60.1
6. LO 8.1 Amanda is being seen today for her hypothyroidism, which was induced when she took sulfonamide as prescribed by her physician, initial encounter. What is/are the correct code(s) for this condition?
   a. E03.2, T37.0X1A   b. T37.0X5A, E03.2   c. E03.2, T37.0X5A   d. T37.0X5A
7. LO 8.1 When a patient has _____, the thyroid converts energy more slowly than normal, resulting in an otherwise unexplained weight gain and fatigue.
   a. hypothroidism   b. myxedema   c. hyperthyroidism   d. thyroidits
8. LO 8.4 Which of the following conditions is a disorder of water metabolism that is the result of an ADH deficiency?
   a. Type I DM   b. Diabetes insipidus   c. Secondary DM   d. Gestational DM
9. LO 8.5 When the patient is diagnosed with obesity, his or her body mass will be between
   a. 20 and 24.9   b. 25 and 29.9   c. 30 and 38.9   d. 40 and 45.0
10. LO 8.6 Which of the following is a metabolic diagnosis?
    a. G6PD deficiency   b. Mucopolysaccharidoses   c. Hyperoxaluria   d. All of these

Let's Check It! Guidelines

Refer to the Official Guidelines and fill in the blanks according to the Chapter 4, Endocrine, Nutritional and Metabolic Diseases, Chapter-Specific Coding Guidelines.

T85.6-	not	T85.6-	E08–E13
body system	E13	T38.3x6-	age
E09	T38.3x1-	combination	Z79.4
puberty	E89.1	temporarily	E11.-
Z79.84	type	E08	

1. The diabetes mellitus codes are _____ codes that include the type of diabetes mellitus, the _____ affected, and the complications affecting that body system.
2. Assign as many codes from categories _____ as needed to identify all of the associated conditions that the patient has.
3. The _____ of a patient is not the sole determining factor, though most type 1 diabetics develop the condition before reaching _____.
4. If the _____ of diabetes mellitus is not documented in the medical record, the default is _____, type 2 diabetes mellitus.

CHAPTER 8 REVIEW

5. An underdose of insulin due to an insulin pump failure should be assigned to a code from subcategory _____, Mechanical complication of other specified internal and external prosthetic devices, implants and grafts, that specifies the type of pump malfunction, as the principal or first-listed code, followed by code _____, Underdosing of insulin and oral hypoglycemic [antidiabetic] drugs.

6. The principal or first-listed code for an encounter due to an insulin pump malfunction resulting in an overdose of insulin should also be _____, Mechanical complication of other specified internal and external prosthetic devices, implants and grafts, followed by code _____, Poisoning by insulin and oral hypoglycemic [antidiabetic] drugs, accidental (unintentional).

7. Codes under categories _____, Diabetes mellitus due to underlying condition, _____, Drug or chemical induced diabetes mellitus, and _____, Other specified diabetes mellitus, identify complications/manifestations associated with secondary diabetes mellitus.

8. For patients who routinely use insulin or hypoglycemic drugs, code _____, Long-term (current) use of insulin, or _____, Long term (current) use of oral hypoglycemic drugs should also be assigned.

9. Code Z79.4 should _____ be assigned if insulin is given _____ to bring a patient's blood sugar under control during an encounter.

10. For postpancreatectomy diabetes mellitus (lack of insulin due to the surgical removal of all or part of the pancreas), assign code _____, Postprocedural hypoinsulinemia.

Let's Check It! Rules and Regulations

Please answer the following questions from the knowledge you have gained after reading this chapter.

1. LO 8.1 Discuss Graves' disease. When you look up Graves' disease in the Alphabetic Index, where does it send you?

2. LO 8.2 Explain the difference between diabetes mellitus type 1 and diabetes mellitus type 2; include the ICD-10-CM category code for each.

3. LO 8.3 How would you code an overdose of insulin caused by a malfunction of an insulin pump?

4. LO 8.4 Explain Cushing's syndrome, including the ICD-10-CM code category as well as an example of another diagnosis that may result from having Cushing's.

5. LO 8.6 What is cystic fibrosis and what gene is defective? Include an example of where manifestations can appear.

YOU CODE IT! Basics

First, identify the main term in the following diagnoses; then code the diagnosis.

Example: Diabetes mellitus, type 1, with dermatitis:
    a. main term: *diabetes* **b.** diagnosis *E10.620*

1. Endemic hypothyroid cretinism:
    a. main term: _____ **b.** diagnosis: _____

2. Diabetes mellitus with hyperglycemia:
    a. main term: _____ **b.** diagnosis: _____

3. Abscess of the thyroid:
    a. main term: _____ **b.** diagnosis: _____

4. Type I glycogen storage disease:
    a. main term: _____ **b.** diagnosis: _____

5. Urea cycle metabolism disorder:
    a. main term: _____ **b.** diagnosis: _____

6. Thyroid nodules with thyrotoxicosis:
    a. main term: _____ **b.** diagnosis: _____

7. Hashimoto's disease:
   a. main term: _____   b. diagnosis: _____
8. 5-alpha-reductase deficiency:
   a. main term: _____   b. diagnosis: _____
9. Wernicke's encephalopathy:
   a. main term: _____   b. diagnosis: _____
10. Hartnup's disease:
    a. main term: _____   b. diagnosis: _____
11. Beta hyperlipoproteinemia:
    a. main term: _____   b. diagnosis: _____
12. Cystic fibrosis with intestinal manifestations:
    a. main term: _____   b. diagnosis: _____
13. Respiratory acidosis:
    a. main term: _____   b. diagnosis: _____
14. Postprocedural hypoparathyroidism:
    a. main term: _____   b. diagnosis: _____
15. Dysmetabolic syndrome X:
    a. main term: _____   b. diagnosis: _____

YOU CODE IT! Practice

Using the techniques described in this chapter, carefully read through the case studies and determine the most accurate ICD-10-CM code(s) and external cause code(s), if appropriate, for each case study.

1. Jason Peak, a 33-year-old male, comes to see Dr. James with the complaint that he is having difficulty sleeping, is sweating a lot, and has diarrhea. Dr. James completes an examination and notes muscle weakness and skin warmth with moistness. Dr. James also notes eyelid retraction with exophthalmos. Jason is diagnosed with Graves' disease.

2. Pauline Allyson, a 2-week-old female, is brought in by her mother to see her pediatrician, Dr. Goldburg. Pauline is having feeding difficulties with vomiting. She also has diarrhea. Dr. Goldburg notes the child is failing to thrive, as well as hepatosplenomegaly and abdominal distention. Pauline is admitted to the hospital, where lab tests confirm the absence of lysosomal lipase acid (LIPA). Pauline is diagnosed with Wolman's disease.

3. Joyce Meadows, a 42-year-old female, was found unconscious by her husband, George, who rushed his wife to the nearest ED. Dr. Herald asked about her medical history and George said she was diagnosed with type 2 diabetes about 3 years ago. After lab work, Joyce is admitted in a diabetic hypoglycemic coma.

4. Richard Sullivan, a 12-year-old male, presents with the complaint of tiredness. Richard is accompanied by his mother. Mrs. Sullivan tells Dr. Gilbert that Richard has been clumsy lately and seems confused. After a thorough examination, Dr. Gilbert notes slight muscle stiffness and Kayser–Fleischer rings bilaterally. Richard is admitted to Weston Hospital, where a liver biopsy confirmed the diagnosis of Wilson's disease.

5. April Sundell, a 48-year-old female, presents today with the complaint of generally being "out of sorts" or a feeling of uneasiness. Dr. Loveichelle notes muscle weakness and mild hyperventilation. The laboratory results confirm the diagnosis of hyperkalemia.

6. Latoya Nexsen, a 61-year-old female with diabetes type 1, presents today with the complaint that her left lower leg is cold and she has a sore that won't heal. Dr. Benson notes gangrene in Latoya's left extremity and admits her to Weston Hospital. After a thorough physical exam, lab workup, and an angiography, Latoya is diagnosed with atherosclerosis and gangrene of the left lower extremity due to type 1 diabetes mellitus.

CHAPTER 8 REVIEW

7. Lee Summers, a 3-year-old male, is brought in by his parents for a checkup. The parents have no specific concerns. Lee does have a history of ear infections and colds. Dr. Shirley, his pediatrician, notes a prominent forehead, a flattened nose bridge, and a slightly enlarged tongue. Dr. Shirley completes a urine test, which reveal the presence of mucopolysaccharides. Lee is admitted to the hospital, where further laboratory tests confirm the diagnosis of Hunter's syndrome.

8. Loretta Sims, a 14-year-old female, presents today with the complaint of abdominal bloating and cramps with vomiting. Mrs. Sims, her mother, says this usually occurs shortly after Loretta has drunk milk or eaten yogurt. Dr. Albany completes an examination and the hydrogen breath test confirms the diagnosis of primary lactose intolerance.

9. Billy Siau, an 8-month-old male with a congenital cataract, was referred to an ophthalmologist by his pediatrician, Dr. Wilberly. Billy and his mother present today to discuss the results of Billy's tests. Dr. Wilberly also notes that Billy has hypotonia and below-normal reflexes. The ophthalmologist's report confirms glaucoma. Dr. Wilberly diagnoses Billy with Lowe's syndrome.

10. Anita Kucherin, a 27-year-old female, is at 29 weeks gestation. This is Anita's first baby and she has not felt the baby move all day, so she presents to the ED. Anita was diagnosed with diabetes type 2 approximately 3 years ago. Anita states she has tried to keep her diabetes under control. Anita is admitted to the hospital for observation.

11. James Bucklew, a 38-year-old male, presents for the results of the blood tests taken last week. Dr. Walter documents central obesity, hypertension, decreased serum HDL cholesterol (fasting), elevated serum triglyceride level (fasting), and pre-diabetes. James's BMI is 35.4. Dr. Walter diagnoses James with Dysmetabolic syndrome X.

12. Diana Gamble, a 56-year-old female, had her pancreas removed and is now experiencing headaches, blurred vision, and weight loss. Diana admits she has not been taking her medications as prescribed. Dr. Caldwell notes a blood sugar of 305 mg/dL postprandial and admits Diana. After a complete workup, Diana is diagnosed with postpancreatectomy hyperglycemia.

13. Mark Hennecy, a 32-year-old male, presents today with the complaints of feeling tired all the time, difficulty concentrating, and abdominal pain. Dr. Mather notes mild jaundice. After a thorough examination and review of the laboratory results, Mark is diagnosed with Gilbert's syndrome.

14. Erica Lamotte, a 63-year-old female, has been diagnosed with insulin-dependent (type 1) diabetic nephropathy and chronic renal failure, stage 4. She is now requiring regular dialysis treatments.

15. Sue Pittman, a 46-year-old female, presents today with the complaints of tiredness and numbness. Sue was diagnosed with hypertension 2 years ago. Dr. Charmers notes muscle weakness with slight paralysis. Sue is admitted to the hospital, where blood tests reveal a high level of calcium. After a complete workup, Sue is diagnosed with familial aldosteronism, type I.

YOU CODE IT! Application

The following exercises provide practice in abstracting physicians' documentation from our health care facility, Prader, Bracker, & Associates. These case studies are modeled on real patient encounters. Using the techniques described in this chapter, carefully read through the case studies and determine the most accurate ICD-10-CM code(s) and external cause code(s), if appropriate, for each case study.

PRADER, BRACKER, & ASSOCIATES
A Complete Health Care Facility
159 Healthcare Way • SOMEWHERE, FL 32811 • 407-555-6789

PATIENT: FUENTES, GILES

ACCOUNT/EHR #: FUENGI001

DATE: 09/16/18

Attending Physician: Renee O. Bracker, MD

This 61-year-old male returns today to review the results of his blood tests, ordered last week. Patient had come in with complaints of hyperactive deep tendon reflexes, muscle cramps, and carpopedal spasm.

Pathology report shows abnormally decreased blood calcium levels. I discussed the details of this condition and reviewed treatment options. He wants to discuss this with his wife, and he will call within the next few days.

DX: Hypocalcemia

ROB/pw   D: 09/16/18 09:50:16   T: 09/18/18 12:55:01

Determine the most accurate ICD-10-CM code(s).

PRADER, BRACKER, & ASSOCIATES
A Complete Health Care Facility
159 Healthcare Way • SOMEWHERE, FL 32811 • 407-555-6789

PATIENT: MOLINAZZI, JAMES

ACCOUNT/EHR #: MOLIJA001

DATE: 09/16/18

Attending Physician: Oscar R. Prader, MD

S: Pt is a 52-year-old male, comes in for a 6-week follow-up since his diagnosis of secondary diabetes mellitus due to hyperthyroidism. Patient states he has been taking his methimazole, as prescribed.

O: H: 6'0", W: 168, T: 99.1, BP: 125/82; HEENT: unremarkable. Heart rhythm is regular and steady. Lung sounds are also normal. EKG unremarkable. I emphasized the importance of medication and diet. I reviewed the plan to control the secondary diabetes with diet and exercise as first treatment choice.

A: Hyperthyroidism with secondary diabetes mellitus

P: 1. Rx: Propranolol to manage tachycardia. Methimazole continued

   2. Rx: TSH blood test. Patient to go to lab for test within the week.

   3. Patient to return in 10–14 days.

ORP/pw   D: 09/16/18 09:50:16   T: 09/18/18 12:55:01

Determine the most accurate ICD-10-CM code(s).

CHAPTER 8 REVIEW

PRADER, BRACKER, & ASSOCIATES

A Complete Health Care Facility

159 Healthcare Way • SOMEWHERE, FL 32811 • 407-555-6789

PATIENT: CARTER, KIMBERLY

ACCOUNT/EHR #: CARTKI001

DATE: 09/16/18

Attending Physician: Renee O. Bracker, MD

Pt, a 61-year-old female, comes in for her regular checkup. She has insulin-dependent diabetes mellitus, type 2, with bilateral, mild, nonproliferative retinal edema and chronic kidney disease, stage I. In addition, she suffers from hypertensive heart disease with episodes of congestive heart failure. After the exam, some time is spent talking about her day-to-day activities, her diet and overall eating habits, whether or not she is engaging in regular exercise, and her overall mental attitudes as well as physical well-being. The patient states it can be difficult to get around by herself due to the problems with her eyes, and she is finding it more and more difficult to give herself the insulin injections. I provided her with some information about an insulin pump and she states she will go over it and discuss it with her son.

ROB/pw   D: 09/16/18 09:50:16   T: 09/18/18 12:55:01

Determine the most accurate ICD-10-CM code(s).

PRADER, BRACKER, & ASSOCIATES

A Complete Health Care Facility

159 Healthcare Way • SOMEWHERE, FL 32811 • 407-555-6789

PATIENT: WILLRODT, VICTORIA

ACCOUNT/EHR #: WILLVI001

DATE: 09/16/18

Attending Physician: Oscar R. Prader, MD

S: Pt is a 28-year-old female complaining of discoloration of her right lower eyelid. She states the discoloration is of 4 weeks duration with no evidence of healing despite multiple home remedies and over-the-counter treatments. Pt is a type 1 diabetic for 10 years.

O: Wt: 146 lb, Ht: 5′5″ T: 98.6, BP: 131/58; HEENT: unremarkable. Dr. Prader notes premature graying of the right eyelashes and eyebrows and discoloration of the right lower eyelid. Ultraviolet light treatment and micropigmentation are discussed as treatment options.

A: Type 1 diabetes; Vitiligo

P: RX: 0.1% Tacrolimus ointment, b.d

   Pt to return in 2 weeks for follow-up

ORP/pw   D: 09/16/18 09:50:16   T: 09/18/18 12:55:01

Determine the most accurate ICD-10-CM code(s).

WESTON HOSPITAL

629 Healthcare Way • SOMEWHERE, FL 32811 • 407-555-6541

PATIENT: HAWKINS, TYRONE

ACCOUNT/EHR #: HAWKTY001

DATE: 09/16/18

Attending Physician: Renee O. Bracker, MD

S: Patient is a 46-year-old male with insulin-dependent type 2 diabetic nephropathy and end-stage renal disease. He presents today for an arteriovenous shunt for dialysis. Tyrone complains of shortness of breath and extreme fatigue.

PE: H: 5'10", Wt: 164, T: 99.2, R: 24, P: 106, BP: 175/63. Dr. Bracker notes some confusion and admits Tyrone for an emergency hemodialysis treatment. Once patient was stabilized, a Cimino-type direct arteriovenous anastomosis is performed by incising the skin of the left antecubital fossa. Vessel clamps are placed on the vein and adjacent artery. The vein is dissected free, and the downstream portion of the vein is sutured to an opening in the artery using an end-to-side technique. The skin incision is closed in layers.

ROB/pw   D: 09/16/18 09:50:16   T: 09/18/18 12:55:01

Determine the most accurate ICD-10-CM code(s).

9 Coding Mental, Behavioral, and Neurological Disorders

Key Terms

Abuse
Acute
Anxiety
Behavioral Disturbance
Chronic
Dependence
Depressive
Manic
Phobia
Schizophrenia
Somatoform Disorder
Use

Learning Outcomes

After completing this chapter, the student should be able to:

LO 9.1 Determine underlying conditions that affect mental health.
LO 9.2 Distinguish mood and nonmood disorders.
LO 9.3 Apply the guidelines for reporting nonpsychotic mental conditions.
LO 9.4 Identify conditions affecting the central nervous system.
LO 9.5 Interpret details regarding peripheral nervous system conditions into accurate codes.
LO 9.6 Assess the diagnosis of pain and report it with accurate codes.

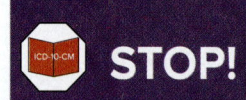

STOP! Remember, you need to follow along in your ICD-10-CM code book for an optimal learning experience.

9.1 Conditions That Affect Mental Health

Mental and behavioral disorders have long been a mystery to the average person, and the lack of understanding has fed fear of patients with these disorders. The dysfunction of a person's brain is often the result of many of the same things that cause other bodily health concerns, including genetics, congenital anomalies, traumatic injury, or the invasion of a pathogen. Any of these, along with other conditions and circumstances, have the ability to impact the health and function of the brain. Scientific research has evidenced shared signs and symptoms between psychiatric illness and neurological illness.

The accepted understanding of mental illness is a condition that negatively affects an individual's thoughts, emotions, behaviors, ability to maintain effective social interactions, and ability to appropriately carry out the activities of daily living.

Mental Disorders Due to Known Physiological Conditions

In some cases, a mental disorder is caused by another condition in the body. The physiological condition may be any of various diagnoses, including an infarction of the brain, hypertensive cerebrovascular disease, or a disease such as Creutzfeldt-Jakob disease, Parkinson's disease, or trypanosomiasis (a condition commonly known as *sleeping sickness*). Moreover, some endocrine disorders, exogenous hormones, and toxic substances can cause cognitive and/or intellectual malfunction, including signs and symptoms of problematic memory, impaired judgment, and diminished intellect.

Dementia is included in this subsection of the chapter on mental and behavioral disorders in ICD-10-CM. This diagnosis can be identified by evidence of both neurologic and psychological signs and symptoms, such as differences in personality, altered thoughts and feelings, and behavioral changes.

When it comes to reporting diagnoses for mental disorders that are manifestations of physiological conditions, you need to identify from the documentation the specific known etiology in cerebral disease, brain injury, or other insult leading to this cerebral dysfunction.

Vascular Dementia

A patient may develop vascular dementia after having experienced an infarction of the brain that is known to be a manifestation of a previously existing vascular disease. In ICD-10-CM, code category F01 also includes a diagnosis of hypertensive cerebrovascular disease as well as arteriosclerotic dementia. A cerebrovascular disease and ischemic or hemorrhagic brain injury can often result in cognitive impairment known as vascular dementia.

> **EXAMPLE**
>
> At the code category F01, you can see the definition, along with some important notations:
>
> ☑4 **F01 Vascular dementia**
>
> Vascular dementia as a result of infarction of the brain due to vascular disease, including hypertensive cerebrovascular disease.
>
> INCLUDES arteriosclerotic dementia
>
> *Code first* the underlying physiological condition or sequelae of cerebrovascular disease.

Therefore, the notation to "*Code first* **the underlying physiological condition or sequelae of cerebrovascular disease**" logically supports your correct sequencing of codes that may be involved in the reporting of this diagnosis.

> **EXAMPLES**
>
> F01.50   Vascular dementia without behavioral disturbance
> F01.51   Vascular dementia with behavior disturbance
>
> *Use additional code*, if applicable, to identify wandering in vascular dementia (Z91.83).

As you read down this code category listing, you can see that, in addition to identifying the underlying physiological condition, you will also need to identify whether or not the patient is documented as having **behavioral disturbance**. If so, has the patient also been documented as having episodes of "wandering"? These details will guide you toward the correct code or codes to accurately report this patient's condition.

Amnestic Disorder Due to Known Physiological Condition

Reporting amnestic disorder due to known physiological condition will take you to code category F04 Amnestic disorder, with the additional descriptions of Korsakov's psychosis and Syndrome, nonalcoholic. You can see that the *Code first* **underlying condition** notation requires that the underlying condition be physiological, thereby eliminating any psychological underlying conditions from qualifying for this code.

Behavioral Disturbance
A type of common behavior that includes mood disorders (such as depression, apathy, and euphoria), sleep disorders (such as insomnia and hypersomnia), psychotic symptoms (such as delusions and hallucinations), and agitation (such as pacing, wandering, and aggression).

Note that ICD-10-CM reporting of this diagnosis has an **EXCLUDES1** notation. An **EXCLUDES1** notation identifies other diagnoses that are mutually exclusive to the diagnosis above the notation (in this case, F04). This is the absolute statement that the excluded code can never be used at the same time because the two conditions cannot occur together in one patient at one time.

> **EXCLUDES1** amnesia NOS (R41.3)
> anterograde amnesia (R41.1)
> dissociative amnesia (F44.0)
> retrograde amnesia (R41.2)

F04 also carries an **EXCLUDES2** notation identifying several amnestic disorders that are not included in F04, therefore requiring either a different code or an additional code:

> **EXCLUDES2** alcohol-induced or unspecified Korsakov's syndrome (F10.26, F10.96)
> Korsakov's syndrome induced by other psychoactive substances (F13.26, F13.96, F19.16, F19.26, F19.96)

Mood Disorder Due to Known Physiological Condition

A mood disorder is a daily issue of dealing with one's emotional state. This category of mental illnesses includes major depressive disorder, dysthymic disorder, and bipolar disorder. Code subcategory F06.3- differentiates itself from other diagnoses under "Mood [affective] disorders," which includes bipolar disorder (F30–F39), because this diagnosis (reported with F06.3-) includes a documented physiological underlying cause.

EXAMPLES

F06.30	Mood disorder due to known physiological condition, unspecified
F06.31	Mood disorder due to known physiological condition, with depressive features
F06.32	Mood disorder due to known physiological condition, with major depressive-like episode
F06.33	Mood disorder due to known physiological condition, with manic features
F06.34	Mood disorder due to known physiological condition, with mixed features

As you abstract documentation related to a mood disorder, you must be alert to mentions of any additional signs and symptoms.

Depressive features include decrease in interest in hobbies or favorite activities, hypersomnia, or insomnia virtually every day.

Manic features are identified by documented episodes of intensely disruptive and exaggerated behaviors of heightened mood.

Mixed features refer to documented and regular (virtually every day within 1 week) meeting of the criteria of both depressive and manic features. Also known as roller-coastering.

Beneath F06.3 is an **EXCLUDES2** notation, indicating specific diagnoses that are not included in this subcategory:

> **EXCLUDES2** mood disorders due to alcohol and other psychoactive substances (F10-F19 with .14, .24, .94)
> mood disorders, not due to known physiological condition or unspecified (F30-F39)

Personality and Behavioral Disorders Due to Known Physiological Condition

There have been known physiological conditions that manifest personality changes or behavioral disorders. Traumatic brain injury—specifically, damage to the patient's frontal lobe—can be evidenced by apathy, a lack of ability to formulate plans, emotional bluntness, and inability to perform abstract thinking. In this code category, you will find a *Code first* **underlying physiological condition** notation applicable to all codes within.

Beneath F07.0 are two EXCLUDES notations, which further clarify which diagnoses are reported with this code and which require the coder to look elsewhere in the code set:

EXAMPLE

F07.0	Personality change due to known physiological condition (Frontal lobe syndrome) (Organic pseudopsychopathic personality) (Postleucotomy syndrome)
	Code first **underlying physiological condition**
EXCLUDES1	mild cognitive impairment (G31.84) postconcussional syndrome (F07.81) postencephalitic syndrome (F07.89) signs and symptoms involving emotional state (R45.-)
EXCLUDES2	specific personality disorder (F60.-)
F07.81	Postconcussion syndrome (Postcontusion syndrome or encephalopathy) (Posttraumatic brain syndrome, nonpsychotic)
	Use additional code **to identify associated post-traumatic headache, if applicable (G44.3-)**
EXCLUDES1	Current concussion (brain) (S06.0-) Postencephalitic syndrome (F07.89)

Remember that an EXCLUDES1 notation in ICD-10-CM identifies diagnoses that are mutually exclusive—that cannot be reported for the same patient at the same time. Also, don't forget to read the notation at the top of this code category, directly beneath F07 . . . this applies to all codes within this code category.

Code first **underlying physiological condition**

LET'S CODE IT! SCENARIO

Eboni O'Neal, a 37-year-old female, came with her husband, Carl, to see Dr. Annikah, a psychiatrist, on a referral from her regular physician. She complains about unusual fatigue and problems remembering things. Her husband has complained that she has been unusually irritable. Carl stated that he has found Eboni wandering the neighborhood several times over the last few weeks. Eboni admitted to being on a new dairy-free, animal product–free diet. After a complete physical examination, Dr. Annikah performed a complete psychology exam and ordered blood work, which confirmed his diagnosis of dementia caused by vitamin B_{12} deficiency.

(continued)

Let's Code It!

Dr. Annikah diagnosed Eboni with *dementia caused by vitamin B_{12} deficiency.* You also read that she did have incidents of *wandering.* When you turn to the Alphabetic Index, you see

> **Dementia (degenerative (primary)) (old age) (persisting)** F03.90
> In (due to)
> Vitamin B12 deficiency E53.8 *[F02.80]*
> With behavioral disturbance E53.8 *[F02.81]*

You should remember from the chapter *The Coding Process* that the second code, in italicized brackets, tells you that you will need two codes for this diagnosis and in which order to report these two codes. Turn to the Tabular List to read the first suggested code:

> ✔4 **E53**   **Deficiency of other B group vitamins**

Read down and review all of the fourth-character choices to determine the most accurate code:

> **E53.8**   **Deficiency of other specified B group vitamins**

Next, you know that you will need to follow this code with a code from F02—either F02.80 or F02.81. Let's take a look at both codes and see what exactly is meant by **behavioral disturbance**:

> **F02.80**   Dementia in other diseases classified elsewhere without behavioral disturbance
> **F02.81**   Dementia in other diseases classified elsewhere with behavioral disturbance

Did you notice the notation beneath F02.81?

> *Use additional code*, if applicable, to identify wandering in dementia in conditions classified elsewhere (Z91.83)

Aha! This tells you that "wandering" is considered a behavioral disturbance. Dr. Annikah documented that Eboni had been wandering, so you will need one more code:

> **Z91.83**   **Wandering in conditions classified elsewhere**

Good job! You determined the three codes required to accurately report Dr. Annikah's encounter with Eboni.

Check the top of all three chapters in ICD-10-CM. Check them all for an INCLUDES notation, a *Use additional code* note, an EXCLUDES1 notation, and an EXCLUDES2 notation. Read carefully. Do any relate to Dr. Annikah's diagnosis of Eboni? No. Turn to the Official Guidelines and read Section 1.c.4, 1.c.5, and 1.c.21. There is nothing specifically applicable here either.

Now you can report these three codes with confidence.

> **E53.8**   Deficiency of other specified B group vitamins
> **F02.81**   Dementia in other diseases classified elsewhere with behavioral disturbance
> **Z91.83**   Wandering in conditions classified elsewhere

Good coding!

Mental and Behavioral Disorders Due to Psychoactive Substance Use

Reporting Alcohol-Related and Drug-Related Disorders

When a patient is diagnosed with an alcohol- or drug-related disorder, the diagnosis is often more complex, as such conditions are susceptible to both psychological and physiological signs, symptoms, manifestations, and co-morbidities. Alcohol use doesn't damage the actual brain cells, but it does damage the ends of neurons, which are called *dendrites.* This results in problems conveying messages between the neurons.

EXAMPLES

NOTE: All codes in this example require additional characters.

F10.1	Alcohol abuse
F10.2	Alcohol dependence
F10.9	Alcohol use, unspecified
F11.1	Opioid abuse
F11.2	Opioid dependence
F11.9	Opioid use, unspecified
F12.1	Cannabis abuse
F12.2	Cannabis dependence
F12.9	Cannabis use, unspecified
F13.1	**Sedative, hypnotic or anxiolytic**-related abuse
F13.2	Sedative, hypnotic or anxiolytic-related dependence
F13.9	Sedative, hypnotic or anxiolytic-related use, unspecified
F14.1	Cocaine abuse
F14.2	Cocaine dependence
F14.9	Cocaine use, unspecified

Sedative
A tranquilizer; a drug used to calm or soothe.

Hypnotic
A drug that induces sleep.

Anxiolytic
A drug used to reduce anxiety.

The first thing you might notice about these codes is that details are required from the documentation to identify *use* of, *abuse* of, or *dependence* on the psychoactive substance. Also, there are codes for specifically reporting the *use* of alcohol and drugs that enable the tracking of the patient's behavior, which often will ultimately have a negative impact on his or her health. These details can give providers and researchers a great deal of useful information as they look for better ways to care for patients and their maladies.

What is the clinical difference between these terms?

Use: Consumption of a substance without significant clinical manifestations.

Abuse: Ongoing, regular consumption of a substance with resulting clinical manifestations.

Dependence: Ongoing, regular consumption of a substance with resulting significant clinical manifestations and a dramatic decrease in the effect of the substance with continued use, therefore requiring an increased quantity of the substance to achieve intoxication. In addition, the patient will require continued consumption of the substance to avoid withdrawal symptoms and other serious behavioral effects, occurring at any time in the same 12-month period.

All of these codes require additional characters to identify details from the documentation about manifestations and co-morbidities. Let's take *alcohol abuse* as an example of what details you may need to abstract from the clinical documentation.

Use
Occasional consumption of a substance without clinical manifestations.

Abuse
Regular consumption of a substance with manifestations.

Dependence
Ongoing, regular consumption of a substance with resulting significant clinical manifestations, and a dramatic decrease in the effect of the substance with continued use, therefore requiring an increased quantity of the substance to achieve intoxication.

EXAMPLES

F10.1	Alcohol abuse
F10.10	Alcohol abuse, uncomplicated
F10.120	Alcohol abuse with intoxication, uncomplicated
F10.121	Alcohol abuse with intoxication delirium
F10.14	Alcohol abuse with alcohol-induced mood disorder
F10.150	Alcohol abuse with alcohol-induced psychotic disorder with delusions
F10.180	Alcohol abuse with alcohol-induced anxiety disorder
F10.181	Alcohol abuse with alcohol-induced sexual dysfunction
F10.182	Alcohol abuse with alcohol-induced sleep disorder
F10.188	Alcohol abuse with other alcohol-induced disorder

> **GUIDANCE CONNECTION**
>
> Read the ICD-10-CM Official Guidelines for Coding and Reporting, section **I. Conventions, General Coding Guidelines and Chapter Specific Guidelines,** subsection **C. Chapter-Specific Coding Guidelines,** chapter **5. Mental, Behavioral, and Neurodevelopmental disorders (F01–F99),** subsection **b. Mental and behavioral disorders due to psychoactive substance use, 2) Psychoactive substance use, abuse and dependence** and **3) Psychoactive substance use.**

As you can see, ICD-10-CM requires an understanding of the psychological and behavioral impacts of the use, abuse, or dependence. Signs, symptoms, manifestations, and co-morbidities such as delirium, mood disorder, and hallucinations will be reported with one combination code from this subsection.

In the subcategories for alcohol use and dependence, you will also find codes including a state of withdrawal, again providing one combination code to report this condition.

EXAMPLE

F10.231   Alcohol dependence with withdrawal delirium

The extended descriptions and combination-code choices include those codes used to report the use of other nontherapeutic substances as well. Take, for example, caffeine use, hallucinogens, and inhalant use.

EXAMPLES

F15.120	Other stimulant abuse with intoxication, uncomplicated
F15.920	Other stimulant use, unspecified with intoxication, uncomplicated
F16.1-	Hallucinogen abuse
F16.2-	Hallucinogen dependence
F16.9-	Hallucinogen use, unspecified
F18.1-	Inhalant abuse
F18.9-	Inhalant use, unspecified

ICD-10-CM code descriptions separate inhalant abuse and dependence into its own specific code category (F18), and caffeine (yes, this is considered a substance) is included in the "Other" code category, now combined with amphetamine-related disorders.

As with the previous code categories in this subsection, the additional characters required for these ICD-10-CM codes include abstracting documentation for details on accompanying intoxication, delirium, perceptual disturbance, mood disorder, psychotic disorder with delusions or hallucinations, **anxiety** disorder, flashbacks, and other manifestations.

Anxiety
The feelings of apprehension and fear, sometimes manifested with physical manifestations such as sweating and palpitations.

One more addition to this subsection of ICD-10-CM's *Chapter 5, Mental, Behavioral, and Neurodevelopmental disorders*, is code category *F17 Nicotine dependence*. The **EXCLUDES1** note reminds you that nicotine dependence is not the same diagnosis as tobacco use (Z72.0) or history of tobacco dependence (Z87.891). Therefore, the documentation will need to specifically discern between tobacco use and nicotine dependence.

EXAMPLES

F17.210	Nicotine dependence, cigarettes, uncomplicated
F17.211	Nicotine dependence, cigarettes, in remission
F17.213	Nicotine dependence, cigarettes, with withdrawal
F17.218	Nicotine dependence, cigarettes, with other nicotine-induced disorders
F17.220	Nicotine dependence, chewing tobacco, uncomplicated
F17.221	Nicotine dependence, chewing tobacco, in remission

F17.223	Nicotine dependence, chewing tobacco, with withdrawal
F17.228	Nicotine dependence, chewing tobacco, with other nicotine-induced disorders
F17.290	Nicotine dependence, other tobacco product, uncomplicated
F17.291	Nicotine dependence, other tobacco product, in remission
F17.293	Nicotine dependence, other tobacco product, with withdrawal
F17.298	Nicotine dependence, other tobacco product, with other nicotine-induced disorders

The bottom line is that ICD-10-CM has organized these codes in a logical and efficient order and provided you with many combination codes.

LET'S CODE IT! SCENARIO

Jason Hurst, a 63-year-old male, has been a salesman for the last 30 years. He travels throughout the Midwest and has had a less-than-stellar career. Very often, he has come close to being fired for not making quota, but his supervisor takes pity on him because he has been with the company for so long. He is at the medical office today by court order after being arrested for his third DUI in the last 6 months. Seeking treatment is part of his plea deal so he doesn't lose his driver's license. He needs to be able to drive to see his customers.

Jason states he has tried to stop drinking but can't because it is part of his job. He must take customers out for a drink. And when he is back at his office, all the guys go out for drinks after work. When he is on the road, he finds nothing to do in the motel at night, so he drinks away the loneliness. The one time he tried to quit drinking, he got really sick. The only thing that helped him feel better was a little "hair of the dog."

He states that at times he is very sad and hopeless, while other times, especially when he is with clients, he is the life of the party and knows some of the best jokes. He pleads for help and begins to cry.

Dr. Walkowicz diagnoses Jason with alcohol dependence with alcohol-induced mood disorder.

Let's Code It!

Dr. Walkowicz diagnosed Jason with *alcohol dependence with alcohol-induced mood disorder*. Turn in the Alphabetic Index to find

Dependence (on) (syndrome) F19.20
    Alcohol (ethyl) (methyl) (without remission) F10.20
      With
        Mood disorder F10.24

Now let's turn to find this suggested code in the Tabular List:

☑4 **F10**   **Alcohol related disorder**

Use additional code for blood alcohol level, if applicable (Y90.-)

This is not applicable in Jason's case, so continue reading to review all of the options for the required fourth character. Did you choose this code?

☑5 **F10.2**   **Alcohol dependence**

Don't skip over the EXCLUDES1 and EXCLUDES2 notations. You must read them all carefully, and then determine whether they apply to the specific case you are coding. In this case, they do not. Keep reading all of the fifth-character choices to determine the most accurate code. You can see the code that matches Dr. Walkowicz's notes perfectly!

    F10.24   **Alcohol dependence with alcohol-induced mood disorder**

Good work!

> **GUIDANCE CONNECTION**
>
> Read the ICD-10-CM Official Guidelines for Coding and Reporting, section **I. Conventions, General Coding Guidelines and Chapter Specific Guidelines,** subsection **C. Chapter-Specific Coding Guidelines,** chapter **5. Mental, Behavioral, and Neurodevelopmental disorders (F01–F99),** subsection **b. Mental and behavioral disorders due to psychoactive substance use, 1) In remission.**

Manic
An emotional state that includes elation, excitement, and exuberance.

Depressive
An emotional state that includes sadness, hopelessness, and gloom.

In Remission

The determination of whether a patient who has been diagnosed with a mental or behavioral disorder due to the use of a psychoactive substance is in remission is in the judgment of the attending physician. Therefore, report the appropriate character identifying the state of remission only when the physician has specifically documented this condition.

> **EXAMPLES**
>
> F11.21   Opioid dependence, in remission
> F14.21   Cocaine dependence, in remission

9.2 Mood (Affective) and Nonmood (Psychotic) Disorders

Mood (Affective) Disorders

Bipolar Disorders

The etiology of bipolar disorders is uncertain and complex. The strongest evidence leads to the belief that many factors act together to activate the signs and symptoms. While some evidence exists that the condition tends to have familial connections, there have been studies of identical twins in which only one twin is affected.

Bipolar disorder is categorized as a "mood disorder" identified by acute swings exhibited by the patient, ranging from euphoria and hyperactivity to depression and lethargy. An overly elated or overexcited state is called a **manic** episode, and an acute sad or hopeless state is known as a **depressive** episode. Bipolar disorder may also be present in a *mixed* state, during which the patient experiences both mania and depression simultaneously.

Bipolar disorder is a chronic illness, therefore requiring long-term, continuous treatment to control symptoms. Mood stabilizers (e.g., lithium carbonate), atypical antipsychotics (e.g., clozapine), and antidepressants are most commonly prescribed in combination.

This diagnosis is categorized into two types: Type I bipolar disorder is identified as alternating between manic episodes and depressive episodes, while type II bipolar patients deal with recurring depressive episodes with occasional mania.

> **EXAMPLES**
>
> F31   Bipolar disorder
> F31.0   Bipolar disorder, current episode hypomanic
> F31.11   Bipolar disorder, current episode, manic without psychotic features, mild
> F31.12   Bipolar disorder, current episode, manic without psychotic features, moderate
> F31.13   Bipolar disorder, current episode, manic without psychotic features, severe
> F31.2   Bipolar disorder, current episode, manic, severe, with psychotic features
> F31.31   Bipolar disorder, current episode, depressed, mild
> F31.32   Bipolar disorder, current episode, depressed, moderate
> F31.4   Bipolar disorder, current episode, depressed, severe, without psychotic features

> F31.5   Bipolar disorder, current episode, depressed, severe, with psychotic features
> F31.6- Bipolar disorder, current episode, mixed
> F31.81 Bipolar II disorder
> F31.89 Other bipolar disorder (recurrent manic episodes NOS)
>
> When you abstract the documentation regarding a current episode, you need to be on the lookout for details regarding the aspects:
>
> - Manic means that the patient reports periods of high energy and an inability to sleep.
> - Depressed mood regards periods of low energy, disinterest in favorite activities, and feeling sad for no apparent reason.
> - Psychotic features include the patient experiencing either auditory or visual hallucinations.

The categorization of those patients in partial or full remission is also available, so you will need to check the documentation for this detail or query the physician.

> **EXAMPLES**
>
> F31.7- Bipolar disorder, currently in remission
> F31.71 Bipolar disorder, in partial remission, most recent episode hypomanic
> F31.72 Bipolar disorder, in full remission, most recent episode hypomanic
> F31.73 Bipolar disorder, in partial remission, most recent episode manic
> F31.74 Bipolar disorder, in full remission, most recent episode manic
> F31.75 Bipolar disorder, in partial remission, most recent episode depressed
> F31.76 Bipolar disorder, in full remission, most recent episode depressed
> F31.77 Bipolar disorder, in partial remission, most recent episode mixed
> F31.78 Bipolar disorder, in full remission, most recent episode mixed
>
> A patient in full remission has not experienced any significant mood fluxuataion for at least 2 months, virtually always during treatment.
>
> A patient in partial remission has experienced reduced episodes or has had no episodes for less than 60 days.

Major Depressive Disorder

Everyone feels sad or depressed at times. It is part of life. However, major depressive disorder causes patients to feel hopeless, guilty, and worthless. The typical activities of life (work, study, sleep, and fun) become difficult and, for some, nearly impossible. Some patients may experience ongoing (recurrent) episodes, while others suffer only a one-time (single) episode. Additional diagnostic terms used by some psychiatrists include *agitated depression, depressive reaction, major depression, psychogenic depression, reactive depression,* and *vital depression*.

Major depressive disorder may be mild, moderate, or severe and may be described as with or without psychotic features. Patients diagnosed with this illness may also experience partial or full remission. As the professional coding specialist, it is your job to ensure that your physician documents all of these details.

> **EXAMPLES**
>
> F32.- Major depressive disorder, single episode
> F33.- Major depressive disorder, recurrent
>
> *(continued)*

> You will need an additional character to identify the current episode as mild, moderate, severe without psychotic features, or severe with psychotic features.
>
> F32.4 Major depressive disorder, single episode, in partial remission
> F33.41 Major depressive disorder, recurrent, in partial remission
>
> A patient in partial remission has experienced reduced episodes or has had no episodes for less than 60 days.
>
> F32.5 Major depressive disorder, single episode, in full remission
> F33.42 Major depressive disorder, recurrent, in full remission
>
> A patient in full remission has not experienced any significant depressive symptoms for at least 2 months, virtually always during treatment.

YOU CODE IT! CASE STUDY

Sherri L., a 23-year-old female, came in to see Dr. Keel, a psychiatrist. She has a very demanding and high-stress life, being a second-year law student. In addition, she is clerking for a judge, and she is planning her wedding for this coming summer. She states that she has always been highly motivated to achieve her goals. After graduating with top honors from college, she went on to achieve a 3.95 GPA in her first year in law school. She admits that she can be very self-critical when she is not able to achieve perfection, even though, intellectually, she knows that perfection is not necessary for success. Recently, she has been struggling with considerable feelings of worthlessness and shame due to her inability to perform as well as she has in the past.

For the past few weeks, Sherri has noticed that she is constantly feeling fatigued, no matter how much she has slept. She also states that it has been increasingly difficult to concentrate at work and pay attention in class. Her best friend, RaeAnn, who works with her at the courthouse, stated that, recently, Sherri is irritable and withdrawn, not at all her typical upbeat and friendly disposition. While she has always prided herself on perfect attendance at school and at work, Sherri has called in sick on several occasions. On those days she stayed in bed all day, watching TV and sleeping.

At home, Sherri's fiancé has noticed changes in her as well. He states that, in the last 6 months, it seems that she has lost interest in sex despite a very healthy sex life during the previous 2 years they had been together. He also has noticed that she has had difficulties falling asleep at night. Her tossing and turning for an hour or two after they go to bed has been keeping him awake. He confesses that he overheard her having tearful phone conversations with RaeAnn and her sister that have worried him. When he tries to get her to open up, she denies anything is wrong, emphatically stating, "I'm fine," and walking away.

Sherri states that she has found herself increasingly dissatisfied with her life. She admits to having frequent thoughts of wishing she was dead, yet denies ever considering suicide. She gets frustrated with herself because she feels that she has every reason to be happy yet can't seem to shake the sense of a heavy dark cloud enshrouding her. Dr. Keel diagnosed Sherri with major depressive disorder, single episode, moderate severity.

You Code It!

Go through the steps of coding, and determine the code or codes that should be reported for this encounter between Dr. Keel and Sherri.

Step #1: Read the case carefully and completely.

Step #2: Abstract the scenario. Which main words or terms describe why the physician cared for the patient during this encounter?

Step #3: Are there any details missing or incomplete for which you would need to query the physician? [If so, ask your instructor.]

Step #4: Check for any relevant guidance, including reading all of the symbols and notations in the Tabular List and the appropriate sections of the Official Guidelines.

> Step #5: Determine the correct diagnosis code or codes to explain why this encounter was medically necessary.
>
> Step #6: Double-check your work.
>
> **Answer:**
>
> Did you determine this to be the correct code?
>
> F32.1   Major depressive disorder, single episode, moderate

Nonmood (Psychotic) Disorders

Schizophrenia

There is no known cause of **schizophrenia** (a psychotic disorder); however, evidence does exist that it may have an etiology of genetic, biological, cultural, and/or psychological foundations. The belief of a genetic predisposition is supported with statistical research showing that the close relatives of a schizophrenic are 50 times more likely to develop the condition. There is also a widely held belief of a biochemical imbalance, specifically excessive activity of dopaminergic synapses, encouraging the signs and symptoms of schizophrenia. Five types of schizophrenia are recognized by psychiatric professionals:

- *Paranoid,* also known as *paraphrenic schizophrenia* [F20.0]
- *Disorganized,* also known as *hebephrenic schizophrenia* or *hebephrenia* [F20.1]
- *Catatonic,* also known as *schizophrenic catalepsy, catatonia,* or *flexibilitas cerea* [F20.2]
- *Undifferentiated,* also known as *atypical schizophrenia* [F20.3]
- *Residual,* also known as *restzustand* [F20.5]

Schizophrenia
A psychotic disorder with no known cause.

The signs and symptoms of schizophrenia are generally categorized into three groups: positive symptoms, negative symptoms, and cognitive symptoms. The specific behaviors related to this diagnosis will vary depending upon the type and phase of the disorder.

> **EXAMPLES**
>
> | Code | Description |
> |---|---|
> | F20.0 | Paranoid schizophrenia |
> | F20.1 | Disorganized schizophrenia |
> | F20.2 | Catatonic schizophrenia |
> | F20.3 | Undifferentiated schizophrenia (Atypical schizophrenia) |
> | F20.5 | Residual schizophrenia |
> | F20.81 | Schizophreniform disorder |
> | F20.89 | Other schizophrenia (Simple schizophrenia) |
> | F21 | Schizotypal disorder (Latent schizophrenia) |
> | F25.0 | Schizoaffective disorder, bipolar type |
> | F25.1 | Schizoaffective disorder, depressive type |
> | F25.8 | Other schizoaffective disorders |

Coders working with health care professionals caring for patients diagnosed with schizophrenia should be aware of the known adverse effects of the antipsychotic drugs most often used to treat this condition. Also known as *neuroleptic drugs,* antipsychotics (such as haloperidol) are known to result in a high incident rate of extrapyramidal effects, including

- Drug-induced parkinsonism [G21.11] with signs of propulsive gait, stooped posture, muscle rigidity, tremors
- Drug-induced acute dystonia [G24.02] showing signs of severe muscle contractions
- Drug-induced akathisia [G25.71] showing signs of restlessness and pacing

Some low-potency drugs in this category have been known to cause orthostatic hypotension [I95.2]—a sudden drop in blood pressure when the patient changes position quickly, such as standing up. A development of malignant neuroleptic syndrome [G21.0] has been reported in as many as 1% of patients taking antipsychotics.

Remember that when these adverse effects have been diagnosed, you will need to include an external cause code to identify the "drug taken for therapeutic purposes" as the reason for this condition. You would choose a code from category T43 Poisoning by, adverse effect of and underdosing of psychotropic drugs, not elsewhere classified in ICD-10-CM.

Schizoid Personality Disorder

There may appear to be some overlap in the signs and symptoms of schizophrenia (a psychotic disorder) and schizoid personality disorder; however, they are very different conditions.

Patients diagnosed with schizoid personality disorder exhibit a limited range of emotions and an aversion to social relationships and personal interactions. These patients have little to no interest in sex and are indifferent to both praise and criticism. Overall, these patients have a flat affect. Report this diagnosis with code F60.1 Schizoid personality disorder.

YOU CODE IT! CASE STUDY

Gary R., a 20-year-old male, is a junior at a state university. Over the past month, his parents have noticed that his behavior has become quite peculiar. Several times, his mother has overheard him speaking in a quiet yet angry tone, even though no one was in the room with him. Over the past 7 to 10 days, Gary has refused to answer or make calls on his cell phone, stating that he knows if he uses the phone, it will activate a deadly chip that has been implanted in his brain by evil men from space.

Gary's parents, as well as his brother and his best friend, have attempted to convince him to join them at an appointment with a psychiatrist for an evaluation, but he adamantly refused, until today. Several times, Gary has accused his parents of conspiring with the aliens to steal his brain. He no longer attends classes and will soon flunk out unless he can get some help.

Other than a few beers with his friends, Gary denies abusing alcohol or drugs. There is a family history of psychiatric illness; an estranged aunt has been in and out of psychiatric hospitals over the years due to erratic and bizarre behavior.

Dr. Zavakos diagnosed Gary with paranoid schizophrenia.

You Code It!

Go through the steps of coding, and determine the code or codes that should be reported for this encounter between Dr. Zavakos and Gary.

Step #1: Read the case carefully and completely.

Step #2: Abstract the scenario. Which main words or terms describe why the physician cared for the patient during this encounter?

Step #3: Are there any details missing or incomplete for which you would need to query the physician? [If so, ask your instructor.]

Step #4: Check for any relevant guidance, including reading all of the symbols and notations in the Tabular List and the appropriate sections of the Official Guidelines.

Step #5: Determine the correct diagnosis code or codes to explain why this encounter was medically necessary.

Step #6: Double-check your work.

Answer:

Did you determine this to be the correct code?

F20.0 Paranoid schizophrenia

9.3 Anxiety, Dissociative, Stress-Related, Somatoform, and Other Nonpsychotic Mental Disorders

Phobias

Are you terrified of something, with no real rationale? The definition of a **phobia** is the excessive and irrational fear of an object, activity, or situation. Of course, a slight fear of a spider or of flying would not typically result in a physician encounter or documented diagnosis. Therefore, for the most part, the code categories for phobias will be used to report the condition in which this fear has risen to the level at which it actually interferes with daily life and, therefore, requires treatment.

Phobia
Irrational and excessive fear of an object, activity, or situation.

Somatoform Disorder
The sincere belief that one is suffering an illness that is not present.

> **EXAMPLES**
> | | |
> |---|---|
> | F40.0- | Agoraphobia |
> | F40.1- | Social phobia |
> | F40.23- | Blood, injection, injury type phobia |
> | F41.0 | Panic disorder [episodic paroxysmal anxiety] |
> | F41.1 | Generalized anxiety disorder |

Somatoform Disorders

The term **somatoform disorders** may be new to you; however, you have probably heard of one type, *hypochondria (hypochondriacal disorder)*, in which patients have an ongoing belief that they have an illness that they do not have. This group of psychological disorders causes the patient to exhibit, or believe he or she exhibits, physical signs and symptoms.

> **EXAMPLES**
> | | |
> |---|---|
> | F45.0 | Somatization disorder (Multiple psychosomatic disorder) |
> | F45.22 | Body dysmorphic disorder |
> | F45.41 | Pain disorder exclusively related to psychological factors |
> | F45.42 | Pain disorder with related psychological factors |
> | | *Code also* associated acute or chronic pain (G89.-) |

GUIDANCE CONNECTION

Read the ICD-10-CM Official Guidelines for Coding and Reporting, section **I. Conventions, General Coding Guidelines and Chapter Specific Guidelines,** subsection **C. Chapter-Specific Coding Guidelines,** chapter **5. Mental, Behavioral, and Neurodevelopmental disorders (F01–F99),** subsection **a. Pain disorders related to psychological factors.**

YOU CODE IT! CASE STUDY

Brian B., a 52-year-old divorced father of two teenagers, states he has a successful, financially rewarding career. He has been with this company for the last 15 years, the last 5 as vice president of his division. Even though his job performance evaluations are good and he has been lauded by his boss, he is overwrought with worry constantly

(continued)

about losing his job and being unable to provide for his children. This worry has been troubling him for about the last 8 or 9 months. Despite really trying, he can't seem to shake the negative thoughts.

Over these last months, he noticed that he feels restless, tired, and stressed out. He often paces in his office when he's alone, especially when not deeply engaged in tasks. He's found difficulty in expressing himself and has been humiliated in a few meetings when this has occurred. At night, when attempting to go to sleep, he often finds that his brain won't shut off. Instead of resting, he finds himself obsessing over all the worst-case scenarios, including losing his job and ending up homeless.

Dr. Burnett diagnoses Brian with generalized anxiety disorder and discusses a treatment plan with him.

You Code It!

Go through the steps of coding, and determine the code or codes that should be reported for this encounter between Dr. Burnett and Brian.

Step #1: Read the case carefully and completely.

Step #2: Abstract the scenario. Which main words or terms describe why the physician cared for the patient during this encounter?

Step #3: Are there any details missing or incomplete for which you would need to query the physician? [If so, ask your instructor.]

Step #4: Check for any relevant guidance, including reading all of the symbols and notations in the Tabular List and the appropriate sections of the Official Guidelines.

Step #5: Determine the correct diagnosis code or codes to explain why this encounter was medically necessary.

Step #6: Double-check your work.

Answer:

Did you determine this to be the correct code?

F41.1   Generalized anxiety disorder

Stress-Related Disorders

Post-traumatic stress disorder (PTSD) is a condition in which a horrible experience leaves a lasting imprint on the patient's sense of danger. Normally, when an individual senses danger, a "fight or flight" response initiates feelings of worry and fear. For those suffering from PTSD, the harmful or dangerous situation is gone, yet the sensation of fear continues.

Situations that may ignite PTSD can affect more individuals than just our wonderful military personnel returning from the horrors of war. Sadly, it has become far too typical to read about a shooting at a school or restaurant, rape, abuse (child, spouse, elder), transportation accidents (car, truck, train, airplane), natural disasters (hurricane, earthquake, flood), or other terrifying ordeals occurring in an all-American neighborhood. As health information management professionals and professional coding specialists, we should be aware, empathetic, and accurate. PTSD affects an estimated 7.5 million adults in the United States.

Signs and symptoms typically appear within 3 months of the event; however, in some cases, they can be internalized and take longer to recognize. Flashbacks, hyperarousal (overreactions), and avoidance are the most frequently experienced behaviors. When the symptoms are acute but then dissipate after a few weeks, this may be diagnosed as acute stress disorder (ASD), reported with ICD-10-CM code F43.0 Acute stress reaction, also known as crisis state or psychic shock.

When the patient experiences at least one flashback or "re-experiencing" symptom (including diaphoresis (sweating) and tachycardia (rapid heart rate)), at least two hyperarousal symptoms (patients may feel edgy, easily startled, or overly nervous), and at least three avoidance symptoms (avoid locations that are reminiscent of the event) that last longer than 1 month, it may be PTSD. Additionally, these patients often experience depression and anxiety as well as frequent attempts to self-medicate, resulting in substance abuse. PTSD is reported with one of these ICD-10-CM codes:

F43.10	Post-traumatic stress disorder, unspecified
F43.11	Post-traumatic stress disorder, acute
F43.12	Post-traumatic stress disorder, chronic

> **CODING BITES**
>
> NOTE: There is a difference between acute PTSD and chronic PTSD. If the documentation is ambiguous or unclear, query the physician.

When reporting PTSD, remember to include external cause codes to explain the specifics about the traumatic event. This is important to both treatment and reimbursement.

- *Cause of the injury,* such as an earthquake or a multicar accident.

EXAMPLES

All of these codes require additional characters to complete a valid code.

X34.xxx-	Earthquake
X37.0xx-	Hurricane (storm surge) (typhoon)
X96.3xx-	Assault by fertilizer bomb
X99.1xx-	Assault by knife
Y36.-	Operations of war
Y37.-	Military Operations

- *Place of the occurrence,* such as the park or the kitchen.

EXAMPLES

Y92.133	Barracks on military base as the place of occurrence of the external cause
Y92.212	Middle school as the place of occurrence of the external cause
Y92.26	Movie house or cinema as the place of occurrence of the external cause
Y92.821	Forest as the place of occurrence of the external cause

- *Activity during the occurrence,* such as almost drowning while SCUBA diving or being involved in a construction accident.

EXAMPLE

Y93.15	Activity, underwater diving and snorkeling
Y93.34	Activity, bungee jumping
Y93.H3	Activity, building and construction

- *Patient's status,* such as paid employment, on-duty military, or leisure activity.

The patient's status at the time must also be included in analysis for research purposes, in addition to the determination of financial liability for treatment. For example, reporting Y99.0 Civilian activity done for income or pay would connect to a workers' compensation liability, while Y99.1 Military activity would tie the diagnosis to military service.

9.4 Physiological Conditions Affecting the Central Nervous System

Inflammatory Conditions of the Central Nervous System

Bacteria and viruses can invade the nervous system and cause infection, malfunction, and, in some cases, death. Examples include encephalitis (inflammation of the brain tissue), myelitis (inflammation of the spinal cord), intracranial abscess, and, probably the most well-known condition, meningitis.

Meningitis is an inflammatory disease of the CNS. However, as a professional coder, you must know more than the fact that the patient is diagnosed with meningitis. Meningitis can be caused by a virus or a bacterial invader that you will need to identify from the documentation; this may be a virus such as enterovirus, herpes zoster, or leptospira or a bacteria such as *Haemophilus influenzae,* streptococcus, pneumococcus, staphylococcus, or *E. coli,* to name just a few. Each specific detail may lead you to a different code or require a second code.

EXAMPLES

G00.1	Pneumococcal meningitis
G00.8	Other bacterial meningitis (Meningitis due to Escherichia coli)
G03.0	Nonpyogenic meningitis

LET'S CODE IT! SCENARIO

Lamonte Millwood went to see Dr. Vaughn after returning home from college on spring break. He stated that his new dorm room is a small suite and he has three roommates. He said that the last couple of days before he left to come home, two of his roommates were coughing and sneezing. Lamonte tells Dr. Vaughn that he has been nauseous and vomiting, he has become very sensitive to light, and he feels a bit confused, having trouble concentrating on his school work. Tests confirmed Dr. Vaughn's diagnosis of bacterial meningitis caused by Neisseria meningitidis.

Let's Code It!

Dr. Vaughn confirmed Lamonte's diagnosis of "*bacterial meningitis caused by* Neisseria meningitidis," so let's begin with the first part and turn to the Alphabetic Index to look up "Meningitis." You can see a long, long list of additional descriptors indented below this entry. Take a minute to review the elements listed to see if any of them match what the physician wrote in the documented diagnosis.

> **Meningitis**
> bacterial G00.9

Now, there is another indented list beneath the term "bacterial" that offers many different names of bacteria . . . except *Neisseria meningitidis (N. meningitidis).* There are many possibilities including: gram-negative [G00.0] and specified organism NEC [G00.8]. Do you know if *N. meningitidis* is gram-negative or gram-positive?

According to the Centers for Disease Control and Prevention, *Neisseria meningitidis* is a gram-negative bacterium.

Let's go to the Tabular List and begin reading at the three-character code category suggested here:

> ☑4 **G00**   Bacterial meningitis, not elsewhere classified

Read the INCLUDES and EXCLUDES1 notations directly below this code. You are good to continue reading down and review the two choices:

> **G00.8**   **Other bacterial meningitis**
> *Use additional code* to further identify organism (B96.-)
>
> **G00.9**   **Bacterial meningitis, unspecified (Meningitis due to gram-negative bacteria, unspecified)**

Even though G00.9 includes gram-negative bacteria, which is accurate for Lamonte's diagnosis, it is not true that the bacterium is unspecified. It <u>was</u> specified as *Neisseria meningitidis*. So, you cannot honestly and accurately report G00.9.

Turn to B96 in your Tabular List to see if you can find a code to specify that *Neisseria meningitidis* is the specific bacterium involved. It appears that the only code that could be used truthfully would be

> **B96.89**   **Other specified bacterial agents as the cause of diseases classified elsewhere**

This doesn't quite add any details, does it? Not really. Before you make a decision, check one more time in the Alphabetic Index under meningitis, only this time check for any mention of *Neisseria meningitidis*.

> **Meningitis**
>   Neisseria A39.0

This points us to a code in the Infectious diseases chapter of ICD-10-CM. Let's take a look at it.

> ✓4 **A39**   **Meningococcal infection**
>   **A39.0**   **Meningococcal meningitis**

Two choices to report this diagnosis: A39.0 or G00.8, B96.89

And still you are unable to provide the specific details you know are important. Therefore, you should append a special report, such as the pathology report, with this claim to provide these additional details.

Check the head of this chapter in ICD-10-CM. There is an EXCLUDES2 notation. Read carefully. Do any relate to Dr. Vaughn's diagnosis of Lamonte? No. Turn to the Official Guidelines and read Section 1.c.6. There is nothing specifically applicable here either.

For this encounter between Dr. Vaughn and Lamonte, you can confidently report these codes:

> **G00.8**   **Other bacterial meningitis**
> **B96.89**   **Other specified bacterial agents as the cause of diseases classified elsewhere**

Great job!

Hereditary and Degenerative Diseases of the Central Nervous System

Some nervous system conditions that affect the function of the CNS are linked to genetics or degeneration but not trauma. The patient may have a condition that is well known, such as Alzheimer's disease or dementia, or a lesser-known condition such as parkinsonism or Huntington's chorea.

As you have seen before, a diagnosis may seem to be complete but actually may not include enough information for a professional coder. For example, it is not enough to know the patient was diagnosed with dementia. To determine the most accurate code, you need more details, such as

Frontotemporal dementia (Pick's disease) G31.01
Dementia with Lewy bodies (Lewy body dementia) G31.83

You may remember we discussed coding some forms of dementia in the *Conditions That Affect Mental Health* section of this chapter. The good news here is that the coding process you learned will help you get to the correct ICD-10-CM chapter, know which specific descriptors to look for in the documentation, and then lead you directly to the most accurate code.

> ## 🛑 LET'S CODE IT! SCENARIO
>
> *Nate Mercado, an 81-year-old male, came to see Dr. Bronson with complaints of increasing forgetfulness and difficulty remembering new information. He states virtually no ability to focus or concentrate. His presentation confirms a deterioration in personal hygiene, and his appearance is somewhat disheveled. Nate's daughter insisted that he come to the doctor. After a neurologic exam, psychometric testing, a PET scan, and an EEG, Dr. Bronson diagnosed Nate with late-onset Alzheimer's disease.*
>
> ### Let's Code It!
>
> Dr. Bronson diagnosed Nate with *Alzheimer's disease*. Let's turn to the Alphabetic Index in the ICD-10-CM book and find
>
> > **Disease**
> > > **Alzheimer's** G30.9 *[F02.80]*
>
> Read the list of additional descriptors indented below this. The specific code to report will change on the basis of documentation of behavioral disturbance, early onset, and/or late onset. What did Dr. Bronson document?
>
> > **Disease**
> > > **Alzheimer's** G30.9 *[F02.80]*
> > > > late onset G30.1 *[F02.80]*
>
> Dr. Bronson stated nothing about behavioral disturbances, so this matches the notes. Let's turn to the Tabular List and begin reading at the three-character code:
>
> > ☑4 **G30   Alzheimer's disease**
>
> Take a look at the **INCLUDES** note here, which identifies Alzheimer's dementia senile and presenile forms, as well as the **Use additional code** notation, which directs you to the second code suggested in the Alphabetic Index listing, and an **EXCLUDES1** note citing three diagnoses that are not reported from this code category. Do you see any of these diagnoses included in Dr. Bronson's documentation? No. Read all of the choices for the fourth character available in this code category and determine which one best matches what Dr. Bronson wrote in Nate's notes:
>
> > **G30.1   Alzheimer's disease with late onset**
>
> This matches the documentation exactly! Good job! Now you must go and investigate the second code suggested by the Alphabetic Index: F02.80. Remember, even though the Alphabetic Index gave us five characters, you must always begin reading at the three-character level:
>
> > ☑4 **F02   Dementia in other diseases classified elsewhere**
>
> Directly below this entry, you can see a notation to **Code first** the underlying physiological condition, such as Alzheimer's disease. This is a great confirmation that you will need these two codes, and now you know the order in which to report them: G30.1 first, followed by the F02 code. Also, read carefully both the **EXCLUDES1** and **EXCLUDES2** notations. For Nate's encounter with Dr. Bronson, none of these apply. However, the next case you code may involve one of these diagnoses. Now is the best time to establish good coding habits.
>
> Review the fourth-character choices. You will notice there is only one:
>
> > ☑5 **F02.8   Dementia in other diseases classified elsewhere**
>
> Now review the fifth-character choices. You have two. Which one matches Dr. Bronson's notes about Nate? Dr. Bronson makes no mention at all about any behavioral disturbance.
>
> > **F02.80   Dementia in other diseases classified elsewhere without behavioral disturbance**
>
> You have done a great job determining the two codes to report for Dr. Bronson's diagnosis of Nate:
>
> > **G30.1   Alzheimer's disease with late onset**
> > **F02.80   Dementia in other diseases classified elsewhere without behavioral disturbance**

Hydrocephalus

When too much CSF accumulates in the ventricles of the brain, and the body cannot absorb it back into the vascular system fast enough, the brain tissues can be damaged and lose the ability to function properly. This can occur in infants (a congenital anomaly: ICD-10-CM code category Q03 Congenital hydrocephalus), or it can develop in adults (code category G91 Hydrocephalus).

You will find that, again, a diagnostic statement of "hydrocephalus" is insufficient to determine an accurate code, as there are several different types, each with its own specific code.

Communicating hydrocephalus, also referred to as secondary normal pressure hydrocephalus, is a condition in which the CSF is still able to flow out of the ventricles but then encounters an obstruction preventing it from moving further. This results in a flooding of the brain tissues in and around the ventricles. This is reported with code G91.0 Communicating hydrocephalus.

Noncommunicating hydrocephalus, also referred to as obstructive hydrocephalus, most commonly is caused by aqueductal stenosis, a narrowing of one or more of the aqueducts (narrow passageways) that connect the ventricles. This is reported with code G91.1 Obstructive hydrocephalus.

(Idiopathic) normal pressure hydrocephalus (NPH) is an abnormal increase in the quantity of CSF flowing into the ventricles. This is reported with code G91.2 (Idiopathic) normal pressure hydrocephalus.

Post-traumatic hydrocephalus, also known as hydrocephalus ex-vacuo, is the result of damage to the brain after a cerebrovascular accident (CVA) or a traumatic injury, such as traumatic brain injury (TBI). This is reported with code G91.3 Post-traumatic hydrocephalus, unspecified.

Hydrocephalus may also occur as a manifestation of another condition, such as a neoplasm or congenital syphilis. As you have learned in these situations before, you will need to report that underlying condition's code first, followed by code G91.4 Hydrocephalus in diseases classified elsewhere.

Migraine Headaches

Medical researchers have been trying to determine the cause of migraine headaches for quite a long time. According to the U.S. National Library of Medicine, currently the theory is that genes related to the control of some brain cell function are the cause.

While the genetic potential for having migraines may be congenital, generally, this pain is not constant, but caused by specific actions or events in one's life. These are known as triggers, and they include

- Stress or anxiety
- Insufficient sleep
- Lack of food
- Fluctuations in hormone levels (specifically in females)

There are several different types of migraine headaches, and these details should be available to you when you abstract the documentation.

Aura: The aura connected with a migraine is actually a sequence of neurologic symptoms that occur within the hour prior to the onset of the migraine itself (in adults). These experiences may affect their vision, such as the appearance of dark or colored spots; their physical sensations, such as tingling or numbness, possibly vertigo; or their senses, such as difficulty with speech or hearing.

Intractable: An intractable migraine may also be described in the documentation as pharmacologically resistant, treatment resistant, medically induced (refractory), and/or poorly controlled by treatment.

Status migrainosus: This term is used to identify that the patient's migraine headache has lasted more than 72 continuous hours.

Chronic: A diagnosis of chronic migraine is documented as the patient reporting more than 15 headache days within a 30-day period, with more than half of these described as migraines.

Other types of migraines: There are many more categories of migraine headaches that you may abstract from the documentation, such as cyclical vomiting, abdominal, or menstrual. Each of these has its own specific code within code category G43 Migraine.

Be alert to these terms, in connection with a migraine diagnosis. The absence of a term, such as aura or intractable, can be used as an indicator that the patient was "without" that aspect of the condition. What this means is that, if the physician does not specifically document that the patient *had* aura with his or her migraine, you are permitted to use a code that states, "without aura." It is not expected that the physician would necessarily document elements that are not present. However, if the detail is documented, a code that includes that detail must be reported.

LET'S CODE IT! SCENARIO

Jeffrey Himes was referred to Dr. Jonas, a neurosurgeon, after his last brain MRI came back showing signs of an abundance of cerebrospinal fluid (CSF) in the ventricles of his brain. After taking a full history and examination, Dr. Jonas determined that there was malabsorption of CSF in the brain—an official diagnosis of communicating hydrocephalus. Dr. Jonas discussed the treatment options with Jeffrey and his family.

Let's Code It!

Dr. Jonas diagnosed Jeffrey with *hydrocephalus*. Let's turn to the Alphabetic Index in the ICD-10-CM book and find

Hydrocephalus (acquired) (external) (internal) (malignant) (noncommunicating) (obstructive) (recurrent) G91.9

This seems to match the notes, except included in the parenthetical nonessential modifiers is the term *noncommunicating*. When you look back at the notes, you can see that Dr. Jonas diagnosed Jeffrey with *communicating*—the opposite. So, you know that this code cannot be correct. There is still a long list of additional modifying terms indented below *hydrocephalus*. Read through all of the choices and see if you can determine which one matches the documentation. Did you find this?

Hydrocephalus
  communicating G91.0

This matches the notes, so let's turn to the Tabular List and begin reading at the three-character code:

✓4 **G91   Hydrocephalus**

Carefully read the INCLUDES note that identifies acquired hydrocephalus and the EXCLUDES1 note citing three diagnoses that are not reported from this code category. Do you see any of these diagnoses included in Dr. Jonas's documentation? No. Read all of the choices for the fourth character available in this code category and determine which one best matches what Dr. Jonas wrote in Jeffrey's notes:

G91.0   Communicating hydrocephalus

This matches the documentation exactly! Good job!

9.5 Physiological Conditions Affecting the Peripheral Nervous System

Disorders that affect the peripheral nervous system may interfere with only one nerve, or multiple nerves. In an earlier chapter, you learned that conditions such as diabetes mellitus may cause the development of manifestations affecting the peripheral nervous system, such as diabetic neuropathy. There are various types of underlying causes, such as infection, compression, or injury.

Dominant and Nondominant Sides

Are you right-handed? If so, the right side of your body is considered your dominant side. Individuals who are left-handed have the left side of their bodies considered the dominant side. Then there are those who are ambidextrous (use both hands equally).

Patients suffering with *hemiplegia* (paralysis of one side of the body) or *hemiparesis* (weakness of one side of the body)—code category G81—will need documentation of whether the dominant side or nondominant side is affected. The same is required for a patient diagnosed with *monoplegia* (paralysis of one extremity, e.g., one arm or one leg)—code category G83.

You may have no memory of a physician ever asking you whether you are right- or left-handed—I don't. While neurologists are trained to consider this, you may find this detail missing from the documentation. For such cases, querying the physician may not help because he or she may not know. *ICD-10-CM Official Guidelines* are here to help you determine the correct code when the affected (weakened or paralyzed) side is documented yet there is no indication of whether or not this is the patient's dominant side. Here is how the guidelines direct you:

- If the documentation states the right side is affected—report as dominant.
- If the documentation states the left side is affected—report as nondominant.

For those patients documented to be ambidextrous, whichever side is documented as affected should be reported as the patient's dominant side.

> **GUIDANCE CONNECTION**
>
> Read the ICD-10-CM Official Guidelines for Coding and Reporting, section **I. Conventions, General Coding Guidelines and Chapter Specific Guidelines,** subsection **C. Chapter-Specific Coding Guidelines,** chapter **6. Diseases of the Nervous System,** subsection **a. Dominant/nondominant side.**

> **EXAMPLES**
>
> G81.12 Spastic hemiplegia affecting left dominant side
> G83.14 Monoplegia of lower limb affecting left nondominant side
>
> Remember that the laterality refers to the patient's right or left, not that of the writer of the documentation.

Carpal Tunnel Syndrome

Many people know about carpal tunnel syndrome, when the nerve that feeds through the carpal tunnel within the wrist becomes painful, and sometimes incapacitating. The ligaments and tendons become swollen and compress the nerves threaded through the tunnel from the hand to the arm. In addition to having a confirmed diagnostic statement, you will need documentation of laterality to determine a specific code: G56.01 Carpal tunnel syndrome, right upper limb **or** G56.02 Carpal tunnel syndrome, left upper limb **or** G56.03 Carpal tunnel syndrome, bilateral upper limbs.

Plexus Disorders

Many plexus disorders are the result of a specific point in the peripheral neural pathway for that plexus becoming compressed. Typically, something causes the nerve to be pinched between muscle and bone, such as the thoracic outlet syndrome (brachial

> **CODING BITES**
>
> Four nerve plexuses branch from the spinal cord off into the peripheral nerve network:
>
> - The **cervical plexus** branches nerves to the head, neck, and shoulder.
> - The **brachial plexus** branches nerves to the chest, shoulders, upper arms, forearms, and hands.
> - The **lumbar plexus** branches nerves to the back, abdomen, groin, thighs, knees, and calves.
> - The **sacral plexus** branches nerves to the pelvis, buttocks, genitals, thighs, calves, and feet.

plexus disorder) occurring from the muscles of the neck and shoulder squeezing down on the nerve. See code G54.0 Brachial plexus disorders **or** G54.1 Lumbosacral plexus disorders.

Complex Regional Pain Syndrome

After a traumatic injury, complex regional pain syndrome (CRPS) may develop in the damaged extremity (arm/hand, leg/foot). Signs and symptoms include chronic (ongoing) pain; dramatic changes to the color, texture, or temperature of the epidural surface; a burning sensation; and edema and stiffness in involved joints, which often results in decreased mobility.

There are two types of CRPS: CRPS-I and CRPS-II.

CRPS-I used to be called reflex sympathetic dystrophy syndrome. Physicians classify this diagnosis when the patient denies the occurrence of any nerve injury.

G90.511	Complex regional pain syndrome I of right upper limb
G90.512	Complex regional pain syndrome I of left upper limb
G90.513	Complex regional pain syndrome I of upper limb, bilateral
G90.521	Complex regional pain syndrome I of right lower limb
G90.522	Complex regional pain syndrome I of left lower limb
G90.523	Complex regional pain syndrome I of lower limb, bilateral

CRPS-II has been previously documented as causalgia, for patients who have a confirmed nerve injury prior to this diagnosis.

G56.41	Causalgia of right upper limb
G56.42	Causalgia of left upper limb
G56.43	Causalgia of bilateral upper limbs
G57.71	Causalgia of right lower limb
G57.72	Causalgia of left lower limb
G57.73	Causalgia of bilateral lower limbs

YOU CODE IT! CASE STUDY

Simon Clossberg is a 37-year-old architect. While on a business trip to Los Angeles, Simon and guys on his team decided to have some fun and rented some motorcycles. Taking a turn too wide, Simon was involved in a one-vehicle motorcycle accident. In the accident, Simon was pinned and slid between the bike and the pavement, ultimately landing on his back. A police officer witnessed the accident and immediately called for medical assistance.

EMTs arrived within minutes and immediately immobilized Simon's neck and secured him to a rigid board prior to transporting him to the emergency department of the nearest hospital. Upon arrival at the ED, Simon was conscious and complained of pain in his lower back. ED physician Dr. NeJame examined Simon and found numerous abrasions and contusions, in addition to a loss of both sensation and motor control of his legs. After he was stabilized, Dr. NeJame admitted Simon and called for a neurologic consult. Dr. Cheslea completed the neurologic assessment.

The neurologic exam revealed the following: Simon demonstrated normal or near normal strength in flexing and extending his elbows, in extending his wrists, and when flexing his middle finger and abducting his little finger on both hands. However, he exhibited no movement when medical personnel tested his ability to flex his hips, extend his knees, and dorsiflex his ankles.

Stretch reflexes involving the biceps, brachioradialis, and triceps muscles were found to be normal, while those involving the patella and ankle were absent. In addition, Simon was found to have normal sensitivity to pin prick and light touch in areas of his body above the level of his inguinal (groin) region, but not below that region of the body.

Dr. Cheslea diagnosed Simon with lumbosacral plexus disorder.

> **You Code It!**
>
> Go through the steps of coding, and determine the code or codes that should be reported for this encounter between Dr. Cheslea and Simon.
>
> Step #1: Read the case carefully and completely.
>
> Step #2: Abstract the scenario. Which main words or terms describe why the physician cared for the patient during this encounter?
>
> Step #3: Are there any details missing or incomplete for which you would need to query the physician? [If so, ask your instructor.]
>
> Step #4: Check for any relevant guidance, including reading all of the symbols and notations in the Tabular List and the appropriate sections of the Official Guidelines.
>
> Step #5: Determine the correct diagnosis code or codes to explain why this encounter was medically necessary.
>
> Step #6: Double-check your work.
>
> **Answer:**
>
> Did you determine this to be the correct code?
>
>   **G54.1**   **Lumbosacral plexus disorder**
>
> Good work!

9.6 Pain Management

Neurologists are among the health care professionals who most often treat pain because neurologic conditions involve the nerve endings and electrical impulses within the nervous system. There are physicians who specialize in pain management, although specialized training is not mandatory. **Acute** pain is determined by the severity of the pain and its impact on the patient's ability to function. The most common types of **chronic** pain include headache, low back pain, cancer pain, arthritis pain, neurogenic pain, and psychogenic pain. There is no specific time measurement to determine chronic pain. Therefore, the judgment of the physician, as stated in the documentation, is what differentiates acute pain from chronic pain. You must be careful not to assume a diagnosis of *chronic pain syndrome*. This condition is different from chronic pain, and its diagnosis may be reported (code G89.4) only when the attending physician specifically documents this condition.

Pain can be a very difficult thing to deal with clinically because it is not the same for every patient. Medically speaking, pain is an unpleasant sensation often initiated by tissue damage that results in impulses being transmitted to the brain via specific nerve fibers. It can be challenging for the patient to describe the level of intensity, and each individual patient's ability to cope with pain will vary greatly. Clinically speaking, pain can be diagnosed as acute, chronic, or both acute and chronic.

Most health care facilities use some type of pain scale from 0 to 10 (see Table 9-1) to help improve communication with patients. The zero indicates no pain at all, and the scale increases up to the number 10, representing excruciating, intolerable pain. Some facilities use a scale that includes illustrations to help patients accurately communicate what they are feeling.

Acute
Severe; serious.

Chronic
Long duration; continuing over an extended period of time.

TABLE 9-1 Numeric Rating Scale for Pain

Numeric Rating	Meaning
0	No pain
1–3	Mild pain (nagging, annoying, interfering little with ADLs)
4–6	Moderate pain (interferes significantly with ADLs)
7–10	Severe pain (disabling; unable to perform ADLs)

Source: National Institutes of Health

Reporting Pain Separately

When the physician has documented a confirmed diagnosis and this condition is the underlying cause of the pain, pain should not be reported with a separate code. In these circumstances, the pain is considered to be an inclusive symptom. The exceptions to this guideline occur when

- The principal purpose of the encounter is pain management and the encounter does not include treatment or management of the underlying condition.
- The pain is noted as acute and/or chronic, documenting that the pain suffered by the patient is above and beyond the level typical of the underlying condition.

ICD-10-CM provides code category G89 Pain, not elsewhere classified, from which to choose an appropriate code.

> **EXAMPLES**
>
> 1. Megan slipped during ice skating practice and broke her right ankle. After x-raying the ankle and applying the cast, Dr. Hustey gave her a prescription for pain medication. In this case, only the fractured ankle would be reported (**S82.64xA, Nondisplaced fracture of lateral malleolus of right fibula, initial encounter for closed fracture**). The pain is an inclusive symptom of the fracture.
> 2. Megan came back to Dr. Hustey 10 days later complaining of unbearable pain and stating that the prescribed medication was not "doing the trick." Dr. Hustey discussed with Megan several management treatments for the acute pain, and she agreed to try a different medication. This encounter was only for pain management. Dr. Hustey did not attend to the fracture at all. Therefore, this encounter would be reported with two codes:
>
>   G89.11   Acute pain due to trauma
>   S82.64xD   Nondisplaced fracture of lateral malleolus of right fibula, subsequent encounter for fracture with routine healing
>
>   A code from category G89 is reported to add details about the reason for this encounter with Dr. Hustey. The code for the fracture explains why Megan had pain.
> 3. Phillip is diagnosed with chronic tension headaches due to the extreme pressures of his job. He told the doctor he could not stand the pain anymore and he needed help. This diagnosis would be reported with both of these codes:
>
>   G89.29   Other chronic pain
>   G44.229   Chronic tension-type headache, not intractable

The official guidelines state that if the pain is not specifically documented as acute or chronic, it should not be reported separately. The exceptions to this guideline include

- *Post-thoracotomy pain:* G89.12 Acute post-thoracotomy pain (post-thoracotomy pain NOS); G89.22 Chronic post-thoracotomy pain.
- *Postprocedural pain:* G89.18 Other acute postprocedural pain (postprocedural pain NOS); G89.28 Other chronic postprocedural pain.
- *Neoplasm-related pain:* G89.3 Neoplasm related pain (acute) (chronic).
- *Central pain syndrome:* G89.0 Central pain syndrome.

In these four situations, the code from category G89 should be reported in addition to any other conditions related to the encounter.

Postprocedural Pain

As stated above, postprocedural pain would be reported with either G89.18 or G89.28, depending upon the physician's documentation of the pain as either acute or chronic. One of these codes may be reported only when the pain is documented as

- More intense or lasting longer than the expected level of pain that is considered normal immediately after a surgical procedure.
- Not related to a detailed complication of the surgical procedure.

Site-Specific Pain Codes

There are many other code categories within ICD-10-CM used to report pain located in a specific anatomical site. Code category G89 Pain, not elsewhere classified, does not include any site-specific information. Anatomical site-specific code categories include

M54.5	Low back pain (lumbago)
M79.602	Pain in left arm
M79.672	Pain in left foot

Sequencing Pain Codes with Other Codes

To determine the proper sequencing of a code from category G89 with codes for site-specific pain or underlying conditions, the first question to be answered from the documentation is, "Why was this encounter necessary?" If the answer is for pain management, the code from category G89 should be first-listed or the principal diagnosis reported. If the encounter is for any other reason and the attention to pain management is secondary to the purpose for the encounter, then the first-listed or principal diagnosis code would report that other reason and the code from category G89 would be reported afterward.

> **GUIDANCE CONNECTION**
>
> Read the ICD-10-CM Official Guidelines for Coding and Reporting, section **I. Conventions, General Coding Guidelines and Chapter Specific Guidelines,** subsection **C. Chapter-Specific Coding Guidelines,** chapter **6. Diseases of the Nervous System,** subsection **b. Pain—category G89.**

LET'S CODE IT! SCENARIO

Patti Moscowicz came in to see Dr. Levine with complaints of extreme pain in her head. She stated that she was nauseous and irritable and that light made the pain even worse. Patti stated that these headaches seemed to happen every month, right before she got her menstrual period, and she couldn't take it anymore. She begged for something to help with the pain. After a full examination, Dr. Levine diagnosed her with chronic premenstrual migraine.

Let's Code It!

Dr. Levine diagnosed Patti with *premenstrual migraine headaches,* and pain management was the purpose of this visit to the physician. Let's turn to the ICD-10-CM Alphabetic Index and find

Migraine (idiopathic) G43.909

(continued)

There is a list of additional descriptors indented below this. Go back to the physician's notes. Did he describe the migraine with more detail? Yes, he stated her migraine was premenstrual. So look down the list and see if you can find a suggested code:

> Migraine (idiopathic) G43.909
>> Premenstrual—*see* Migraine, menstrual
>
> Menstrual G43.829

Perfect! Now, let's turn to code category G43 in the Tabular List:

> ☑4 **G43** **Migraine**

Did you notice the notation below this code?

> *Use additional code* for adverse effect, if applicable, to identify drug (T36-T50 with fifth or sixth character 5)

There is no mention of any drugs or adverse reactions in Dr. Levine's documentation, so let's continue. Read the **EXCLUDES1** and **EXCLUDES2** notes. Nothing there matches the physician's notes, so continue down the column and review *all* of the choices for the mandatory fourth character. Which one matches what Dr. Levine wrote?

> ☑5 **G43.8** **Other migraine**

There are fifth-character choices listed below this code, so you will have to look down the column and find the box containing the fifth-character choices. You will see the box directly below the three-character code category. Review the four choices. Which one matches?

> ☑6 **G43.82** **Menstrual migraine, not intractable**

Good. There was no mention that Patti was having an intractable migraine. Read the notation beneath this code classification:

> *Code also* associated premenstrual tension syndrome (N94.3)

There was no mention of this in Dr. Levine's notes on Patti. Review the choices for the sixth character:

> **G43.829** **Menstrual migraine, not intractable, without mention of status migrainosus**

Do you also need to include a code from the G89 code category? Check the Official Guidelines, specifically Section 1.c.6.b.1)(b), **Use of category G89 codes in conjunction with site specific pain codes.** You will see that it states, *"If the code describes the site of the pain, but does not fully describe whether the pain is acute or chronic, then both codes should be assigned."* Terrific! Dr. Levine documented that Patti's pain was chronic, and code G43.829 does not include that specific detail. That's the answer to that question, so go and review all of the possible codes from code category G89 to determine the most accurate code to report:

> **G89.29** **Other chronic pain**

You have one last task to complete. Now that you have two codes to report Dr. Levine's reasons for caring for Patti during this encounter, you need to determine the correct sequence in which to report these codes. Refer again to that guideline, and the next part tells you, *"If the encounter is for pain control or pain management, assign the code from category G89 followed by the code identifying the specific site of pain."* You know from the notes that the reason for this encounter was pain management, so now you know the correct codes and the correct order in which to report the reason why Dr. Levine cared for Patti during this encounter:

> **G89.29** **Other chronic pain**
> **G43.829** **Menstrual migraine, not intractable, without mention of status migrainosus**

Good job!

Chapter Summary

Due to an increase in available care, more patients are receiving treatment for mental and behavioral disorders. Therefore, it is important for professional coding specialists to understand both psychological and physiological concerns. Through education and understanding, these patients can receive treatment and their providers can receive accurate reimbursement.

Many different circumstances and situations can be the cause of malfunction anywhere in the nervous system. As with any other organ system or diagnosis, professional coding specialists should never assume. Everything you need to report these conditions accurately is in the physician's documentation. If it is not, you must query the physician.

CODING BITES

Did you know there are hundreds of named phobias . . . such as

- Acrophobia = fear of high places
- Aerophobia = fear of air travel
- Apiphobia = fear of bees
- Bromidrosiphobia = fear of body odor
- Claustrophobia = fear of enclosed places
- Gephyrophobia = fear of bridges
- Haemophobia = fear of blood
- Kakorrhaphiaphobia = fear of failure
- Linonophobia = fear of string
- Phasmophobia = fear of ghosts
- Scotophobia = fear of the dark
- Taphephobia = fear of being buried alive
- Triskaidekaphobia = fear of the number 13

CHAPTER 9 REVIEW
Coding Mental, Behavioral, and Neurological Disorders

Let's Check It! Terminology

Match each key term to the appropriate definition.

1. LO 9.2 An emotional state that includes sadness, hopelessness, and gloom. **E**
2. LO 9.1 Ongoing, regular consumption of a substance with resulting significant clinical manifestations, and a dramatic decrease in the effect of the substance with continued use, therefore requiring an increased quantity of the substance to achieve intoxication. **D**
3. LO 9.2 An emotional state that includes elation, excitement, and exuberance. **F**
4. LO 9.1 The feelings of apprehension and fear, sometimes manifested with physical manifestations such as sweating and palpitations. **B**
5. LO 9.3 The sincere belief that one is suffering an illness that is not present. **I**
6. LO 9.1 Consumption of a substance without significant clinical manifestations. **J**
7. LO 9.1 Common behaviors include mood disorders, sleep disorders, psychotic symptoms, and agitation. **C**

A. Abuse
B. Anxiety
C. Behavioral Disturbance
D. Dependence
E. Depressive
F. Manic
G. Phobia
H. Schizophrenia
I. Somatoform Disorders
J. Use

8. LO 9.3 Irrational and excessive fear of an object, activity, or situation.
9. LO 9.1 Ongoing, regular consumption of a substance with resulting clinical manifestations.
10. LO 9.2 A psychotic disorder with no known cause.

Let's Check It! Concepts

Choose the most appropriate answer for each of the following questions.

1. LO 9.1 When a patient is diagnosed with an alcohol- or drug-related disorder, such condition is susceptible to _____ signs, symptoms, manifestations, and co-morbidities.
   a. psychological
   b. physiological
   c. psychological and physiological
   d. none of these

2. LO 9.2 All of the following are mood disorders *except*
   a. depression. b. apathy. c. euphoria. d. hallucinations.

3. LO 9.1 Pete smokes marijuana on a regular basis and it takes a little more each time to achieve the full effect. Pete is beginning to have some problems with his memory and gets irritable when he doesn't smoke pot. Pete is _____ marijuana.
   a. using b. abusing c. dependent on d. withdrawing from

4. LO 9.3 Which of the following is a somatoform disorder?
   a. panic disorder
   b. bipolar disorder
   c. hypochondriacal disorder
   d. schizophreniform disorder

5. LO 9.2 The patient has been diagnosed with Bipolar disorder, current episode, manic, severe, with psychotic features. The correct code is
   a. F31 b. F31.2 c. F31.4 d. F31.5

6. LO 9.4 Huntington's chorea is an example of a(n)
   a. inflammatory disease of the CNS.
   b. trauma of the CNS.
   c. hereditary disease of the CNS.
   d. disease of the PNS.

7. LO 9.4 The Official Guidelines state that if the pain is not specifically documented as acute or chronic, it should not be reported separately. The exceptions to this guideline include all of the following *except*
   a. neoplasm-related pain.
   b. tension headaches.
   c. central pain syndrome.
   d. post-thoracotomy pain.

8. LO 9.3 _____ is a condition in which a horrible experience leaves a lasting imprint on the patient's sense of danger.
   a. Fear
   b. Anxiety
   c. Post-traumatic stress disorder
   d. Reactive depression

9. LO 9.5 The _____ plexus branches nerves to the chest, shoulders, upper arms, forearms, and hands.
   a. brachial b. cervical c. lumbar d. sacral

10. LO 9.6 To determine the proper sequencing of a code from category G89 with codes for site-specific pain or underlying conditions, the first question to be answered from the documentation is
    a. Where did the encounter take place?
    b. How was the service provided?
    c. When did the encounter take place?
    d. Why was the encounter necessary?

Let's Check It! Guidelines

Refer to the Official Guidelines and fill in the blanks according to the Chapter 5, Mental, Behavioral, and Neurodevelopmental Disorders, and Chapter 6, Diseases of the Nervous System, Chapter-Specific Coding Guidelines.

G89	default	G89.2	cancer	psychological
relationship	one	acute	pain	associated
G89.4	G89.0	F45.41	G89.3	only
documentation	F45.42	mental	appropriate	

1. Assign code _____, for pain that is exclusively related to _____ disorders. As indicated by the Excludes 1 note under category G89, a code from category G89 should not be assigned with code F45.41.

2. Code _____, Pain disorders with related psychological factors, should be used with a code from category _____, Pain, not elsewhere classified, if there is documentation of a psychological component for a patient with acute or chronic pain.

3. The _____ codes for "in remission" are assigned only on the basis of provider _____ (as defined in the Official Guidelines for Coding and Reporting).

4. When the provider documentation refers to use, abuse and dependence of the same substance, only _____ code should be assigned to identify the pattern of use.

5. The codes are to be used only when the psychoactive substance use is _____ with a _____ or behavioral disorder, and such a _____ is documented by the provider.

6. Codes in category G89, Pain, not elsewhere classified, may be used in conjunction with codes from other categories and chapters to provide more detail about acute or chronic _____ and neoplasm-related pain, unless otherwise indicated below.

7. The _____ for post-thoracotomy and other postoperative pain not specified as acute or chronic is the code for the _____ form.

8. Chronic pain is classified to subcategory _____.

9. Code _____ is assigned to pain documented as being related, associated or due to _____, primary or secondary malignancy, or tumor.

10. Central pain syndrome _____ and chronic pain syndrome _____ are different than the term "chronic pain," and therefore codes should _____ be used when the provider has specifically documented this condition.

Let's Check It! Rules and Regulations

Please answer the following questions from the knowledge you have gained after reading this chapter.

1. **LO 9.1** What is the clinical difference between use, abuse, and dependence?

2. **LO 9.2** Explain schizoid personality disorder.

3. **LO 9.3** What is a phobia?

4. **LO 9.4** Differentiate between an inflammatory and a hereditary/degenerative type of disease of the nervous system. Give an example of each type.

5. **LO 9.5** Why is it important to know which side is dominant when coding weakness or paralysis? How do the guidelines help us if the dominant side is not documented in the patient's chart? How do the guidelines direct the coder for a patient who has been documented as being ambidextrous?

YOU CODE IT! Basics

First, identify the main term in the following diagnoses; then code the diagnosis.

Example: Korsakoff's alcoholic psychosis

a. main term: *psychosis*   b. diagnosis *F10.96*

1. Nicotine dependence:
   a. main term: _____   b. diagnosis: _____
2. Generalized anxiety disorder:
   a. main term: _____   b. diagnosis: _____
3. Vascular dementia:
   a. main term: _____   b. diagnosis: _____
4. Mild cognitive impairment:
   a. main term: _____   b. diagnosis: _____
5. Cocaine abuse:
   a. main term: _____   b. diagnosis: _____
6. Schizoaffective manic type disorder:
   a. main term: _____   b. diagnosis: _____
7. Delirium with multiple etiologies:
   a. main term: _____   b. diagnosis: _____
8. Infantile autism:
   a. main term: _____   b. diagnosis: _____
9. Bacterial meningitis, E. coli:
   a. main term: _____   b. diagnosis: _____
10. Acute disseminated encephalitis:
    a. main term: _____   b. diagnosis: _____
11. Early-onset cerebellar ataxia:
    a. main term: _____   b. diagnosis: _____
12. Amyotrophic lateral sclerosis:
    a. main term: _____   b. diagnosis: _____
13. Postencephalitic parkinsonism:
    a. main term: _____   b. diagnosis: _____
14. Generalized idiopathic epilepsy:
    a. main term: _____   b. diagnosis: _____
15. Congenital dystonic cerebral palsy:
    a. main term: _____   b. diagnosis: _____

YOU CODE IT! Practice

Using the techniques described in this chapter, carefully read through the case studies and determine the most accurate ICD-10-CM code(s) and external cause code(s), if appropriate, for each case study.

1. Albert Goings, a 54-year-old male, presents today with abdominal cramping and diarrhea. Albert had knee surgery 6 months ago and the surgeon prescribed oxycodone for pain control. Albert has stopped taking the medication but is having difficulty. Dr. Kenneth documents dilated pupils as well as goose bumps. Albert is diagnosed with oxycodone dependence, uncomplicated.

2. Charles Homer, a 6-year-old male, is brought in by his parents to see his pediatrician, Dr. Freibert. Mrs. Homer is concerned because Charles has been eating dirt and sand and he has tried to eat paper for approximately 1 month. Dr. Freibert completes a thorough examination and notes paleness and failure to thrive. Charles is admitted to Weston Hospital for a full workup. After reviewing the laboratory and developmental test results, Charles is diagnosed with pica.

3. Kelley Dumont, a 19-year-old female, comes in to see Dr. Molusky. Kelley complains that she feels powerless and depressed. Kelley is accompanied by her mother. Mrs. Dumont states that Kelley has given up activities and has become fearful. Dr. Molusky completes a psychological examination and diagnoses Kelley with chronic paranoid reaction.

4. Kevin Genutis, a 24-year-old male, presents with the complaint of experiencing early orgasm and ejaculation, usually a minute or two after beginning sexual activity. Dr. Fox completes an examination and diagnoses Kevin with premature ejaculation.

5. April Carter, a 56-year-old female, was brought to the emergency department by a friend who found her in a stupor. After Dr. Hoogenboom completed a thorough examination and after documenting posturing, echolalia, and echopraxia, April is admitted for further psychological testing. After reviewing the test results, Dr. Hoogenboom diagnoses April with schizophrenic catatonia.

6. Brent Brooke, an 18-year-old male, presents for immunizations before joining the army. Brent passes out when given an injection. Dr. Meetze diagnoses Brent with fear of injections.

7. Melissa Roxburgh, a 21-year-old female, presents for a checkup. Melissa states she is deliberately trying to lose weight, exercises strenuously, and uses appetite suppressants. Dr. Fritz documents a BMI of 16.5, hypotension, and tachycardia as well as Melissa's inability to concentrate. Dr. Fritz decides to admit Melissa. After reviewing the laboratory results and a psychological evaluation, Melissa is diagnosed with anorexia nervosa, restricting type.

8. Gregory Abreu, a 37-year-old male, was previously diagnosed with African rhodesiense trypanosomiasis infection due to *Trypanosoma bruceri*. Greg presents today with the complaint of a severe headache and a stiff neck. Greg says he feels so bad that it actually hurts to walk. Dr. Crumpler notes a fever of 102F and shivering. Greg is admitted to Weston Hospital, where the results of a lumbar puncture confirm an elevated CSF pressure of 24 cm H_2O. Gregory is diagnosed with meningitis.

9. Carol Abuelo, a 39-year-old female, presents today with general restlessness. Dr. Sabbagha documents unintentional and uncontrollable movements as well as slowed saccadic eye movements. Carol is admitted. An MRI scan reveals atrophy of the caudate nuclei and genetic tests confirmed the diagnosis of Huntington's chorea.

10. Harold Darden, a 5-month-old male, is brought in by his parents for a checkup. Dr. Hottel notes muscle weakness and a weak cry. Mrs. Darden says that Harold seems to have some difficulty swallowing. Harold is admitted to Weston Hospital. The genetic blood tests, EMG, and NCV all confirm a diagnosis of infantile spinal muscular atrophy, type I.

11. Ruby Jenkins, a 26-year-old female, presents with popping or clicking sounds in her ears. After a thorough examination and the appropriate tests, Dr. Thompson diagnoses Ruby with palatal myoclonus.

12. Joe Frances, a 47-year-old male, presents with weakness and a numb feeling in his legs. Dr. Wigley notes hypertonia and orders an MRI, which reveals a thoracic spinal cord lesion. Joe is diagnosed with acute transverse myelitis.

13. Daniela Wiebenga, an 11-year-old female, is brought in by her mother. Mrs. Wiebenga is concerned because Daniela is starting to knock over objects and drop things, mostly in the morning. Daniela says it's hardest in the morning and seems to get better as the day progresses. Dr. Jefferson orders an EEG, which reveals spikes and waves, and admits Daniela. After a full workup, Daniela is diagnosed with juvenile absence epilepsy.

14. Eric Lewter, a 56-year-old male, presents with the feeling of tiredness but has been sleeping a lot over the last 3 to 4 months. Eric is accompanied by his wife, Peggy, who states she has noticed some mild mood changes as well. Dr. Shealy completes a thorough examination and the appropriate tests and diagnoses Eric with Kleine-Levin syndrome (KLS).

15. Paige Henderson, a 42-year-old female, comes in today with the complaint of numbness in her left little finger. Dr. McKenna notes Paige has difficulty performing fine motor movements with her left hand and fingers. After an examination and the appropriate tests, Dr. McKenna diagnoses Paige with tardy ulnar nerve palsy, left arm.

YOU CODE IT! Application

The following exercises provide practice in abstracting physicians' notes and learning to work with documentation from our health care facility, Prader, Bracker, & Associates. These case studies are modeled on real patient encounters. Using the techniques described in this chapter, carefully read through the case studies and determine the most accurate ICD-10-CM code(s) and external cause code(s), if appropriate, for each case study.

CHAPTER 9 REVIEW

PRADER, BRACKER, & ASSOCIATES

A Complete Health Care Facility

159 Healthcare Way • SOMEWHERE, FL 32811 • 407-555-6789

PATIENT: PORTER, KELSEY

ACCOUNT/EHR #: PORTKE001

DATE: 10/16/18

Attending Physician: Oscar R. Prader, MD

Kelsey is a straight "A" student at the state university. He is well liked and respected, handsome, tall, and personable. However, he is finding it increasingly difficult to socialize with his friends without the need to, unobtrusively, wash his hands for fear of contamination. He began carrying antibacterial wipes for those occasions when he could not get to a sink. He had difficulty tolerating medication to help defuse these feelings, and he has found talk therapy to be of little benefit. He stated that he came to my office with his parents, desperately hoping to get some relief.

After a thorough 2½-hour evaluation, I diagnosed Kelsey with OCD.

Diagnosis: Obsessive-compulsive disorder (OCD).

ORP/pw   D: 10/16/18 09:50:16   T: 10/18/18 12:55:01

Determine the most accurate ICD-10-CM code(s).

PRADER, BRACKER, & ASSOCIATES

A Complete Health Care Facility

159 Healthcare Way • SOMEWHERE, FL 32811 • 407-555-6789

PATIENT: MYRICK, JULIE

ACCOUNT/EHR #: MYRIJU001

DATE: 10/16/18

Attending Physician: Oscar R. Prader, MD

S: Julie, a 47-year-old female, came to see me because her youngest son was getting married, leaving her alone. She stated that, over the last several weeks, she had begun having panic attacks whenever she thought about the upcoming separation. Patient has tried cognitive behavioral therapy and different medications without success.

O: CBC results showed the size of her red blood cells (MCV) was slightly abnormal. The range was 80–100, and she was 101. Evidence-based medicine has documented an elevated MCV could indicate a B_{12} deficiency, so I had Julie do a Schilling test, which was positive.

A: Panic disorder without agoraphobia, vitamin B_{12} deficiency.

P: Rx B_{12} injections; patient to return in 10–14 days.

ORP/pw   D: 10/16/18 09:50:16   T: 10/16/18 12:55:01

Determine the most accurate ICD-10-CM code(s).

PRADER, BRACKER, & ASSOCIATES

A Complete Health Care Facility

159 Healthcare Way • SOMEWHERE, FL 32811 • 407-555-6789

PATIENT: FALCONE, ANTONIO

ACCOUNT/EHR #: FALANT001

DATE: 10/16/18

Attending Physician: Renee O. Bracker, MD

Antonio, a 43-year-old male, was referred by his therapist of 3 years, Ms. Benton, for psychiatric evaluation and consideration of medication to treat worsening depression. At the initial interview, Antonio's wife, Marie, an attorney, was present to provide some history and perceptions. She was quite cooperative yet strangely detached. She answered all of the questions that I asked in a genuine manner. All pathological causes of sadness have been ruled out. A complete workup is performed.

It gradually became clear that the source of Antonio's persistent depression was his wife's lack of accountability and responsibility in the marriage. She was frequently late for sessions, with no notice. Antonio always wanted to be a family man. Marie refuses to work at the marriage, crushing Antonio's expectations of a satisfying marriage.

Antonio checked into a hotel 500 miles away from home and threatened suicide 2 days ago. When Antonio returned, he came directly to my office. This episode was due to his wife's lack of therapy participation. Antonio stated he feels like a failure because he can't make the marriage work. Suicide seemed to be a viable exit strategy from the pain.

My recommendations were that an environment change was needed to recover from the suicidal ideation. Antonio was experiencing continued depression caused by this environment in which his level of control over the outcome was minimal. This led to more severe and frequent depression. I advised him to stay out of the house.

Diagnosis: Major depressive disorder, recurrent, moderate

ROB/pw   D: 10/16/18 09:50:16   T: 10/18/18 12:55:01

Determine the most accurate ICD-10-CM code(s).

WESTON HOSPITAL

629 Healthcare Way • SOMEWHERE, FL 32811 • 407-555-6541

PATIENT: LYNCH, VICTOR

ACCOUNT/EHR #: LYNVIC001

DATE: 10/16/18

Attending Physician: Renee O. Bracker, MD

S: This is a 3-year-old male who is recovering from a mild case of the Flu and suddenly began vomiting. The babysitter may have given him aspirin by accident instead of acetaminophen. Luke's mother brought him to the ED for unexplained irritability and restlessness. He later develops convulsions, which are treated with anticonvulsants. He is admitted to PICU.

O: T: 36.7, P: 102, R 48, BP 115/69, oxygen saturation 99% in room air. Height, weight, and head circumference are all at the 50th percentile. PERRLA. No signs of external trauma. Sclera nonicteric. EOMs cannot be fully tested, but they are conjugate. TMs are normal. Neck reveals no adenopathy. He is agitated and uncooperative. Heart regular without murmurs or gallops. Lungs are clear. Abdomen—normal bowel sounds. No definite tenderness. No inguinal hernias are present. He moves all extremities.

LABS: Serum bilirubin: normal. Serum AST and ALT: increased. Serum ammonia: increased. Prothrombin time: prolonged. A CT scan of the brain shows cerebral edema. Neurologic symptoms rapidly deteriorate and he becomes unresponsive. Patient is intubated and put on mechanical ventilation and IV fluid is started. A liver biopsy reveals diffuse, small lipid deposits in the hepatocytes (microvesicular steatosis) without significant necrosis or inflammation.

A: Reye's syndrome.

P: Continue to follow and treat.

ROB/pw   D: 10/16/18 09:50:16   T: 10/18/18 12:55:01

Determine the most accurate ICD-10-CM code(s).

WESTON HOSPITAL

629 Healthcare Way • SOMEWHERE, FL 32811 • 407-555-6541

PATIENT: YAN, MARANDA

ACCOUNT/EHR #: YANMAR001

DATE: 10/16/18

Attending Physician: Oscar R. Prader, MD

S: This is a 23-year-old female who presents with a chief complaint of clumsiness and blurred vision. Patient states she had been feeling fine until about 10 days ago when she noticed some numbness and weakness in her right leg, and suddenly her vision became blurry.

O: VS are normal. She is alert but subdued, afebrile with some ataxia noted. HEENT exam is notable for severe visual loss and pale optic discs on funduscopy. Her heart, lungs, and abdomen are normal. She is noted to have a hyporeflexive paraparesis noted on the right.

I decided to admit her to the hospital. An MRI scan shows multiple lesions in the periventricular white matter and cerebellum. Pattern visual evoked responses showed markedly delayed latencies. Corticosteroids are prescribed. Prognosis—a full recovery within 10–14 days.

A: Multiple sclerosis (MS)

P: Continue to follow and treat with traditional medication.

ORP/pw   D: 10/16/18 09:50:16   T: 10/18/18 12:55:01

Determine the most accurate ICD-10-CM code(s).

Coding Dysfunction of the Optical and Auditory Systems

10

Learning Outcomes

After completing this chapter, the student should be able to:

LO 10.1 Identify conditions affecting the external eye.
LO 10.2 Interpret the details documented about diseases of the internal optical system to report accurate code.
LO 10.3 Determine the accurate code to report other conditions of the eye.
LO 10.4 Abstract documentation accurately to report conditions affecting the auditory system.
LO 10.5 Enumerate the causes, signs, and symptoms of hearing loss.

Key Terms

Accommodation
Blepharitis
Bulbar Conjunctiva
Cataract
Choroid
Ciliary Body
Cone
Conjunctivitis
Cornea
Corneal Dystrophy
Dacryocystitis
Extraocular Muscles
Glands of Zeis
Glaucoma
Iris
Keratitis
Lacrimal Apparatus
Lens
Meibomian Glands
Moll's Glands
Orbit
Palpebrae
Palpebral Conjunctiva
Proptosis
Pupil
Retina
Retinal Detachment
Retinopathy
Rod
Sclera
Uveal Tract
Vitreous Chamber

STOP! Remember, you need to follow along in your ICD-10-CM code book for an optimal learning experience.

10.1 Diseases of the External Optical System

The Exterior of the Eye

The **palpebrae** (eyelids) cover the eyeballs to protect them from injury and environmental invaders as well as to maintain the proper level of moisture. Some people think eyelids are made of epidermis, like regular skin; however, they are really composed of connective tissue. The *levator palpebrae muscle superioris* (*levator* = lift; *palpebrae* = eyelids; muscle; *superioris* = above) is responsible for opening and closing the upper eyelid, while the fascia behind the orbicularis oculi muscle (the orbital septum) creates a barrier between the lids and the **orbit**. There is a thin mucous membrane that lines the inside of the eyelid, known as the **palpebral conjunctiva**; this lines the eyelid internally, creasing over at the fornix, and covers the surface of the eyeball. At that point, it becomes known as the **bulbar conjunctiva** (see Figure 10-1).

Within the palpebrae (eyelids), there are three types of glands:

- **Moll's glands**: ordinary sweat glands.
- **Meibomian glands**: sebaceous glands that secrete a tear film component that prevents tears from evaporating so that the area stays moist.
- **Glands of Zeis**: altered sebaceous glands that are connected to the eyelash follicles.

Palpebrae
The eyelids; singular *palpebra*.

Orbit
The bony cavity in the skull that houses the eye and its ancillary parts (muscles, nerves, blood vessels).

Palpebral Conjunctiva
A mucous membrane that lines the palpebrae.

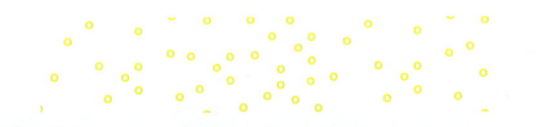

263

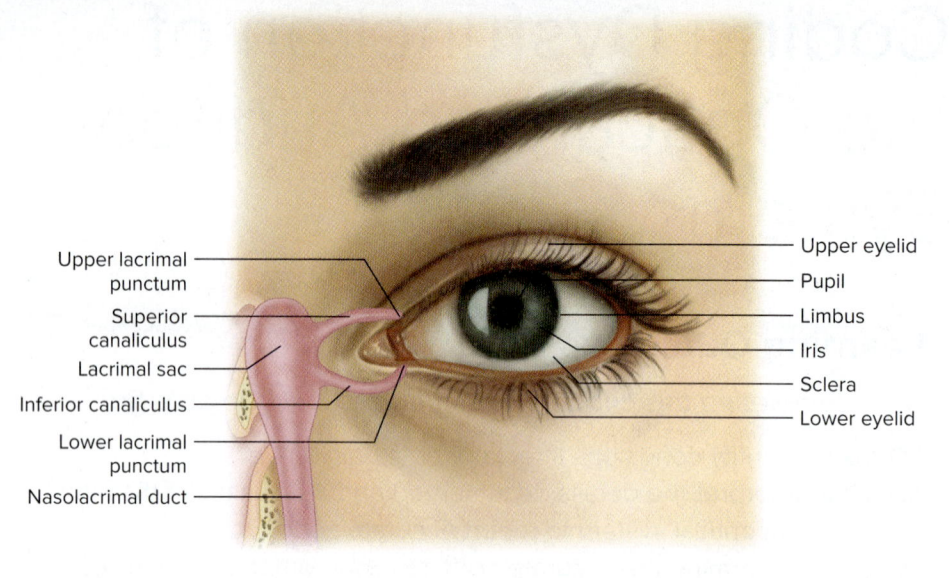

FIGURE 10-1 The anatomical components of the external eye

Bulbar Conjunctiva
A mucous membrane on the surface of the eyeball.

Moll's Glands
Ordinary sweat glands.

Meibomian Glands
Sebaceous glands that secrete a tear film component that prevents tears from evaporating so that the area stays moist.

Glands of Zeis
Altered sebaceous glands that are connected to the eyelash follicles.

Blepharitis
Inflammation of the eyelid.

EXAMPLES

H00.024	Hordeolum internum left upper eyelid
H00.15	Chalazion left lower eyelid
H01.112	Allergic dermatitis of right lower eyelid
H02.031	Senile entropion of right upper eyelid
H02.131	Senile ectropion of right upper eyelid

You may be thinking, "Hey, wait a minute. You just taught us that palpebra is the medical term for eyelid. And yet here in the code descriptions, they each state 'eyelid,' the English word." That's very true. However, the reason you need to learn that the term *palpebra* means eyelid is because when your physician is writing operative notes or procedure notes, he or she may use the term *palpebra*, and if you're not familiar with that and you don't know what it means, you won't know how to code this.

Blepharitis

Staphylococcal blepharitis, also known as ulcerative **blepharitis**, is a condition in which the rims of the eyelids become inflamed and appear red. Most often, this condition is chronic and affects bilaterally, as well as simultaneously to the upper and lower lids. In addition to the redness, dry scales and ulcerations may form.

Squamous blepharitis is similar, with inflammation of the glands of Zeis. Signs and symptoms include itching, burning, photophobia, mucous discharge, and a crusty formation on the eyelids.

As you abstract documentation with a confirmed diagnosis of blepharitis, you will need to confirm the specific eye involved (right or left) as well as the specific lid (upper or lower). Code subcategory H01.0- Blepharitis.

YOU CODE IT! CASE STUDY

Rosemary Seaborn, a 25-year-old female, came to see Dr. Spencer, an ophthalmologist, with complaints of itching and a burning sensation in both of her eyes. She stated her upper eyelids looked like they had "dandruff" with a crusty appearance, and she noted an increased sensitivity to light. After examinations and testing, Dr. Spencer documented a confirmed case of bilateral squamous blepharitis on her upper palpebrae.

> **You Code It!**
>
> Review the details of this documentation, and determine the accurate code or codes to report Dr. Spencer's diagnosis for Rosemary.
>
> Step #1: Read the case carefully and completely.
>
> Step #2: Abstract the scenario. Which main words or terms describe why the physician cared for the patient during this encounter?
>
> Step #3: Are there any details missing or incomplete for which you would need to query the physician? [If so, ask your instructor.]
>
> Step #4: Check for any relevant guidance, including reading all of the symbols and notations in the Tabular List and the appropriate sections of the Official Guidelines.
>
> Step #5: Determine the correct diagnosis code or codes to explain why this encounter was medically necessary.
>
> Step #6: Double-check your work.
>
> **Answer:**
>
> Did you determine these to be the correct codes?
>
> | H01.021 | Squamous blepharitis right upper eyelid |
> | H01.024 | Squamous blepharitis left upper eyelid |

Exophthalmic Conditions

Exophthalmos, also known as **proptosis**, is an abnormal displacement of the eyeball. Most often, ophthalmic Graves' disease is the underlying condition that results in the eyeball bulging outward while the eyelids retract backward, bilaterally. Trauma, such as ethmoid bone fracture, may cause a unilateral diagnosis. Edema, hemorrhage, thrombosis, or varicosities may also cause exophthalmos, either unilaterally or bilaterally.

As you abstract the documentation, note the difference between the displacement of the orbit, or eyeball, and whether or not the exophthalmos is constant, intermittent, or pulsating so you can determine the accurate code:

H05.21-	Displacement (lateral) of globe
H05.24-	Constant exophthalmos
H05.25-	Intermittent exophthalmos
H05.26-	Pulsating exophthalmos

Proptosis
Bulging out of the eye; also known as *exophthalmos.*

> **CODING BITES**
>
> NOTE: All of these codes [in the H05 code category] require a sixth character to specify right eye, left eye, or bilateral (both eyes) involved.

Disorders of the Lacrimal Apparatus

The *lacrimal glands,* the *upper canaliculi,* the *lower canaliculi,* the *lacrimal sac,* and the *nasolacrimal duct* are together known as the **lacrimal apparatus**. Tears are created in the main lacrimal gland and then flow through several excretory ducts, pass through the canaliculi and the lacrimal sac, and continue down the nasolacrimal duct into the nasal cavity—the nose. This is why when you cry, your nose runs.

Signs and symptoms of an obstructed lacrimal apparatus include recurring conjunctivitis (pink eye), discharge of pus or mucus from the eyelids and/or the conjunctiva, blurred vision, and excessive tearing.

Congenital nasolacrimal duct anomalies: A neonate may be born with a duct abnormality, an obstruction, or a lacrimal apparatus that is not fully developed. This is reported with one of these codes:

| Q10.4 | Absence and agenesis of lacrimal apparatus |

or

Lacrimal Apparatus
A system in the eye that consists of the lacrimal glands, the upper canaliculi, the lower canaliculi, the lacrimal sac, and the nasolacrimal duct

	Q10.5	Congenital stenosis and stricture of lacrimal duct

or

	Q10.6	Other congenital malformations of lacrimal apparatus

Neonatal lacrimal duct (passages) obstruction: An infant born with a healthy lacrimal apparatus may still develop an obstruction of the nasolacrimal duct. As you are abstracting the documentation, confirm that this condition is acquired and not congenital so you can determine the accurate code:

	H04.531	Neonatal obstruction of right nasolacrimal duct

or

	H04.532	Neonatal obstruction of left nasolacrimal duct

or

	H04.533	Neonatal obstruction of bilateral nasolacrimal ducts

Dacryops, also known as lacrimal gland cyst or lacrimal duct cyst, is reported with one of these codes:

	H04.111	Dacryops of right lacrimal gland

or

	H04.112	Dacryops of left lacrimal gland

or

	H04.113	Dacryops of bilateral lacrimal glands

Dacryocystitis

Dacryocystitis
Lacrimal gland inflammation.

Dacryocystitis is lacrimal gland inflammation (*dacry/o* = lacrimal sac or duct + *cyst* = sac + *itis* = inflammation). This may be a manifestation of a nasolacrimal duct obstruction and can be acute and/or chronic. Research shows that *Staphylococcus aureus*—or, on occasion, beta-hemolytic streptococci—is the pathogen responsible for acute dacryocystitis inflammation, whereas the chronic condition is more often caused by *Streptococcus pneumoniae* or, on occasion, a fungal infection such as *Actinomyces* or *Candida albicans.*

Signs and symptoms include pain, redness, and swelling over the inner aspect of the lower eyelid and epiphora. As you are abstracting the documentation, confirm whether the patient is a neonate or not, so you can determine the accurate code:

	H04.321	Acute dacryocystitis of right lacrimal passage

or

	H04.322	Acute dacryocystitis of left lacrimal passage

or

	H04.323	Acute dacryocystitis of bilateral lacrimal passages

or

	P39.1	Neonatal conjunctivitis and dacryocystitis

YOU CODE IT! CASE STUDY

Raven Mercado, a 27-year-old female, came in to see Dr. Garner complaining of swelling, pain, and redness on her left eyelid. She was pretty certain it was a stye, but it was so painful, she had to ask for help. Dr. Garner examined her and confirmed a diagnosis of hordeolum externum of the left lower eyelid (commonly known as a stye).

> **You Code It!**
>
> Go through the steps of coding, and determine the code or codes that should be reported for this encounter between Dr. Garner and Raven.
>
> Step #1: Read the case carefully and completely.
>
> Step #2: Abstract the scenario. Which main words or terms describe why the physician cared for the patient during this encounter?
>
> Step #3: Are there any details missing or incomplete for which you would need to query the physician? [If so, ask your instructor.]
>
> Step #4: Check for any relevant guidance, including reading all of the symbols and notations in the Tabular List and the appropriate sections of the Official Guidelines.
>
> Step #5: Determine the correct diagnosis code or codes to explain why this encounter was medically necessary.
>
> Step #6: Double-check your work.
>
> **Answer:**
>
> Did you determine this to be the correct code?
>
> **H00.015**   Hordeolum externum left lower eyelid

10.2 Diseases of the Internal Optical System

Interior of the Eye

The organ that is commonly referred to as the *eye* (see Figure 10-2) consists of the eyeball, the optic nerves, the **extraocular muscles**, the cranial nerves, the blood vessels, orbital adipose (fat), and the lacrimal system.

Extraocular Muscles
The muscles that control the eye.

Disorders of the Conjunctiva

Conjunctivitis, commonly known as *pink eye,* actually refers to an inflammation of the conjunctiva of the eye. The most common signs and symptoms include swelling, itching, burning, and redness of the conjunctiva as well as the palpebral conjunctiva (lining of the eyelids).

Conjunctivitis
Inflammation of the conjunctiva.

A pathogen (bacterium or virus), allergic reactions, environmental irritants, a contact lens product, eyedrops, or eye ointments may all be an underlying cause of conjunctivitis. This condition is highly contagious (easily spread from one person to another). Viral conjunctivitis is reported from the infectious disease chapter of ICD-10-CM. You will need to check the pathology report to determine an accurate code:

B00.53	Herpesviral conjunctivitis
B30.1	Conjunctivitis due to adenovirus
B30.3	Acute epidemic hemorrhagic conjunctivitis (enteroviral)
	Conjunctivitis due to coxsackievirus 24
	Conjunctivitis due to enterovirus 70
	Hemorrhagic conjunctivitis (acute) (epidemic)
B30.8	Other viral conjunctivitis
	Newcastle conjunctivitis

Mucopurulent conjunctivitis is evident by mucus and pus produced by the inflammation, whereas *atopic conjunctivitis* is most often caused by allergies. Yet, be careful:

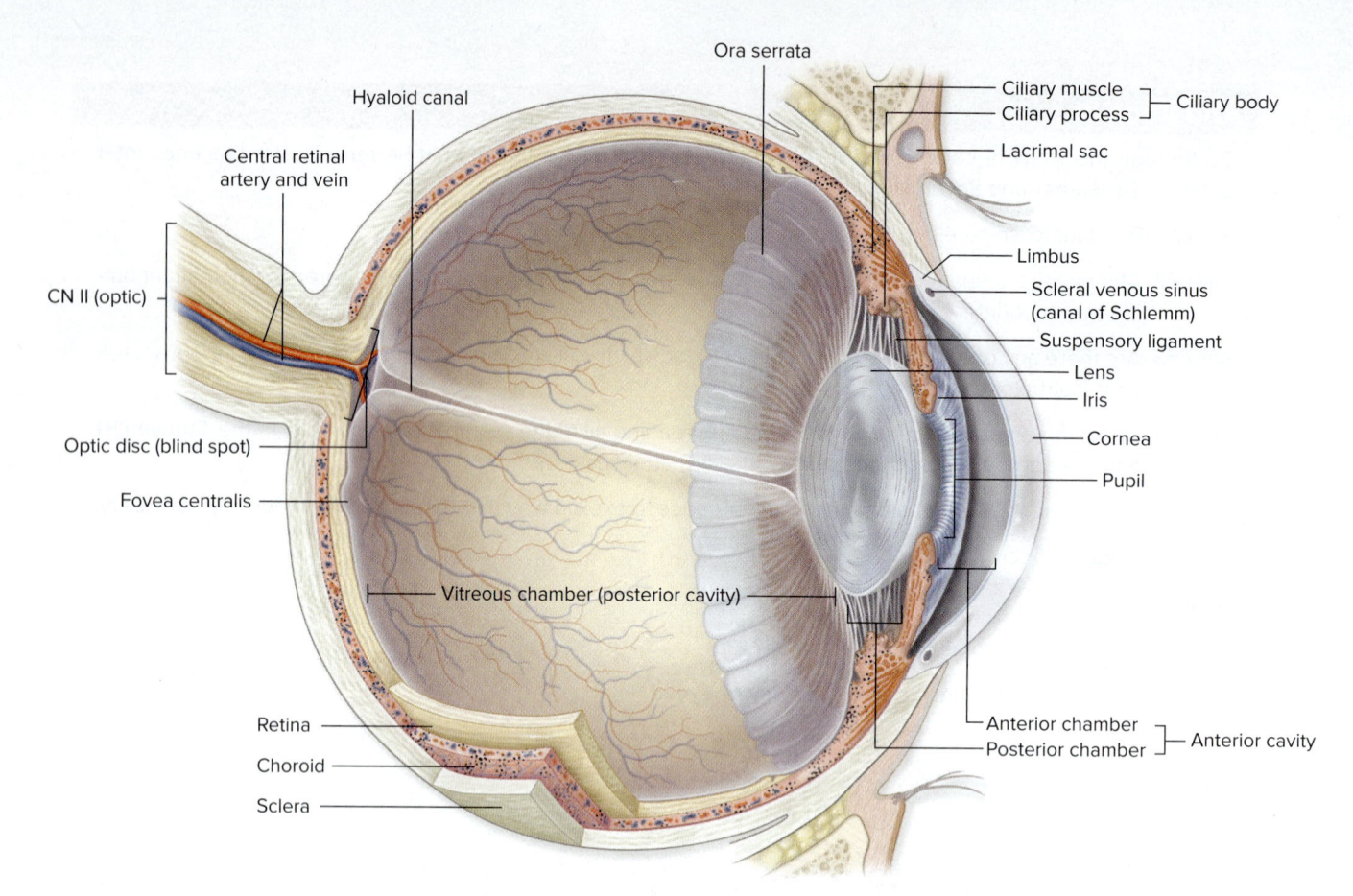

FIGURE 10-2 The anatomical components of the orbital septum (view from the right side)

Vernal conjunctivitis is the result of an allergic reaction to seasonal allergens, such as pollen or mold. Abstract the specific details about the conjunctivitis, as well as the laterality for the eye involved (right, left, or bilateral), from the documentation.

H10.01-	**Acute follicular conjunctivitis**
H10.02-	**Other mucopurulent conjunctivitis**
H10.1-	**Acute atopic conjunctivitis**
	Acute papillary conjunctivitis
H10.21-	**Acute toxic conjunctivitis**
H10.22-	**Pseudomembranous conjunctivitis**
H10.23-	**Serous conjunctivitis, except viral**

NOTE: All of the codes in code category H10 Conjunctivitis require a fifth or sixth character to report laterality.

Disorders of the Sclera, Cornea, Iris, and Ciliary Body

The portion of the **sclera** at the medial anterior aspect (the middle of the front) of the eyeball is called the **cornea**. It is a curved, multilayer, transparent, and avascular (no blood vessels) segment of this structure (see Figure 10-3). The cornea's only function within the eye is to refract light rays. There are five layers that make up the cornea:

- *Epithelium:* the location of sensory nerves.
- *Bowman's membrane:* the location of epithelial cells.
- *Stroma:* the supporting tissue that makes up 90% of the corneal structure.

Sclera
The membranous tissue that covers all of the eyeball (except the cornea); also known as *the white of the eye*.

Cornea
Transparent tissue covering the eyeball; responsible for focusing light into the eye and transmitting light.

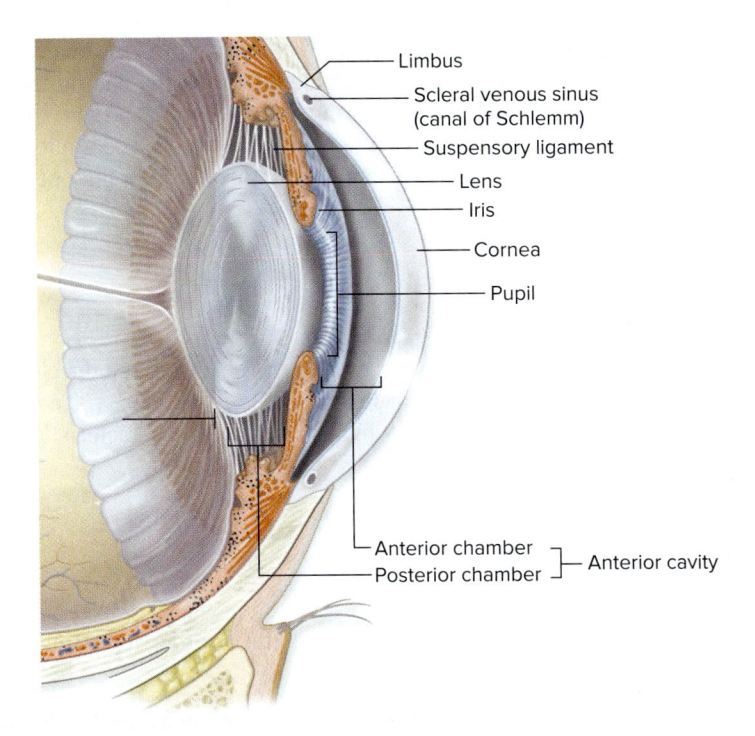

FIGURE 10-3 An illustration showing the sclera, iris, and cornea

- *Descemet's membrane:* elastic fibers.
- *Endothelium:* cells that help to maintain proper hydration of the cornea to keep it moist.

The posterior (back) surface of the cornea is coated in an aqueous humor that keeps intraocular pressure at a consistent volume and rate of outflow.

Keratitis, an inflammation and ulceration of the cornea, may be instigated by any type of pathogen: bacterium, virus, or fungus. You will need to abstract two additional details from the documentation: the location of the ulcer on the cornea, as well as the laterality affected (right, left, bilateral).

H16.11-	Macular keratitis
H16.12-	Filamentary keratitis
H16.13-	Photokeratitis
H16.14-	Punctate keratitis

NOTE: All of the codes in code subcategory H16.1 Other and unspecified superficial keratitis without conjunctivitis require a fifth or sixth character to report laterality.

When reporting a corneal ulcer, you will need to abstract two additional details from the documentation: the location of the ulcer on the cornea, as well as the laterality affected (right, left, bilateral).

H16.01-	Central corneal ulcer
H16.02-	Ring corneal ulcer
H16.03-	Corneal ulcer with hypopyon
H16.04-	Marginal corneal ulcer
H16.05-	Mooren's corneal ulcer
H16.06-	Mycotic corneal ulcer
H16.07-	Perforated corneal ulcer

NOTE: All of the codes in code subcategory H16.0 Corneal ulcer require a fifth or sixth character to report laterality.

Keratitis
An inflammation of the cornea, typically accompanied by an ulceration.

CODING BITES

Hypopyon is an inflammation in the anterior chamber of the eye.

Mooren's ulcer is also known as peripheral ulcerative keratitis.

Mycotic corneal ulcer is also known as fungal ulcerative keratitis.

When caused by herpes simplex virus, type 1, the diagnosis is dendritic corneal ulcer (herpesviral keratitis). Typically it is a unilateral condition, and initial signs and symptoms include reduced visual clarity, tearing, photophobia, and varying levels of pain (anywhere from mild discomfort to acute pain). As you can see, there are several different viruses that cause keratitis. You should find this detail in the documentation and the pathology report.

B00.52	Herpesviral keratitis
B01.81	Varicella keratitis
B02.33	Zoster keratitis

Corneal dystrophy occurs when one or more parts of the cornea develop an accumulation of cloudy material, resulting in the loss of normal clarity. There are over 20 varieties of corneal dystrophies, all of which share several characteristics:

- Genetic (inherited)
- Bilateral
- Not the result of external causes, such as injury or diet
- Develop gradually
- Onset limited to a single layer of the cornea, with the disorder spreading later to the others

Some of the most common corneal dystrophies include Fuchs' dystrophy (endothelial corneal dystrophy), keratoconus, lattice dystrophy, and map-dot-fingerprint (epithelial corneal) dystrophy.

H18.51	Endothelial corneal dystrophy
	Fuchs' dystrophy
H18.52	Epithelial (juvenile) corneal dystrophy
H18.53	Granular corneal dystrophy
H18.54	Lattice corneal dystrophy
H18.55	Macular corneal dystrophy

Corneal Dystrophy
Growth of abnormal tissue on the cornea, often related to a nutritional deficiency.

LET'S CODE IT! SCENARIO

Jessica Harvey, a 41-year-old female, came in to see Dr. Loughlin with complaints of pain in her left eye upon blinking, photophobia, and increased tearing. She has also noticed some blurring. She states she hasn't been able to put her contact lenses in for several days. Dr. Loughlin examined Jessica and dropped fluorescein dye into the conjunctival sac, which stained the outline of the ulcer, the entire outer rim of the cornea. Dr. Loughlin diagnosed Jessica with a ring corneal ulcer of the left eye.

Let's Code It!

Dr. Loughlin diagnosed Jessica with a *ring corneal ulcer* of the *left eye*. In the Alphabetic Index, let's look at the main term—*ulcer:*

Ulcer, ulcerated, ulcerating, ulceration, ulcerative

Find the term *cornea* in the long list below. Then, in the list indented beneath *cornea,* determine the most accurate match to Dr. Loughlin's notes:

Ulcer, ulcerated, ulcerating, ulceration, ulcerative
- Cornea H16.00-
-- Ring H16.02-

Now to the Tabular List—let's check out the top of the code category:

☑4 **H16**   **Keratitis**

Are you in the wrong place? Remember that earlier, when you learned about keratitis, you learned it is an inflammation and ulceration of the cornea. Double-check, though, to be certain. Do you see a confirmation that you are in the correct location?

☑5 **H16.0**   **Corneal ulcer**

Whew! Now review the options for the fifth and sixth characters to see if you can determine an accurate code:

H16.022   **Ring corneal ulcer, left eye**

That matches perfectly!

Check the top of this subsection and the head of this chapter in ICD-10-CM. There are notations at the beginning of this chapter: a **NOTE** and an **EXCLUDES2** notation. Read carefully. Do any relate to Dr. Loughlin's diagnosis of Jessica? No. Turn to the Official Guidelines and read Section 1.c.7. There is nothing specifically applicable here either.

Now you can report H16.022 for Jessica's diagnosis with confidence.

Good coding!

Disorders of the Lens

The **lens** of the eye is located at the anterior of the **vitreous chamber** (see Figure 10-3). The lens is a semipermeable membrane that is transparent, avascular (contains no blood vessels), and biconvex. The lens goes through what's called **accommodation**, which is the process of changing shape to accomplish seeing objects both near and far. To view objects that are close (near vision), the lens reshapes to a spherical body, the **pupil** contracts, and the eyes converge (come toward the middle). When looking at something at a distance (far vision), the lens flattens out, the eyes straighten, and the pupils dilate (open wider). As individuals get older, the lens gets tired of accommodating and is not as flexible as it used to be. This makes it more likely the lens may get stuck in the near-vision shape, meaning the individual is nearsighted and may need corrective lenses (eyeglasses or contact lenses) to enable him or her to see far away. When somebody is farsighted, the lens gets stuck in the flattened position and the individual will need corrective lenses to see close up.

A **cataract** is the gradual opacity (clouding) of the lens or lens capsule of the eye, which causes a reduction of vision. Many individuals perceive this to be a condition of the elderly; however, cataracts can occur at any age, including being present at birth. Patients with diabetes mellitus are especially prone to developing cataracts. Complicated cataracts are most often an idiopathic condition, caused by a preexisting condition such as diabetes mellitus or hypoparathyroidism. However, this condition can also be caused by trauma, especially after a foreign body has injured the lens.

Ophthalmoscopy examination, or a slit-lamp exam, can be used to confirm the presence of a cataract by enabling the observation of a dark area in the normally consistent red reflex of the lens.

H25.11	Age-related nuclear cataract, right eye
H26.012	Infantile and juvenile cortical, lamellar, or zonular cataract, left eye
Q12.0	Congenital cataract

Lens
A transparent, crystalline segment of the eye, situated directly behind the pupil, that is responsible for focusing light rays as they enter the eye and travel back to the retina.

Vitreous Chamber
The interior segment of the eye that contains the vitreous body.

Accommodation
Adaptation of the eye's lens to adjust for varying focal distances.

Pupil
The opening in the center of the iris that permits light to enter and continue on to the lens and retina.

Cataract
Clouding of the lens or lens capsule of the eye.

> # 🛑 YOU CODE IT! CASE STUDY
>
> Nicholas McCord, a 45-year-old male, was tightening the rope holding a load on the bed of his pickup truck when the rope broke suddenly. His fist, clenching the rope, snapped backward, hitting him in the right eye. The pain was difficult for him to deal with, so his friends brought him to the emergency department. After examination, Dr. Espinal diagnosed Nicholas with an anterior dislocation of his right eye lens. He was taken up to the procedure room.
>
> ### You Code It!
>
> Go through the steps of coding, and determine the code or codes that should be reported for this encounter between Dr. Espinal and Nicholas.
>
> Step #1: Read the case carefully and completely.
>
> Step #2: Abstract the scenario. Which main words or terms describe why the physician cared for the patient during this encounter?
>
> Step #3: Are there any details missing or incomplete for which you would need to query the physician? [If so, ask your instructor.]
>
> Step #4: Check for any relevant guidance, including reading all of the symbols and notations in the Tabular List and the appropriate sections of the Official Guidelines.
>
> Step #5: Determine the correct diagnosis code or codes to explain why this encounter was medically necessary.
>
> Step #6: Double-check your work.
>
> **Answer:**
>
> Did you determine this to be the correct code?
>
> H27.121   Anterior dislocation of lens, right eye

Disorders of the Choroid and Retina

The Uveal Tract

The **uveal tract** is the middle layer of the eye; it has three sections: the **iris** (in the anterior), followed by the **ciliary body**, and **choroid** in the posterior. Together, the parts of the uvea improve the contrast of the image created by the retina. The uvea accomplishes this by reducing the light reflected within the eye while absorbing outside light as it is transmitted. The uvea is also responsible for providing nutrition to the eye structure and exchanging gases (see Figure 10-4).

The Retina

The **retina**, the area of the eye that contains nerve endings, is responsible for receiving visual images and forwarding these images to the brain for analysis (see Figure 10-4). The choroid is lightly attached to the retinal pigment epithelium (RPE) and is adjacent to the rods and cones that function as light receptors. The **rods** are located throughout the retina and are responsible for detecting movement so that you can see when something in front of you is moving. There are three types of **cones** that, together, provide designation for up to 150 shades of color: one type of cone reacts to red light, one to blue-violet light, and the third to green light. Isn't it amazing that you can go into a paint store and see 500 different colors, yet the eye can

Uveal Tract
The middle layer of the eye, consisting of the iris, ciliary body, and choroid.

Iris
The round, pigmented muscular curtain in the eye.

Ciliary Body
The vascular layer of the eye that lies between the sclera and the crystalline lens.

Choroid
The vascular layer of the eye that lies between the retina and the sclera.

Retina
A membrane in the back of the eye that is sensitive to light and functions as the sensory end of the optic nerve.

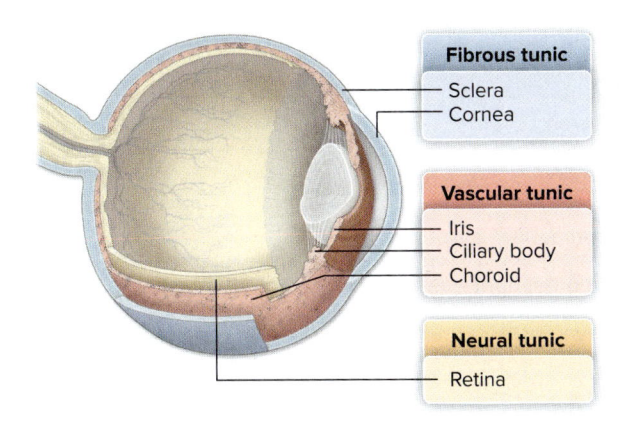

FIGURE 10-4 The anatomical components of the interior of the eye

really only interpret up to 150? The eye combines the light wavelengths to enable perception of a multitude of colors.

Retinal detachment is the separation of the outer RPE from the neural retina, creating a space immediately beneath the retina. This subretinal space then fills with fluid (liquid vitreous) and obstructs the flow of choroidal blood (which supplies oxygen and nutrients to the retina). Signs and symptoms include floaters (floating black spots) as well as photopsia (recurring flashes of light).

H33.012	Retinal detachment with single break, left eye
H33.021	Retinal detachment with multiple breaks, right eye
H33.21	Serous retinal detachment, right eye

10.3 Other Conditions Affecting the Eyes

Glaucoma

Glaucoma is a malfunction of the fluid pressure within the eye; the pressure rises to a level that can cause damage to the optic disc and nerve. Glaucoma is essentially categorized as either open angle or closed angle:

- *Open angle:* a slowly developing, chronic condition that typically has no signs or symptoms until very advanced.
- *Closed angle:* a painful condition with a sudden onset and rapidly progressing vision loss.

In addition to abstracting the documented diagnosis of glaucoma, you will need to confirm the current stage of development of this condition to accurately report the seventh character:

- *mild* stage (evidence of changes in the aqueous outflow system of the eye)
- *moderate* stage (elevated intraocular pressure)
- *severe* stage (atrophy of the optic nerve and loss of the visual field)
- *indeterminate* stage (for unusual circumstances, when the physician documented being unable to determine the stage; this is *not* the same as unspecified)

H40.1113	Primary open-angle glaucoma, right eye, severe stage
H40.2221	Chronic angle-closure glaucoma, left eye, mild stage

rod
An elongated, cylindrical cell within the retina that is photosensitive in low light.

Cone
A receptor in the retina that is responsible for light and color.

Retinal Detachment
A break in the connection between the retinal pigment epithelium layer and the neural retina.

Glaucoma
The condition that results when poor draining of fluid causes an abnormal increase in pressure within the eye, damaging the optic nerve.

> **GUIDANCE CONNECTION**
>
> Read the ICD-10-CM Official Guidelines for Coding and Reporting, section **I. Conventions, General Coding Guidelines and Chapter Specific Guidelines,** subsection **C. Chapter-Specific Coding Guidelines,** chapter **7. Diseases of the Eye and Adnexa,** subsection **a. Glaucoma.**

YOU CODE IT! CASE STUDY

PATIENT NAME: Peter Calvern

DATE OF OPERATION: 10/05/2018

PREOPERATIVE DIAGNOSIS: Narrow-angle glaucoma, right eye.

POSTOPERATIVE DIAGNOSIS: Narrow-angle glaucoma, right eye.

OPERATION PERFORMED: Laser iridotomy, right eye.

SURGEON: JoAnn Hannigan, MD

ANESTHESIA: Topical proparacaine.

INDICATIONS FOR PROCEDURE: The patient is a 67-year-old male with a history of narrow-angle glaucoma, at high risk for blindness or angle-closure glaucoma, diagnosed on physical examination by gonioscopy. Risks, benefits, and alternatives of laser iridotomy were discussed with the patient preoperatively. The patient agreed and signed appropriate consent preoperatively.

DESCRIPTION OF PROCEDURE: On the day of the procedure, the right eye was identified as the operative eye. The patient received 3 sets q. 5 minutes of the following drops: proparacaine, pilocarpine, and Iopidine. Appropriate constriction and anesthesia were achieved. The patient was then brought back to the laser suite, where first the argon laser was used to pretreat the iris superiorly in an area that was covered by the lid with the following settings: 800 milliwatts, 0.06 second duration and 50 micron spot size. Then, the YAG laser was used to complete the iridotomy with the following settings: 5 millijoules, 2 pulses and a total of 2 pulses applied. Good flow of aqueous was noted from the posterior chamber to the anterior chamber and a patent iridotomy was obtained. The patient was given the following postoperative instructions: No bending, coughing, lifting, straining, or sneezing. Return to the clinic for further followup care, and the patient is to use prednisolone acetate 1 drop, left eye, 4 times a day for 1 week.

You Code It!

Review this documentation about the procedure that Dr. Hannigan performed on Peter, and determine the correct code or codes to report the reason why this procedure was medically necessary.

Step #1: Read the case carefully and completely.

Step #2: Abstract the scenario. Which main words or terms describe why the physician cared for the patient during this encounter?

Step #3: Are there any details missing or incomplete for which you would need to query the physician? [If so, ask your instructor.]

Step #4: Check for any relevant guidance, including reading all of the symbols and notations in the Tabular List and the appropriate sections of the Official Guidelines.

Step #5: Determine the correct diagnosis code or codes to explain why this encounter was medically necessary.

Step #6: Double-check your work.

Answer:

Did you determine this to be the correct code?

    H40.031   Anatomical narrow angle, right eye

Good work!

Diabetic Retinopathy

Patients diagnosed with diabetes mellitus are at risk for ophthalmic manifestations of their improper glucose levels. Diabetic **retinopathy** is the most common; it is a condition that causes damage to the tiny blood vessels inside the retina (*retina* + *-pathy* = disease). Signs and symptoms include

- Blurry or double vision.
- Rings around lights.
- Flashing lights.
- Blank spots.
- Dark or floating spots (commonly known as *floaters*).
- Pain in one or both eyes.
- Sensation of pressure in one or both eyes.
- Difficulty in seeing things peripherally (out of the corners of the eyes).
- Macular edema, which occurs when fluid and protein deposits collect on or beneath the macula (a central area of the retina), resulting in swelling (edema). The swelling then causes the macula to thicken, distorting the person's central vision.

Retinopathy
Degenerative condition of the retina.

Diabetic retinopathy progresses through four stages of development:

1. Mild nonproliferative retinopathy (microaneurysms).
2. Moderate nonproliferative retinopathy (blockage in some retinal vessels).
3. Severe nonproliferative retinopathy (more vessels are blocked, depriving the retina of blood supply).
4. Proliferative retinopathy (most advanced stage).

When diagnosis and treatment are implemented in the early stages, vision loss can be reduced. Therefore, individuals with diabetes mellitus are encouraged to get regular eye exams. Diabetic retinopathy is one of the leading causes of blindness in U.S. adults, affecting more than 4 million Americans.

EXAMPLES

E10.321   Type 1 diabetes mellitus with mild nonproliferative diabetic retinopathy with macular edema

E11.36   Type 2 diabetes mellitus with diabetic cataract

Remember, whenever a combination code is available that includes the underlying condition and the manifestation in one code, you must use this to report the diagnosis. If no combination code is accurate, then you will probably need to report multiple codes to provide the whole picture.

Hypertensive Retinopathy

Patients with hypertension (high blood pressure) can develop damage to the retina because of the unusually high pressure of the blood traveling through the vessels. This condition is known as *hypertensive retinopathy*. The higher the pressure and the longer this condition has been ongoing, the more severely the retina may be harmed. Signs and symptoms most evident for those with hypertensive retinopathy include

- Double vision
- Dimmed vision
- Blindness (vision loss)
- Headaches

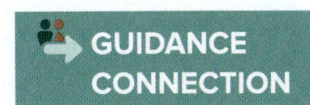

GUIDANCE CONNECTION

Read the ICD-10-CM Official Guidelines for Coding and Reporting, section **I. Conventions, General Coding Guidelines and Chapter Specific Guidelines**, subsection **C. Chapter-Specific Coding Guidelines**, chapter **9. Diseases of the Circulatory System**, subsection **a. 5) Hypertensive retinopathy.**

> **EXAMPLES**
>
> H35.031   Hypertensive retinopathy, right eye
> H35.032   Hypertensive retinopathy, left eye
>
> Did you notice that, with diabetic retinopathy, the combination codes are available to you in the subsection for the underlying condition, diabetes mellitus? However, with hypertensive retinopathy, these combination codes are with the ophthalmic codes—the manifestation. You always need to read carefully and completely.

LET'S CODE IT! SCENARIO

PATIENT'S NAME: Arlene Masconetti

MRN: ALMAS0122

DATE OF PROCEDURE: 07/22/2018

PRE/POSTOPERATIVE DIAGNOSIS: Cataract, traumatic and mature, right eye.

PROCEDURE PERFORMED: Phacoemulsification and implantation of intraocular lens, right eye.

SURGEON: Jason Britemann, MD

ANESTHESIA: MAC with retrobulbar

PREPROCEDURE: Patient is a 37-year-old female who had been playing softball with co-workers and got hit by a ball in the right eye, causing a total traumatic cataract. She tried to ignore the discomfort, but it was interfering with her doing her work, and she was afraid to drive. Patient was given the complete information on this procedure, possible outcomes, and projected outcomes, and she signed consent. Prior to bringing the patient to the operating room, the patient received three sets of topical dilating, antibiotic drops.

DESCRIPTION OF OPERATION: The patient was brought to the procedure room and placed in a supine position on the operating table, and was prepped and draped in a sterile manner. She was sedated and retrobulbar injection of 0.75% Marcaine and 1% lidocaine was made. No complications were evident. A lid speculum was inserted to part the eyelid. A paracentesis was made infratemporally. The anterior chamber was filled with air and then indocyanine green to stain the anterior capsule. The cataract was noted to be extremely mature. A small capsulorrhexis was initiated. Immediately, milky white fluid extruded from the capsulorrhexis opening. A 27-gauge cannula was then used to aspirate this fluid. The cystotome was then used to complete the capsulorrhexis. The nucleus was gently rocked to facilitate mobility. The phacoemulsification apparatus was introduced into the eye. The nucleus was phacoemulsified and removed without any complications. The remaining cortex was removed with irrigation and aspiration. An SA60 AC 21-diopter lens was placed in the bag and the remaining viscoelastic was removed. One interrupted 10-0 nylon suture was placed in the cornea. The patient tolerated the procedure well. The lid speculum was removed. One drop of Betadine, one drop of Ciloxan, and bacitracin ointment were placed into the eye and patch and shield were applied. The patient was returned to postanesthesia care in satisfactory condition. The patient was instructed to take the eye patch off at 6 p.m. and use the topical Vigamox and Pred Forte eye drops every 2 hours until bedtime.

Let's Code It!

Dr. Britemann performed cataract surgery on Arlene to treat her traumatic and mature cataract of her right eye. Open your ICD-10-CM code book to the Alphabetic Index and find

Cataract (cortical) (immature) (incipient) H26.9

Hmm. The first thing you might notice is that this included a nonessential modifier of "immature," and Dr. Britemann documented that Arlene's cataract is mature. What is the difference? This is why it is always such a great idea to have a medical dictionary nearby. A *mature cataract* is one that produces swelling and opacity of the entire lens. In this case, mature is not the same as senile (an age-related cataract). As you look down the indented list, notice there is no specific listing for Cataract, mature. However, keep reading and you will find:

Cataract (cortical) (immature) (incipient) H26.9
    traumatic H26.10-

Let's take a look at this code and see what additional information the Tabular List might offer. You can always come back here to the Alphabetic Index.

    ☑4 H26   Other cataract
           EXCLUDES1 *congenital cataract (Q12.0)*

Before you review the fourth character options, scan this entire subsection, code categories H25, H26, H27, and H28. Do you see any description that suits Dr. Britemann's diagnosis of Arlene? Neither do I, so continue investigating the options available within H26.

    ☑5 H26.1   Traumatic cataract
        Use additional code (Chapter 20) to identify external cause

The required fifth character will explain if the trauma was localized, partially resolved, or total. Go back to the documentation and determine which is the accurate character:

    ☑6 H26.13   Total traumatic cataract

You are making good progress. The sixth character will report which eye, or both eyes, are injured.

    H26.131   Total traumatic cataract, right eye

Check the top of this subsection and the head of this chapter in ICD-10-CM. A **NOTE** and an **EXCLUDES2** notation are at the head of this chapter. Read carefully. Do any relate to Dr. Britemann's diagnosis of Arlene? No. Turn to the Official Guidelines and read Section 1.c.7. There is nothing specifically applicable here, either.
    Now you can report H26.131 for Arlene's diagnosis with confidence.

    H26.131   **Total traumatic cataract, right eye**

Wait one minute. You are not done yet. Remember the **Use Additional Code** notation? External cause codes are required. Turn to the Index to External Causes. Arlene was hit, or struck, by a ball. So, find

    Struck (accidentally) **by**
        ball (hit) (thrown) W21.00-
            softball W21.07-

Now, turn in the Tabular List, to find:

    ☑4 W21   **Striking against or struck by sports equipment**
        EXCLUDES1 assault with sports equipment (Y08.0-)
            striking against or struck by sports equipment with subsequent fall (W18.01)

    ☑5 W21.0   Struck by hit or thrown ball
        ☑xx7 W21.07   Struck by softball

You will learn more about external cause codes in this book's chapter **Coding Injury, Poisoning, and External Causes**.

    H26.131   **Total traumatic cataract, right eye**
    W21.07   **Struck by softball**
    Y93.64   **Activity, baseball (activity, softball)**
    Y99.8   **Other external cause status**

Good coding!

10.4 Dysfunctions of the Auditory System

Auditory Diseases

Otitis media is the inflammation of the middle ear. There are various types of this condition: suppurative and nonsuppurative, acute and chronic. While otitis media is common in children, it is not exclusively a childhood condition. Interestingly, the cases of this diagnosis increase during the winter, while there is an increase of otitis externa (inflammation of the external ear) in the summer. ICD-10-CM code category H66.- Suppurative and unspecified otitis media requires additional characters to report details including acute or chronic, suppurative or nonsuppurative, and with or without rupture of the eardrum, as well as laterality.

Endolymphatic hydrops (Ménière's disease) is a dysfunction of the labyrinth (semicircular canals). Signs and symptoms include vertigo, sensorineural hearing loss, and tinnitus. A feeling of fullness within the ear is not uncommon. Report this diagnosis with ICD-10-CM code H81.0- Ménière's disease, with an additional character to identify laterality.

LET'S CODE IT! SCENARIO

Kaitlyn Logan, a 27-year-old female, was at a club and met a guy doing ear piercings. She got a piercing through the cartilage of her upper left ear. Now, 3 days later, her ear is erythematous (red), swollen, and painful to the touch. Dr. Sweeting examined her ear and diagnosed her with acute perichondritis of the left pinna. He prescribed fluoroquinoline with a semisynthetic penicillin and told her to come back in 2 weeks.

Let's Code It!

Dr. Sweeting diagnosed Kaitlyn with *acute perichondritis of the left pinna*. Let's turn in the Alphabetic Index to find

Perichondritis

Read down the indented list, and you will see that *pinna* is listed:

Perichondritis
  Pinna — *see* Perichondritis, ear

However, this is giving us a directive, not a code, to look back up the list to

Perichondritis
  Ear (external) H61.00
    Acute H61.01-
    Chronic H61.02-

OK, now we have a suggested code to get us started. Turn to the three-digit code category suggested here:

☑4 **H61**   **Other disorders of external ear**

You remember from earlier in this chapter that the pinna is a part of the external ear, so this may be the correct code category. Go ahead and review the fourth and fifth characters available and see if any match Dr. Sweeting's diagnosis.

☑5 **H61.0**   **Chondritis and perichondritis of external ear**
☑6 **H61.01**   **Acute perichondritis of external ear**

That is great. Now review the choices for the sixth character, and determine the complete code to report for Dr. Sweeting's encounter with Kaitlyn.

H61.012   **Acute perichondritis of left external ear**

Good job!

Otosclerosis is a condition of increasing growth of spongy bone in the otic capsule. This growth interferes with the travel of sound vibrations from the tympanic membrane to the cochlea, causing a progressive deterioration of hearing. This condition is seen most frequently in adults between the ages of 18 and 35, and it is more prevalent in females. Report this condition with ICD-10-CM code category H80.- Otosclerosis, with additional characters to identify the specific location within the ear as well as laterality.

LET'S CODE IT! SCENARIO

Alexis Acosta, a 33-year-old female, was having a terrible time with dizziness. She states that she has also had a problem keeping her balance. A complete examination by Dr. McQuaig confirmed a diagnosis of bilateral aural vertigo.

Let's Code It!

Dr. McQuaig confirmed a diagnosis of *bilateral aural vertigo*. Turn to the Alphabetic Index and find

> Vertigo R42

Wait. Before you turn to the Tabular List, review the additional terms shown in the indented list.

> Vertigo R42
> Aural H81.31-

This matches the diagnosis documented by Dr. McQuaig much closer, doesn't it? Let's check this out in the Tabular List, of course, beginning at the code category:

> ✓4 H81   Disorders of vestibular function

Directly below this is an EXCLUDES1 notation. Does either of these diagnoses relate to Dr. McQuaig's notes about Alexis? No. Good. Continue reading to review the available choices for the fourth and fifth characters. Did you find this?

> ✓6 H81.31   Aural vertigo

Perfect! Just one more thing: Take a look at Dr. McQuaig's documentation and determine which ear or ears are affected. Now you can report with confidence that Alexis's diagnosis is

> H81.313   Aural vertigo, bilateral

Good work!

Tumors of the ear canal include osteomas and sebaceous cysts and can grow large enough to interfere with hearing. Should the growth become infected, the patient may develop a fever and other signs of inflammation, including pain. While these tumors rarely become malignant, pain might indicate a malignancy. Examination with an otoscope can typically confirm this diagnosis, although a biopsy would be required to confirm benign or malignant status.

EXAMPLES

C30.1	Malignant neoplasm of middle ear (malignant neoplasm of inner ear)
C44.212	Basal cell carcinoma of skin of right ear and external auricular canal
D14.0	Benign neoplasm of middle ear, nasal cavity and accessory sinuses
D23.22	Other benign neoplasm of skin of left ear and external auricular canal

Labyrinthitis is an infection within the inner ear's labyrinth. The most evident symptom is incapacitating vertigo that may last as long as 5 days. Sensorineural hearing loss may also occur. Viral labyrinthitis can be a manifestation of some upper respiratory tract infections, or caused by trauma or toxic drug ingestion. In some cases, cholesteatoma may form on the bone of the labyrinth and erode it. Labyrinthitis may be described as circumscribed, destructive, diffused, latent, purulent, or suppurative. Report H83.0- Labyrinthitis with an additional character to identify laterality.

YOU CODE IT! CASE STUDY

Rebekka Keith, a 9-year-old female, was brought to her pediatrician, Dr. Granberry, because her right ear was very painful and inflamed, and there was presence of both blood and fluid in her ear canal. She had suffered with the Flu (upper respiratory infection), which had resolved last week. Physical examination revealed blebs and evidence that one or two had ruptured spontaneously causing the presence of fluid and blood. Culture identified the pathogen as Haemophilus influenzae. Dr. Granberry diagnosed Rebekka with acute infectious bullous myringitis of the right ear and prescribed antibiotic ear drops.

You Code It!

Go through the steps of coding, and determine the diagnosis code or codes that should be reported for this encounter between Dr. Granberry and Rebekka.

Step #1: Read the case carefully and completely.

Step #2: Abstract the scenario. Which main words or terms describe why the physician cared for the patient during this encounter?

Step #3: Are there any details missing or incomplete for which you would need to query the physician? [If so, ask your instructor.]

Step #4: Check for any relevant guidance, including reading all of the symbols and notations in the Tabular List and the appropriate sections of the Official Guidelines.

Step #5: Determine the correct diagnosis code or codes to explain why this encounter was medically necessary.

Step #6: Double-check your work.

Answer:

Did you determine these to be the correct codes?

H73.011	Acute bullous myringitis, right ear
B96.3	Hemophilus influenzae (H. influenzae) as the cause of diseases classified elsewhere

10.5 Causes, Signs, and Symptoms of Hearing Loss

There are several things that might contribute to loss of hearing: genetics and congenital anomalies, pathogens, and external causes that may be traumatic or environmental.

Signs and Symptoms of Hearing Loss

While each individual will notice loss of hearing in a different way, these are the most common complaints:

- Hearing speech and other sounds as muffled.
- Having difficulty understanding conversations, particularly when in a crowd or in a noisy place (e.g., a restaurant).

- Frequently asking others to speak more slowly, clearly, and loudly.
- Turning up the volume of the television or radio.
- No longer engaging in conversation.
- Avoiding some social settings.

The degrees of hearing loss are measured in decibels (dB). This part of the assessment identifies the volume heard—from soft sounds to loud. The horizontal lines of the audiogram track the patient's acknowledged sounds. Audiologists tend to measure volumes from zero dB (soft sounds) up to 120 dB (extremely loud sounds). Hearing loss is classified in degrees of hearing from normal to profound. This determination is evaluated using the standard hearing thresholds—the softest a sound was heard at a specific frequency (see Table 10-1).

TABLE 10-1 Degrees of Hearing Loss

Indication of Hearing Loss	Hearing Threshold (dB)
Normal hearing	0–20
Mild hearing loss	21–40
Moderate hearing loss	41–55
Moderately severe hearing loss	56–70
Severe hearing loss	71–90
Profound hearing loss	91 and above

http://www.hopkinsmedicine.org/hearing/hearing_testing/understanding_audiogram.html
Source: "Understanding Your Audiogram" *Johns Hopkins Medicine*, The Johns Hopkins University, hopkinsmedicine.org

EXAMPLES

Z01.10 Encounter for examination of ears and hearing without abnormal findings
Z13.5 Encounter for screening for eye and ear disorders

Here are two examples of code you might report to explain the reason *why* the physician or audiologist met with the patient for this encounter.

Genetics and Congenital Anomalies Causing Hearing Loss

During gestation, some infections, such as rubella, herpes, or toxoplasmosis, are known to possibly cause deafness in the fetus. In addition, congenital anomalies may cause a malformation of any of the ear structures, and there are over 400 genetic conditions that have been identified as causing genetic hearing loss. Most often, these circumstances result in sensorineural hearing loss.

EXAMPLES

P00.2 Newborn (suspected to be) affected by maternal infectious and parasitic diseases
Q16.5 Congenital malformation of inner ear
H91.1- Presbycusis
H93.25 Central auditory processing disorder (Congenital auditory imperception)

Psychogenic (Hysterical) Hearing Loss

Sometimes a traumatic event can be so upsetting to an individual that it results in neurologic symptoms that have no organic cause. This is a psychiatric disorder that was formerly called "hysteria."

> **EXAMPLE**
>
> F44.6 Conversion disorder with sensory symptom or deficit (psychogenic deafness)

Idiopathic Causes of Hearing Loss

Cerumen (earwax) serves an important function within the ear canal. It protects the skin of the ear canal; protects the middle ear from bacteria, fungi, insects, and water; and enables cleaning and lubrication. However, too much cerumen can build up in the canal and form an obstruction, blocking the entrance of sound waves and causing sudden conductive hearing loss. Recurrent ear infections can result in scarring of the tympanic membrane, reducing its ability to transmit sounds into the middle ear.

Presbycusis is the deterioration of the ability to hear that naturally occurs for about a third of adults as they get into their late 60s to mid 70s. Report this diagnosis from code category H91.1 with a fifth character to report laterality.

> **EXAMPLES**
>
> H61.22 Impacted cerumen, left ear
> H91.21 Sudden idiopathic hearing loss, right ear

YOU CODE IT! CASE STUDY

Tatiana Clayton, a 39-year-old female, felt something in her ear. She was having problems hearing in her left ear and felt very uncomfortable. When Dr. Silver asked her, she stated that it felt like something was inside her ear. Upon inspection with the otoscope, Dr. Silver diagnosed a polyp in her middle ear.

You Code It!

Go through the steps of coding, and determine the code or codes that should be reported for this encounter between Dr. Silver and Tatiana.

Step #1: Read the case carefully and completely.

Step #2: Abstract the scenario. Which main words or terms describe why the physician cared for the patient during this encounter?

Step #3: Are there any details missing or incomplete for which you would need to query the physician? [If so, ask your instructor.]

Step #4: Check for any relevant guidance, including reading all of the symbols and notations in the Tabular List and the appropriate sections of the Official Guidelines.

Step #5: Determine the correct diagnosis code or codes to explain why this encounter was medically necessary.

> Step #6: Double-check your work.
>
> **Answer:**
>
> Did you determine this to be the correct code?
>
> **H74.42**   **Polyp of left middle ear**
>
> Terrific!

Traumatic (External) Causes of Hearing Loss

The ear is well protected, for the most part, by the skull; however, trauma can still damage it and interfere with the proper transmission of sound. Fireworks set off too close to a person's ear, explosions, and even standing too close to the amplifiers at a rock concert can result in a loss of hearing. A skull fracture might also cause injury to the ear structures or nerves. While you might not have thought about this, some medications and drugs can result in ototoxic hearing loss. Ototoxic medications—including gentamicin (an aminoglycoside antibiotic) and cisplatin and carboplatin (both cancer chemotherapy drugs)—may cause permanent hearing loss. Others—such as aspirin and other salicylate pain relievers, quinine (which is used to treat malaria), and some loop diuretics—are known to result in temporary hearing loss.

> **EXAMPLES**
>
> H83.3x1   Noise effects on right inner ear
> H91.03   Ototoxic hearing loss, bilateral
> S09.21xA   Traumatic rupture of right ear drum

Remember, whenever an external cause is documented, you must include the additional codes to explain how the injury or poisoning occurred.

> **EXAMPLES**
>
> T36.8x5A   Adverse effect of other systemic antibiotics, initial encounter
> W36.1xxA   Explosion and rupture of aerosol can, initial encounter

Sound Levels Causing Hearing Loss

Walk down the street and you can hear construction equipment or the siren from a passing ambulance that may cause you to cover your ears to lessen the discomfort. Your neighbor revs his motorcycle as he drives past your house, or you go to the airport to see your parents off on a flight for vacation and you wait as the jet takes off into the sky. What is "loud"? And what is so loud that it could damage your hearing? Take a look at Table 10-2 to see the decibel (dB) levels of some of the sounds of everyday life.

> **EXAMPLE**
>
> When the physician documents that sound has caused the patient's hearing loss, you may report an external cause code from the ☑ **W42 Exposure to noise** code category.

TABLE 10-2 Common Sounds

Sound	Noise Level (dB)	Effect
Boom cars	145	
Jet engines (near)	140	
Shotgun firing Jet takeoff (100–200 ft)	130	
Rock concerts (varies)	110–140	Threshold of pain begins around 125 dB.
Oxygen torch	121	
Discotheque/boom box Thunderclap (near)	120	Threshold of sensation begins around 120 dB.
Stereos (over 100 watts)	110–125	
Symphony orchestra Power saw (chainsaw) Pneumatic drill/jackhammer	110	**Regular exposure to sound over 100 dB for more than 1 minute risks permanent hearing loss.**
Snowmobile	105	
Jet flyover (1,000 ft.)	103	
Electric furnace area Garbage truck/cement mixer	100	No more than 15 minutes of unprotected exposure recommended for sounds between 90 and 100 dB.
Farm tractor	98	
Newspaper press	97	
Subway, motorcycle (25 ft)	88	Very annoying.
Lawn mower, food blender Recreational vehicles, TV	85–90 70–90	**85 dB is the level at which hearing damage (8 hr) begins.**
Diesel truck (40 mph, 50 ft)	84	
Average city traffic Garbage disposal	80	Annoying; interferes with conversation; constant exposure may cause damage.
Washing machine	78	
Dishwasher	75	
Vacuum cleaner, hair dryer	70	Intrusive; interferes with telephone conversation.
Normal conversation	50–65	

Source: Decibel table developed by the National Institute on Deafness and Other Communication Disorders, National Institutes of Health. January 1990. nidcd.nih.gov

GUIDANCE CONNECTION

Read the ICD-10-CM Official Guidelines for Coding and Reporting, section **I. Conventions, General Coding Guidelines and Chapter Specific Guidelines,** subsection **C. Chapter-Specific Coding Guidelines,** chapter **20. External Causes of Morbidity.**

Chapter Summary

One of the five senses, vision is involved in virtually every aspect of one's life. This incredible complex organ system captures light and transmits it via interactive anatomical sites to the optic nerve and into the brain for evaluation and interpretation. Even though it is protected by the skull, the optical system is still susceptible to the invasions of pathogens (bacteria, viruses, fungi); can be damaged by trauma; and can be impacted by other environmental issues, such as UV light rays from the sun.

The auditory (hearing) system enables the human body to hear—one of only two senses that have their own organ systems. The auditory system passes along sound vibrations captured by the external ear, through the middle ear and the inner ear, to the cerebellum for interpretation.

CODING BITES

There are many abbreviations related directly to the optical and auditory systems that may be used by your health care providers in their documentation. Some of the most common abbreviations are shown below:

Optical System–Related Abbreviations

OD = right eye
OS = left eye
OU = each eye
ACC = accommodation
PERRLA = pupils equal, round, reactive to light and accommodation
VA = visual acuity
VF = visual field
REM = rapid eye movements
ARMD = age-related macular degeneration

Audiology-Related Abbreviations

AD = right ear
AS = left ear
AC audiometry = air conduction audiometry
BC audiometry = bone conduction audiometry
dB = decibel
dBHL = decibel hearing level
dBSPL = decibel sound pressure level
dBHTL = decibel hearing threshold level
HF = high frequency
HL = hearing level
Hz = hertz (and kHz: kilohertz)
LF = low frequency
PTA = pure tone audiometry

CHAPTER 10 REVIEW
Coding Dysfunction of the Optical and Auditory Systems

Let's Check It! Terminology

Match each key term to the appropriate definition.

Part I

1. LO 10.2 A membrane in the back of the eye that is sensitive to light and functions as the sensory end of the optic nerve.
2. LO 10.2 An elongated, cylindrical cell within the retina that is photosensitive in low light.
3. LO 10.2 A receptor in the retina that is responsible for light and color.
4. LO 10.2 The membranous tissue that covers the entire eyeball (except the cornea); also known as *the white of the eye*.
5. LO 10.2 Transparent tissue covering the eyeball; responsible for focusing light into the eye and transmitting light.

A. Choroid
B. Cones
C. Cornea
D. Iris
E. Lens

CHAPTER 10 REVIEW

6. LO 10.2 The vascular layer of the eye that lies between the retina and the sclera. **A**
7. LO 10.1 A transparent, crystalline segment of the eye, situated directly behind the pupil, that is responsible for focusing light rays as they enter the eye and travel back to the retina. **E**
8. LO 10.2 The opening in the center of the iris that permits light to enter and continue on to the lens and retina. **G**
9. LO 10.1 The bony cavity in the skull that houses the eye and its ancillary parts (muscles, nerves, and blood vessels). **F**
10. LO 10.2 The round, pigmented muscular curtain in the eye. **D**

F. Orbit
G. Pupil
H. Retina
I. Rod
J. Sclera

Part II

1. LO 10.1 The eyelids. **J**
2. LO 10.1 Sebaceous glands that secrete a tear film component that prevents tears from evaporating so that the area stays moist. **G**
3. LO 10.2 The vascular layer of the eye that lies between the sclera and the crystalline lens. **C**
4. LO 10.2 The interior segment of the eye that contains the vitreous body. **L**
5. LO 10.1 Altered sebaceous glands that are connected to the eyelash follicles. **E**
6. LO 10.1 A system in the eye that consists of the lacrimal glands, the upper canaliculi, the lower canaliculi, the lacrimal sac, and the nasolacrimal duct. **F**
7. LO 10.1 A mucous membrane that lines the palpebrae. **I**
8. LO 10.1 Adaptation of the eye's lens to adjust for varying focal distances. **A**
9. LO 10.1 Ordinary sweat glands. **H**
10. LO 10.2 The muscles that control the eye. **D**
11. LO 10.1 A mucous membrane on the surface of the eyeball. **B**
12. LO 10.2 The middle layer of the eye, consisting of the iris, ciliary body, and choroid. **K**

A. Accommodation
B. Bulbar Conjunctiva
C. Ciliary body
D. Extraocular Muscles
E. Glands of Zeis
F. Lacrimal Apparatus
G. Meibomian Glands
H. Moll's Glands
I. Palpebral Conjunctiva
J. Palpebrae
K. Uveal Tract
L. Vitreous Chamber

Part III

1. LO 10.1 Inflammation of the eyelid. **A**
2. LO 10.3 Degenerative condition of the retina. **I**
3. LO 10.2 A break in the connection between the retinal pigment epithelium layer and the neural retina. **H**
4. LO 10.2 An inflammation of the cornea, typically accompanied by an ulceration. **F**
5. LO 10.1 Bulging out of the eye; also known as *exophthalmos*. **G**
6. LO 10.2 Inflammation of the conjunctiva. **B**
7. LO 10.1 Lacrimal gland inflammation. **D**
8. LO 10.3 The condition that results when poor draining of fluid causes an abnormal increase in pressure within the eye, damaging the optic nerve. **E**
9. LO 10.2 Growth of abnormal tissue on the cornea, often related to a nutritional deficiency. **C**

A. Blepharitis
B. Conjunctivitis
C. Corneal Dystrophy
D. Dacryocystitis
E. Glaucoma
F. Keratitis
G. Proptosis
H. Retinal Detachment
I. Retinopathy

Let's Check It! Concepts

Choose the most appropriate answer for each of the following questions.

1. LO 10.1 All of the following are layers of the cornea *except*
   a. epithelium. **b. conjunctiva.** c. stroma. d. endothelium.

2. LO 10.1 Tears are created in the main
   a. lacrimal gland. b. upper canaliculi. c. lacrimal sac. d. lower canaliculi.

3. LO 10.2 _____ is commonly known as *pink eye.*
   a. Keratitis b. Dacryocystitis **c. Conjunctivitis** d. Blepharitis

4. LO 10.2 The muscles that control the eye are known as
   a. intraocular. b. palpebrae. c. vitreous. **d. extraocular.**

5. LO 10.3 What is the correct diagnosis code for intermittent angle-closure glaucoma, left eye?
   a. H40.23 b. H40.231 **c. H40.232** d. H40.233

6. LO 10.3 Signs and symptoms of diabetic retinopathy include all of the following *except*
   a. double vision. b. flashing lights. c. rings around lights. **d. headaches.**

7. LO 10.4 Auditory dysfunction of the labyrinth is known as
   a. otitis media. b. otosclerosis. **c. endolymphatic hydrops.** d. tumors of the ear canal.

8. LO 10.4 _____ is an infection within the inner ear's labyrinth.
   a. Labyrinthitis b. Otitis media c. Chondritis d. Perichondritis

9. LO 10.5 Too much cerumen can build up in the canal and form an obstruction, blocking the entrance of sound waves and causing sudden
   a. inner ear hearing loss. b. sensorineural hearing loss. c. organ of Corti hearing loss. **d. conductive hearing loss.**

10. LO 10.5 The hearing threshold for moderately severe hearing loss is
    a. 20 dB and below. b. 40 to 55 dB. **c. 56 to 70 dB.** d. 90 dB and above.

Let's Check It! Guidelines

Refer to the Official Guidelines and fill in the blanks according to the Chapter 7, Diseases of the Eye and Adnexa, Chapter-Specific Coding Guidelines.

glaucoma	different	seventh
highest	each	admitted
laterality	H40	clinical
4	bilateral	progresses
stage one	both	type

1. Assign as many codes from category _____, Glaucoma, as needed to identify the type of _____, the affected eye, and the glaucoma stage.

2. When a patient has _____ glaucoma and both eyes are documented as being the same type and _____, and there is a code for bilateral glaucoma, report only the code for the type of glaucoma, bilateral, with the seventh character for the stage.

CHAPTER 10 REVIEW

3. When a patient has bilateral glaucoma and _____ eyes are documented as being the same _____ and stage, and the classification does not provide a code for bilateral glaucoma report only _____ code for the type of glaucoma with the appropriate seventh character for the stage.

4. When a patient has bilateral glaucoma and each eye is documented as having a _____ type or stage, and the classification distinguishes _____, assign the appropriate code for _____ eye rather than the code for bilateral glaucoma.

5. If a patient is _____ with glaucoma and the stage _____ during the admission, assign the code for _____ stage documented.

6. Assignment of the _____ character "_____" for "indeterminate stage" should be based on the _____ documentation.

Let's Check It! Rules and Regulations

Please answer the following questions from the knowledge you have gained after reading this chapter.

1. LO 10.1 What are the three types of glands within the palpebrae, including their function?
2. LO 10.2 Explain the difference between rods and cones.
3. LO 10.3 What is hypertensive retinopathy? Include some of the most common signs and symptoms.
4. LO 10.4 Explain otosclerosis, including the ICD-10-CM category code.
5. LO 10.5 List five signs and symptoms of hearing loss.

YOU CODE IT! Basics

First, identify the condition in the following diagnoses; then code the diagnosis.

Example: *Hordeolum externum, left upper eye*
  a. main term: <u>Hordeolum</u>   b. diagnosis: <u>H00.014</u>

1. Stenosis of lacrimal sac, bilateral:
   a. main term: _____   b. diagnosis: _____
2. Transient ischemic deafness, bilateral:
   a. main term: _____   b. diagnosis: _____
3. Retinal telangiectasis, bilateral:
   a. main term: _____   b. diagnosis: _____
4. Ulcerative blepharitis, right upper eyelid:
   a. main term: _____   b. diagnosis: _____
5. Cholesteatoma of attic, left ear:
   a. main term: _____   b. diagnosis: _____
6. Subluxation of lens, left eye:
   a. main term: _____   b. diagnosis: _____
7. Granuloma of right orbit:
   a. main term: _____   b. diagnosis: _____
8. Chronic perichondritis of external ear, left:
   a. main term: _____   b. diagnosis: _____
9. Labyrinthine dysfunction, right ear:
   a. main term: _____   b. diagnosis: _____
10. Bullous keratopathy, left ear:
    a. main term: _____   b. diagnosis: _____
11. Mechanical entropion of eyelid, right lower:
    a. main term _____   b. diagnosis: _____
12. Total attic perforation of tympanic membrane, right ear:
    a. main term: _____   b. diagnosis: _____
13. Recurrent bilateral mastoiditis:
    a. main term: _____   b. diagnosis: _____
14. Senile ectropion of eyelid, left lower:
    a. main term: _____   b. diagnosis: _____
15. Vestibular neuronitis, left ear:
    a. main term: _____   b. diagnosis: _____

YOU CODE IT! Practice

Using the techniques described in this chapter, carefully read through the case studies and determine the most accurate ICD-10-CM code(s) and external cause code(s), if appropriate, for each case study.

1. George McKeown, a 65-year-old male, presents with pain around his right eye and sensitivity to bright light. Dr. Zabawa notes redness of the eye and sagging skin around the lower eyelid. George is diagnosed with entropion of the right eye, lower eyelid.

2. Sheila Friday, a 17-year-old female, presents with the complaint that her left upper eyelid is swollen but doesn't hurt. This is the third time it has happened. Dr. Moss completes a thorough examination and diagnoses Sheila with blepharochalasis, left upper eyelid.

3. John Di Toma, a 10-month-old male, was diagnosed with congenital bilateral cataracts several weeks ago. John is admitted today for the surgical removal of the cataracts.

4. Robert Gould, a 42-year-old male, presents today complaining of pain and lack of vision in his left eye. Robert states that he was playing in a baseball game at the local baseball field and was accidentally struck in the face by the ball. Dr. Beck notes visual acuity of 20/200 (OS), a protruding eyeball, and an intraocular pressure of 42 mm Hg. Normal right eye exam. Robert is admitted, where the CT scan confirms the diagnosis of subarachnoid hematoma.

5. Fred Grossman, a 36-year-old male, presents with the complaint of blurred vision and difficulty seeing at night. Dr. Cole, an ophthalmologist, takes a complete medical history and completes a thorough examination. The results of the slit lamp examination of the cornea confirm a diagnosis of stable keratoconus, right eye.

6. Jill Pruitt, a 9-year-old female, is brought in today by her mother. Jill was jumping on her bed in her bedroom at home when she fell off and struck her head on the floor; now she is seeing double. Dr. Brownder completes an examination and decides to admit Jill for observation. After CT scan results were reviewed, Jill is diagnosed with temporary diplopia.

7. Donald McShane, a 32-year-old male, presents with the complaints of headaches, blurred vision, and eye pain. Dr. Clayton notes redness of the eyes and irregular pupils. Don has been having recurrent episodes and his condition has worsened. The oral steroid treatment does not seem to be effective. After an examination, Dr. Clayton makes the decision to admit Don for a complete workup. Don is diagnosed with acute recurrent iridocyclitis, bilaterally.

8. Streeta Frederick, a 31-year-old female, presents with the complaints of headaches, hearing loss, and dizziness. Dr. Molair completes an examination and admits Streeta. The MRI confirms a diagnosis of primary malignant neoplasm of inner ear, left.

9. Micah Fullmore, a 17-year-old male, comes in today with a swollen left ear lobe that is painful. Dr. Wiccetta notes a red pus-filled lump and, after an examination, Micah is diagnosed with furuncle of external left ear.

10. Rosa Fuller, a 24-year-old female, presents with ear pain. Dr. Rider documents a thick greyish-white matter. After a thorough examination, Rosa is diagnosed with diffuse otomycosis, external ear.

11. Mark Gamble, a 57-year-old male, presents with a low fever and right ear pain. Dr. Martin completes an examination with otoscope, which confirmed a moderately bulging, nonperforated, right tympanic membrane; left tympanic membrane is noted to be within normal limits. Dr. Martin also notes this is the third bout this year. Mark is diagnosed with acute suppurative otitis media, recurrent, right ear.

12. Latoya Simpkins, a 36-year-old female, presents with the complaint of right ear pain. Dr. Herauf also documents a low-grade fever, cough, and nasal drainage. Dr. Herauf completes an examination with otoscope, which visualizes a cloudy bulging eardrum with blisters. Latoya is diagnosed with bullous myringitis.

13. Ken Medlock, a 37-year-old male, presents today with the complaint of ringing in his ears and the feeling of being unbalanced. Ken also states he is having difficulty with his hearing and has pressure in both ears. Dr. Burgos completes an examination and decides to admit Ken for a full workup. Sensorineural

CHAPTER 10 REVIEW

hearing loss is verified by audiometry; MRI scan and electrocochleography confirm the final diagnosis of bilateral Ménière's disease.

14. Tamika Robinson, a 12-year-old female, is having difficulty hearing at school. Dr. Zaprzalka uses an otoscope to visualize the tympanic membrane, noting left and right are within normal range without indication of inflammation. The results of audiometry suggest conductive hearing loss. The CT scan confirms the diagnosis of cochlear otosclerosis, right ear.

15. Rodney Sabido, a 49-year-old male, is suddenly having difficulty with his hearing. Rod describes it as the pitch is higher in one ear than the other. Dr. Butterfield completes an examination and the audiometry confirms a diagnosis of diplacusis, right ear.

YOU CODE IT! Application

The following exercises provide practice in abstracting physicians' notes and learning to work with documentation from our health care facility, Prader, Bracker, & Associates. These case studies are modeled on real patient encounters. Using the techniques described in this chapter, carefully read through the case studies and determine the most accurate ICD-10-CM code(s) and external cause code(s), if appropriate, for each case study.

WESTON EYE CENTER

658 Healthcare Way • SOMEWHERE, FL 32811 • 407-555-7892

PATIENT: OLDENBERG, KYLE

ACCOUNT/EHR #: OLDEKY001

DATE: 10/17/18

Attending Physician: Renee O. Bracker, MD

Kyle Oldenberg, 65-year-old male, presents today with the complaints of gradual loss of vision OD of a 2-month duration. Kyle states it doesn't hurt, "just getting to where I can't see." Kyle saw his ophthalmologist and was diagnosed with angle closure glaucoma and was referred to us for treatment.

PMH: Healthy, no medications

FH: Noncontributory with no history of glaucoma

SH: Drinks alcohol socially and denies use of tobacco.

Eye Exam:

- Best corrected visual acuities: 20/20 OS, barely hand motion vision OD.
- Pupils: >2.9 LU RAPD OD
- EOM: full OU
- IOP: 17 mmHg OS, 66 mmHg OD
- DFE: retina exam—normal macula, vessels, and periphery OU. Optic nerves: 0.3 C/D OS, complete cup OD.

Gonioscopy: moderately open angles OD. (+) Sampaolesi's line OD.

Dx: Pseudoexfoliation glaucoma, moderate stage

P: Selective laser trabeculoplasty (ALT or SLT).

ROB/pw D: 10/17/18 09:50:16   T: 10/19/18 12:55:01

Determine the most accurate ICD-10-CM code(s).

PRADER, BRACKER, & ASSOCIATES
A Complete Health Care Facility
159 Healthcare Way • SOMEWHERE, FL 32811 • 407-555-6789

PATIENT: TRUDELL, LEONARD

ACCOUNT/EHR #: TRUDLE001

DATE: 10/17/18

Attending Physician: Renee O. Bracker, MD

S: Leonard presents today with a red, irritated right eye and decreased vision.

O: History of Present Illness: A 69-year-old male presented to our office with a 1-day history of conjunctival injection and mild discomfort in his right eye (OD). He had a known history of pigmentary glaucoma that was treated with PCIOL and trabeculectomy with mitomycin C in the right eye 5 years earlier. His visual acuity had decreased from 20/120 to 20/250 OD.

Past Ocular History: Pigmentary glaucoma (OD), age-related macular degeneration in both eyes (OU). The patient had suffered a severe retinal detachment in the left eye (OS).

Medical History: Hypertension, thyroidectomy.

Medications: Latanoprost OD qhs, Synthroid, and Buspar.

Family History: Noncontributory.

Social History: The patient denies alcohol and tobacco use.

Exam, Ocular:

- Visual acuity, with correction: OD—20/250; OS—Light perception.
- Intraocular pressure: OD—8 mmHg.
- External and anterior segment examination, OD: Conjunctival hyperemia with papillary reaction. There were 4+ cells (per high-power field) visible in the anterior chamber with a small (0.75-mm) hypopyon. The right eye had an elevated, thin avascular bleb with a small infiltrate visible within the bleb. The bleb had a positive Seidel test.
- Dilated fundus exam (DFE), OD: 3+ vitreous cell with a hazy view. Visible retina appeared to be normal.

Course: Performed aqueous and vitreous taps; administered intravitreal vancomycin and ceftazidime; and prescribed hourly topical, fortified gentamycin and vancomycin drops.

The patient responded well to treatment. His visual acuity has returned to baseline, and the bleb leak resolved in 6 weeks.

A: Bleb-related endophthalmitis

P: Next appointment 2 months or earlier prn

ROB/pw D: 10/17/18 09:50:16 T: 10/18/18 12:55:01

Determine the most accurate ICD-10-CM code(s).

WESTON HOSPITAL

629 Healthcare Way • SOMEWHERE, FL 32811 • 407-555-6541

PATIENT: SIMONSON-WALKER, SIERRA

ACCOUNT/EHR #: SIMOSI001

DATE: 10/17/18

Attending Physician: Oscar R. Prader, MD

S: Sierra Simonson-Walker, a 61-year-old woman, presented with left ear discharge with some bleeding. Sierra has a 4-year history of progressive hearing loss in the left ear. She denied any pain, numbness, or weakness.

O: Upon examination, her right ear is within normal limits and the left ear canal is completely blocked with skin debris not consistent with cerumen. An attempt was made to remove the debris in the office, but the patient could not tolerate the severe discomfort.

Medical History: Progressive hearing loss, no ear surgery, no reoccurring ear infections, no prolonged exposure to sun, no head and neck malignancies.

Family History: Noncontributory

Social History: The patient denies alcohol and tobacco use.

Maximum conductive hearing loss on the left and normal hearing on the right is verified by the audiometry.

CT scan showed opacification of the external ear canal with no evidence of bone erosion.

The patient is admitted and taken to the operating room; the debris is visualized to be flaky and keratinaceous. A portion of this was traced back to the anterior portion of the cartilaginous ear canal, where it appeared to be adherent to the skin. This lesion was removed en block and sent to frozen pathology, resulting in no identified carcinoma. There was also some irregular-appearing tissue along the tympanic membrane, which was also removed and sent with the specimen. The patient underwent a tympanoplasty without complication.

Final pathology, however, shows squamous cell carcinoma. The patient was then taken for a lateral temporal bone resection and external ear canal closure.

A: Squamous cell carcinoma of the external ear canal, left

P: Will continue to follow patient closely

ORP/pw   D: 10/16/18 09:50:16   T: 10/18/18 12:55:01

Determine the most accurate ICD-10-CM code(s).

WESTON HOSPITAL

629 Healthcare Way • SOMEWHERE, FL 32811 • 407-555-6541

PATIENT: RIVERA, WALTER

ACCOUNT/EHR #: RIVEWA001

DATE: 10/16/18

Attending Physician: Renee O. Bracker, MD

S: Walter Rivera, a 57-year-old male, presents today with ear pain and loss of hearing. Dr. Wiccetta notes some facial paralysis and slurred speech. Walter is admitted for a full workup.

O: H: 5.10", Wt: 176, T: 97.3 F, HR: 86, R: 25, BP: 176/92. Patient is in obvious pain. Right pupil is 2.6 mm and left is 3.1 mm. Left auricle shows erythematous and is tender and swollen; tympanic membrane is not visible. Chest is clear; heart is regular without murmurs, rubs, or gallops; abdomen is soft and nontender; normal bowel sounds; no hepatosplenomegaly. Extremities are within normal range; skin is clear. Patient is alert and oriented.

Laboratory results:

Sodium 135 mEq/L, potassium 4.6 mEq/L, chloride 91 mEq/L, creatinine 0.6 mg/dL, glucose 274 mg/dL, calcium 9.3 mg/dL, total protein 6.7 g/dL, albumin 3.6 g/dL, total bilirubin 0.7 mg/dL, hemoglobin 15.3 g/dL, WBC 22.4 × $10^3/\mu L$, hematocrit 48.0, platelet count 288 × $10^3/\mu L$.

CT scan shows thickened tissue of the external auditory canal. Brain appears normal from MRI scan.

A: Diabetes, type 2, and malignant otitis externa, right.

P: Antipseudomonal therapy

ROB/pw D:10/16/18 09:50:16   T: 10/18/18 12:55:01

Determine the most accurate ICD-10-CM code(s).

PRADER, BRACKER, & ASSOCIATES

A Complete Health Care Facility

159 Healthcare Way • SOMEWHERE, FL 32811 • 407-555-6789

PATIENT: BARDARO, LYNNE

ACCOUNT/EHR #: BARDLY001

DATE: 10/16/18

Attending Physician: Renee O. Bracker, MD

S: Lynne, a 37-year-old female, presents today with the complaint that her right ear is throbbing.

O: T: 101, BP: 137/83, R: 21, P: 78. PERRLA. Lynne is in moderate discomfort. She admits to a pain level of 4 on a scale of 0–10.

Past medical history: noncontributory.

Review of systems: negative.

Medications: none.

Ear exam: Left is within normal range. Right pinna: a lump is noted, as well as swelling and inflammation. It appears to be a localized pool of blood. Dr. Bracker evacuates the blood and applies a pressure bandage.

A: Auricle hematoma

P: Rx: antibiotics

Follow up with patient in 10–14 days.

ROB/pw D: 10/16/18 09:50:16   T: 10/18/18 12:55:01

Determine the most accurate ICD-10-CM code(s).

11 Coding Cardiovascular Conditions

Key Terms

Angina Pectoris
Atherosclerosis
Atrium
Cerebral Infarction
Cerebrovascular Accident (CVA)
Edema
Elevated Blood Pressure
Embolus
Gestational Hypertension
Hypertension
Hypotension
Infarction
Myocardial Infarction (MI)
NSTEMI
Secondary Hypertension
STEMI
Thrombus
Vascular
Ventricle

Learning Outcomes

After completing this chapter, the student should be able to:

LO 11.1 Abstract the documentation accurately to report heart dysfunction.
LO 11.2 Discern the specifics of cardiovascular disease.
LO 11.3 Evaluate documentation to determine details about abnormal blood pressure diagnoses.
LO 11.4 Identify known manifestations of hypertension.
LO 11.5 Interpret the details of cerebrovascular disease.
LO 11.6 Distinguish the sequelae of cerebrovascular disease and report them accurately.

STOP! Remember, you need to follow along in your ICD-10-CM code book for an optimal learning experience.

11.1 Heart Conditions

At the center of your body is the heart. Like the engine in a car, this small organ pumps oxygen-rich blood through your arteries to every cell in your body, from your head to your toes. The heart beats approximately once every second (60 beats per minute). Each beat is a compression—the heart contracting to force blood through it and out through the aorta to travel through the body delivering oxygen (see Figure 11-1).

Heart Disorders

Cardiac Arrest

Cardiac arrest means the heart actually stops beating. Typically, this happens suddenly. The key factor that you need to know about this condition is that it must be caused by something else. Possible causes of cardiac arrest include an underlying condition such as a myocardial infarction (dead tissue within the heart), an arrhythmia (abnormal heartbeat), electric shock (such as from wiring or lightning), a drug interaction, a drug overdose, a medical procedure, or a trauma. Therefore, along with abstracting this specific diagnosis, you will also need to look for the underlying cause (Figure 11-2).

There are several codes available to report this condition, specifying the underlying cause; here are some of the codes shown in the Tabular List:

I46.2	Cardiac arrest due to underlying cardiac condition
	Code first **underlying cardiac condition**
I46.8	Cardiac arrest due to other underlying condition
	Code first **underlying condition**
I97.710	Intraoperative cardiac arrest during cardiac surgery

I97.711	Intraoperative cardiac arrest during other surgery
I97.120	Postprocedural cardiac arrest during cardiac surgery
I97.121	Postprocedural cardiac arrest during other surgery
O75.4	Other complications of obstetric surgery and procedures

As you can interpret from these code descriptions, you would have to go back to the physician's documentation and specifically identify the underlying condition (that caused

> **CODING BITES**
>
> In reality, there is a code available with no specific underlying cause:
>
> **I46.9 Cardiac arrest, cause unspecified**
>
> As you learned in *Abstracting Clinical Documentation*, you are required to query the physician to obtain the details about the cause of this patient's cardiac arrest to be added to the documentation so the code you report is accurate.

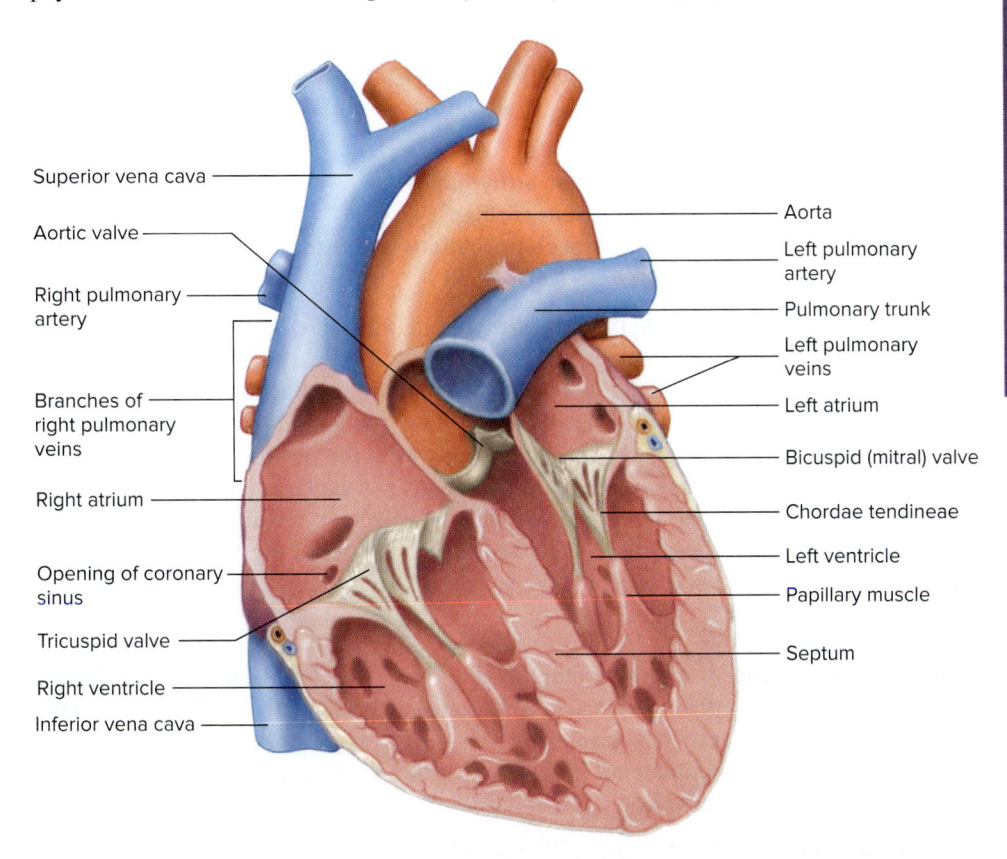

FIGURE 11-1 The anatomical components of the heart David Shier et al., *HOLE'S HUMAN ANATOMY & PHYSIOLOGY,* 12/e. ©2010 McGraw-Hill Education. Figure 15.6b, p. 558. Used with permission.

Arrest, arrested

- cardiac I46.9
-- complicating
--- abortion — *see* Abortion, by type, complicated by, cardiac arrest
--- anesthesia (general) (local) or other sedation — *see* Table of Drugs and Chemicals, by drug,
---- in labor and delivery O74.2
---- in pregnancy O29.11-
---- postpartum, puerperal O89.1
--- delivery (cesarean) (instrumental) O75.4
-- due to
--- cardiac condition I46.2
--- specified condition NEC I46.8
-- intraoperative I97.71-

FIGURE 11-2 ICD-10-CM, Alphabetic Index, partial, from Cardiac Arrest to Intraoperative Arrest Source: *ICD-10-CM Official Guidelines for Coding and Reporting* The Centers for Medicare and Medicaid Services (CMS) and the National Center for Health Statistics (NCHS)

> **GUIDANCE CONNECTION**
>
> Read the ICD-10-CM Official Guidelines for Coding and Reporting, section **II. Selection of Principal Diagnosis,** as well as section **III. Reporting Additional Diagnoses.**

the cardiac arrest). You need this information so you can determine which of these two codes to report, and so you will know what that other (principal) diagnosis code should be.

Dysrhythmia/Arrhythmia

Dysrhythmia, or *arrhythmia,* refers to an irregular heartbeat. Signs include *tachycardia* (rapid heartbeat, more than 100 beats per minute) or *bradycardia* (abnormally slow heartbeat, less than 60 beats per minute). A short-term version of tachycardia may be *palpitations,* a condition in which the patient feels a very rapid heartbeat that lasts only a few minutes. Palpitations are a temporary condition that may be caused by another condition, such as anxiety, whereas tachycardia is an ongoing malfunction of the heart.

R00.0	Tachycardia, unspecified
R00.1	Bradycardia, unspecified
I49.8	Other specified cardiac arrhythmias
I49.9	Cardiac arrhythmia, unspecified
I97.89	Other postprocedural complications and disorders of the circulatory system, not elsewhere classified

When you search for dysrhythmia or arrhythmia, the ICD-10-CM Alphabetic Index directs you to I49.9. You can see that there are no codes specific to dysrhythmia. Notice that other codes are suggested when this condition is diagnosed in a newborn or occurring postoperatively. These details are a tip for you to go back to the documentation and check the patient's age or if the patient was in the postoperative period when the dysrhythmia occurred. Essentially, this diagnosis is vague, as it expresses what is wrong (irregular heartbeat) but does not relate the reason or reasons why the heartbeat is abnormal. You will need more specific information about the patient's condition, from either the documentation or the physician, to determine the correct code(s).

Mitral Valve Prolapse

Mitral valve prolapse is a rather common abnormality that prevents the mitral valve from closing properly (the mitral valve is the gateway between the left **atrium** and the left **ventricle**). A prolapse may develop or be influenced by other conditions, including hyperthyroidism, congenital heart lesions, or Marfan syndrome.

In the Alphabetic Index, find

Prolapse, prolapsed
   mitral (valve) I34.1

When you turn to the code category in the Tabular List, you will see

☑4 I34	Nonrheumatic mitral valve disorders
I34.1	Nonrheumatic mitral (valve) prolapse

The inclusion of the term "nonrheumatic" is a tip to go back into the documentation to ensure that the physician did not state that the patient's condition was caused by rheumatic fever. Rheumatic fever can manifest heart inflammation as well as affect joints and other parts of the body. Rheumatic fever with heart involvement as well as chronic rheumatic heart diseases are reported from code categories I01–I09.

Atrial Fibrillation

Atrial fibrillation is a condition in which atria shudder or tremble in the heart instead of contracting to push blood through to the ventricles. This results in incomplete emptying of the atria, leaving blood to collect and sometimes clot. Episodes of paroxysmal atrial tachycardia (PAT), a rapid heart rate that can go as high as 150 or 200 beats per minute, can occur. Anticoagulants (drugs that prevent clotting) and/or thrombolytics (clot-dissolving drugs) are often prescribed.

I48.2	Chronic atrial fibrillation
I47.1	Supraventricular tachycardia (Atrial (paroxysmal) tachycardia)

Atrium
A chamber that is located in the top half of the heart and receives blood.

Ventricle
A chamber that is located in the bottom half of the heart and receives blood from the atrium.

When the atrial fibrillation is chronic and the patient is prescribed anticoagulants or antithrombotics, this additional information may need to be reported. The following diagnosis codes explain the medical necessity for more frequent blood tests or office visits.

Z79.01   **Long term (current) use of anticoagulants**
Z79.02   **Long term (current) use of antithrombotics/antiplatelets**
Z79.82   **Long term (current) use of aspirin**

And when the reason, or one of the reasons, for the encounter is regular blood testing, you will also need to report:

Z51.81   **Encounter for therapeutic drug level monitoring**

LET'S CODE IT! SCENARIO

Sara Cohen, a 73-year-old woman, was brought to the ED via ambulance after a witnessed cardiac arrest at the local airport.

Past medical history included hypertension, elevated cholesterol, and obstructive sleep apnea. She wore CPAP nightly but continued to experience daytime somnolence. She has smoked half a pack of cigarettes a day for the past 40 years and drank no alcohol. She had a chronic daily cough. She walked 2 miles daily without dyspnea or other limitation. She had never experienced chest pain, palpitations, presyncope, or syncope and had no known history of CAD. Current medications included nifedipine 30 mg orally once daily and simvastatin 20 mg orally once daily.

On the day of presentation, she was at the airport waiting for a flight to visit her grandchildren. Bystanders at the airport reported that they saw her suddenly drop to the floor while walking in the terminal. At a subsequent interview, the first lay responder described that the woman collapsed abruptly without any vocalization and was found to be unresponsive, pulseless, and without respirations. This lay responder, along with another bystander who was a nurse without formal training in advanced resuscitation, began CPR. This particular airport had recently instituted a policy of providing public access defibrillators in the terminals. Bystanders notified airport security staff, who brought a defibrillator to the scene and also called the EMTs. The woman was revived and brought to the hospital.

After examination, Dr. Troy diagnosed Sara with sudden cardiac arrest. He admitted her to the hospital for further testing to determine the cause of this event.

Let's Code It!

Dr. Troy diagnosed Sara with *sudden cardiac arrest*. Turn in your ICD-10-CM Alphabetic Index and find

Arrest, arrested
    cardiac I46.9

There is no mention of "sudden," but the rest matches, so let's turn in the Tabular List to find this code, and we can read from there.

☑4 **I46 Cardiac arrest**
EXCLUDES1 cardiogenic shock (R57.0)

I46.2	Cardiac arrest due to underlying cardiac condition
	Code first underlying cardiac condition
I46.8	Cardiac arrest due to other underlying condition
	Code first underlying condition
I46.9	Cardiac arrest, cause unspecified

Let's go back and read Dr. Troy's documentation carefully. Did he identify the cause of Sara's cardiac arrest? No, actually he specifically stated that he was admitting Sara with the express purpose of determining the underlying condition. Therefore, this is the code you must report:

I46.9   **Cardiac arrest, cause unspecified**

Good work!

> **CODING BITES**
>
> To determine the diagnosis code for heart failure, you need to know:
>
> - What type of heart failure?
> - Is it acute or chronic?

Heart Failure

A diagnosis of heart failure is serious; however, it does not mean the heart has totally "failed" to function. This condition, also known as *congestive heart failure (CHF)*, is characterized by the inability of an individual's heart to pump a sufficient quantity of blood throughout the body. Congestive heart failure can cause fluid to back up into the lungs, resulting in respiratory problems such as shortness of breath and fatigue. In addition, fluid might build up in the lower extremities, causing edema (swelling) in the feet, ankles, and legs. In some patients, the edema can become so acute (severe) that they may have pain and trouble walking.

The National Heart, Lung, and Blood Institute reported in November 2015 that approximately 5.7 million people in the United States currently have a diagnosis of heart failure. The institute estimates that this condition contributes to as many as 30,000 deaths each year.

The Types of Heart Failure

Left heart failure, also known as *pulmonary edema* or cardiac asthma, indicates an insufficiency of the heart's left ventricle. This malfunction results in the accumulation of fluid in the lungs. When this happens, patients may also develop respiratory problems.

I50.1	Left ventricular failure, unspecified

Right heart failure, secondary to left heart failure, is diagnosed when the heart cannot pump and circulate the blood needed throughout the body. Patients with this diagnosis may develop hypertension, congestion, edema, and fluid collection in the lungs.

I50.814	Right heart failure (due to left heart failure)

Systolic heart failure occurs when the contractions of the ventricles are too weak to push the blood through the heart. The documentation should include the specific detail that the condition is acute, chronic, or acute on chronic.

I50.21	Acute systolic (congestive) heart failure
I50.22	Chronic systolic (congestive) heart failure
I50.23	Acute on chronic systolic (congestive) heart failure

Diastolic heart failure is the result of a ventricle of the heart being unable to fill as it should. The documentation should include the specific detail that the condition is acute, chronic, or acute on chronic.

I50.31	Acute diastolic (congestive) heart failure
I50.32	Chronic diastolic (congestive) heart failure
I50.33	Acute on chronic diastolic (congestive) heart failure

Combined systolic and diastolic heart failure means that the function of the heart is weak and unable to process blood properly. The documentation should include the specific detail that the condition is acute, chronic, or acute on chronic.

I50.41	Acute combined systolic (congestive) and diastolic (congestive) heart failure
I50.42	Chronic combined systolic (congestive) and diastolic (congestive) heart failure
I50.43	Acute on chronic combined systolic (congestive) and diastolic (congestive) heart failure

Secondary Hypertension
The condition of hypertension caused by another condition or illness.

> **CODING BITES**
>
> When a condition, such as right heart failure, causes the patient to develop another condition, such as hypertension, that other condition may be referred to as a *secondary* condition.
>
> For example, if Ralph developed hypertension due to his right heart failure, you would report the hypertension as **secondary hypertension**.

> # YOU CODE IT! CASE STUDY
>
> *Judith Patriko, a 78-year-old female, came to see her cardiologist, Dr. Fillmari, to follow up on her CHF. The edema (swelling) of her legs has improved, but she continues to have dyspnea (shortness of breath) with mild exertion. No syncope (fainting) at this time. Dx: Chronic diastolic congestive heart failure.*
>
> ## You Code It!
>
> Look at Dr. Fillmari's notes for Judith Patriko, and determine the best, most appropriate code or codes.
>
> Step #1: Read the case carefully and completely.
>
> Step #2: Abstract the scenario. Which main words or terms describe why the physician cared for the patient during this encounter?
>
> Step #3: Are there any details missing or incomplete for which you would need to query the physician? [If so, ask your instructor.]
>
> Step #4: Check for any relevant guidance, including reading all of the symbols and notations in the Tabular List and the appropriate sections of the Official Guidelines.
>
> Step #5: Determine the correct diagnosis code or codes to explain why this encounter was medically necessary.
>
> Step #6: Double-check your work.
>
> Answer:
>
> Did you determine this to be the diagnosis code?
>
> **I50.32**   Chronic diastolic (congestive) heart failure
>
> Good job!

Myocardial Infarction

When a part of the heart muscle deteriorates, or actually dies, that muscle can no longer function properly. This malfunction within a person's heart, known as a **myocardial infarction (MI)**, will cause persistent pain in the chest, left arm, jaw, and neck; fatigue; nausea; vomiting; and shortness of breath. A preliminary diagnosis of MI, based on these signs and symptoms, can be confirmed by an electrocardiogram (EKG or ECG), blood tests measuring the serial serum enzyme levels, and/or an echocardiogram.

An ST elevation myocardial infarction (**STEMI**) is a heart event during which the coronary artery is completely blocked by a **thrombus** or **embolus**. The ST segment is a specific range seen in an EKG (ECG). A nontransmural ST elevation myocardial infarction (**NSTEMI**) indicates that only a portion of the artery is occluded (blocked).

To determine the code for a diagnosis of MI, you will need to know

- What specific part of the heart was affected by the infarction?
- Has this patient been treated for an MI before? If so, how long ago?
- Is this infarction a STEMI or an NSTEMI?

Anatomical Site of the AMI

An infarction can occur in almost any location within the heart, and it is important that you identify the specific site from the documentation to support the accurate code to report. You will see that the individual codes in the code category for STEMI infarctions include different locations, specifically identified by the fourth character:

Myocardial Infarction (MI)
Malfunction of the heart due to necrosis or deterioration of a portion of the heart muscle; also known as a *heart attack*.

STEMI
An ST elevation myocardial infarction—a heart event during which the coronary artery is completely blocked by a thrombus or embolus.

Thrombus
A blood clot in a blood vessel; plural = *thrombi*.

Embolus
A thrombus that has broken free from the vessel wall and is traveling freely within the vascular system.

NSTEMI
A nontransmural elevation myocardial infarction—a heart event during which the coronary artery is partially occluded (blocked).

GUIDANCE CONNECTION

Read the ICD-10-CM Official Guidelines for Coding and Reporting, section **I. Conventions, General Coding Guidelines and Chapter Specific Guidelines,** subsection **C. Chapter-Specific Coding Guidelines,** chapter **9. Diseases of the Circulatory System,** subsection **e. Acute myocardial infarction (AMI).**

CODING BITES

A thrombus is a blood clot that has attached itself to the wall of a blood vessel. If left untreated, it may cause a blockage, preventing blood from flowing through the artery or vein. In addition, there is always concern that the clot will detach and float through the vessel and pass through an organ. A detached clot is known as an *embolus;* it can get stuck as it passes through an organ and can completely prevent blood from moving through. The greatest danger occurs when an embolus travels into the lung or the heart, potentially causing death.

I21.01   ST elevation (STEMI) myocardial infarction involving left main coronary artery
I21.02   ST elevation (STEMI) myocardial infarction involving left anterior descending coronary artery
I21.11   ST elevation (STEMI) myocardial infarction involving right coronary artery
I21.21   ST elevation (STEMI) myocardial infarction involving left circumflex coronary artery

Subsequent MI

Another important aspect of a diagnosis of MI is whether or not this is the first time a patient has experienced this event. When a patient is documented as having had an acute myocardial infarction (AMI) within the last 4 weeks (28 days) and is at your facility for a second event, this current MI is reported with a code describing a "subsequent" MI:

I22.0   Subsequent ST elevation (STEMI) myocardial infarction of anterior wall
I22.1   Subsequent ST elevation (STEMI) myocardial infarction of inferior wall
I22.2   Subsequent non-ST elevation (NSTEMI) myocardial infarction
I22.8   Subsequent ST elevation (STEMI) myocardial infarction of other sites

When the previous MI is documented either as a "healed MI" or as a past MI without any current signs or symptoms, it is reported with this code:

I25.2   Old myocardial infarction

CODING BITES

If the physician documents this encounter has focused on the patient's subsequent or second MI and the . . .

- Previous MI was within the last 4 weeks = code from category I22
- Previous MI was more than 4 weeks ago = code I25.2

GUIDANCE CONNECTION

Read the ICD-10-CM Official Guidelines for Coding and Reporting, section **I. Conventions, General Coding Guidelines and Chapter Specific Guidelines,** subsection **C. Chapter-Specific Coding Guidelines,** chapter **9. Diseases of the Circulatory System,** subsection **e. Acute myocardial infarction (AMI), 4) Subsequent acute myocardial infarction.**

YOU CODE IT! CASE STUDY

Mark is sitting in the stands watching his son play softball when all of a sudden he feels a severe pain in his chest. He is having difficulty taking a breath, and the pain is radiating down his left arm. He arrives at the ED via ambulance, and Dr. Constantine and nurses work on him, taking blood and doing an EKG. Dr. Constantine determines that Mark had an ST elevation myocardial infarction (STEMI) of the inferolateral wall. Once he is stabilized, Mark is admitted into the hospital and transferred to the ICU.

You Code It!

Go through the steps of coding, and determine the code or codes that should be reported for this encounter between Dr. Constantine and Mark.

Step #1: Read the case carefully and completely.

Step #2: Abstract the scenario. Which main words or terms describe why the physician cared for the patient during this encounter?

Step #3: Are there any details missing or incomplete for which you would need to query the physician? [If so, ask your instructor.]

Step #4: Check for any relevant guidance, including reading all of the symbols and notations in the Tabular List and the appropriate sections of the Official Guidelines.

Step #5: Determine the correct diagnosis code or codes to explain why this encounter was medically necessary.

Step #6: Double-check your work.

Answer:

Did you determine this to be the correct code?

I21.19   ST elevation (STEMI) myocardial infarction involving other coronary artery of inferior wall (Inferolateral transmural (Q wave) infarction (acute))

11.2 Cardiovascular Conditions

The circulatory (cardiovascular) system (Figure 11-3) includes the heart, arteries, and veins. It has the job of circulating blood to carry oxygen to cells throughout the body and to move waste products away from those cells. The circulatory network touches and affects every area of the body, from hair and tissues to organ function.

Circulatory conditions are very serious because they affect the flow of blood and, therefore, the delivery of oxygen. While problems with circulation can affect a patient of any age, older individuals are more susceptible to such conditions. As the body ages, the strength and elasticity of blood vessels decrease and they become less efficient. In addition, long-term poor nutrition and insufficient cardiovascular exercise take their toll and contribute to the circulatory system's inability to do its job.

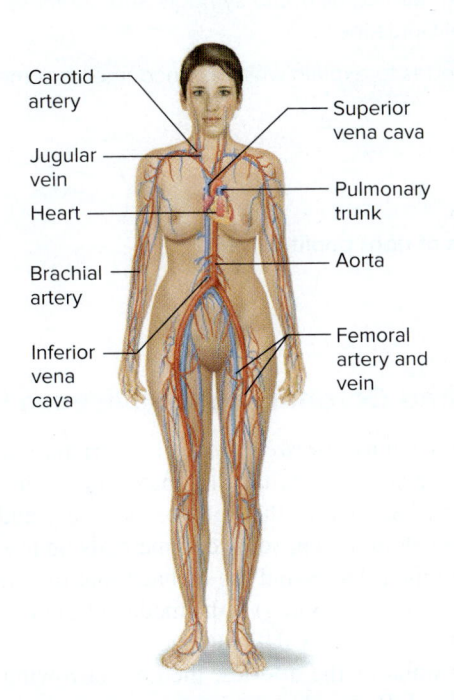

FIGURE 11-3 The cardiovascular system, highlighting major vessels   Booth et al., *Medical Assisting*, 5e. Copyright ©2013 by McGraw-Hill Education. Figure 22-6b, p. 479. Used with permission.

> **CODING BITES**
>
> Cardiovascular: *cardio* = heart + *-vascular* = vessels (veins and arteries)
>
> **Arteries** = blood vessels that carry oxygenated blood from the heart to the tissues and cells throughout the body.
>
> **Veins** = blood vessels that carry deoxygenated blood, along with carbon dioxide and cell waste, away from the tissues and cells throughout the body and back to the heart.

Deep Vein Thrombosis

Earlier in this chapter, you learned about thrombi and emboli—blood clots that develop within the blood vessels. Deep vein thrombi can block the blood flow, causing venous insufficiency and affecting the ability of oxygen to get to the tissues throughout the body. A lack, or reduction, of blood flow can cause edema, congestion, necrosis, and pain. In addition, there is the danger that the blood clot can break loose and travel within the veins and arteries (embolism), causing damage to internal organs, blocking oxygen from the lungs (pulmonary embolism), or blocking off blood flow through the heart.

Reporting a diagnosis of deep vein thrombosis (DVT) [the presence of a blood clot attached to the wall of an interior vein] will require you to know a few specifics to determine the most accurate code:

- Is the condition identified as acute or chronic?
- Where (the specific anatomical site) has the thrombus been located?

I82.412	Acute embolism and thrombosis of left femoral vein
I82.543	Chronic embolism and thrombosis of tibial vein, bilateral

YOU CODE IT! CASE STUDY

Dr. Victorelli examined Carter Franchez and diagnosed him with a chronic thrombosis of the right popliteal vein.

You Code It!

Review the notes about why Dr. Victorelli provided care to Carter Franchez and determine the accurate diagnosis code or codes.

Step #1: Read the case carefully and completely.

Step #2: Abstract the scenario. Which main words or terms describe why the physician cared for the patient during this encounter?

Step #3: Are there any details missing or incomplete for which you would need to query the physician? [If so, ask your instructor.]

Step #4: Check for any relevant guidance, including reading all of the symbols and notations in the Tabular List and the appropriate sections of the Official Guidelines.

Step #5: Determine the correct diagnosis code or codes to explain why this encounter was medically necessary.

Step #6: Double-check your work.

Answer:

Did you determine this to be the accurate code?

I82.531   Chronic embolism and thrombosis of right popliteal vein

Good job!

Atherosclerosis and Coronary Artery Disease (CAD)

Atherosclerosis
A condition resulting from plaque buildup on the interior walls of the arteries, causing reduced blood flow; also known as *arteriosclerosis*.

Atherosclerosis, also known as *arteriosclerosis*, is a stricture or stenosis of an artery (e.g., code I70.0 Atherosclerosis of aorta) that may require the placement of a stent (a wire mesh tube inserted to support the walls of the artery and to keep them open). You have probably heard about this in some commercials on television that talk about the buildup of plaque in the arteries and the damage that may result. Atherosclerosis (*athero* = artery + *sclerosis* = hardening) is the medical term for plaque-lined arteries. You may also see the abbreviation ASHD (arteriosclerotic heart disease). The plaque builds up on the inner walls of the arteries, thereby narrowing the passageway and reducing the flow of blood. Remember that arteries carry oxygenated blood from the heart to the tissues and cells throughout the body.

In coronary artery disease (CAD), plaque collects specifically within the coronary arteries (arteries within the heart); the heart itself becomes oxygen-deprived. This means there will be a greater potential for a stroke (cerebrovascular accident [CVA]), a heart attack, or death. According to the National Heart, Lung, and Blood Institute, CAD is the number-one cause of death in the United States.

When you look in the ICD-10-CM Alphabetic Index, you will read:

Disease, diseased
- coronary (artery) — *see* Disease, heart, ischemic, atherosclerotic
- heart (organic) I51.9
-- ischemic (chronic or with a stated duration of over 4 weeks) I25.9
--- atherosclerotic (of) I25.10
---- with angina pectoris — *see* Arteriosclerosis, coronary (artery)
---- coronary artery bypass graft — *see* Arteriosclerosis, coronary (artery)

A patient may first be alerted to reduced flow of blood to the heart muscle by angina. **Angina pectoris** is an event of acute chest pain caused by an insufficient supply of oxygen to an area of the heart. This condition may be treated with drugs categorized as vasodilators, such as Isordil or Nitrostat (sublingual nitroglycerin), that dilate arterial walls, making it easier for blood to flow smoothly. When hypertension is also present, a calcium channel blocker, such as Norvasc or Vascor, may be prescribed instead. Report angina pectoris with a code from category I20.- Angina pectoris, with a required additional character for the specific type of angina, and be certain to pay attention to the notation directly above this code category that applies to this whole range of codes I20–I25:

Use additional code **to identify presence of hypertension (I10–I16)**

In addition to diet and exercise modification, antilipemic drugs, such as Lipitor or Zocor, may be prescribed to decrease the lipid (fat) blood level. If these actions are not sufficient, a percutaneous transluminal coronary angioplasty (PTCA) may be performed. During a PTCA, a catheter is threaded through the artery to the site of the plaque buildup. A balloon on the tip of the catheter is expanded, compacting the plaque against the walls of the artery, thereby reducing the blockage.

Angina Pectoris
Chest pain.

> **GUIDANCE CONNECTION**
>
> Read the ICD-10-CM Official Guidelines for Coding and Reporting, section **I. Conventions, General Coding Guidelines and Chapter Specific Guidelines,** subsection **C. Chapter-Specific Coding Guidelines,** chapter **9. Diseases of the Circulatory System,** subsection **b. Atherosclerotic coronary artery disease with angina.**

YOU CODE IT! CASE STUDY

PATIENT: Basti, Carl

REASON FOR CONSULTATION: Surgical evaluation for coronary artery disease.

HISTORY OF PRESENT ILLNESS: The patient is a 47-year-old male who has a known history of coronary artery disease. He underwent previous PTCA and stenting procedures in December and most recently in August. Since that time, he has been relatively stable with medical management. However, in the past several weeks, he started to notice some exertional dyspnea with chest pain.

For the most part, the pain subsides with rest. For this reason, he was reevaluated with a cardiac catheterization. This demonstrated 3-vessel coronary artery disease with a 70% lesion to the right coronary artery; this was a proximal lesion. The left main had a 70% stenosis. The circumflex also had a 99% stenosis. Overall left ventricular function was mildly reduced with an ejection fraction of about 45%. The left ventriculogram did note some apical hypokinesis. In view of these findings, surgical consultation was requested and the patient was seen and evaluated by Dr. Isaacson.

PAST MEDICAL HISTORY:

1. Coronary artery disease as described above with previous PTCA and stenting procedures.
2. Dyslipidemia.
3. Hypertension.

ALLERGIES: None.

(continued)

MEDICATIONS: Aspirin 81 mg daily, Plavix 75 mg daily, Altace 2.5 mg daily, metoprolol 50 mg b.i.d., and Lipitor 10 mg q.h.s.

SOCIAL HISTORY: He quit smoking approximately 8 months ago. Prior to that time, he had about a 35- to 40-pack-per-year history. He does not abuse alcohol.

FAMILY MEDICAL HISTORY: Mother died prematurely of breast cancer. His father died prematurely of gastric carcinoma.

REVIEW OF SYSTEMS: There is no history of any CVAs, TIAs, or seizures. No chronic headaches. No asthma, TB, hemoptysis, or productive cough. There is no congenital heart abnormality or rheumatic fever history. He has no palpitations. He notes no nausea, vomiting, constipation, diarrhea, but immediately prior to admission, he did develop some diffuse abdominal discomfort. He says that since then, this has resolved. No diabetes or thyroid problem. There is no depression or psychiatric problems. There are no musculoskeletal disorders or history of gout; no hematologic problems or blood dyscrasias; no bleeding tendencies; and no recent fevers, malaise, changes in appetite, or changes in weight.

PHYSICAL EXAMINATION: His blood pressure is 120/70; pulse is 80. He is in a sinus rhythm on the EKG monitor. Respirations are 18 and unlabored. Temperature is 98.2 degrees Fahrenheit. He weighs 260 pounds and is 5 feet 10 inches. In general, this was a pleasant male who currently is not in acute distress. Skin color and turgor are good. Pupils were equal and reactive to light. Conjunctivae clear. Throat is benign. Mucosa was moist and noncyanotic. Neck veins not distended at 90 degrees. Carotids had 2+ upstrokes bilaterally without bruits. No lymphadenopathy was appreciated. Chest had a normal AP diameter. The lungs were clear in the apices and bases; no wheezing or egophony appreciated. The heart had a normal S1, S2. No murmurs, clicks, or gallops. The abdomen was soft, nontender, nondistended. Good bowel sounds present. No hepatosplenomegaly was appreciated. No pulsatile masses were felt. No abdominal bruits were heard. His pulses are 2+ and equal bilaterally in the upper and lower extremities. No clubbing is appreciated. He is oriented x3. Demonstrated a good amount of strength in the upper and lower extremities. Face was symmetrical. He had a normal gait.

IMPRESSION: This is a 47-year-old male with significant multivessel coronary artery disease. The patient also has a left main lesion. He has undergone several PTCA and stenting procedures within the last year to year and a half. At this point, in order to reduce the risk of any possible ischemia in the future, surgical myocardial revascularization is recommended.

PLAN: We will plan to proceed with surgical myocardial revascularization. The risks and benefits of this procedure were explained to the patient. All questions pertaining to this procedure were answered.

Vaughn Pronder, MD

You Code It!

Carefully review Dr. Pronder's documentation after his evaluation of Carl Basti, and determine the correct diagnosis code or codes to report.

Step #1: Read the case carefully and completely.

Step #2: Abstract the scenario. Which main words or terms describe why the physician cared for the patient during this encounter?

Step #3: Are there any details missing or incomplete for which you would need to query the physician? [If so, ask your instructor.]

Step #4: Check for any relevant guidance, including reading all of the symbols and notations in the Tabular List and the appropriate sections of the Official Guidelines.

Step #5: Determine the correct diagnosis code or codes to explain why this encounter was medically necessary.

Step #6: Double-check your work.

Answer:

Did you determine these to be the correct codes?

I25.10	Atherosclerotic heart disease of native coronary artery without angina pectoris
I10	Essential (primary) Hypertension
Z87.891	Personal history of nicotine dependence
Z79.82	Long term (current) use of aspirin

Good work!

11.3 Hypertension

The average adult has approximately 10 pints (5 liters) of blood in his or her cardiovascular system. Together, the components of the cardiovascular system will pump these 10 pints through the body every minute. The level of pressure at which the blood travels through the vessels is very important.

Blood Pressure

The force with which blood travels through your veins and arteries must create enough pressure to ensure the cycle of oxygenation and carbon dioxide is maintained properly. Blood pressure that is too low—a condition known as **hypotension** (*hypo* = low or under + *tension* = pressure)—can result in organs and tissue cells being unable to function. In hypotension, the patient has lower-than-normal blood pressure. Low blood pressure indicates an inadequate flow of blood and, therefore, inadequate oxygen to the brain, heart, and other vital organs. Lightheadedness and dizziness can occur in a person with hypotension. Some medications, such as antianxiety drugs and diuretics, can cause hypotension, as can alcohol and narcotics. Conditions such as advanced diabetes, dehydration, or arrhythmia can also result in a patient suffering from hypotension. Code category I95 will provide you with the details you will need to abstract from the documentation about this diagnosis:

> **Hypotension**
> Low blood pressure; systolic blood pressure below 90 mmHg and/or diastolic measurements of lower than 60 mmHg.

I95.0	Idiopathic hypotension
I95.1	Orthostatic hypotension
I95.2	Hypotension due to drugs
	Use additional code for adverse effect, if applicable, to identify drug
I95.3	Hypotension of hemodialysis
I95.81	Postprocedural hypotension
I95.89	Other hypotension

Hypertension (*hyper* = high or over + *tension* = pressure) is a condition when blood pressure is too high. The increased force of the blood's pressure moving through the vessels can actually damage organs and tissues as the blood rushes through.

A health care professional will use a sphygmomanometer (blood pressure machine) to measure a patient's blood pressure and will document the results in two numbers. For example: A patient's blood pressure is documented in the chart as 125/85. The number 125 represents the systolic pressure and the number 85 is the diastolic pressure (see Table 11-1).

Systolic pressure (SP) is the measure of the maximum push of blood being forced into an artery from the ventricle during a cardiac contraction. This is the top number of a reported blood pressure.

> **Hypertension**
> High blood pressure, usually a chronic condition; often identified by a systolic blood pressure above 140 mmHg and/or a diastolic blood pressure above 90 mmHg.

TABLE 11-1 Blood Pressure Levels

Systolic/Diastolic Measurement (mmHg)	Diagnosis
< 90/60	Hypotension
90–120/60–80	Normal
120–139/80–89	Prehypertension
140–159/90–99	Hypertension stage 1
160–179/100–109	Hypertension stage 2
180–209/110–119	Hypertension stage 3
210/120 +	Hypertension stage 4

Diastolic pressure (DP) is the measure of the pressure of blood left in the arteries in between ventricular contractions. This is the bottom number of a reported blood pressure.

Hypertension is a condition that millions of people must deal with every day and is a major cause of death. According to the Centers for Disease Control and Prevention (CDC), 29% of all American adults—70 million people—have high blood pressure. These numbers include more women than men and a greater prevalence in individuals over 65 years of age. There are estimates that only about one-third of hypertensive people have been officially diagnosed and are getting treatment. It is believed that as many as 50% of all people over age 60 are included in these numbers.

The CDC also determined that high blood pressure was a primary or contributing cause of death for more than 360,000 people in the United States in 2013. The risk of heart disease is increased 300% by the presence of hypertension, and the risk of stroke is increased 700%. Research also proves that African-Americans are at a much higher risk of hypertension and its effects than any other racial or ethnic group.

Elevated Blood Pressure

Elevated blood pressure is not the same as a diagnosis of *hypertension*. Almost anyone might have a single measure above the norm. Some individuals get nervous when visiting a health care facility, while others may have just eaten something with a great deal of salt, causing an unusual measure one time. For his or her own reasons, the physician may want to document a reading of elevated blood pressure and therefore include this as a diagnosis to be reported.

> R03.0   Elevated blood-pressure reading, without diagnosis of hypertension

Hypertension is a chronic state of elevated blood pressure. Therefore, without the specific diagnosis of hypertension, you, as the professional coder, cannot report a code for hypertension.

Primary Hypertension

Hypertension frequently shows no signs and symptoms, other than continuous high blood pressure measurements, until the condition alters **vascular** function in the heart, brain, and/or kidneys. This effect is similar to what would happen if the pressure level at which water flows through the pipes in your home increased: High pressure can break a dish in your kitchen sink and make a mess. Patients with high blood pressure specifically diagnosed as *hypertension* are known to suffer manifestations of this condition, including damage to the heart and kidneys. Hypertension causes the heart to work harder than normal and can result in left ventricular hypertrophy, which can subsequently cause left-sided heart failure or right-sided heart failure as well as pulmonary **edema** (excess fluid in the tissues).

There are many risk factors that promote the development of hypertension. Here are a few of the most common:

- An underlying disorder such as renal disease or Cushing's syndrome
- Chronic emotional stress
- A sedentary lifestyle
- Excessive sodium in diet
- Family history of hypertension
- Postmenopausal state
- Advancing age
- Excessive use of alcohol
- Obesity
- African-American ancestry

Elevated Blood Pressure
An occurrence of high blood pressure; an isolated or infrequent reading of a systolic blood pressure above 140 mmHg and/or a diastolic blood pressure above 90 mmHg.

Vascular
Referring to the vessels (arteries and veins).

Edema
An overaccumulation of fluid in the cells of the tissues.

A diagnosis will typically come from trending—charting the blood pressure readings over time (an excellent tool in most electronic health record software programs). In addition, a physician can support a diagnosis of hypertension with other data derived from a variety of sources:

- *Auscultation* (listening to sounds with a stethoscope) over the abdominal aorta as well as the carotid, renal, and femoral arteries may reveal bruits (an abnormal sound created by blood flowing past an obstruction; also known as *turbulent flow*).
- *Ophthalmoscopy* (examination of the interior of the eye) may reveal arteriovenous nicking.
- *Patient history* may include a family history of hypertension.
- *Chest x-ray* may reveal cardiomegaly (enlargement of the heart).
- *Echocardiography* may show left ventricular hypertrophy (*hyper* = high or over + *-trophy* = growth).
- *Electrocardiogram* (ECG or EKG) may show ischemia (shortage of oxygen due to reduced or restricted blood flow).

When the documentation includes a specific diagnosis of hypertension, you, the coder, will need more information to accurately report this diagnosis.

Essential Hypertension

Essential (primary) hypertension is the usual type of hypertension. Code category I10 is used for any diagnosis written by the physician that is stated as high blood pressure, arterial hypertension, benign hypertension, malignant hypertension, primary hypertension, or systemic hypertension.

Most often, essential hypertension can be kept under control with diet (including avoiding high-sodium foods) and medication (e.g., angiotensin-converting enzyme, or ACE, inhibitors, diuretics, and beta-blockers).

> **CODING BITES**
>
> Hypertension is a systemic disease, meaning it can affect every part of the body, throughout the patient's entire system. With this in mind, a diagnosis of hypertension will affect treatment of almost any other condition, disease, or injury. Therefore, a code for the hypertension is almost always included, regardless of the reason for the encounter and even if treatment of the hypertension is not performed directly.

LET'S CODE IT! SCENARIO

Anna Epstein, a 63-year-old female, came to see Dr. Tanner. She was complaining of occasional dizziness and a headache. After a complete examination, Dr. Tanner diagnosed Anna with idiopathic systemic hypertension.

Let's Code It!

Dr. Tanner diagnosed Anna with *idiopathic systemic hypertension*. Let's turn to the Alphabetic Index and find the main term *hypertension* and begin reading. If you look down the alphabetic listing under *hypertension*, you will see no listing for *idiopathic* or *systemic*. So go back to the very first entry for this key term, "Hypertension, hypertensive," and read the words shown in parentheses following that entry.

Do you see the words *(idiopathic)* and *(systemic)* included? Both of the adjectives used by Dr. Tanner in his diagnostic statement are in the listing. Therefore, the diagnosis code for Anna's current diagnosis is I10. Turn to the Tabular List to double-check.

One more stop: Let's turn to the Official Guidelines and check chapter 9. Diseases of the Circulatory System (I00-I99), subsection a. Hypertension. There don't seem to be any guidelines that relate to Dr. Tanner's diagnosis for Anna.

> **I10**   **Essential (primary) hypertension**
>   INCLUDES high blood pressure
>   hypertension (arterial) (benign) (essential) (malignant) (primary) (systemic)

Perfect!

Secondary Hypertension

There are occasions when another condition or a medication may cause hypertension instead of hypertension causing other conditions (manifestations) in the patient. Medications, such as corticosteroids (e.g., prednisone), antidepressants (e.g., Sinequan), and hormones (e.g., Estrace), or diseases, such as Cushing's syndrome or scleroderma, may trigger a hypertensive condition. When the hypertensive condition is generated by, or secondary to, another disease or medication, the condition is called **secondary hypertension**.

The involvement of renal disease as an underlying cause of hypertension, also known as *renovascular hypertension,* may be diagnosed as a result of testing including:

- *Urinalysis,* which shows protein levels and red and white blood cells indicating glomerulonephritis (inflammation of small blood vessels in the kidneys).
- *Excretory urography,* which reveals renal atrophy (wasting away of a kidney), pointing to chronic renal disease, or a shortening of one kidney, which may indicate unilateral renal disease.
- *Blood tests for serum potassium levels* (measuring the levels of potassium in the blood), which show levels below the normal measure of 3.5 mEq/L, which can indicate primary hyperaldosteronism (*hyper* = high or over + *aldosterone* = a hormone produced by the adrenal cortex that prompts the kidney to preserve sodium and water).

Hypertension is coded as secondary when the physician uses terms such as "due to" an underlying disease, "resulting from" another condition, or other descriptors that point to another disease or condition. In such cases, you will need two codes:

1. The underlying condition
2. The type of secondary hypertension (I15.*x*)

There is a notation to "*Code also underlying condition*." Note that sequencing is not identified in this notation. Therefore, you will need to report the two codes based on the sequencing guidelines in the Official Guidelines, Section II, which will guide you in determining the principal diagnosis code. So the order in which you will list the two codes is determined by the answer to the question, "Why did the patient come to see the physician today?"

EXAMPLES

I15.0	Renovascular hypertension
I15.1	Hypertension secondary to other renal disorders
I15.2	Hypertension secondary to endocrine disorders
I15.8	Other secondary hypertension
I15.9	Secondary hypertension, unspecified

Secondary Hypertension
The condition of hypertension caused by another condition or illness.

GUIDANCE CONNECTION

Read the ICD-10-CM Official Guidelines for Coding and Reporting, section **I. Conventions, General Coding Guidelines and Chapter Specific Guidelines,** subsection **C. Chapter-Specific Coding Guidelines,** chapter **9. Diseases of the Circulatory System,** subsection **a.6) Hypertension, secondary.**

LET'S CODE IT! SCENARIO

Breanna Payne, a 67-year-old female, came to see Dr. Lebonna in his office. She was having headaches and bouts of dizziness. After a physical examination, a urinalysis, and blood work, he diagnosed her with benign hypertension. Dr. Lebonna's notes stated that Breanna's hypertension was the result of her existing diagnosis of pituitary-dependent Cushing's disease.

Let's Code It!

Dr. Lebonna diagnosed Breanna with *benign hypertension due to pituitary-dependent Cushing's disease*. This means that Cushing's disease caused Breanna's hypertension. First, go to the Alphabetic Index and look under *hypertension*. Look down the indented column until you see "due to" (which is the same as "result of" stated in the physician's notes). Now, look at the indented listing under "due to"; you will see no listing for "Cushing's disease." So "specified disease" is a strong consideration. You can also keep looking down the column until you see "secondary" specified disease NEC I15.8. Both paths take you to the same suggested code:

> Hypertension
> > Due to
> > > Endocrine disorders I15.2

Now let's check this code in the Tabular List:

> I15.2   Hypertension secondary to endocrine disorders

Did you remember that the pituitary gland is a component of the endocrine system? Now, one more thing: Is there a notation beneath I15 alerting you that something is missing?

Code also underlying condition

That's right—a code for the Cushing's disease. In the Alphabetic Index, you see the following under *Cushing's:*

> Cushing's
> > Syndrome or disease E24.9
> > > Pituitary-dependent E24.0

In the Tabular List, you will see

> ☑4 E24   Cushing's syndrome

Next, there is an **EXCLUDES1** note:

> **EXCLUDES1** *congenital adrenal hyperplasia (E25.0)*

Just because Breanna is 67 years old does not mean this isn't a congenital condition. However, Dr. Lebonna provides no documentation stating that her Cushing's disease is congenital, so this **EXCLUDES1** note does not apply to this patient for this encounter.

> E24.0   Pituitary-dependent Cushing's disease

Check for any relevant guidance, including reading all of the symbols and notations in the Tabular List and the appropriate sections of the Official Guidelines. Nothing is directed to this specific case, so you will report these two codes for this encounter between Dr. Lebonna and Breanna:

> I15.2   Hypertension secondary to endocrine disorders
> E24.0   Pituitary-dependent Cushing's disease

How should these codes be sequenced? List the hypertension first (I15.2) because it was the symptoms of the hypertension (headaches, dizziness) that brought Breanna to Dr. Lebonna's office for this encounter.

Hypertensive Crisis

Code category I16 provides three codes for reporting a hypertensive crisis. This is when a patient suffers an acute and dramatic increase in blood pressure, measuring approximately 180/120. This situation can result in blood vessels becoming damaged and leaking, as well as dysfunction of the heart's ability to pump blood through the body.

A hypertensive crisis is categorized as either urgent or emergency.

CODING BITES

Code category I16 includes a notation applicable to all codes in this category:

Code also any identified hypertensive disease (I10-I15)

- **I16.0 Hypertensive urgency** identifies a patient with an extremely high spike of blood pressure, with the belief that the vessels have not yet been damaged.
- **I16.1 Hypertensive emergency** documents that the patient's extraordinarily high blood pressure has caused damage to blood vessels and/or organs. This diagnosis can be associated with life-threatening complications.
- **I16.9 Hypertensive crisis, unspecified** is a code that should rarely be reported. Instead, as you have learned, you should query the physician to determine what type of crisis it is and have the documentation amended.

Hypertension and Pregnancy

When a pregnant woman has a diagnosis of hypertension, you will first need to determine from the documentation whether she developed hypertension before or after conception.

A woman with a preexisting diagnosis of hypertension who then becomes pregnant will be reported with the appropriate code from the O10 Pre-existing hypertension complicating pregnancy, childbirth, and the puerperium code category. A code from the O10 code category reports this situation clearly with additional details, provided by the fourth character, to report the specific hypertensive manifestation, if any:

Gestational Hypertension Hypertension that develops during pregnancy and typically goes away once the pregnancy has ended.

O10.0-	Pre-existing essential hypertension complicating pregnancy, childbirth, and the puerperium
O10.1-	Pre-existing hypertensive heart disease complicating pregnancy, childbirth, and the puerperium
O10.2-	Pre-existing hypertensive chronic kidney disease complicating pregnancy, childbirth, and the puerperium
O10.3-	Pre-existing hypertensive heart and chronic kidney disease complicating pregnancy, childbirth, and the puerperium
O10.4-	Pre-existing secondary hypertension complicating pregnancy, childbirth, and the puerperium

GUIDANCE CONNECTION

Read the ICD-10-CM Official Guidelines for Coding and Reporting, section **I. Conventions, General Coding Guidelines and Chapter Specific Guidelines,** subsection **C. Chapter-Specific Coding Guidelines,** chapter **9. Diseases of the Circulatory System,** subsection **a.7) Hypertension, transient.**

However, if the hypertension is diagnosed as **gestational hypertension**, or transient hypertension, you will report a code from O13 Gestational [pregnancy-induced] hypertension without significant proteinuria. This is not unusual and generally means that the hypertension will go away after the baby is born.

O13.1	Gestational [pregnancy-induced] hypertension without significant proteinuria, first trimester
O13.2	Gestational [pregnancy-induced] hypertension without significant proteinuria, second trimester
O13.3	Gestational [pregnancy-induced] hypertension without significant proteinuria, third trimester

Should the woman's diagnosed hypertension cause problems directly related to the pregnancy or complicating the pregnancy, you will choose the best, most appropriate code from ICD-10-CM's *Chapter 15, Pregnancy, Childbirth, and the Puerperium (O00–O9A)*.

LET'S CODE IT! SCENARIO

Zena Browning, a 23-year-old female, is 20 weeks pregnant. Dr. Shinto diagnoses her with gestational hypertension. Even though there is no evidence of proteinuria, he is concerned about the effect of the condition on her pregnancy and writes a prescription.

Let's Code It!

Zena Browning has *gestational hypertension*. Her hypertensive condition is complicating her pregnancy. Turn to the term *hypertension* in the Alphabetic Index and look down the column of adjectives below the primary term *hypertension*. You see

> **Hypertension**
>   **complicating**
>   **pregnancy**
>   **gestational (pregnancy-induced) (transient) (without proteinuria) O13.-**
>
> That matches Dr. Shinto's notes. Now you must turn to the Tabular List to confirm the code *and* determine the correct fourth character:
>
> **O13**   **Gestational [pregnancy-induced] hypertension without significant proteinuria**
>
> Now turn to the first page of Chapter 15 in ICD-10-CM to see the definitions of the trimesters. You can see the information:
>
> **1st trimester—less than 14 weeks, 0 days**
> **2nd trimester—14 weeks, 0 days to less than 28 weeks, 0 days**
> **3rd trimester—28 weeks, 0 days until delivery**
>
> Zena is in her 20th week, so she is in her 2nd trimester. This points us to the correct fourth character of 2. The code to be used for this visit between Dr. Shinto and Zena Browning is
>
> **O13.2**   **Gestational [pregnancy-induced] hypertension without significant proteinuria, second trimester**
>
> Before you report this code, be certain to carefully check for any relevant guidance, including reading all of the symbols and notations in the Tabular List and the appropriate sections of the Official Guidelines. Confirmed! Good job!

11.4 Manifestations of Hypertension

Hypertensive Heart Disease

When a patient has heart disease or heart failure and also has hypertension, you must carefully examine the words used by the physician in the description.

1. Heart condition *due to* hypertension
2. *Hypertensive* heart condition
3. Heart condition *with* hypertension

If the physician states that the patient has both hypertension and heart disease, a combination code from code category I11 Hypertensive heart disease must be recorded.

I11.0   Hypertensive heart disease with heart failure
             Use additional code to identify type of heart failure (I50.-)
I11.9   Hypertensive heart disease without heart failure

Hypertensive Heart Disease with Heart Failure

In cases where a physician states that a patient has heart failure due to hypertension, you will need to

1. Use the appropriate fourth character, as shown in the Tabular List under category I11.
2. *Use additional code* to specify the type of heart failure from category I50.-.

ICD-10-CM includes a notation directing you to "*Use additional code* **to identify type of heart failure (I50.-)**" to remind you.

> **GUIDANCE CONNECTION**
>
> Read the ICD-10-CM Official Guidelines for Coding and Reporting, section **I. Conventions, General Coding Guidelines and Chapter Specific Guidelines,** subsection **C. Chapter-Specific Coding Guidelines,** chapter **9. Diseases of the Circulatory System,** subsection **a.1) Hypertensive with heart disease.**

> **CODING BITES**
>
> Determine what type of heart failure the patient has so you can report it with an additional code. You learned about the different types of heart failure earlier in this chapter.

> **EXAMPLE**
>
> *Acute congestive heart failure due to benign hypertension*
>
> You will report two codes, in this sequence: I11.0, I50.31
>
> I11.0   Hypertensive heart disease with heart failure
> I50.31   Acute diastolic (congestive) heart failure

LET'S CODE IT! SCENARIO

Colin Fahey, a 53-year-old male, was diagnosed with chronic diastolic congestive heart failure due to benign hypertension. Dr. Engman wrote a prescription for medication and scheduled follow-up tests.

Let's Code It!

Colin was diagnosed with *congestive heart failure due to benign hypertension.*
Turn in the Alphabetic Index to find

Failure, failed
    heart (acute) (senile) (sudden) I50.9
        hypertensive—*see* Hypertension, heart

OK, turn to . . .

Hypertension, hypertensive (accelerated) (benign) (essential) (idiopathic) (malignant) (systemic) I10
    heart (disease) (conditions in I51.4-I51.9 due to hypertension) I11.9

Remember from earlier in this chapter that when the diagnostic statement is written "heart condition *due to* hypertension," the guidelines state that only one code, from category I11, is used. Turn to the Tabular List for I11:

I11   **Hypertensive heart disease**
       INCLUDES any condition in I51.4-I51.9 due to hypertension

This description fits perfectly. Now we must look at the fourth character. Dr. Engman wrote "congestive heart failure," bringing us to

I11.0   **Hypertensive heart disease with heart failure**
        Use additional code to identify type of heart failure (I50.-)

Does the documentation identify the specific type of heart failure? Yes, Dr. Engman indicated that Colin has congestive heart failure. Let's turn to

I50   **Heart failure**

Read the notation under the code:

Code first:
    heart failure due to hypertension (I11.0)

This is the book's way of reinforcing the guideline as well as the notation that you found beneath I11. Continue reading, and you see that the second code you need to include for Colin's diagnosis is this:

I50.32   **Chronic diastolic (congestive) heart failure**

Be certain to check for any relevant guidance, including reading all of the symbols and notations in the Tabular List and Section 1.c.9 of the Official Guidelines. There is nothing that alters the determination of these codes.
    You need to show both codes for the visit between Colin and Dr. Engman:

I11.0   **Hypertensive heart disease with heart failure**
I50.32   **Chronic diastolic (congestive) heart failure**

Good work!

Hypertensive Chronic Kidney Disease

When a diagnosis of hypertensive chronic kidney disease is documented, you will report a combination code, as appropriate. In such cases, a cause-and-effect relationship between the hypertension and the kidney disease does *not* need to be specifically stated by the physician. The mere existence of both conditions in the same body at the same time is enough to report them together. You will need the documentation to specify the stage of the chronic kidney disease to determine the correct code in ICD-10-CM. Code category I12 is to be used for reporting a patient with a diagnosis of hypertensive chronic kidney disease.

> ☑4 **I12** Hypertensive chronic kidney disease

The fourth-character choices are

I12.0 Hypertensive chronic kidney disease with stage 5 chronic kidney disease or end stage renal disease
Use additional code to identify the stage of chronic kidney disease (N18.5, N18.6)

I12.9 Hypertensive chronic kidney disease with stage 1 through stage 4 chronic kidney disease or unspecified chronic kidney disease
Use additional code to identify the stage of chronic kidney disease (N18.1-N18.4, N18.9)

You can see that beneath each of these codes is a notation:

- Beneath I12.20:

    Use additional code to identify the stage of chronic kidney disease (N18.5, N18.6)

- Beneath I12.29:

    Use additional code to identify the stage of chronic kidney disease (N18.1-N18.4, N18.9)

> **CODING BITES**
>
> If you can't find the information in the documentation as to what stage of kidney disease the patient has, query the doctor.

> **GUIDANCE CONNECTION**
>
> Read the ICD-10-CM Official Guidelines for Coding and Reporting, section **I. Conventions, General Coding Guidelines and Chapter Specific Guidelines,** subsection **C. Chapter-Specific Coding Guidelines,** chapter **9. Diseases of the Circulatory System,** subsection **a.2) Hypertensive chronic kidney disease.**

YOU CODE IT! CASE STUDY

Matthew Spencer, a 69-year-old male, is admitted to Franklin General Hospital for observation with a diagnosis of stage 3 chronic renal disease due to benign hypertension.

You Code It!

Go through the steps of coding, and determine the code or codes that should be reported for Matthew Spencer's admission into the hospital.

Step #1: Read the case carefully and completely.

Step #2: Abstract the scenario. Which main words or terms describe why the physician cared for the patient during this encounter?

Step #3: Are there any details missing or incomplete for which you would need to query the physician? [If so, ask your instructor.]

Step #4: Check for any relevant guidance, including reading all of the symbols and notations in the Tabular List and the appropriate sections of the Official Guidelines.

Step #5: Determine the correct diagnosis code or codes to explain why this encounter was medically necessary.

Step #6: Double-check your work.

(continued)

Answer:

Did you determine these to be the diagnosis codes?

I12.9   Hypertensive chronic kidney disease with stage 1 through stage 4 chronic kidney disease or unspecified chronic kidney disease

N18.3   Chronic kidney disease, stage 3 (moderate)

Hypertensive Heart and Chronic Kidney Disease

If the patient is diagnosed with both hypertensive heart disease and hypertensive chronic kidney disease, you will choose one combination code from category I13. Now, great emphasis has been placed on the fact that you should never assume. You are permitted to code only what you know for a fact from the documentation. But, as you know, every rule has an exception, and this is it. The Official Guidelines state that you "*may assume the relationship between the hypertensive heart disease and hypertensive renal disease even if the physician does not state this relationship in the diagnosis.*"

You will still need to confirm that a cause-and-effect relationship is specified for the hypertension and the heart condition, even though the cause-and-effect relationship between the hypertension and the kidney disease does not have to be specified. The additional-character choices for code I13 will identify whether the patient is documented to have

- Heart failure or not
- Stage 1, 2, 3, or 4 chronic kidney disease or unspecified stage
- Stage 5 chronic kidney disease, or ESRD

In addition to using this code, you will also need a code for the specific type of heart failure and another to report the stage of the kidney disease. ICD-10-CM includes notations under code I13 to remind you of the additional coding:

Use additional code to identify type of heart failure (I50.-)
Use additional code to identify stage of chronic kidney disease (N18.-)

> **GUIDANCE CONNECTION**
>
> Read the ICD-10-CM Official Guidelines for Coding and Reporting, section **I. Conventions, General Coding Guidelines and Chapter Specific Guidelines,** subsection **C. Chapter-Specific Coding Guidelines,** chapter **9. Diseases of the Circulatory System,** subsection **a.3) Hypertensive heart and chronic kidney disease.**

YOU CODE IT! CASE STUDY

Clarissa Bennelli, a 71-year-old female, is seen at Weston Hospital with a diagnosis of acute systolic congestive heart failure due to hypertensive heart disease. Ms. Bennelli responds positively to Lasix therapy. She is also diagnosed with stage 1 chronic renal disease.

You Code It!

Go through the steps of coding, and determine the code or codes that should be reported for Clarissa Bennelli's admission into the hospital.

Step #1: Read the case carefully and completely.

Step #2: Abstract the scenario. Which main words or terms describe why the physician cared for the patient during this encounter?

Step #3: Are there any details missing or incomplete for which you would need to query the physician? [If so, ask your instructor.]

Step #4: Check for any relevant guidance, including reading all of the symbols and notations in the Tabular List and the appropriate sections of the Official Guidelines.

Step #5: Determine the correct diagnosis code or codes to explain why this encounter was medically necessary.

Step #6: Double-check your work.

Answer:

Did you determine these to be the diagnosis codes?

I13.0	Hypertensive heart and chronic kidney disease with heart failure and stage 1 through stage 4 chronic kidney disease or unspecified chronic kidney disease
I50.21	Acute systolic (congestive) heart failure
N18.1	Chronic kidney disease, stage 1

Good job!

Hypertensive Retinopathy

Retinopathy is a degenerative disease of the eye, most specifically the retina. The condition can be caused by diabetes, hypertension, or other circumstances. In cases where the patient is diagnosed with hypertensive retinopathy due to hypertension, you will need two codes to thoroughly report the patient's condition.

Your first code is from the subcategory H35.03- Hypertensive retinopathy. This code requires a sixth character to identify which eye is affected:

H35.031	Hypertensive retinopathy, right eye
H35.032	Hypertensive retinopathy, left eye
H35.033	Hypertensive retinopathy, bilateral

Then you will need an additional code to identify the type of hypertension that caused the retinopathy. Choose that code from the I10–I15 range. There is a reminder notation for you, shown beneath code H35.0:

Code also any associated hypertension (I10.-)

Hypertensive Cerebrovascular Disease

Patients diagnosed with cerebrovascular disease due to hypertension will have two codes assigned. The first code will report the cerebrovascular disease, a code from the I60–I69 range. The second code will identify the hypertension, using the appropriate code from the I10–I15 range. Both the guidelines and a notation under the category heading shown directly above code I60 remind you of the necessity for a second code. You can see that the notation also instructs you as to in which order to place the codes:

Use additional code to identify presence of hypertension (I10-I15)

> **GUIDANCE CONNECTION**
>
> Read the ICD-10-CM Official Guidelines for Coding and Reporting, section **I. Conventions, General Coding Guidelines and Chapter Specific Guidelines,** subsection **C. Chapter-Specific Coding Guidelines,** chapter **9. Diseases of the Circulatory System,** subsection **a.5) Hypertensive retinopathy.**

YOU CODE IT! CASE STUDY

Denise Argudin, a 53-year-old female, came to see Dr. Fenwick because she was experiencing headaches and problems with her vision. Denise was diagnosed with essential benign hypertension 3 years ago. After a thorough physical examination and further questioning about her visual disturbances, Dr. Fenwick ordered a CT scan of her head and a few other tests. The test results indicate that Denise has hypertensive encephalopathy.

(continued)

> **You Code It!**
>
> Carefully review Dr. Fenwick's notes on his visit with Denise, along with the test results. Determine the best, most appropriate diagnosis code or codes.
>
> Step #1: Read the case carefully and completely.
>
> Step #2: Abstract the scenario. Which main words or terms describe why the physician cared for the patient during this encounter?
>
> Step #3: Are there any details missing or incomplete for which you would need to query the physician? [If so, ask your instructor.]
>
> Step #4: Check for any relevant guidance, including reading all of the symbols and notations in the Tabular List and the appropriate sections of the Official Guidelines.
>
> Step #5: Determine the correct diagnosis code or codes to explain why this encounter was medically necessary.
>
> Step #6: Double-check your work.
>
> **Answer:**
>
> Did you determine these to be the diagnosis codes?
>
> | I67.4 | Hypertensive encephalopathy |
> |---|---|
> | I10 | Essential hypertension |
>
> Good job!

11.5 CVA and Cerebral Infarction

While arteries and veins run through the entire body, special attention is paid to those that service the brain—the cerebellum—the cerebrovascular system.

> **CODING BITES**
>
> Cerebrovascular = *cerebro* = cerebellum (brain)
>
> \+
>
> *-vascular* = blood vessels

A **cerebrovascular accident (CVA)** is technically considered a condition of the neurologic system, yet this diagnosis is reported with codes included in this subsection (codes I60–I67) because a CVA is the result of an obstruction in a cerebral blood vessel. A cerebrovascular accident, also referred to as a *stroke,* is the result of a thrombus or embolism getting lodged in a cerebral vessel and preventing blood from flowing through the area.

There are times when the blockage (occlusion) resolves quickly, either on its own or from the administration of blood-thinning/clot-busting medication (tPA), making the event short-lived. This is known as an *ischemic* attack (code categories I63, I65, and I66) (Figure 11-4).

In some cases, the obstruction causes a backup of blood that subsequently bursts through the vessel wall and a hemorrhage floods the area of the brain. This is known as a *hemorrhagic* attack (code categories I60, I61, I67) (see Figure 11-5).

While a cerebrovascular accident is not technically the same as a **cerebral infarction**, the term *CVA* is frequently used to indicate a cerebral infarction. An **infarction** occurs when the occlusion created by the thrombus deprives surrounding tissue of oxygen and the cells die (necrosis).

GUIDANCE CONNECTION

Read the ICD-10-CM Official Guidelines for Coding and Reporting, section **I. Conventions, General Coding Guidelines and Chapter Specific Guidelines,** subsection **C. Chapter-Specific Coding Guidelines,** chapter **9. Diseases of the Circulatory System,** subsection **a.4) Hypertensive cerebrovascular disease.**

Cerebrovascular Accident (CVA)
Rupture of a blood vessel causing hemorrhaging in the brain or an embolus in a blood vessel in the brain causing a loss of blood flow; also known as *stroke.*

Cerebral Infarction
An area of dead tissue (necrosis) in the brain caused by a blocked or ruptured blood vessel.

Infarction
Tissue or muscle that has deteriorated or died (necrotic).

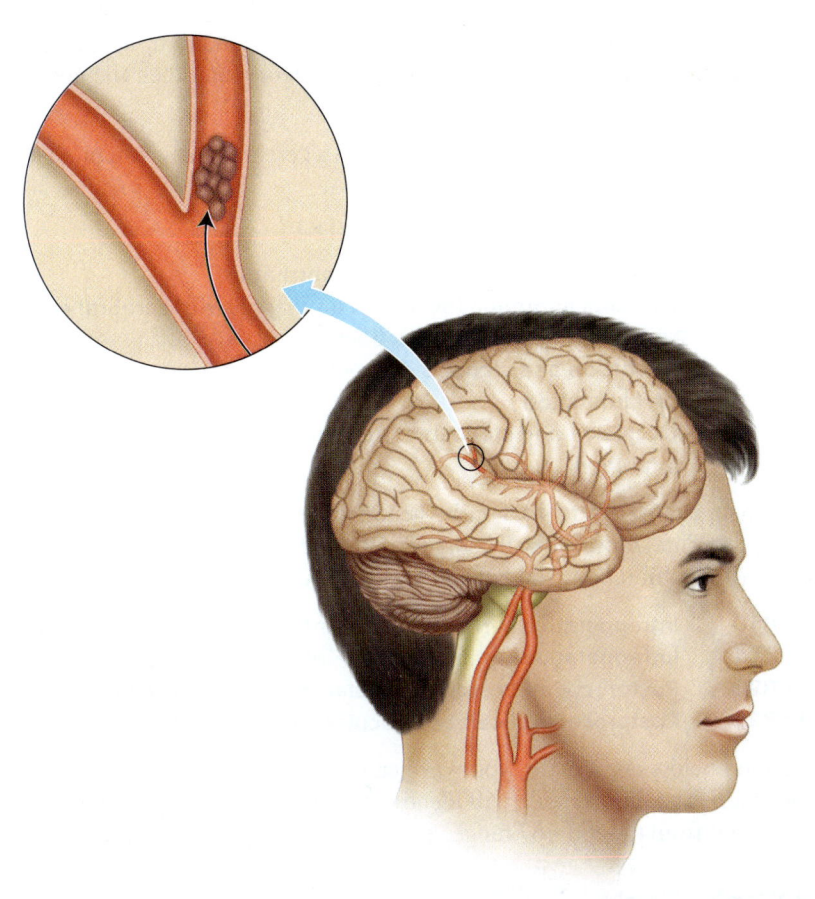

FIGURE 11-4 Illustration highlighting the position of an embolus causing an iscemic stroke

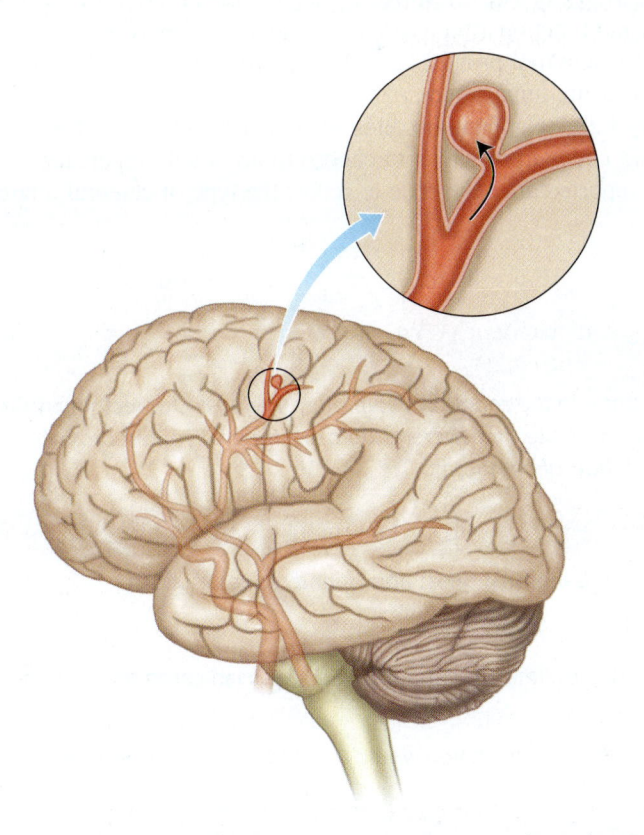

FIGURE 11-5 Illustration highlighting an aneurysm causing a hemorrhagic stroke

> **GUIDANCE CONNECTION**
>
> Read the ICD-10-CM Official Guidelines for Coding and Reporting, section **I. Conventions, General Coding Guidelines and Chapter Specific Guidelines,** subsection **C. Chapter-Specific Coding Guidelines,** chapter **9. Diseases of the Circulatory System,** subsection **c. Intraoperative and postprocedural cerebrovascular accident.**

CHAPTER 11 | **CODING CARDIOVASCULAR CONDITIONS**

You will need specific details about the patient's condition, abstracted from the documentation, to determine the correct code category, and then the correct code to report:

- Was the attack a result of a hemorrhage from a cerebral aneurysm or an obstruction from a thrombus or embolism?
- What is the specific anatomical site of the attack?

I61.-	Nontraumatic intracerebral hemorrhage
I63.-	Cerebral infarction (occlusion and stenosis of cerebral arteries, resulting in cerebral infarction)
I65.-	Occlusion and stenosis of precerebral arteries, not resulting in cerebral infarction
I66.-	Occlusion and stenosis of cerebral arteries, not resulting in cerebral infarction

It can happen that a cerebrovascular hemorrhage or infarction is brought about by a medical procedure, most typically surgery. When the procedure is plainly identified as the cause of the infarction, you have to use two codes. The first code will be

I97.810	Intraoperative cerebrovascular infarction during cardiac surgery
I97.811	Intraoperative cerebrovascular infarction during other surgery
I97.820	Postprocedural cerebrovascular infarction following cardiac surgery
I97.821	Postprocedural cerebrovascular infarction following other surgery

As noted below code I97.8, you will need an additional code to identify the exact complication. The second code will identify the exact nature of the infarction, and you will choose it from the I60–I67 range, as appropriate, according to the documentation.

NIH Stroke Scale

The National Institutes of Health Stroke Scale (NIHSS) is used to assess a patient's cerebral activity and function after a cerebrovascular accident (CVA—also known as a stroke). The assessment tool provides health care professionals with a numeric (quantifiable) way to measure impairment.

Code category R29.7 National Institutes of Health Stroke Scale (NIHSS) score provides you with 43 codes from which to choose to accurately report the score. Notice that this code is reported after the code to report the type of cerebral infarction (code category I63).

> **GUIDANCE CONNECTION**
>
> Read the ICD-10-CM Official Guidelines for Coding and Reporting, section **I. Conventions, General Coding Guidelines and Chapter Specific Guidelines**, subsection **C. Chapter-Specific Coding Guidelines**, chapter **18. Symptoms, signs, and abnormal clinical and laboratory findings, not elsewhere classified**, subsection **i. NIHSS Stroke Scale.**

YOU CODE IT! CASE STUDY

Ruben Sackheim, a 55-year-old male, was brought into the recovery room after having a craniectomy for the drainage of an intracranial abscess. Dr. Turner's notes indicate that Ruben had a postoperative cerebrovascular infarction with intracranial hemorrhage and an acute subdural hematoma.

You Code It!

Look at Dr. Turner's notes for Ruben, and determine the best, most appropriate code or codes.

Step #1: Read the case carefully and completely.

Step #2: Abstract the scenario. Which main words or terms describe why the physician cared for the patient during this encounter?

Step #3: Are there any details missing or incomplete for which you would need to query the physician? [If so, ask your instructor.]

> Step #4: Check for any relevant guidance, including reading all of the symbols and notations in the Tabular List and the appropriate sections of the Official Guidelines.
>
> Step #5: Determine the correct diagnosis code or codes to explain why this encounter was medically necessary.
>
> Step #6: Double-check your work.
>
> **Answer:**
>
> Did you determine these to be the diagnosis codes?
>
> | | |
> |---|---|
> | I97.821 | Postprocedural cerebrovascular infarction following other surgery |
> | I62.01 | Nontraumatic acute subdural hemorrhage |
>
> Good job!

11.6 Sequelae of Cerebrovascular Disease

The sequelae, or late effects, of cerebrovascular disease are coded differently from other sequelae.

ICD-10-CM provides a series of combination codes in category I69 Sequela of cerebrovascular disease. It is not unusual for patients who are status post CVA to suffer with neurologic deficits that last past the initial onset of the condition. In such cases, the physician must connect the dots and specifically identify the current condition as a sequela, or late effect, of the cerebrovascular issue.

Should the patient be diagnosed with neurologic deficits from both a previous cerebrovascular condition *and* a current CVA, you are permitted to use both a code from the I60–I67 range *and* a code from the I69 category.

> **EXAMPLES**
>
> Sometimes a deficit, known as a sequela from a CVA, includes:
> - Cognitive deficit
> - Speech and language deficit including aphasia, dysphasia, dysarthria, and fluency disorders
> - Monoplegia (paralysis) of a limb (arm or leg)
> - Hemiplegia and hemiparesis (paralysis of one side of the body)

When there are no neurologic deficits present and the patient has a personal history of cerebrovascular disease, you should use a code from subcategory Z86.7- Personal history of diseases of the circulatory system, and not code I69. Remember, you will only code that history when it has been documented that the physician addressed the condition during the current encounter.

You will see similar notes in other locations as well. Sometimes, they can be confusing to understand. What the note above means is this: When you read in the patient's chart that he or she was previously diagnosed with a condition that was originally reported with any of the codes in the range I60–I67 and, during this visit, the doctor documents that the patient currently has a neurologic deficit, such as paralysis or dysphasia, that is a result of that earlier condition, you will use a code from category I69 to report the new condition—the neurologic deficit.

CODING BITES

There is a **NOTE** in the Tabular List, directly under code I69, that reads:

NOTE: Category I69 is to be used to indicate conditions in I60–I67 as the cause of sequelae. The "sequelae" include conditions specified as such or as residuals which may occur at any time after the onset of the causal condition.

GUIDANCE CONNECTION

Read the ICD-10-CM Official Guidelines for Coding and Reporting, section **I. Conventions, General Coding Guidelines and Chapter Specific Guidelines,** subsection **C. Chapter-Specific Coding Guidelines,** chapter **9. Diseases of the Circulatory System,** subsection **d. Sequelae of cerebrovascular disease.**

LET'S CODE IT! SCENARIO

Arlene Williams goes to see Dr. McGovern. She was diagnosed with a cerebral embolism 3 months ago that has now been resolved. She explains that she has been having difficulty putting words together to make a sentence and it seems to be getting worse. After examination, Dr. McGovern diagnoses her with post-cerebral embolic dysphasia.

Let's Code It!

Arlene has been diagnosed with *post-cerebral embolic dysphasia*. This is one way the physician may state that the dysphasia is a late effect of the cerebral embolism she had before.

Turn to the ICD-10-CM Alphabetic Index and look up the term *dysphasia*.

There is one code suggested: R47.02. In the Tabular List, find the beginning of this code category:

☑4 **R47   Speech disturbances, not elsewhere classified**

Dysphasia is a speech disturbance—a problem speaking—so that is OK, so far. There is nothing in the EXCLUDES1 note that relates to this patient. As you read down, you see that fourth and fifth characters are required, so continue reading the column until you get to

R47.0   Dysphasia and aphasia
R47.02   Dysphasia

This is where the Alphabetic Index pointed you, so look closely at this code. Below it is another EXCLUDES1 note, which tells you that this code does not include a diagnosis of *dysphasia due to a late effect of cerebrovascular accident* and directs you to the codes in the I69 code category.

EXCLUDES1 dysphasia following cerebrovascular disease (I69. with final characters -21)

Go back to the physician's notes (the scenario). The documentation doesn't state that Arlene had cerebrovascular disease; it states that she had a cerebral embolism. Is this the same thing, or is it unrelated to this notation?

This is the same thing: A cerebral embolism is a type of CVA. When you look it up, you will see that a cerebral embolism is reported with code I66.9, clearly in the range of I60–I67. This means you will report the dysphasia from a code in the I69 category.

Therefore, this EXCLUDES1 note applies to this encounter, and you must turn to code I69 to determine the correct code to report Arlene's diagnosis. The notation directly under **I69 Sequelae of cerebrovascular disease** confirms that you are in the right place now. Read down and determine the code:

I69.821   Dysphasia following other cerebrovascular disease

Before you report this code, remember to check for any relevant guidance, including reading all of the symbols and notations in the Tabular List and the appropriate sections of the Official Guidelines. No additional direction is there and you can now report this code with confidence!

Good work!

CODING BITES

Read carefully! *Dysphasia* (ending in "sia") means impaired speech and *dysphagia* (ending in "gia") means difficulty swallowing. Another word that is close is *dysplasia*, which means abnormal cell growth. Big difference!

Chapter Summary

Cardiovascular conditions may initially be treated within the specialty of a cardiologist. However, the manifestations of heart failure and heart disease can affect the patient anywhere in the body—from the brain to the feet. Blood vessels extend throughout the body, from the large aorta to the tiny capillaries, delivering oxygen and transporting carbon dioxide back to the lungs so it can be released. When something goes awry, the health of the entire body, as well as the patient's quality of life, can be negatively affected.

Hypertension is a condition that you may encounter as a professional coder while working for a family physician, an internist, a gerontologist, or a cardiologist. It can be a very dangerous condition and can cause many co-morbidities and manifestations. As complex as the condition is, so is the coding of the diagnosis. As with all other situations, it must be diagnosed and documented by the attending physician. Read the notes carefully, and query the physician when necessary to get all the specifics that you need to code accurately.

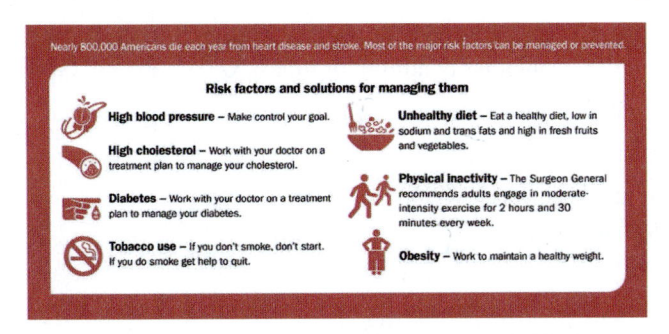

Source: http://www.cdc.gov/vitalsigns/heartdisease-stroke/infographic.html

CHAPTER 11 REVIEW
Coding Cardiovascular Conditions

Enhance your learning by completing these exercises and more at connect.mheducation.com!

Let's Check It! Terminology

Match each key term to the appropriate definition.

Part I

1. LO 11.2 Chest pain. **A**
2. LO 11.3 An occurrence of high blood pressure; an isolated or infrequent reading of a systolic blood pressure above 140 mmHg and/or a diastolic blood pressure above 90 mmHg. **G**
3. LO 11.5 A stroke. **E**
4. LO 11.5 An area of dead tissue (necrosis) in the brain caused by a blocked or ruptured blood vessel. **D**
5. LO 11.2 A condition resulting from plaque buildup on the interior walls of the arteries, causing reduced blood flow. **B**
6. LO 11.1 A thrombus that has broken free and is traveling freely within the vascular system. **H**
7. LO 11.1 A chamber that is located in the top half of the heart and receives blood. **C**
8. LO 11.3 An overaccumulation of fluid in the cells of the tissues. **F**

A. Angina Pectoris
B. Atherosclerosis
C. Atrium
D. Cerebral Infarction
E. Cerebrovascular Accident (CVA)
F. Edema
G. Elevated Blood Pressure
H. Embolus

Part II

1. LO 11.1 A chamber that is located in the bottom half of the heart and receives blood from the atrium.
2. LO 11.3 High blood pressure, usually a chronic condition; often identified by a systolic blood pressure above 140 mmHg and/or a diastolic blood pressure above 90 mmHg. **B**

A. Gestational Hypertension
B. Hypertension

CHAPTER 11 REVIEW

3. LO 11.3 Hypertension that develops during pregnancy and typically goes away once the pregnancy has ended. **A**
4. LO 11.1 A heart event during which the coronary artery is partially occluded (blocked). **F**
5. LO 11.1 A heart event during which the coronary artery is completely blocked by a thrombus or embolus. **H**
6. LO 11.1 A blood clot in a blood vessel. **I**
7. LO 11.1 A heart attack **E**
8. LO 11.3 The condition of hypertension caused by another condition or illness. **G**
9. LO 11.5 Tissue or muscle that has deteriorated or died (necrotic). **D**
10. LO 11.3 Referring to the vessels (arteries and veins). **J**
11. LO 11.3 Low blood pressure; systolic blood pressure below 90 mmHg and/or diastolic measurements of lower than 60 mmHg. **C**

C. Hypotension
D. Infarction
E. Myocardial Infarction (MI)
F. NSTEMI
G. Secondary Hypertension
H. STEMI
I. Thrombus
J. Vascular
K. Ventricle

Let's Check It! Concepts

Choose the most appropriate answer for each of the following questions.

1. LO 11.2 _____ are blood vessels that carry oxygenated blood from the heart to the tissues and cells throughout the body.
   - **a. Arteries**
   - b. Veins
   - c. Venules
   - d. Cardiovascular

2. LO 11.5 The patient is diagnosed with a cerebral infarction due to thrombosis of left anterior cerebral artery. How is this coded?
   - a. I63.321
   - **b. I63.322**
   - c. I63.323
   - d. I63.329

3. LO 11.1 _____ refers to an irregular heartbeat.
   - a. Angina
   - b. Dyspnea
   - **c. Dysrhythmia**
   - d. Edema

4. LO 11.4 If the patient has a diagnosis of heart failure due to hypertension, you will need to
   - a. use the appropriate fourth character, as shown in the Tabular List under category I11.
   - b. use an additional code to specify the type of heart failure from category I50.
   - c. use code I10.
   - **d. use both the appropriate fourth character, as shown in the Tabular List under category I11, and an additional code to specify the type of heart failure from category I50.**

5. LO 11.1 A heart event during which the coronary artery is completely blocked by a thrombus or embolus is called a(n)
   - a. myocardial infarction.
   - b. thrombus.
   - c. nontransmural myocardial infarction.
   - **d. ST elevation myocardial infarction.**

6. LO 11.3 A diagnosis of secondary hypertension means you will code
   - a. the underlying condition only.
   - b. the hypertension only.
   - **c. the underlying condition code and the hypertension code.**
   - d. the hypertension code first and then the underlying condition code.

7. LO 11.3 When a pregnant woman is diagnosed with hypertension, you must determine
   - **a. if it is gestational hypertension.**
   - b. if it is an infarction.
   - c. if it is transient hypertension.
   - d. if it is familial.

8. **LO 11.6** The code for a patient with no neurologic deficits and who had a previous diagnosis of cerebrovascular disease (which has since resolved) should be reported from
   a. the I60–I69 range.
   b. the I69 code category.
   c. the Z86.7- code subcategory.
   d. none of these.

9. **LO 11.3** According to ICD-10-CM Official Guidelines section I.C.9.a.7 "Assign code _____, Elevated blood pressure reading without diagnosis of hypertension, unless patient has an established diagnosis of hypertension."
   a. R03.1
   b. I15.1
   c. R03.0
   d. I10

10. **LO 11.3** A physician can support a diagnosis of hypertension with all of the following data *except*
    a. auscultation over the abdominal aorta.
    b. EKG.
    c. chest x-ray.
    d. ACE.

Let's Check It! Guidelines

Refer to the Official Guidelines and fill in the blanks according to the Chapter 9, Diseases of the Circulatory System, Chapter-Specific Coding Guidelines.

I13	current	Two
site	I60-I69	AMI
I69	STEMI	before
hypertension	secondary	deficits
evolves	admitted	underlying
subendocardial	first	N18
combination	I15	Uncontrolled

1. The appropriate code from category _____ should be used as a _____ code with a code from category I12 to identify the stage of chronic kidney disease.

2. The codes in category _____, Hypertensive heart and chronic kidney disease, are _____ codes that include hypertension, heart disease, and chronic kidney disease.

3. For hypertensive cerebrovascular disease, _____ assign the appropriate code from categories _____, followed by the appropriate _____ code.

4. Secondary hypertension is due to an underlying condition. _____ codes are required: one to identify the _____ etiology and one from category _____ to identify the hypertension. Sequencing of codes is determined by the reason for admission/encounter.

5. _____ hypertension may refer to untreated hypertension or hypertension not responding to current therapeutic regimen.

6. If a patient with coronary artery disease is _____ due to an acute myocardial infarction (AMI), the AMI should be sequenced _____ the coronary artery disease.

7. Codes from category _____ may be assigned on a health care record with codes from I60-I67, if the patient has a _____ cerebrovascular disease and _____ from an old cerebrovascular disease.

8. The ICD-10-CM codes for acute myocardial infarction (AMI) identify the _____, such as anterolateral wall or true posterior wall.

9. If NSTEMI _____ to STEMI, assign the _____ code.

10. If an _____ is documented as nontransmural or subendocardial, but the site is provided, it is still coded as a _____ AMI.

Let's Check It! Rules and Regulations

Please answer the following questions from the knowledge you have gained after reading this chapter.

1. **LO 11.3** Differentiate between systolic pressure and diastolic pressure.

2. **LO 11.3** What is the difference between hypertension and elevated blood pressure?
3. **LO 11.3** What is gestational hypertension?
4. **LO 11.1** Explain the difference between STEMI and NSTEMI.
5. **LO 11.4** Read the ICD-10-CM Official Guidelines for Coding and Reporting, section I. Conventions, General Coding Guidelines and Chapter Specific Guidelines, subsection C. Chapter-Specific Coding Guidelines, chapter 9. Diseases of the Circulatory System, subsection a.1) Hypertensive with heart disease. Explain the coding guideline.

YOU CODE IT! Basics

First, identify the main term in the following diagnoses; then code the diagnosis.

Example: Acute rheumatic myocarditis:

a. main term: <u>myocarditis</u>   b. diagnosis: <u>I01.2</u>

1. Acute diastolic (congestive) heart failure:
   a. main term: _____   b. diagnosis: _____
2. Secondary hypertension due to pheochromocytoma:
   a. main term: _____   b. diagnosis: _____
3. Left posterior fascicular block:
   a. main term: _____   b. diagnosis: _____
4. Aneurysm of heart, 6 weeks' duration:
   a. main term: _____   b. diagnosis: _____
5. Ischemic cardiomyopathy:
   a. main term: _____   b. diagnosis: _____
6. Chronic total occlusion of coronary artery:
   a. main term: _____   b. diagnosis: _____
7. Atherosclerosis of bypass graft of coronary artery of transplanted heart:
   a. main term: _____   b. diagnosis: _____
8. Chronic embolism of superior vena cava:
   a. main term: _____   b. diagnosis: _____
9. Rupture of pulmonary vessels:
   a. main term: _____   b. diagnosis: _____
10. Nonrheumatic pulmonary valve stenosis:
    a. main term: _____   b. diagnosis: _____
11. Arteriosclerotic endocarditis:
    a. main term: _____   b. diagnosis: _____
12. Giant cell myocarditis:
    a. main term: _____   b. diagnosis: _____
13. Cardiac arrest due to cardiac condition:
    a. main term: _____   b. diagnosis: _____
14. Ventricular fibrillation:
    a. main term: _____   b. diagnosis: _____
15. Neurogenic orthostatic hypotension:
    a. main term: _____   b. diagnosis: _____

YOU CODE IT! Practice

Using the techniques described in this chapter, carefully read through the case studies and determine the most accurate ICD-10-CM code(s) and external cause code(s), if appropriate, for each case study.

1. Kitty Hearn, a 63-year-old female, presents today with the complaint of chest tightness. She also states that her left jaw and shoulder hurt. Dr. Kickey notes diaphoresis. Kitty has smoked cigarettes for 40 years. Dr. Kickey completes an examination and reviews blood test results, which reveal a high level of creatine phosphokinase (CPK). Kitty is admitted to the hospital, where a coronary angiography confirms the diagnosis of crescendo angina.
2. Calvin Ballew, an 8-year-old male, is brought in by his parents with the complaint that Calvin has been "out of sorts" for the last day or two and has not been eating well. Dr. Barfield notes a cough and labored

breathing. After a thorough examination, Dr. Barfield decides to admit Calvin to Weston Hospital. The blood tests reveal an increased erythrocyte sedimentation rate (ESR) and ECG confirms a diagnosis of chronic rheumatic myocarditis.

3. Judith Raj, a 49-year-old female, has been diagnosed with hypertension heart disease and stage II chronic kidney disease. Dr. Bennett documents the fact that Judith is not in heart failure at this time.

4. Kay Risinger, a 57-year-old female, presents today with chest pain and shortness of breath on exertion. Kay also admits that it is difficult to breathe at night when lying in bed. Dr. Tate notes a cough and completes a thorough examination. The echocardiogram confirms a diagnosis of rheumatic aortic regurgitation with mitral valve disease.

5. Johnette Barrett, a 27-year-old female, is brought in by her husband, who is concerned because Johnette has been very confused. Johnnette says her chest hurts and it feels like her heart is racing. Dr. Bakker notes labored breathing. Patient is admitted to the hospital, where test results confirm the diagnosis of paroxysmal atrial fibrillation.

6. Richard Grimm, a 57-year-old male, suffered a cerebral infarction 3 months ago due to an occlusion of the left anterior cerebral artery. Richard is having difficulty with his speech and is finding it hard to write. Dr. McManus diagnoses Richard with aphasia due to the cerebral infarction.

7. Vanessa Dostoimov, a 67-year-old female, had a pericardiotomy 6 weeks ago. Dr. Baker last saw Vanessa 2 weeks ago for a fever and chest pain. Today, Dr. Baker notes patient is experiencing similar symptoms today and documents a pericardial rub, tachycardia, and hepatomegaly. Vanessa is admitted to the hospital for a possible pericardiocentesis. After a thorough examination and review of the test results, Vanessa was diagnosed with postcardiotomy syndrome.

8. Jessie Jacobs, a 48-year-old female, presents today with the complaint of shortness of breath and weakness. During the examination, Jessie experiences severe chest pain. Dr. Raley completes an ECG, which confirms a diagnosis of acute transmural myocardial infarction ST elevated inferior diaphragmatic wall. Jessie is admitted to Weston Hospital for stabilization and treatment.

9. Ben Jamison, a 51-year-old obese male, was diagnosed with a chronic embolism of the left subclavian vein.

10. James Tedder, a 62-year-old male, complains of chest tightness with physical activity. Jim also says he has a funny feeling in his neck. Dr. Franklin notes tachycardia and admits him to Weston Hospital. A cardiac CT scan and stress ECG confirm a diagnosis of silent myocardial ischemia.

11. Shirley Hatfield, a 59-year-old female, presents today with the complaint of a tender swollen left leg. Dr. Neal documents a nonpressure ulceration left ankle limited to skin breakdown. After an examination and a Doppler sonography were completed, Shirley was diagnosed with chronic total arterial occlusion of left extremity with atherosclerosis of arteries of the left extremity.

12. Gary Allen, a 59-year-old male, presents today with chest pain and cough. Upon examination, Dr. Rogers documents a low-grade fever, dyspnea, tachypnea, and a pleural friction rub. The decision is made to admit Gary to Weston Hospital, where he is diagnosed with a saddle embolus of pulmonary artery with acute cor pulmonale.

13. Earline Hodges, a 57-year-old female, has a sharp sudden chest pain. Dr. Harper notes a pericardial rub. The laboratory results confirm infective pericarditis due to retrovirus.

14. Donald Ross, a 49-year-old male, presents today with numbness in his fingers and toes. Dr. Jones notes pale coloration in the ring finger of his right hand. Don also states that the numbness is worse with temperature changes. Dr. Jones completes a thorough examination and reviews the laboratory results, which confirm a diagnosis of Raynaud's syndrome without gangrene.

15. Dedrick Andrews, a 43-year-old male, presents today with a cough, fever, and night sweats. Dr. Jamerson completes an examination, the appropriate laboratory tests, and a chest x-ray. Dedrick is diagnosed with septic arterial embolism of thoracic aorta with lung abscess due to MSSA.

CHAPTER 11 REVIEW

YOU CODE IT! Application

The following exercises provide practice in abstracting physicians' notes and learning to work with documentation from our health care facility, Prader, Bracker, & Associates. These case studies are modeled on real patient encounters. Using the techniques described in this chapter, carefully read through the case studies and determine the most accurate ICD-10-CM code(s) and external cause code(s), if appropriate, for each case study.

PRADER, BRACKER, & ASSOCIATES
A Complete Health Care Facility
159 Healthcare Way • SOMEWHERE, FL 32811 • 407-555-6789

PATIENT: PETERS, CHARLENE

ACCOUNT/EHR #: PETECH001

DATE: 08/11/18

Attending Physician: Renee O. Bracker, MD

S: Pt is a 68-year-old female who suffered a cerebral infarction 3 weeks ago. Her son is concerned about the patient's dysarthria, which doesn't seem to be getting any better. The patient understands but is having difficult pronouncing her words. Dr. Bracker also notes a low degree of audibility.

O: Ht. 5'4", Wt. 146 lb., R 18, T 99.6, BP 138/95. Physical examination: unremarkable.

A: Dysarthria, following a cerebral infarction.

P: 1. Pt to return PRN
   2. Referral to speech therapist

ROB/pw   D: 08/11/18 09:50:16   T: 08/13/18 12:55:01

Determine the most accurate ICD-10-CM code(s).

WESTON HOSPITAL
629 Healthcare Way • SOMEWHERE, FL 32811 • 407-555-6541

PATIENT: CROWDER, CHRISTOPHER

ACCOUNT/EHR #: CROWCH001

DATE: 11/04/18

ATTENDING PHYSICIAN: Oscar R. Prader, MD

ADMITTING DIAGNOSES: Deep venous thrombosis (DVT) right leg
   Urinary tract infection (UTI)
   Parkinson's disease

FINAL DIAGNOSES: Acute DVT, right
   UTI
   Parkinson's disease

HOSPITAL COURSE: The patient presented to the office with left leg pain, and uneasiness as well as cloudy urine. He was evaluated, and Doppler studies of the leg confirmed DVT. Urinalysis reveals infection and the patient was started on Levaquin and Lovenox subcu 1 mg per kg twice a day; after 3 days patient asymptomatic for both with his urinary symptoms and calf pain. Patient's vital signs are stable. He is afebrile. Lungs clear. Heart rhythm regular.

Neurologic examination: Tremors and rigidity secondary to Parkinson's disease. Rest is unremarkable. His Doppler studies were positive for left popliteal vein thrombosis and flow abnormalities in superficial femoral vein. The results of the pelvic sonogram reveal an enlarged prostate and questionable intraluminal. Right kidney, normal. Left kidney, cyst lower pole.

PT, INR on the day of discharge was 13.5 and 0.9 His UA was positive for blood, negative for leukocyte esterase, nitrites, and WBC. His CHEM-7 showed sodium of 135, potassium 3.8, chloride 98, CO_2 29, sugar 126, BUN 18 mg/dL, and creatinine 1.1. WBC 6,500, H&H 17.2 and 52. Platelets 150,000. He was discharged home.

DISPOSITION: Arrange for home health.

Follow-up with his primary physician in 7 to 10 days. Arrange for patient evaluation for repeat urinalysis and urology consultation for possible BPH and bladder mass.

ORP/pw   D: 11/04/18 09:50:16   T: 11/07/18 12:55:01

Determine the most accurate ICD-10-CM code(s).

PRADER, BRACKER, & ASSOCIATES
A Complete Health Care Facility
159 Healthcare Way • SOMEWHERE, FL 32811 • 407-555-6789

PATIENT: NOLAN, SHERYESSE

ACCOUNT/EHR #: NOLASH001

DATE: 08/21/18

Attending Physician: Oscar R. Prader, MD

S: Pt is a 53-year-old female who comes in today complaining of fainting, chest pain, and difficulty breathing of approximately 1 week duration. Patient was diagnosed 3 years ago with hypertension. Hypertension has been under control with diet and exercise.

O: Ht. 5'5", Wt. 153 lb., R 19, T 98.4, BP 148/89. Results of blood tests, UA, CBC, ECG, and echocardiogram indicate the development of renal sclerosis (stage 4) with benign hypertension. Tests also reveal left ventricular failure and acute systolic heart failure.

A: Renal sclerosis with benign hypertension; left ventricular failure and acute systolic heart failure

P: 1. Pt to return PRN
   2. Referral for renal dialysis evaluation

ORP/pw   D: 08/21/18 09:50:16   T: 08/23/18 12:55:01

Determine the most accurate ICD-10-CM code(s).

PRADER, BRACKER, & ASSOCIATES
A Complete Health Care Facility
159 Healthcare Way • SOMEWHERE, FL 32811 • 407-555-6789

PATIENT: GUZMANN, EVAN

ACCOUNT/EHR #: GUZMEV001

DATE: 08/23/18

Attending Physician: Renee O. Bracker, MD

S: Pt is a 68-year-old male returning to discuss test results done 2 days ago at our imaging center. Patient is accompanied by his wife, Angie.

O: Ht. 5'10", Wt. 184 lb., R 20, T 98.9, BP 134/86. I explain to the patient and his wife that the test results show a narrowing of the basilar, carotid, and vertebral arteries on his right side, which we believe to be the cause of the symptoms experienced by Mr. Guzmann that we discussed in our last encounter. These arterial strictures account for the headaches, dizziness, and reduced mental acuity. There is currently no cerebral infarction. We discussed a variety of treatment options, and they both agreed to a surgical consultation referral to explore the possibility of a shunt insertion.

A: Stenosis of precerebral arteries, including the basilar, carotid, and vertebral arteries

P: 1. Pt to return PRN

   2. Referral for surgical consult for shunt placement

ROB/pw   D: 08/23/18 09:50:16   T: 08/28/18 12:55:01

Determine the most accurate ICD-10-CM code(s).

WESTON HOSPITAL

629 Healthcare Way • SOMEWHERE, FL 32811 • 407-555-6541

PATIENT: WEINER, PHILLIP

ACCOUNT/EHR #: WEINPH001

DATE: 08/03/18

Attending Physician: Oscar R. Prader, MD

Pt is a 73-year-old male who was admitted to the hospital because of asthenia, xerostomia, fatigue. The patient states he is very weak, drinks a lot of water, but has not been urinating much. His blood pressure was 165/91, and he has been having pain in the left jaw and neck.

PMH: 2003 he had bladder suspension operation and has a history of PVCs.

The patient has had trouble with some edema of the ankles and feet.

The electrocardiogram shows a sinus rhythm with premature ventricular contractions.

FH: Father died of CVA. Mother died of stomach cancer.

CURRENT MEDICATIONS: Inderal; Ativan; Zestril

ALLERGIES: NKA

FINAL DIAGNOSES:

1. Acute myocardial infarction—anterior wall

2. Systemic arterial hypertension

3. Cardiomegaly with chronic systolic CHF

4. Cardiac arrhythmia

ORP/pw   D: 08/03/18 09:50:16   T: 08/05/18 12:55:01

Determine the most accurate ICD-10-CM code(s).

Coding Respiratory Conditions

[Handwritten notes: Cause, Place, Activity, Status. May have external cause codes by trauma or poisoning.]

12

Learning Outcomes

After completing this chapter, the student should be able to:

LO 12.1 Discern the various underlying causes of respiratory disorders.
LO 12.2 Report the different types of respiratory disorders.
LO 12.3 Determine the correct way to report cases of pneumonia and influenza.
LO 12.4 Analyze the details required to report chronic respiratory conditions.
LO 12.5 Accurately code any involvement of tobacco in the patient's respiratory disorder.
LO 12.6 Identify the appropriate use of external cause codes when applicable to respiratory conditions.

Key Terms

Chronic Obstructive Pulmonary Disease (COPD)
Exacerbation
Influenza
Pneumonia
Pneumothorax
Respiratory Disorder
Status Asthmaticus

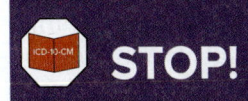

> **STOP!** Remember, you need to follow along in your ICD-10-CM code book for an optimal learning experience.

12.1 Underlying Causes of Respiratory Disease

Respiratory disorders can be caused by many things, including trauma, genetics, environmental concerns, congenital anomalies, and infection. Regardless of the underlying cause, having difficulty bringing oxygen into the lungs and getting carbon dioxide out of the body can interfere with the patient's quality of life—and, actually, the ability to live life at all.

Congenital Anomalies

Respiratory distress and cyanosis are the two most frequent manifestations of congenital anomalies of the lungs and are usually identified within the child's first 24 months. The most common congenital respiratory disorder is *pulmonary hypoplasia,* a situation in which the lung does not form completely or forms improperly. When you are reporting this condition, ICD-10-CM requires you to determine from the documentation whether the pulmonary hypoplasia is a result of short gestation (i.e., prematurity) or not. If the gestation is short, it is reported with code P28.0 Primary atelectasis of newborn (pulmonary hypoplasia associated with short gestation). If it is not, it is reported with code Q33.6 Congenital hypoplasia and dysplasia of lung.

The most common cause of neonate mortality is respiratory distress syndrome (RDS) and it is seen most often in premature births. RDS can be fatal within 72 hours if not treated. Mechanical ventilation improves patient outcomes. Idiopathic RDS is reported with code P22.0 for a *newborn* or code J80 for *acute RDS in a child or adult patient.* Remember, the definition of a neonate (newborn) is one who is age 28 days or younger.

Respiratory Disorder
A malfunction of the organ system relating to respiration.

329

> **CODING BITES**
>
> Congenital anomalies occur during gestation. However, the problem may not be diagnosed until later on in the patient's life.

Genetic Disorders

Alpha-1 antitrypsin deficiency is a genetic condition that may cause respiratory dysfunction as well as liver disease. Individuals with an alpha-1 antitrypsin deficiency often will develop emphysema, with the first signs and symptoms appearing in adulthood (between ages 20 and 50). Cystic fibrosis is another genetic condition that causes malfunction of the mucous glands and results in progressive damage to the lungs. A mutation of the BMPR2 gene causes pulmonary arterial hypertension, a genetic condition with extremely high hypertension specifically in the pulmonary artery. Dyspnea and fainting are symptoms of this condition. *Primary pulmonary arterial hypertension* is reported with code I27.0, while *secondary pulmonary arterial hypertension* is reported with code I27.21.

Manifestations of Another Disease

Measles, as well as the adenovirus, may cause obliterative bronchiolitis (J44.9). Left-sided heart failure can cause pulmonary edema (J81.0 or J81.1), an accumulation of fluid in the lung. The administration of diuretics will help reduce the fluid, while vasodilators are given to decrease vascular resistance. High concentrations of oxygen, via cannula or facemask, will help improve the delivery of oxygen into the tissues.

Pleurisy, an inflammation of the parietal and visceral pleurae, is usually a complication of another condition, such as pneumonia, lupus erythematosus, pulmonary infarction, trauma to the chest, or tuberculosis. *Tuberculous pleurisy,* for example, is reported with combination code A15.6.

Trauma

Car accidents and other activities can result in trauma to the chest, throat, or nose that can interfere with a patient's ability to breathe. Traumatic pneumothorax (S27.0xx-) may result from a penetrating chest wound or can occur due to a medical misadventure during the insertion of a central venous line or during thoracic surgery. During a pneumothorax, air accumulates between the parietal and visceral pleurae, reducing the space in the chest cavity and thereby limiting the room the lungs have to expand during inhalation. When the lungs cannot expand properly, oxygen cannot be brought down into the lungs far enough, so breathing becomes difficult and the exchange of gases (oxygen and carbon dioxide) is hindered. Blunt trauma to the chest, or a penetrating wound, can also cause hemothorax, in which blood (instead of air, as in pneumothorax) fills the pleural cavity. Report this condition with code J94.2 Hemothorax.

LET'S CODE IT! SCENARIO

Vincent Perdimo, a 17-year-old male, decided he wanted to audition for the State Fair. After watching some videos online, he decided that he could do a fire-eating act. As he was practicing in his backyard, he accidentally aspirated some of the isopropyl alcohol he poured in his mouth. After he began having problems breathing, his parents took him to the ED. Dr. Van Hooven documented that Vincent had severe pulmonary complications, and appeared to have pneumonitis with partial respiratory insufficiency. After a workup and testing, Vincent was admitted into the hospital with a diagnosis of acute respiratory distress syndrome.

Let's Code It!

Dr. Van Hooven diagnosed Vincent with acute respiratory distress syndrome.
   In your ICD-10-CM code book, turn to the Alphabetic Index, and find

Syndrome

Read all the way down this long list and find

Syndrome
    respiratory
        distress
            acute J80
                adult J80

This is a great start. Turn to J80 in the Tabular List.

J80 Acute respiratory distress syndrome
    EXCLUDES1 respiratory distress syndrome in newborn (perinatal) (P22.0)

This code's description matches Dr. Van Hooven's documentation perfectly. And the **EXCLUDES1** note does not apply because Vincent is not a newborn.

Check the top of this subsection and the head of this chapter in ICD-10-CM. There are no notations at the beginning of this subsection; however, there are notations at the beginning of this chapter: a **NOTE**, a *Use additional code* note, and an **EXCLUDES2** notation. Read carefully. Do any relate to Dr. Van Hooten's diagnosis of Vincent? No. Turn to the Official Guidelines and read Section 1.c.10. There is nothing specifically applicable here, either.

Now you can report J80 for Vincent's diagnosis with confidence. Hold it! Vincent's respiratory distress syndrome did not just occur; it was the result of an external cause. Turn to the ICD-10-CM *Index to External Causes*. What should you look up? Do you think it has a listing for fire-eating? You never know, so take a look. Nope. Dr. Van Hooten documented that this happened because Vincent "aspirated" isopropyl alcohol. Try looking up Aspiration. Isopropyl alcohol is definitely not food, not a foreign body, and not vomitus. Hmm. What now?

As you think about what actually happened to Vincent, it was the isopropyl alcohol in his lungs that caused the problem. Perhaps this should be reported as a poisoning because this is a chemical. Turn in the Table of Drugs and Chemicals and find

Alcohol
    isopropyl

Look across on this line to the first column. It is documented that this was an accident, so the code T51.2x1 is suggested. Turn to the Tabular List to this code category:

☑4 **T51 Toxic effect of alcohol**

Read all of the fourth character options and you will see:

    ☑5 **T51.2 Toxic effect of 2-Propanol (Toxic effect of isopropyl alcohol)**
        ☑6 **T51.2x Toxic effect of 2-Propanol (Toxic effect of isopropyl alcohol)**
            ☑7 **T51.2x1 Toxic effect of 2-Propanol (Toxic effect of isopropyl alcohol), accidental (unintentional)**

Look back up to the top of this code category. There is a box containing the options for the seventh character. This was the first time Dr. Van Hooven cared for Vincent for this respiratory condition, so use the seventh character: A = Initial encounter.

Now you know, with confidence, what codes to report for Vincent's diagnosis:

J80   **Acute respiratory distress syndrome**
T51.2x1A **Toxic effect of 2-Propanol (Toxic effect of isopropyl alcohol), accidental (unintentional), initial encounter**

Good coding!

Environment

Respiratory dysfunction can be caused by elements in the world around us. Those elements can be natural, like volcanic dust from an erupting volcano or dander from cats, or human-made, such as asbestos in the ceiling (J61). Legionnaires' disease, an aerobic Gram-negative bacillus, is transmitted through the air—for example, through air-conditioning systems (J67.7). Men are more susceptible than women. Administration of antibiotics, specifically erythromycin, is the primary treatment, along with fluid replacement and oxygen administration, if necessary. When a patient is diagnosed with coal worker's pneumoconiosis, another environmentally caused lung disease, this is reported with code J60 Coal worker's pneumoconiosis, along with code Y92.64 Mine or pit as the place of occurrence of the external cause and Y99.0 Civilian activity done for income or pay.

Some patients may suffer respiratory problems from air contaminants at work, which would be reported with a subsequent code; for example: Z57.31 Occupational exposure to environmental tobacco smoke; Z57.39 Occupational exposure to other air contaminants; Z77.110 Contact with and (suspected) exposure to air pollution; or Z77.22 Contact with and (exposure to) environmental tobacco smoke (acute) (chronic).

Lung Infections

Both bacteria and viruses can cause respiratory disorders. Bacterial pneumonia (J15.-), community-acquired pneumonia, nosocomial (originating in a hospital) pneumonia, viral pneumonia (J12.-), and opportunistic pneumonia (affecting individuals with compromised immunities) are common examples of respiratory infection. In addition, bronchitis (inflammation of the bronchi) (J20.-) and influenza (J09.- or J10.-) are also frequently seen, particularly in children and the elderly. Viruses affecting the pulmonary parenchyma result in interstitial pneumonia (J84.9). *Mycobacterium tuberculosis,* acquired by inhaling aerosols, has been seen more often in the last several years, especially in patients who are HIV-positive and have developed AIDS. When an HIV-positive patient is diagnosed with tuberculosis affecting the lungs, this condition would be reported with code B20 HIV, followed by code A15.0 Tuberculosis of the lung.

Lifestyle Behaviors

Smoking cigars and cigarettes is known to cause respiratory disorders, including lung cancer. In addition, sedentary lifestyles can encourage the creation of thrombi in the legs. What does that have to do with the lungs? A dislodged thrombus becomes an embolus that can travel through the pulmonary artery into the lungs, becoming a pulmonary embolus. An acute pulmonary embolism NOS is reported with code I26.99; however, several other details are required for a complete code.

> **GUIDANCE CONNECTION**
>
> At the very beginning of this chapter in ICD-10-CM, there is a *Use additional code* notation. It states:
>
> > *Use additional code*, where applicable, to identify:
> > exposure to environmental tobacco smoke (Z77.22)
> > exposure to tobacco smoke in the perinatal period (P96.81)
> > history of tobacco use (Z87.891)
> > occupational exposure to environmental tobacco smoke (Z57.31)
> > tobacco dependence (F17.-)
> > tobacco use (Z72.0)
>
> This applies to all codes in this chapter of ICD-10-CM, which makes sense, right? It has been proven that inhaling tobacco has a negative effect on the pulmonary system. If the physician's documentation is not clear on this detail, you must query the physician to have it added, if applicable, so you can report this code, as well as the specific respiratory diagnosis.
>
> See more details about this later in this chapter, in the section Reporting Tobacco Involvement.

> **YOU CODE IT! CASE STUDY**
>
> Baby boy Luciano was born vaginally at 33 weeks. Complete physical exam performed. No anomalies were noted with the exception of a perforated nasal septum. He is admitted into the NICU (Neonatal Intensive Care Unit). Dr. Aronson, a pediatrician specializing in congenital respiratory disorders, was called in for a consultation.
>
> **You Code It!**
>
> What ICD-10-CM code or codes will you use to report baby boy Luciano's diagnosis?
>
> Step #1: Read the case carefully and completely.
>
> Step #2: Abstract the scenario. Which main words or terms describe why the physician cared for the patient during this encounter?
>
> Step #3: Are there any details missing or incomplete for which you would need to query the physician? [If so, ask your instructor.]
>
> Step #4: Check for any relevant guidance, including reading all of the symbols and notations in the Tabular List and the appropriate sections of the Official Guidelines.
>
> Step #5: Determine the correct diagnosis code or codes to explain why this encounter was medically necessary.
>
> Step #6: Double-check your work.
>
> **Answer:**
>
> Did you determine this to be the code?
>
> Q30.3   Congenital perforated nasal septum

12.2 Disorders of the Respiratory System

Pleural Disorders

The pleura is made up of two membranes: the visceral pleura, a thin membrane that coats the outside of the lung, and the parietal pleura, a membrane that lines the inside of the thoracic (chest) cavity. *Pleurisy,* also known as *pleuritis,* identifies the presence of inflammation on one or both of the pleural membranes. This condition can cause pain to the patient with each breath. A virus is most often the cause. To report pleurisy, the Alphabetic Index provides a long list of possibilities that lead to a surprisingly short number of codes:

A15.6	Tuberculous pleurisy
J10.1	Influenza due to other identified influenza virus with other respiratory manifestations
R09.1	Pleurisy
J90	Pleurisy with effusion, not elsewhere classified
S27.63XA	Injury to the pleura, laceration of pleura, initial encounter

(*Note:* Of course, you remember that with code S27.63XA, an external cause code should be reported to identify how the injury happened, as well as the place of occurrence.)

The very narrow space between the two pleural membranes is referred to as the *pleural space* or *pleural cavity.* Normally, this space contains a tiny amount of fluid, just enough to enable the visceral pleura and the parietal pleura to move and function without irritation. If excess air or fluid gets into this space, it can cause pressure on the lung and prevent the patient from inhaling because the lung does not have the room required to expand as the oxygen is brought in. Pleural space disorders include pleural effusion, pneumothorax, and hemothorax:

- *Pleural effusion:* The presence of excess fluid in the pleural cavity, frequently a manifestation of congestive heart failure.

J94.0	Chylous effusion
J91.0	Malignant pleural effusion
P28.89	Newborn pleural effusion

Pneumothorax
A condition in which air or gas is present within the chest cavity but outside the lungs.

- *Pneumothorax*: The presence of excess air or gases in the pleural space, typically caused by respiratory disease such as chronic obstructive pulmonary disorder (COPD) or tuberculosis (TB).

J93.81	Chronic pneumothorax
J86.9	Pyothorax without fistula (empyema) [an infection within the pleural space]

- *Hemothorax:* An accumulation of blood in the pleural cavity, most often caused by an injury to the thoracic cavity (the chest).

J94.2	Hemothorax

Pulmonary Embolism

As you probably remember, an embolus is the medical term for a blood clot (thrombus) or other tiny piece of bone marrow fat (most often created by high cholesterol) that travels within the bloodstream. During its passage through the body, this embolus can get stuck in an artery and block the flow of blood through that area. When this occurs in the lungs, it is called a *pulmonary embolism.*

The presence of a pulmonary embolism can create serious problems for the patient, including dyspnea (shortness of breath), pain, and/or hemoptysis (coughing up blood). Over the course of time, a pulmonary embolism can result in permanent damage to the lung as well as damage to the organs being denied oxygen because of the blockage. A pulmonary embolism can also cause an infarction (necrotic tissue) due to the lack of oxygen to the cells. A large clot, or cluster of several clots, can result in the patient's death.

I26.02	Saddle embolus of pulmonary artery with acute cor pulmonale
I27.82	Chronic pulmonary embolism

CODING BITES

Why is a hemothorax coded as a type of pleural effusion? Remember that a pleural effusion is the accumulation of excessive fluid in the pleural space. Blood is a type of fluid.

LET'S CODE IT! SCENARIO

Fawn Springwater, a 3-year-old female, was brought to her pediatrician, Dr. Canterberg, with an odd-sounding cough and chest congestion. She had the measles just a short time prior. After a complete PE and the appropriate tests, Dr. Canterberg diagnosed Fawn with the croup.

Let's Code It!

Fawn was diagnosed with *the croup*. Let's turn to the Alphabetic Index:

Croup, croupous (catarrhal) (infective) (inflammatory) (nondiphtheritic) J05.0

The Tabular List confirms:

☑4 **J05**   Acute obstructive laryngitis [croup] and epiglottitis

You can see a **Use additional code** notation beneath this code category directing you to *"identify the infectious agent."* Notice that *croup* is included, in brackets. This is the common term for the medical diagnosis of acute obstructive laryngitis. However, this is not what Fawn was diagnosed with, so keep reading down the column to review the choices for the required fourth character:

J05.0   Acute obstructive laryngitis

Good job!

Respiratory Syncytial Virus Infections

While most adults and teenagers suffer only mild symptoms (similar to a cold), respiratory syncytial virus infection (RSV) can cause serious problems for infants. Similar to other infectious diseases, RSV can be spread from person to person by touching an infected person or by coming in contact with an infected object like a toy or a tabletop. Upon infection, infants can have difficulty breathing, stuffy noses, and fever. RSV is actually the pathogen that causes respiratory illness in young children such as pneumonia or acute bronchitis.

✓4 **B97**   **Viral agents as the cause of diseases classified elsewhere**

Read down the column to review your choices for the required fourth character.

B97.4   **Respiratory syncytial virus (RSV) as the cause of diseases classified elsewhere**

This code looks perfect except for one thing. Did you read the note directly above code B95 that states:

> **NOTE: These categories are provided for use as supplementary or additional codes to identify the infection agent(s) in diseases classified elsewhere.**

So, if the notes state that the child has pneumonia due to RSV, you would first list the pneumonia followed by B97.4.

Pulmonary Fibrosis

Fibrosis is the creation of extra fibrous tissue (also known as *scar tissue*) in response to inflammation or irritation. When this abnormal process occurs in the lungs, it is called *pulmonary fibrosis*. This development of thickened tissue reduces the flexibility of the lung sac, making it harder for the lungs to expand with inspiration and contract for expiration. Idiopathic pulmonary fibrosis may also be referred to as cryptogenic fibrosing alveolitis, diffuse interstitial fibrosis, idiopathic interstitial pneumonitis, and Hamman-Rich syndrome.

Pulmonary fibrosis may be caused by another disease, such as tuberculosis, or develop as a result of debris inhaled from an environment, such as the dust that may be breathed in by sand blasters or coal miners during their work. Pulmonary fibrosis is also associated as a side effect of certain medications.

J84.10   **Pulmonary fibrosis, unspecified**

🛑 YOU CODE IT! CASE STUDY

Hans Surgesson, a 47-year-old male, has been suffering with chronic inflammation of his left bronchus. He admits to previous crack cocaine use but denies current use. He complains of a dry, hacking, paroxysmal cough and occasional dyspnea lasting at least 5 months. Chest x-ray and pulmonary function tests lead Dr. Mellville to diagnose Hans with idiopathic pulmonary fibrosis due to mucopurulent chronic bronchitis. Hans is placed on oxygen therapy immediately.

You Code It!

Go through the steps of coding, and determine the diagnosis code or codes that should be reported for this encounter between Dr. Mellville and Hans.

Step #1: Read the case carefully and completely.

Step #2: Abstract the scenario. Which main words or terms describe why the physician cared for the patient during this encounter?

(continued)

> Step #3: Are there any details missing or incomplete for which you would need to query the physician? [If so, ask your instructor.]
>
> Step #4: Check for any relevant guidance, including reading all of the symbols and notations in the Tabular List and the appropriate sections of the Official Guidelines.
>
> Step #5: Determine the correct diagnosis code or codes to explain why this encounter was medically necessary.
>
> Step #6: Double-check your work.
>
> **Answer:**
>
> Did you determine these to be the correct codes?
>
> | | |
> |---|---|
> | J84.112 | Idiopathic pulmonary fibrosis |
> | J41.1 | Mucopurulent chronic bronchitis |
>
> Terrific!

Respiratory Failure

Respiratory failure identifies that a patient's lungs are not working efficiently. The result may be a reduced intake of oxygen or an excess of carbon dioxide that is not thoroughly being expelled from the lungs, or both. You have learned throughout this chapter about the problems that can occur in the body when it does not get enough oxygen, a condition called *hypoxemic respiratory failure*, or when there is too much carbon dioxide, a condition called *hypercapnic respiratory failure*.

Respiratory failure can be a manifestation of a respiratory disease, such as COPD. In addition, certain injuries can affect a patient's ability to breathe. For example, a spinal cord injury may involve damage to the nerves that control breathing. A drug or alcohol overdose can also have an impact on the nervous system in a manner that affects the nervous system's ability to properly control respiration. Code choices include

J96.0-	Acute respiratory failure
J96.1-	Chronic respiratory failure
J96.2-	Acute and chronic respiratory failure

The physician may diagnose the patient with acute respiratory failure as a primary diagnosis when it meets the requirements to be first-listed as directed in the Official Guidelines. More typically, you will find that respiratory failure will be a secondary diagnosis, as mentioned previously.

> **GUIDANCE CONNECTION**
>
> Read the ICD-10-CM Official Guidelines for Coding and Reporting, section **I. Conventions, General Coding Guidelines and Chapter Specific Guidelines**, subsection **C. Chapter-Specific Coding Guidelines**, chapter **10. Diseases of the Respiratory System**, subsection **b. Acute Respiratory Failure**.

12.3 Pneumonia and Influenza

Pneumonia

Pneumonia
An inflammation of the lungs.

Pneumonia is a serious infection of the lung parenchyma (tissue) and typically hinders the exchange of gases. When an individual with normal, healthy lungs contracts pneumonia, the expectation of a complete recovery is good. However, early treatment is important. Even with this good news, pneumonia is one of the top 10 leading causes of death in the United States. A virus, bacterium, fungus, or other type of protozoan can cause pneumonia. You have to know which type of pneumonia the patient has contracted in order to code it accurately.

Viral Pneumonia
- Influenza
- Adenovirus
- Respiratory syncytial virus
- Measles (rubeola)
- Chickenpox (varicella)
- Cytomegalovirus

Bacterial Pneumonia
- Streptococcus (*Streptococcus pneumoniae*)
- *Klebsiella*
- Staphylococcus

Protozoan Pneumonia
- *Pneumocystis carinii*

Aspiration pneumonia is a specific type of condition that results from the patient vomiting and then inhaling gastric or oropharyngeal contents into the trachea and/or lungs.

> **EXAMPLES**
>
> J12.0   Adenoviral pneumonia
> J15.0   Pneumonia due to Klebsiella pneumoniae
>
> Note that these examples of pneumonia codes are both combination codes, reporting both the condition (pneumonia) and the pathogen (adenovirus or *Klebsiella*). Not all pneumonia codes are combination codes, so you may need to remember to use an additional code to identify the pathogen.

Pneumonia as a Manifestation of HIV

In some cases, pneumonia *may be* a manifestation of HIV infection. Therefore, if the notes report that the patient has also been diagnosed with HIV-positive status, you have to include

B20   Human immunodeficiency virus (HIV) disease

Code B20 should be listed first, followed by the appropriate pneumonia code. There are other types of pneumonia that may have other underlying diseases. Read the notations carefully.

> **GUIDANCE CONNECTION**
>
> Read the ICD-10-CM Official Guidelines for Coding and Reporting, section **I. Conventions, General Coding Guidelines and Chapter Specific Guidelines**, subsection **C. Chapter-Specific Coding Guidelines**, chapter **10. Diseases of the Respiratory System**, subsection **c. Influenza due to certain identified influenza viruses.**

> **LET'S CODE IT! SCENARIO**
>
> Craig Alaksar, a 13-year-old male, came to see Dr. Winston with a complaint of a sore throat, fever, cough, chills, and malaise. Dr. Winston examined Craig, took a chest x-ray, and did a WBC count. After reviewing the results of the exam and tests, Dr. Winston diagnosed Craig with adenovirus pneumonia.
>
> **Let's Code It!**
>
> Dr. Winston identified Craig's health concern as *adenovirus pneumonia*. The Alphabetic Index will direct you to
>
> Pneumonia
>   Adenoviral J12.0
>
> *(continued)*

Will the Tabular List confirm that it is the correct code? Turn to

☑4 **J12**   **Viral pneumonia, not elsewhere classified**

There are no notations or directions, so keep reading to review all of the choices for the required fourth character:

J12.0   **Adenoviral pneumonia**

You will remember that when there is an infectious organism involved, you must code it. Dr. Winston's notes identify it as the adenovirus. Should you use an additional code or not?

Professional coding specialists are responsible for relating the entire story with all specific details applicable to the diagnosis. This one combination code tells both the condition *and* the infectious organism. There is no reason to provide a second code to repeat the same information. Therefore, the code on Craig's claim form will be J12.0 alone.

GUIDANCE CONNECTION

Read the ICD-10-CM Official Guidelines for Coding and Reporting, section **I. Conventions, General Coding Guidelines and Chapter Specific Guidelines**, subsection **C. Chapter-Specific Coding Guidelines**, chapter **10. Diseases of the Respiratory System**, subsection **d. Ventilator associated Pneumonia**.

Influenza
An acute infection of the respiratory tract caused by the influenza virus.

CODING BITES

Do you know the difference between a cold and the Flu? Colds rarely cause a fever or headaches.

Do you know that what is commonly known as the "stomach flu" is actually gastroenteritis—inflammation in the stomach and small intestines?

Ventilator-Associated Pneumonia

When a patient needs help breathing because of a malfunction in the respiratory system, he or she may be placed on a ventilator, a machine that will essentially complete respiration. While the patient is hooked up to the machine, which uses a tube placed into the patient's throat, pathogens can travel directly into the patient's lungs, potentially resulting in the development of ventilator-associated pneumonia (VAP). The attending physician must specifically document the diagnosis of VAP before you can report code J95.851. Only the physician can link the ventilator with the infection. If the documentation is not clear, you must query the physician for clarification.

Beneath this code is a *Use additional code* notation reminding you that you will need to report a second code to identify the specific organism responsible for this infection. Also, an **EXCLUDES1** notation directs you to report code P27.8 instead if the patient is a newborn.

Influenza

Influenza, the formal term for what is commonly known as the *Flu* or the *grippe,* is a highly contagious and serious illness. It is a respiratory tract infection that can affect individuals of all ages, but it is most dangerous to young children, the elderly, and those who have chronic diseases because these individuals have immune systems that are more sensitive and more susceptible.

The signs and symptoms that are inclusive in a diagnosis of influenza include

- Achy feeling in the muscles, or overall body ache
- Chills
- Fever
- Headache
- Cough
- Sore throat

To code a diagnosis of influenza correctly, you have to know what virus is involved:

J09.X-   Influenza due to identified novel influenza A viruses [Avian influenza] [Bird influenza] [Swine influenza]
J10.-   Influenza due to other identified influenza virus
J11.-   Influenza due to unidentified influenza virus

As you abstract the documentation, you will need to look for mention of any manifestations, such as respiratory, gastrointestinal, encephalopathy, myocarditis, or otitis media, for example. You will need these details to determine the fifth character.

YOU CODE IT! CASE STUDY

Andrea Ignitto, a 21-year-old female, came into the University Clinic with complaints of nasal congestion, cough, sore throat, fatigue, and overall aches. She states that she has had bouts of mild diarrhea for the last 2 days. She indicates that her roommate and about five others on her dorm floor were sick with similar symptoms. She has a low grade fever, chills, and nausea but denies vomiting. She claims loss of appetite and feeling weak with generalized aches and pains. Her cough is mostly nonproductive. She denies chest pain or shortness of breath.

PAST MEDICAL HISTORY: Right knee surgery. [She is a soccer captain.]

CURRENT MEDICATIONS: Birth control pills

ALLERGIES: Sulfa

SOCIAL HISTORY: The patient drinks a couple of beers per week.

REVIEW OF SYSTEMS: Essentially as in the HPI.

OBJECTIVE:

VITAL SIGNS: Blood pressure 116/82, pulse 100, temperature 100.4F, respiratory rate is 18. Pain is 7/10. Saturation is 97% on room air.

GENERAL: The patient is looking unwell, but in no acute distress.

HEENT: Atraumatic and normocephalic. Pupils are equal, round, reactive to light, and accommodation. Extraocular movements are intact. There is no icterus, cyanosis, or pallor of the conjunctivae. Tympanic membranes are dull but not inflamed bilaterally. Nasal turbinates are congested with clear exudates. Sinuses are uncomfortable to percussion. Posterior pharynx is minimally erythematous. No exudates are noted.

CHEST: Air entry is adequate bilaterally with occasional scattered rhonchi. No crackles are appreciated.

HEART: Sounds 1 and 2 are heard and are normal. Regular rate and rhythm, somewhat tachycardic, but no murmurs, gallops, or rubs.

ABDOMEN: Soft and nontender. Bowel sounds are present but somewhat hyperactive. There is no hepatosplenomegaly.

SKIN: Clear, slight pallor.

EXTREMITIES: Without edema, cyanosis, or clubbing.

Specimen taken and tested in our office lab. Novel A influenza virus is confirmed.

ASSESSMENT: Influenza with gastrointestinal manifestations.

PLAN:

1. The patient will be put on Phenergan with Codeine 5 mL p.o. t.i.d. for 7 days.
2. Zyrtec 10 mg p.o. daily for 10 to 14 days.
3. She is instructed to take Tylenol p.r.n. for aches and pains, to drink a lot of liquids, and to stay in the dorm, in bed if possible, and rest.
4. She has been given a note for her coach and any professors.
5. If she does not get any better, she will come back.

Gary H. Mulder, MD

You Code It!

Read carefully about Dr. Mulder's diagnosis of Andrea and determine the correct diagnosis code or codes.

Step #1: Read the case carefully and completely.

Step #2: Abstract the scenario. Which main words or terms describe why the physician cared for the patient during this encounter?

(continued)

> Step #3: Are there any details missing or incomplete for which you would need to query the physician? [If so, ask your instructor.]
>
> Step #4: Check for any relevant guidance, including reading all of the symbols and notations in the Tabular List and the appropriate sections of the Official Guidelines.
>
> Step #5: Determine the correct diagnosis code or codes to explain why this encounter was medically necessary.
>
> Step #6: Double-check your work.
>
> **Answer:**
>
> Did you determine this to be the code?
>
> **J09.X3** Influenza due to identified novel influenza A virus with gastrointestinal manifestations

12.4 Chronic Respiratory Disorders

Chronic Obstructive Pulmonary Disease

Chronic Obstructive Pulmonary Disease (COPD)
An ongoing obstruction of the airway.

One of the most common respiratory disorders that you may code is **chronic obstructive pulmonary disease (COPD)**. It is estimated that as much as 10% of the world population over age 40 has a lung disorder that is on a par with COPD. COPD is distinguished by restricted airflow. It is not fully reversible and, therefore, is a leading cause of disability and death. Clinically, there are three types of COPD:

- Chronic bronchitis
- Emphysema
- Asthma

> **EXAMPLES**
>
> | | |
> |---|---|
> | J40 | Bronchitis, not specified as acute or chronic |
> | J41.- | Simple and mucopurulent chronic bronchitis |
> | J42 | Unspecified chronic bronchitis |
> | J43.- | Emphysema |
> | J44.- | Other chronic obstructive pulmonary disease |
> | J45.- | Asthma |

Diagnoses in the COPD section can be particularly complex. You will need to be very diligent as you read the terms in the physician's notes and those included in the code descriptions. It is, as always, crucial that you refer to the index and then verify the code in the Tabular List.

Let's look at some of the diagnostic statements that might be used in the documentation, by reading through the INCLUDES note under J44.

☑4 **J44** **Other chronic obstructive pulmonary disease**
INCLUDES **asthma with chronic obstructive pulmonary disease**
chronic asthmatic (obstructive) bronchitis
chronic bronchitis with airways obstruction
chronic bronchitis with emphysema

chronic emphysematous bronchitis
chronic obstructive asthma
chronic obstructive bronchitis
chronic obstructive tracheobronchitis

There is also an EXCLUDES1 note that will remind you to read very carefully. You can see that chronic *obstructive* bronchitis is INCLUDED in the J44 code category, while chronic bronchitis is EXCLUDED. This is the ICD-10-CM book's way of reminding you that one word—"obstructive"—makes a big difference as to which code to report.

> **CODING BITES**
>
> *Never, never, never, never* code out of the Alphabetic Index. *Always* confirm the code by reading the complete description in the Tabular List.

LET'S CODE IT! SCENARIO

Tiffany Burnstein, a 57-year-old female, quit smoking 2 years ago after a two-pack-a-day habit that lasted 40 years. She came to see Dr. Mercado with an insidious onset of dyspnea, tachypnea, and malaise. PE showed use of her accessory muscles for respiration. Dr. Mercado took a chest x-ray, EKG, RBC count, and pulmonary function test. The results directed a diagnosis of panlobular emphysema.

Let's Code It!

Dr. Mercado diagnosed Tiffany with *panlobular emphysema*. The Alphabetic Index shows

Emphysema
    Panlobular J43.1

Go to the Tabular List to confirm this code:

☑4 **J43**   **Emphysema**

Read the **Use additional code** notation carefully, as well as the EXCLUDES1 note. Does either of them relate to Tiffany's condition? Yes, the note to **Use additional code** for "history of tobacco use" applies. First, keep reading and review all of the choices for the required fourth character:

J43.1   **Panlobular emphysema**

Now let's follow the lead to the code for "history of tobacco use." Turn to code Z87:

☑4 **Z87**   **Personal history of other diseases and conditions**
Z87.891   **Personal history of nicotine dependence**

Now you have two codes to report the story of why Dr. Mercado cared for Tiffany:

J43.1   **Panlobular emphysema**
Z87.891   **Personal history of nicotine dependence**

Exacerbation and Status Asthmaticus

You may notice that some of the codes in this section have the designation for acute **exacerbation** of asthma, COPD, or other related condition. It is a clinical term and can be assigned only by the attending physician.

Acute exacerbation of asthma indicates an increase in the severe nature of a patient's asthmatic condition. The patient may be suffering from wheezing or shortness of breath, commonly called an *asthma attack*. **Status asthmaticus**, however, is a life-threatening condition and is a diagnosis indicating that the patient is not responding to therapeutic procedures. If a patient is diagnosed with status asthmaticus *and* COPD or acute bronchitis, the status asthmaticus should be the first-listed code. As a life-threatening condition, it is considered to be the diagnosis with the greatest severity

Exacerbation
An increase in the severity of a disease or its symptoms.

Status Asthmaticus
The condition of asthma that is life-threatening and does not respond to therapeutic treatments.

CHAPTER 12 | CODING RESPIRATORY CONDITIONS   **341**

> **CODING BITES**
>
> If both diagnoses are included in the notes—status asthmaticus *and* acute exacerbation of asthma—use only one asthma code, for status asthmaticus. Do not use two asthma codes.

and follows the sequencing rules that you learned earlier. In addition, status asthmaticus, being the more severe condition, will override an additional diagnosis of acute exacerbation of asthma.

> **GUIDANCE CONNECTION**
>
> Read the ICD-10-CM Official Guidelines for Coding and Reporting, section **I. Conventions, General Coding Guidelines and Chapter Specific Guidelines,** subsection **C. Chapter-Specific Coding Guidelines,** chapter **10. Diseases of the Respiratory System,** subsection **a. Chronic Obstructive Pulmonary Disease [COPD] and Asthma.**

LET'S CODE IT! SCENARIO

Isabella LaVelle, a 41-year-old female, has a history of intermittent dyspnea and wheezing. She comes today to see Dr. Slater with complaints of tachypnea, chest tightness, and a cough with thick mucus. The results of Dr. Slater's PE, the chest x-ray, sputum culture, EKG, pulmonary function tests, and an arterial blood gas analysis indicate moderate, persistent asthma with COPD, with exacerbation.

Let's Code It!

Dr. Slater's diagnosis of Isabella's condition is *moderate, persistent asthma with COPD, with exacerbation.* This is also referred to as *chronic obstructive asthma.* Let's turn to the Alphabetic Index and look up

> **Asthma**
>   **With**
>   Chronic obstructive pulmonary disease J44.9
>   **With**
>   Exacerbation (acute) J44.1

That's great, it matches perfectly. Turn in the Tabular List to

   ☑4 **J44**   **Other chronic obstructive pulmonary disease**

You can see "chronic obstructive asthma" in the INCLUDES list. Also notice the instruction to **Code also** type of asthma, if applicable (J45.-).

   J44.0   **Chronic obstructive pulmonary disease with acute lower respiratory infection**
   J44.1   **Chronic obstructive pulmonary disease with (acute) exacerbation**
   J44.9   **Chronic obstructive pulmonary disease, unspecified**

You can see that J44.1 matches. Terrific! Now let's turn to J45 to determine the additional code for the asthma.

Go back to Dr. Slater's notes and determine if Isabella's asthma is documented as mild, moderate, or severe and if her condition is intermittent or persistent. Then match all of the options within code category J45 to determine which code is accurate:

   J45.41   **Moderate persistent asthma with (acute) exacerbation**

One more detail to address: Certainly you saw the **Use additional code** notation regarding tobacco exposure, use, dependence, or history. Is there documentation that Isabella was a smoker? No! Good for her (and good for you). Now you have the codes to report this encounter:

   J44.1   **Chronic obstructive pulmonary disease with (acute) exacerbation**
   J45.41   **Moderate persistent asthma with (acute) exacerbation**

Good job!

> ## YOU CODE IT! CASE STUDY
>
> *Oliver Rockwell, a 61-year-old male, was brought into the emergency department (ED) by ambulance because he was having a severe asthma attack. His wife, Karolyn, stated that he was diagnosed with asthma about 2 years prior. This attack began 5 days ago and has not responded to his inhaler, his regular asthma pills, or any other treatment. Dr. Pressman diagnosed Oliver with acute exacerbation of late-onset severe, persistent asthma with status asthmaticus.*
>
> ### You Code It!
>
> Go through the steps of coding, and determine the diagnosis code or codes that should be reported for this encounter between Dr. Pressman and Oliver.
>
> Step #1: Read the case carefully and completely.
>
> Step #2: Abstract the scenario. Which main words or terms describe why the physician cared for the patient during this encounter?
>
> Step #3: Are there any details missing or incomplete for which you would need to query the physician? [If so, ask your instructor.]
>
> Step #4: Check for any relevant guidance, including reading all of the symbols and notations in the Tabular List and the appropriate sections of the Official Guidelines.
>
> Step #5: Determine the correct diagnosis code or codes to explain why this encounter was medically necessary.
>
> Step #6: Double-check your work.
>
> **Answer:**
>
> Did you determine this to be the correct code?
>
> J45.52   Severe persistent asthma with status asthmaticus
>
> You are really getting good at this!

12.5 Reporting Tobacco Involvement

One set of elements that has become required is the reporting of tobacco use, abuse, and/or dependence. For example, at the start of ICD-10-CM *Chapter 10, Diseases of the Respiratory System (J00–J99)*, there is a notation that applies to all codes within:

> *Use additional code*, where applicable, to identify:
> Exposure to environmental tobacco smoke (Z77.22)
> Exposure to tobacco smoke in the perinatal period (P96.81)
> History of tobacco use (Z87.891)
> Occupational exposure to environmental tobacco smoke (Z57.31)
> Tobacco dependence (F17.-)
> Tobacco use (Z72.0)

Surely you know that tobacco use can be a risk factor to the development of respiratory illness. ICD-10-CM makes it easier to collect data on tobacco use. To do so, you need to understand what the terms *exposure, use, abuse, dependence,* and *history* really mean.

- *Exposure* means that the patient has been in contact with, or in close proximity to, a source of tobacco smoke in such a way that the harmful effects of this agent may impact the patient. When it comes to health care issues, this would apply to an individual who does not use tobacco products but lives or works with someone who smokes, resulting in the patient's breathing in secondhand tobacco smoke on an ongoing basis. If this individual develops a respiratory disease as a result of this environment, you would include a code to report this exposure.

> **EXAMPLE**
>
> Z77.22 Contact with and (suspected) exposure to environmental tobacco smoke (acute) (chronic) [Exposure to second hand tobacco smoke]

- *Use* is the term that identifies that the patient smokes tobacco on a regular basis, taken by his or her own initiative, even though the substance is known to be a detriment to one's health. There are no obvious clinical manifestations.

> **EXAMPLE**
>
> Z72.0 Tobacco use

- *Abuse* describes the patient's habitual smoking of tobacco, taken by his or her own initiative, even though the substance is known to be a detriment to one's health. Clinical manifestations are evident as signs and symptoms develop. The patient deals with a daily fixation on obtaining and smoking tobacco with virtually everything else in life becoming secondary.

> **EXAMPLE**
>
> F17.218 Nicotine dependence, cigarettes, with other nicotine-induced disorders

- *Dependence* indicates the patient's compulsive, continuous smoking of tobacco that has resulted in significant clinical manifestations as well as the physiological need for the substance to function normally. Any interruption results in signs and symptoms of withdrawal, occurring within a continuous 12-month time frame.

> **EXAMPLE**
>
> F17.220 Nicotine dependence, chewing tobacco, uncomplicated

- *History* describes a patient who has successfully quit using tobacco products.

> **EXAMPLE**
>
> Z87.891 Personal history of tobacco dependence

YOU CODE IT! CASE STUDY

Evan Pattison has been smoking cigarettes for more than 10 years. He has tried to quit several times, unsuccessfully. Evan tells the doctor that he has been very stressed and smoking much more than usual and now his throat hurts and his voice is hoarse. Dr. Dieter evaluates Evan and determines acute laryngitis due to tobacco dependence.

You Code It!

Read the scenario and determine what code or codes you need to report why Dr. Dieter cared for Evan.

Step #1: Read the case carefully and completely.

Step #2: Abstract the scenario. Which main words or terms describe why the physician cared for the patient during this encounter?

Step #3: Are there any details missing or incomplete for which you would need to query the physician? [If so, ask your instructor.]

Step #4: Check for any relevant guidance, including reading all of the symbols and notations in the Tabular List and the appropriate sections of the Official Guidelines.

Step #5: Determine the correct diagnosis code or codes to explain why this encounter was medically necessary.

Step #6: Double-check your work.

Answer:

Did you determine these to be the codes?

J04.0	Acute laryngitis
F17.210	Nicotine dependence, cigarettes, uncomplicated

12.6 Respiratory Conditions Requiring External Cause Codes

Earlier in this text, you learned about external cause codes and how to determine whether they are necessary. There are respiratory conditions that may require external cause codes to explain how, and sometimes where, an external condition was involved in causing this health problem. Some of these conditions are

- **J39.8:** Cicatrix of trachea might need an external cause code to identify it as a late effect of an injury or poisoning.
- **J67.0:** Farmer's lung might need an external cause code for a workers' compensation claim.
- **J68.-:** Respiratory conditions due to inhalation of chemicals, gases, fumes, and vapors would need an external cause code to identify the chemical.
- **J70.-:** Respiratory conditions due to other external agents would need an external cause code to identify the external cause of the condition.
- **J95.811:** Postprocedural pneumothorax would need an external cause code to identify that it was a postoperative condition.

External Cause Codes

When a patient has been injured traumatically, has been poisoned, has had an adverse reaction, has been abused or neglected, or has experienced other harm as a result of

> **GUIDANCE CONNECTION**
>
> Read the ICD-10-CM Official Guidelines for Coding and Reporting, section **I. Conventions, General Coding Guidelines and Chapter Specific Guidelines**, subsection **C. Chapter-Specific Coding Guidelines**, chapter **20. External Causes of Morbidity**.

CODING BITES

Refer back to the **Abstracting Clinical Documentation** chapter to remind yourself about reporting external cause codes whenever you are reporting an injury or poisoning.

an external cause, you will need to report the details of the event so that you tell the whole story. In addition to reporting the other codes, you will also need to report codes that explain

- *Cause of the injury,* such as a car accident or a fall off a ladder.
- *Place of the occurrence,* such as the park or the kitchen.
- *Activity during the occurrence,* such as playing basketball or gardening.
- *Patient's status,* such as paid employment, on-duty military, or leisure activity.

LET'S CODE IT! SCENARIO

Amanda Bleigh, a 33-year-old female, works in a veterinary clinic. After a very sick stray animal was brought in, she was instructed by her boss to disinfect the floor of the clinic by mopping it with straight bleach. It was cold outside, so all the doors and windows were closed tightly. Amanda began to have trouble breathing. She went immediately to Dr. Litzkom's office, where, after examination and tests, he diagnosed her with acute chemical bronchitis.

Let's Code It!

Dr. Litzkom diagnosed Amanda with *acute chemical bronchitis*. In the Alphabetic Index:

Bronchitis
    Acute
        chemical (due to gases, fumes, or vapors) J68.0

Will the Tabular List confirm this suggested code?

☑4 **J68**   **Respiratory conditions due to inhalation of chemicals, gases, fumes, and vapors**

Did you notice that there are two notations: **Code first** (T51–T65) to identify cause and **Use additional code** to report the associated respiratory condition. Keep reading down the column to

    J68.0   **Bronchitis and pneumonitis due to chemicals, gases, fumes, and vapors (chemical bronchitis (acute))**

Next, you must report how and where Amanda was exposed to the chemical. Let's go to the Alphabetic Index for external cause codes and look up how Amanda was injured by the bleach—she inhaled the chemical:

Inhalation
    gases, fumes, or vapors NEC T59.9-
        specified agent—see Table of Drugs and Chemicals, by substance

Turn to the Table of Drugs and Chemicals and look down the first column to find *bleach:*

Bleach NEC

Reading across this line, in the column titled "Poisoning, Accidental," you will see the suggested poisoning code. Remember: If the condition was not an adverse reaction to properly prescribed and taken medication, it is reported as a poisoning. The code suggested on the line for bleach is T54.91.

Now turn to the Tabular List to confirm the most accurate code. Let's begin with the poisoning code:

☑4 **T54**   **Toxic effect of corrosive substances**

There are no notations or directives, so keep reading to find the most accurate fourth, fifth, and sixth characters:

> **T54.91xA** Toxic effect of unspecified corrosive substance, accidental (unintentional), initial encounter
>
> This does look like the best choice.
>
> In addition, Amanda was at work when the exposure happened, so you will need an external cause code to report where she was at the time of her injury. The External Cause Code Alphabetic Index will direct you:
>
> **Place of occurrence**
>   hospital Y92.239
>   cafeteria Y92.233
>   corridor Y92.232
>
> There is no specific listing for *veterinary clinic*. However, *hospital* does come the closest. Let's turn to the code in the Tabular List and check the description:
>
> **Y92.232** Corridor of hospital as the place of occurrence of the external cause
>
> Well, that really does hit the target. Remember, the code is being included to explain that Amanda was hurt at work; such information is most often required to support a workers' compensation claim.
>
> These are the three codes on Amanda's report:
>
> **J68.0** Bronchitis and pneumonitis due to chemicals, gases, fumes and vapors (chemical bronchitis (acute))
> **T54.91xA** Toxic effect of unspecified corrosive substance, accidental (unintentional), initial encounter
> **Y92.232** Corridor of hospital as the place of occurrence of the external cause

Chapter Summary

Sadly, most people take breathing for granted . . . until they cannot do it without difficulty or pain. You have to know how to code respiratory conditions accurately whether you are working for a family physician, a pediatrician, respiratory therapist, or a pulmonologist. In addition, respiratory conditions might be present in a patient of an immunologist; allergist; or ear, nose, and throat (ENT) specialist.

> **CODING BITES**
>
> Did you know . . . ?
> - The average healthy adult's respiration rate is 12 to 15 per minute. Adult men breathe more slowly than adult women. Neonates breathe 30 to 60 times per minute.
> - The entire surface area of both lungs combined is approximately the same surface area as a tennis court.
> - Expiration (breathing out) not only expels carbon dioxide from the body, but water as well—an estimated 12 ounces a day.
> - A yawn is an autonomic response when your brain determines the body needs more oxygen.
> - The left lung is smaller than the right lung to accommodate the placement of the heart in the thoracic cavity.

CHAPTER 12 REVIEW
Coding Respiratory Conditions

Let's Check It! Terminology

Match each key term to the appropriate definition.

1. LO 12.4 An increase in the severity of a disease or its symptoms. **B**
2. LO 12.3 An acute infection of the respiratory tract caused by the influenza virus. **C**
3. LO 12.4 An ongoing obstruction of the airway. **A**
4. LO 12.1 A malfunction of the organ system relating to respiration. **F**
5. LO 12.3 An inflammation of the lungs. **D**
6. LO 12.4 The condition of asthma that is life-threatening and does not respond to therapeutic treatments. **G**
7. LO 12.2 A condition in which air or gas is present within the chest cavity but outside the lungs. **E**

A. Chronic Obstructive Pulmonary Disease (COPD)
B. Exacerbation
C. Influenza
D. Pneumonia
E. Pneumothorax
F. Respiratory Disorder
G. Status Asthmaticus

Let's Check It! Concepts

Choose the most appropriate answer for each of the following questions.

1. LO 12.4 COPD stands for
   a. chronic obstructive pneumonia dyspnea.
   b. chronic olfactory pharyngitis disease.
   c. chronic other pneumonic disease.
   d. chronic obstructive pulmonary disease.
2. LO 12.4 One of the three types of COPD is
   a. sinusitis.   b. pneumonia.   **c. emphysema.**   d. pharyngitis.
3. LO 12.3 When the cause of pneumonia is an underlying disease such as HIV, the codes should be sequenced
   a. pneumonia first, underlying disease second.
   b. pneumonia only.
   c. underlying disease only.
   d. underlying disease first, pneumonia second.
4. LO 12.1 Respiratory disorders can be
   a. genetic.   b. environmental.   c. congenital.   **d. all of these.**
5. LO 12.3 When a known infectious organism is involved in a respiratory condition,
   a. code only the infectious organism.
   b. code both the known organism and the respiratory condition.
   c. code only the respiratory condition.
   d. use a personal history code.
6. LO 12.4 If the diagnostic statement includes both status asthmaticus and acute exacerbation of asthma,
   a. code only the status asthmaticus. *overrides all other codes as it is more severe!*
   b. code only the acute exacerbation of asthma.

348   PART II | REPORTING DIAGNOSES

c. code both status asthmaticus and acute exacerbation with two codes.

d. these two diagnoses cannot be in the same patient at the same time.

7. **LO 12.2** Jake Phillipson, a 59-year-old male, presents with dyspnea, tachypnea, and chest pain. After an examination, Jake is diagnosed with a saddle embolus of pulmonary artery with acute cor pulmonale. How would this be coded?

   a. I26.09   b. Z86.711   c. I26.92   d. I26.02

8. **LO 12.6** Respiratory conditions need external cause codes

   a. never.
   b. sometimes.
   c. always.
   d. only if there is an external cause for the condition.

9. **LO 12.5** _____ is the term that identifies that the patient smokes tobacco on a regular basis, taken by his or her own initiative, even though the substance is known to be a detriment to one's health. There are no obvious clinical manifestations.

   a. Exposure   b. Use   c. Abuse   d. Dependence

10. **LO 12.3** Code the diagnosis of pneumonitis due to inhalation of lubricating oil, unintentional, initial encounter.

    a. T52.0X1A   b. J69.1   c. T52.0X1A, J69.1   d. J69.1, T52.0X1A

Let's Check It! Guidelines

Refer to the Official Guidelines and fill in the blanks according to the Chapter 10, Diseases of the Respiratory System, Chapter-Specific Coding Guidelines.

secondary	principal	documentation	mechanical
all	J95.851	not	J96.0
J96.2	exacerbation	confirmed	one
admission			

1. An acute _____ is a worsening or a decompensation of a chronic condition.

2. A code from subcategory _____, Acute respiratory failure, or subcategory _____, Acute and chronic respiratory failure, may be assigned as a principal diagnosis when it is the condition established after study to be chiefly responsible for occasioning the admission to the hospital, and the selection is supported by the Alphabetic Index and Tabular List.

3. Respiratory failure may be listed as a _____ diagnosis if it occurs after admission, or if it is present on admission, but does not meet the definition of _____ diagnosis.

4. Code only _____ cases of influenza due to certain identified influenza viruses (category J09), and due to other identified influenza virus (category J10).

5. As with _____ procedural or postprocedural complications, code assignment is based on the provider's _____ of the relationship between the condition and the procedure.

6. Code _____, Ventilator associated pneumonia, should be assigned only when the provider has documented ventilator associated pneumonia (VAP).

7. Code J95.851 should _____ be assigned for cases where the patient has pneumonia and is on a _____ ventilator and the provider has not specifically stated that the pneumonia is ventilator-associated pneumonia.

8. A patient may be admitted with _____ type of pneumonia (e.g., code J13, Pneumonia due to Streptococcus pneumonia) and subsequently develop VAP. In this instance, the principal diagnosis would be the appropriate code from categories J12-J18 for the pneumonia diagnosed at the time of _____.

Let's Check It! Rules and Regulations

Please answer the following questions from the knowledge you have gained after reading this chapter.

1. **LO 12.2** What is pleural effusion? What is the correct ICD-10-CM code for malignant pleural effusion?
2. **LO 12.3** Explain what ventilator-associated pneumonia is. Include the correct ICD-10-CM code you would use to report VAP.
3. **LO 12.4** Differentiate between exacerbation and status asthmaticus.
4. **LO 12.5** In relation to tobacco involvement, explain the difference between *exposure, use, abuse, dependence,* and *history.*
5. **LO 12.6** Explain why a respiratory condition might require an external cause code. Include an example.

YOU CODE IT! Basics

First, identify the condition in the following diagnoses; then code the diagnosis.

Example: Acute nasopharyngitis:

   a. main term: <u>Nasopharyngitis</u>   b. diagnosis: <u>J00</u>

1. Vasomotor rhinitis:
   a. main term: _____   b. diagnosis: _____
2. Nasal catarrh, acute:
   a. main term: _____   b. diagnosis: _____
3. Acute recurrent empyema of sphenoidal sinus:
   a. main term: _____   b. diagnosis: _____
4. Hypertrophy of tonsils:
   a. main term: _____   b. diagnosis: _____
5. Obstructive laryngitis:
   a. main term: _____   b. diagnosis: _____
6. Chronic laryngotracheitis:
   a. main term: _____   b. diagnosis: _____
7. Aspiration pneumonia due to solids and liquids:
   a. main term: _____   b. diagnosis: _____
8. Bronchitis due to rhinovirus:
   a. main term: _____   b. diagnosis: _____
9. Cellulitis of nose:
   a. main term: _____   b. diagnosis: _____
10. Polypoid sinus degeneration:
    a. main term: _____   b. diagnosis: _____
11. Adenoid vegetations:
    a. main term: _____   b. diagnosis: _____
12. Abscess of lung:
    a. main term: _____   b. diagnosis: _____
13. Bronchiectasis with exacerbation:
    a. main term: _____   b. diagnosis: _____
14. Seropurulent pleurisy with fistula:
    a. main term: _____   b. diagnosis: _____
15. Pulmonary gangrene:
    a. main term: _____   b. diagnosis: _____

YOU CODE IT! Practice

Using the techniques described in this chapter, carefully read through the case studies and determine the most accurate ICD-10-CM code(s) and external cause codes, if appropriate, for each case study.

1. Fred Draper, a 39-year-old male, is HIV-positive, asymptomatic. Fred was just admitted with organic pneumonia.
2. Rebecca Key, a 21-year-old female, presents with a fever and sore throat. Dr. Brice notes large lymph nodes. The throat culture confirms a diagnosis of streptococcal pharyngitis.

3. Larry Ligon, a 58-year-old male, presents today with severe chest congestion. Dr. Snell also notes difficulty breathing and wheezing. Larry is admitted to the hospital, where further laboratory tests confirm the diagnosis of streptococcus, group B, pneumonia.

4. Sally Griffith, a 13-year-old female, was brought to the ED by her mother. Sally had a cough and fever, and her eyes were tearing. She was complaining that her eyes were itchy and burning. After a thorough examination and chest x-ray, Dr. Minister diagnosed her with an upper respiratory infection with bilateral acute conjunctivitis.

5. Chris Fravel, a 13-year-old male, is brought in by his mother with the complaints of sore throat, fever, and that it hurts when he swallows. Dr. Dennis documents white pus-filled spots on the tonsils and large lymph nodes. After completing an examination and an optical fiber endoscopy, Chris is diagnosed with chronic tonsillitis and adenoiditis.

6. Allison Mabry, a 6-year-old female, is brought in by her parents with a fever and hoarseness. Allison says it hurts when she swallows and it's hard to breath. Dr. Macon completes an examination noting drooling; culture is positive for haemophilus influenza. Allison is diagnosed with acute epiglottitis.

7. Benjamin Fulkenbury, a 46-year-old male, comes in today with cough, runny nose, sneezing, and body aches. Dr. Pruessner completes a thorough examination and notes a temperature of 104 F. Ben is admitted, where a CXR and laboratory tests confirm the diagnosis of influenza virus A/H5N1 with pleural effusion.

8. Sandra Busbee, a 43-year-old female, comes in today with a cough and chest pain. Dr. Lindsey completes a thorough examination, the appropriate tests, and a chest x-ray. Sandra is diagnosed with acute bronchitis due to parainfluenza virus.

9. Dale Hunter, a 52-year-old male, was diagnosed with chronic bronchitis 3 months ago and is on medication. This morning, he came to see Dr. Teasdale because he began to cough and is having difficulty breathing. Dr. Teasdale admitted him into the hospital with a diagnosis of chronic obstructive pulmonary disease with acute exacerbation.

10. Monica Adams, a 65-year-old female, comes in today with hoarseness and neck pain. Dr. Fazio completes a thorough examination and the appropriate tests and notes that Monica smokes cigarettes. Monica undergoes a laryngoscopy, which confirms the diagnosis of vocal cord nodules.

11. Caitlyn Joy, a 12-year-old female, comes in today with a nosebleed. She was playing a pickup game of basketball at the local sports area and was struck in the face by the basketball. After an examination, Dr. Jordan diagnoses Caitlyn with a deviated nasal septum.

12. Randy Prescott, a 56-year-old male, presents today with a cough and shortness of breath. Dr. Holden documents notable weight loss from Randy's last visit 6 months ago. Randy admits to joint aches and some chest pain. After a thorough examination and the appropriate tests, Dr. Holden diagnoses Randy with berylliosis.

13. Larry Crosstree, a 29-year-old male, presents today concerned about vocal pitch changes he has been experiencing for approximately 2 weeks. Dr. Leonard notes the frequent need for breath while Larry is speaking as well as hoarseness. Larry is admitted to the hospital, where an MRI scan of the neck and chest confirms a diagnosis of complete bilateral paralysis of the laryngeal nerve.

14. Nakeisha Dittman, a 27-year-old female, presents today with a cough, fever, shortness of breath, and night sweats, 2 weeks duration. Dr. Mokeba completes a thorough examination and decides to admit Nakeisha to the hospital. Further laboratory tests confirm the diagnosis of eosinophilic pneumonia with secondary spontaneous pneumothorax.

15. Beth Northing, a 25-year-old female, was diagnosed 6 months ago with asthma. She presents today with the complaint of shortness of breath and a tight chest. Dr. Hayden completes an examination, noting cyanosis of the lips and confusion. Dr. Hayden diagnoses Beth with a severe persistent asthma attack and admits her into the hospital.

YOU CODE IT! Application

The following exercises provide practice in abstracting physicians' notes and learning to work with documentation from our health care facility, Prader, Bracker, & Associates. These case studies are modeled on real patient encounters. Using the techniques described in this chapter, carefully read through the case studies and determine the most accurate ICD-10-CM code(s) and external cause code(s), if appropriate, for each case study.

WESTON HOSPITAL

629 Healthcare Way • SOMEWHERE, FL 32811 • 407-555-6541

PATIENT: YOUNG, ELIAS

ACCOUNT/EHR #: YOUNEL001

DATE: 07/16/18

Attending Physician: Oscar R. Prader, MD

Elias Young, a 71-year-old male, is brought to the ED by EMS. Elias is on ACUD mode on ventilator with a respiration of 11 breaths per minute. No cyanosis is noted. Pt is currently alert and oriented and able to answer some questions. Dr. Prader notes as time progresses patient is showing signs of confusion and disorientation. He is admitted to the hospital.

The patient's blood gases showed a compensated respiratory acidosis, VS are stable, and patient is afebrile. BP: 148/83. Sinus tachycardia on the monitor at about 131 beats per minute. Lung fields are clear to auscultation and percussion.

DIAGNOSES: 1. Respiratory failure, chronic

2. Sinus tachycardia

PLAN/RECOMMENDATIONS:

1. 100% ventilator support for the time being
2. Nutrition with PulmoCare at 60 cc an hour
3. Follow up laboratory

ORP/pw   D: 07/16/18 09:50:16   T: 07/18/18 12:55:01

Determine the most accurate ICD-10-CM code(s).

PRADER, BRACKER, & ASSOCIATES

A Complete Health Care Facility

159 Healthcare Way • SOMEWHERE, FL 32811 • 407-555-6789

PATIENT: NADER, ERICK

ACCOUNT/EHR #: NADEER001

DATE: 08/11/18

Attending Physician: Oscar R. Prader, MD

S: Erick Nader, an 18-month-old male, is brought in today by his parents because of shortness of breath and a cough that has grown worse over the last 24 hours.

O: H: 32.5", W: 25 lb., T: 103 F, P: 138, R: 37, SpO2: 96% on room air, BP: 95/62. A "bark-like" cough is noted and upon auscultation stridor is heard. A lateral neck x-ray is taken.

A: Stridulous croup

P: 0.5 mL of racemic epinephrine via small volume nebulizer is administered

ORP/pw   D: 08/11/18 09:50:16   T: 08/13/18 12:55:01

Determine the most accurate ICD-10-CM code(s).

WESTON HOSPITAL

629 Healthcare Way • SOMEWHERE, FL 32811 • 407-555-6541

PATIENT: SMUTH, SARAH

ACCOUNT/EHR #: SMUTSA001

DATE: 07/16/18

Attending Physician: Renee O. Bracker, MD

Sarah Smuth, a 52-year-old female, underwent total knee replacement surgery 5 days ago. Patient is alert and oriented, but began to complain of chest pain and dyspnea 3 days after surgery. Laboratory tests reveal a WBC of 15, HR: 101, R: 20 and shallow, P: 56, BP: 135/85, T: 98.9 F, SpO2 is 95% receiving oxygen via nasal cannula at 2 Lpm. VS have remained stable. Diminished sounds and fine crackles are noted on auscultation. Post-op day 3—CXR confirms atelectasis; pneumonia is ruled out. Post-op day 4—patient has not improved; a repeat CXR shows no improvement of atelectasis and a bronchoscopy was performed and mucus plugs were removed. Post-op day 5—patient begins to show improvement and full resolution is expected.

A: Atelectasis, post-op complication

P: Albuterol nebulizer every 4 hours and prn

Deep breathing exercises and coughing. Monitor via continuous capnography.

ROB/pw   D: 07/16/18 09:50:16   T: 07/18/18 12:55:01

Determine the most accurate ICD-10-CM code(s).

CHAPTER 12 REVIEW

WESTON HOSPITAL

629 Healthcare Way • SOMEWHERE, FL 32811 • 407-555-6541

PATIENT: ALBERTSON, JONAH

ACCOUNT/EHR #: ALBEJO001

DATE: 09/15/18

Attending Physician: Renee O. Bracker, MD

Jonah Albertson, a 62-year-old male, was transported to the ED by EMS after an MVA. Patient was involved in a three-car accident while driving home. Patient does not appear to have any injuries. Patient denies any pain or discomfort at this time. Patient is alert and oriented, but appears anxious.

VS: H: 6' 1", W: 192 lb., P: 94, R: 24, T: 99.1 F, BP: 90/60, SpO2 100% on room air.

Laboratory results 25 minutes after arrival:

pH: 7.5
PaO2: 195 mmHg
PaCO2: 32 mmHg
SaO2: 90%
HCO3: 20 mEq
Hgb: 13.9 gms
COHgb: 11.2%

With the level of carbon monoxide on the hemoglobin, the patient is placed on a nonrebreathing mask. COHgb has decreased to 7.1% and patient is breathing comfortably 4 hours after arrival. Patient is admitted for observation.

Three hours later, respiration becomes more rapid and labored. Patient shows extreme fatigue. Auscultation reveals fine crackles throughout both lungs. CXR shows bilateral infiltrates extending into all four lung quadrants.

Arterial blood gases are rechecked:

pH: 7.31
PaO2: 71 mmHg
PaCO2: 43 mmHg
SaO2: 89%
HCO3: 22 mEq
COHgb: 3.9%

Heart Rate: 79
Blood Pressure: 88/57

Dx: ARDS

P: Intubation and mechanical ventilation

ROB/pw   D: 09/15/18 09:50:16   T: 09/17/18 12:55:01

Determine the most accurate ICD-10-CM code(s).

PRADER, BRACKER, & ASSOCIATES

A Complete Health Care Facility

159 Healthcare Way • SOMEWHERE, FL 32811 • 407-555-6789

PATIENT: MASHEN, CYRUS

ACCOUNT/EHR #: MASHCY001

DATE: 11/25/18

Attending Physician: Oscar R. Prader, MD

S: This new Pt is a 57-year-old male complaining of a stabbing chest pain and shortness of breath. Patient states the pain is worse when he breathes in.

PMH: Noncontributory

PFH: Noncontributory

O: VS: within normal range. Chest: Pleural rub on auscultation. Dullness upon percussion. Chest x-ray shows approximately 2.75 liters of fluid in the pleural space.

A: Interlobar pleurisy

P: Schedule aspiration of pleural fluid

ORP/pw   D: 11/25/18 09:50:16   T: 11/27/18 12:55:01

Determine the most accurate ICD-10-CM code(s).

13 Coding Digestive System Conditions

Key Terms

Accessory Organs
Anus
Ascending Colon
Cecum
Cholelithiasis
Common Bile Duct
Descending Colon
Duodenum
Edentulism
Esophagus
Fundus
Gallbladder
Gangrene
Hemorrhage
Hernia
Ileum
Jejunum
Liver
Mesentery
Obstruction
Oral Cavity
Pancreas
Pancreatic Islets
Perforation
Rectum
Salivary Glands
Sigmoid Colon
Sphincter
Stomach
Teeth
Transverse Colon
Vermiform Appendix

Learning Outcomes

After completing this chapter, the student should be able to:

LO 13.1 Analyze the documentation for applicable details needed to report diseases affecting the mouth and salivary glands accurately.

LO 13.2 Interpret documentation to determine necessary details to report conditions affecting the esophagus and stomach correctly.

LO 13.3 Apply your knowledge to identify main terms relating to intestinal disorders.

LO 13.4 Evaluate the specifics from the documentation related to digestive accessory organs and malabsorption disorders accurately.

LO 13.5 Determine when additional codes are required to report the involvement of alcohol.

STOP! Remember, you need to follow along in your ICD-10-CM code book for an optimal learning experience.

13.1 Diseases of Oral Cavity and Salivary Glands

Oral Cavity

Virtually all nourishment enters the body at the mouth, also referred to as the **oral cavity**. The components within this area include the lips, cheeks, tongue, lingual tonsils, hard and soft palates, uvula, palatine tonsils, pharyngeal tonsils, and teeth (Figure 13-1).

Teeth are components of the mouth, required for proper digestion. Typically, as you probably know from your own experiences, they have their very own specialists, dentists, to care for them. Teeth are small, calcified protrusions consisting of multiple tissues of varying density and hardness. Rooted in the jaws (maxillary [upper jaw] and mandibular [lower jaw]), the bases of the teeth are protected and secured by the gums. Their job is to grind and crush food and food particles so they can combine with saliva for easier movement through the rest of the digestive system.

Oral Cavity
The opening in the face that begins the alimentary canal and is used for the input of nutrition; also known as the *mouth*.

Teeth
Small, calcified protrusions with roots in the jaw. (singular: Tooth)

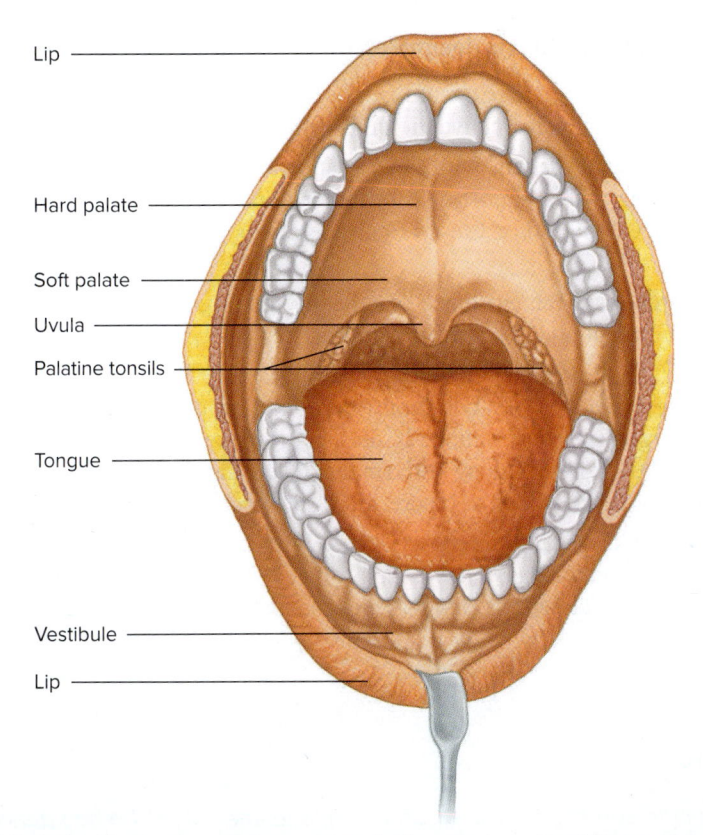

FIGURE 13-1 An illustration of the anatomical components of the oral cavity (human mouth) David Shier et al., *HOLE'S HUMAN ANATOMY & PHYSIOLOGY*, 12/e. ©2010 McGraw-Hill Education. Figure 17.5, p. 657. Used with permission.

> **EXAMPLE**
>
> Perry brought his 8-month-old son, Benjamin, to Dr. Reddington, his pediatrician, because he had been crying all night long. It seemed nothing he or his wife did calmed him. After examination, Dr. Reddington diagnosed Benjamin with teething syndrome and provided Perry with several ways to help the family through this experience. This diagnosis is reported with the following code:
>
> **K00.7**   Teething syndrome

Diagnoses, related to the teeth, range from everything from baby's first tooth to dental caries (commonly known as a dental cavity) to issues of the surrounding tissue, such as gingivitis and other periodontal diseases, to **edentulism** (tooth loss).

When you are abstracting the documentation regarding acquired loss of teeth, you will need to identify three specified details from the notes:

1. **Is the loss complete or partial?**
   - ✓4 K08.1   Complete loss of teeth
   - ✓4 K08.4   Partial loss of teeth

2. **What is the cause of this loss?**
   - ✓5 K08.11   Complete loss of teeth due to trauma
   - ✓5 K08.12   Complete loss of teeth due to periodontal diseases
   - ✓5 K08.13   Complete loss of teeth due to caries
   - ✓5 K08.41   Partial loss of teeth due to trauma
   - ✓5 K08.42   Partial loss of teeth due to periodontal diseases
   - ✓5 K08.43   Partial loss of teeth due to caries

Edentulism
Absence of teeth.

3. **What class classification is documented?**

- *Class I* describes the stage of edentulism believed to have the best prognosis to have successful treatment using conventional prosthodontic techniques.
- *Class II* identifies a patient with deterioration of the gums and other supporting structures, along with systemic disease interactions, soft tissue concerns, as well as patient management and/or lifestyle considerations affecting the prognosis of the treatment.
- *Class III* establishes the existence of other factors significantly affecting the outcomes of treatment and the need for surgical revision of the supporting structures (gums and bone) to create an opportunity for prosthodontics.
- *Class IV* reports a severely compromised condition of the supporting structures requiring surgical reconstruction. If due to the patient's health, personal preferences, past dental history, along with financial considerations, a customized prosthodontic technique may need to be created for an acceptable outcome.

Remember that ICD-10-CM diagnosis codes provide the explanation of why a particular procedure, treatment, or service is provided. You can see that the descriptions of each of these class classifications provides the justification for the treatment plan.

LET'S CODE IT! SCENARIO

Hannah Kim, a 49-year-old female, comes in to see her dentist, Dr. Morrison. She knew that she had periodontitis for a while, but now the teeth on the lower right side of her mouth are really bothering her. Dr. Morrison did a full evaluation and found that five teeth on the lower right were so loose that they came out with little encouragement. Dr. Morrison determined that Hannah has partial loss (edentulism) of teeth due to periodontal disease, class I.

Let's Code It!

Hannah lost five teeth due to periodontal disease. Let's turn to the Alphabetic Index and find the key term of the diagnosis:

Edentulism — *see* Absence, teeth, acquired

Turn to:

Absence
    teeth, tooth (congenital) K00.0
        acquired (complete) K08.109
        partial K08.409
            class I K08.401
            class II K08.402
            class III K08.403
            class IV K08.404

Also take note of the listings within this long list for the loss of teeth due to caries (dental cavities), periodontal disease, trauma, or another specified cause. These will take you to other specific codes.

Refer to the physician's documentation and read that Hannah was diagnosed with *partial class I edentulism*, so let's turn to the Tabular List and find

    ✓4 **K08**   **Other disorders of teeth and supporting structures**

Read the EXCLUDES2 notation carefully. Does it have anything to do with this encounter? No! Great, so now review all the choices for the required fourth character and determine which one most accurately reports the diagnosis:

    ✓5 **K08.4**   **Partial loss of teeth**

There are EXCLUDES1 and EXCLUDES2 notes here. Read them carefully, and reread Dr. Morrison's documentation. Nothing there matches. Next, you must review the options for the fifth character.

> ✓6 **K08.42** Partial loss of teeth due to periodontal diseases
>
> Check the documentation. Dr. Morrison wrote that Hannah's loss of teeth was caused by the periodontitis, and it was class I. Review all of the choices, and determine the most accurate code:
>
> K08.421   Partial loss of teeth due to periodontal diseases, class I
>
> Good work!

Salivary Glands

As the teeth and tongue are breaking down food in preparation for the journey down the alimentary canal, three sets of major **salivary glands** (the parotid, submandibular, and sublingual glands) secrete saliva to moisten and bind the food particles. This begins the chemical digestion of carbohydrates, dissolves foods so their flavor can be appreciated, and helps enable swallowing of the food particles. In addition, saliva helps to clean the teeth and mouth after the particles leave the oral cavity.

As with almost any other part of the body, these glands can become infected. The salivary glands may be negatively impacted by either a bacterium or a virus, so be alert to check the pathology report.

Sialoadenitis, also known as parotitis, is described as acute, acute recurrent, or chronic. Note that *chronic* means ongoing (typically lasting more than 3 months), whereas *acute recurrent* means that the condition is severe, it clears up, and everything is fine for a while, but then it comes back again.

K11.21   Acute sialoadenitis
K11.22   Acute recurrent sialoadenitis
K11.23   Chronic sialoadenitis

Salivary Glands
Three sets of bilateral exocrine glands that secrete saliva: parotid glands, submaxillary glands, and sublingual glands.

YOU CODE IT! CASE STUDY

Isaac McNealy, a 37-year-old male, came in with complaints of pain in his face and mouth. He states that the pain becomes worse just before and during meals. He also claims that he has trouble swallowing and when he went to the dentist, he couldn't open his mouth very wide at all. Dr. Randolph did an ultrasound of Isaac's face and neck and confirmed that he was suffering with calculus of the salivary duct.

You Code It!

Read this documentation, and determine the correct ICD-10-CM diagnosis code or codes to report Dr. Randolph's diagnosis of Isaac's condition.

Step #1: Read the case carefully and completely.

Step #2: Abstract the scenario. Which main words or terms describe why the physician cared for the patient during this encounter?

Step #3: Are there any details missing or incomplete for which you would need to query the physician? [If so, ask your instructor.]

Step #4: Check for any relevant guidance, including reading all of the symbols and notations in the Tabular List and the appropriate sections of the Official Guidelines.

Step #5: Determine the correct diagnosis code or codes to explain why this encounter was medically necessary.

Step #6: Double-check your work.

(continued)

> **Answer:**
>
> Did you determine this to be the code?
>
> **K11.5   Sialolithiasis**
>   **(Calculus of salivary gland or duct)**

13.2 Conditions of the Esophagus and Stomach

Esophagus

The tubelike structure that connects the hypopharynx to the stomach is known as the **esophagus**. As you can see in Figure 13-2, the esophagus lies parallel and posterior to the trachea. Just as the epiglottis blocks food and liquid from entering the trachea, the esophagus has its own gateway, called the *upper esophageal sphincter,* to restrict the entrance of air into the stomach. A **sphincter** is a circular muscle that can open or close an opening. There are several sphincters along the alimentary canal.

A second esophageal sphincter is located at the juncture between the esophagus and the stomach (the lower esophageal sphincter). This sphincter is designed to prevent the contents of the stomach from splashing back up into the esophagus. When this sphincter does not function properly, the patient might experience chronic heartburn, nausea, and possibly a sore throat. This may lead to a diagnosis of gastroesophageal reflux disease (GERD).

Gastroesophageal Reflux Disease (GERD)

Heartburn may not seem like a big concern; however, for many patients with persistent heartburn, one of the first symptoms of GERD (gastroesophageal reflux disease) is an increased intensity of that burning or painful sensation when bending down, lying

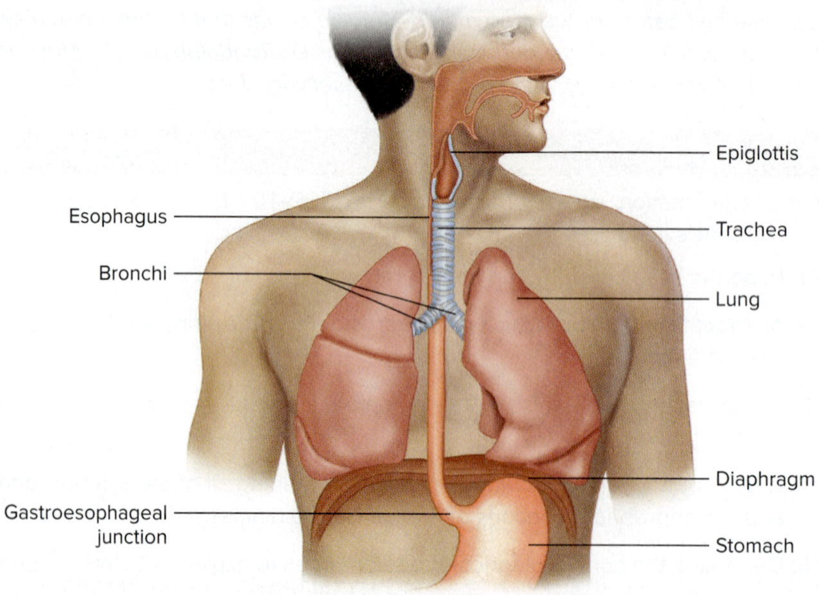

Esophagus
The tubular organ that connects the pharynx to the stomach for the passage of nourishment.

Sphincter
A circular muscle that contracts to prevent passage of liquids or solids.

FIGURE 13-2 An illustration showing the anatomical sites from the epiglottis to the gastroesophageal junction

down, or vigorously exercising. Dysphagia (difficulty with swallowing) and/or esophagitis may also occur.

GERD may be caused by a slacking lower esophageal sphincter, which separates the stomach from the esophagus and is designed to prevent backflow from the stomach upward.

> **EXAMPLES**
>
> K21.0   Gastro-esophageal reflux disease with esophagitis
>
> K21.9   Gastro-esophageal reflux disease without esophagitis

Stomach

The next organ along the alimentary canal is the **stomach**. As stated earlier, the stomach connects to the esophagus at the lower esophageal sphincter in the cardiac region of the stomach, also known as the *cardia*. To the left, the stomach curves upward, creating the fundic region, or **fundus**. A fundus is defined as a domed portion of a hollow organ that sits the farthest from, above, or opposite an opening. As you can see in Figure 13-3, the fundus of the stomach is located superior to (above) the opening to the esophagus.

The lining of the stomach, a mucous membrane, contains gastric glands that secrete gastric juices. As with the function of saliva in the processing of food in the mouth, the gastric juices support the extraction of nutritional elements in the contents that entered from the esophagus. Mucous cells coat the internal wall of the stomach to prevent the gastric juices from digesting it. When this coating is flawed, the patient might develop a gastric (peptic) ulcer, a condition in which the acids in the stomach actually eat a hole in the lining and wall of the stomach. This diagnosis is reported with code K25.9 Gastric ulcer, unspecified as acute or chronic, without hemorrhage or perforation.

As the shape of the stomach's body curves downward, the inside of the curve on the side of the cardia is referred to as the *lesser curvature,* and the outside curve, coming down from the fundus, is referred to as the *greater curvature*. The lower portion of the stomach narrows as it nears the duodenum and connects to the small intestine. The pyloric sphincter is located here to control the emptying of the contents of the stomach into the lower half of the digestive system.

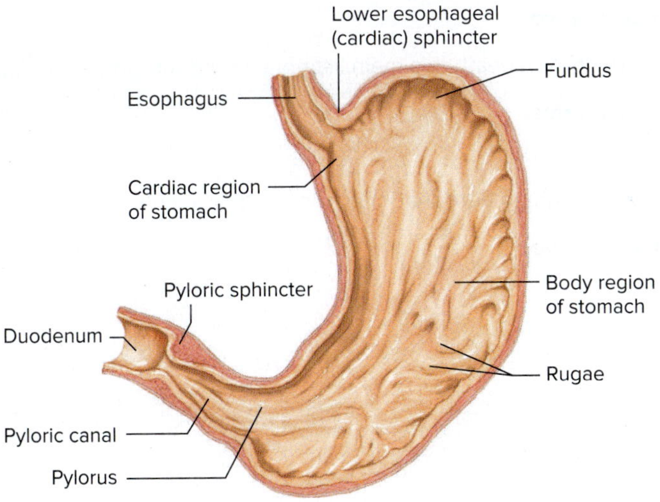

Stomach
A saclike organ within the alimentary canal designed to contain nourishment during the initial phase of the digestive process.

Fundus
The section of an organ farthest from its opening.

FIGURE 13-3 An illustration identifying the specific anatomical sites of the stomach

David Shier et al., *HOLE'S HUMAN ANATOMY & PHYSIOLOGY*, 12/e. ©2010 McGraw-Hill Education. Figure 17.17, p. 666. Used with permission.

> **EXAMPLES**
>
> K31.1   Adult hypertrophic pyloric stenosis
>
> K31.3   Pylorospasm, not elsewhere classified

Perforation
An atypical hole in the wall of an organ or anatomical site.

Hemorrhage
Excessive or severe bleeding.

Ulcers

An ulcer is a sore or hole in the tissue. Ulcers can occur externally, such as a decubitus ulcer, or they can form internally. The terms used to document an internal ulcer in the digestive system may include

- Ulcer of esophagus
- Gastric ulcer (in the lining of the stomach)
- Duodenal ulcer
- Gastrojejunal ulcer

You will notice that these descriptors identify the location of the ulcer, such as the esophagus, the stomach, or the jejunum.

Further description of these ulcers may include known complications resulting from an ulcer in this segment of the upper digestive system: **perforation** and **hemorrhage**.

> **CODING BITES**
>
> If a medication caused the ulcer, an external cause code will be required to identify the specific drug and whether or not it was taken for therapeutic purposes.

LET'S CODE IT! SCENARIO

Pauline Ochoa had been taking aspirin several times a day every day for pain in her knees. Her husband, John, came home and found her lying on the kitchen floor. Emergency medical services (EMS) brought her to the ED. Tests revealed an acute perforated, hemorrhaging peptic ulcer due to chronic use of aspirin.

Let's Code It!

Pauline was diagnosed with an *acute perforated, hemorrhaging peptic ulcer,* so let's turn to the Alphabetic Index of ICD-10-CM and find

    Ulcer, ulcerated, ulcerating, ulceration, ulcerative

There is a very long list of additional terms indented beneath this main listing, so read through it and find

    Ulcer, ulcerated, ulcerating, ulceration, ulcerative
        peptic (site unspecified) K27.9

Beneath *peptic* is another indented list. Is there anything here that matches the physician's notes?

    Ulcer, ulcerated, ulcerating, ulceration, ulcerative
        peptic (site unspecified) K27.9
            with
            hemorrhage K27.4
            and perforation K27.6
        acute K27.3
            with
            hemorrhage K27.0
            and perforation K27.2

Hmmm. The good news is that all of these choices are within one code category, K27, so let's turn to the Tabular List and begin reading at

> ☑4 **K27** Peptic ulcer, site unspecified
>
> *Use additional code* to identify alcohol abuse and dependence (F10.-)

Read the INCLUDES and EXCLUDES1 notes, as well as the *Use additional code* notation. Then read down and review all of the choices for the required fourth character. Which one matches the physician's notes the best?

> **K27.2** Acute peptic ulcer, site unspecified, with both hemorrhage and perforation

Excellent!

Are you done? No. Remember that notation beneath the code category?

> *Use additional code* to identify alcohol abuse and dependence (F10.-)

Was there any mention of alcohol abuse or alcohol dependence in the documentation? No. However, you do know that aspirin caused this ulcer. There is no notation, but remember that your job is to tell the *whole* story. So you will need to find an external cause code to report which drug caused Pauline's peptic ulcer. Aspirin is a drug, so let's turn to the *Table of Drugs and Chemicals* and find the name of the drug that caused Pauline's peptic ulcer in the first column ("Substance"): aspirin. Look across the line to the code listed in the column under "Adverse Effect." Remember that Pauline was taking the aspirin for therapeutic use—a medical reason. This shows code T39.015.

Let's turn to the T codes in the Tabular List and begin reading at

> ☑4 **T39** Poisoning by, adverse effect of and underdosing of nonopioid analgesics, antipyretics and antirheumatics

Notice that beneath this code category is a notation:

> **The appropriate 7th character is to be added to each code from category T39**
> **A** initial encounter
> **D** subsequent encounter
> **S** sequela

Remember, this is here for reference later. But first you need the fourth, fifth, and sixth characters. Read down and review all of the choices. Which one matches most accurately?

> ☑7 **T39.015-** Adverse effect of aspirin

Great! Now you need that seventh character. Go back to the documentation. Is this the first time that Pauline is being treated by this physician for this diagnosis? She is in the emergency department, so, yes, this is the initial encounter. Now you have two codes to report Pauline's condition:

> **K27.2** Acute peptic ulcer, site unspecified, with both hemorrhage and perforation
> **T39.015A** Adverse effect of aspirin, initial encounter

Hernias

A **hernia** is a condition that is created when a tear or opening in a muscle permits a part of an internal organ to push through. Due to the nature of one anatomical part squeezing through a hole in another site, the blood supply can be cut off to the section stuck in that opening. When that happens, the tissue might become necrotic (deteriorate and die) and/or develop **gangrene**. In addition, this condition can create an **obstruction** in the structure or organ, preventing the normal flow of material.

Hernia
A condition in which one anatomical structure pushes through a perforation in the wall of the anatomical site that normally contains that structure.

Gangrene
Necrotic tissue resulting from a loss of blood supply.

Obstruction
A blockage or closing.

> **CODING BITES**
>
> If an activity, such as lifting something very heavy, causes an inguinal hernia, or if a surgical procedure causes an incisional hernia, additional codes may be required to tell the whole story.

There are several types of hernias, or anatomical sites that can be susceptible to herniation:

- *Hiatal* (esophageal) hernia may occur when a portion of the stomach pokes through an opening in the diaphragm; congenital diaphragmatic hernias are considered birth defects and reported from the congenital malformations section of ICD-10-CM.
- *Umbilical* hernia may occur when the muscle around the navel (belly button) does not close completely, permitting an internal organ to protrude.
- *Incisional* hernia is a defect that may occur at the site of a previous abdominal surgical opening (scar tissue).
- *Inguinal* hernias, more common in men, appear in the groin area.
- *Femoral* hernias, more common in women, appear in the upper thigh.

YOU CODE IT! CASE STUDY

Jeffrey Gilberts, a 3-hours-old male, is brought in for Dr. Gensin to surgically repair his diaphragmatic hernia. He was born with this abnormal fistula in the diaphragm, diagnosed at 28 weeks gestation, but it was determined that he was not a candidate for in utero surgery.

You Code It!

Go through the steps of coding, and determine the code or codes that should be reported for this encounter between Dr. Gensin and Jeffrey Gilberts.

Step #1: Read the case carefully and completely.

Step #2: Abstract the scenario. Which main words or terms describe why the physician cared for the patient during this encounter?

Step #3: Are there any details missing or incomplete for which you would need to query the physician? [If so, ask your instructor.]

Step #4: Check for any relevant guidance, including reading all of the symbols and notations in the Tabular List and the appropriate sections of the Official Guidelines.

Step #5: Determine the correct diagnosis code or codes to explain why this encounter was medically necessary.

Step #6: Double-check your work.

Answer:

Did you determine this to be the correct code?

> Q79.0   Congenital diaphragmatic hernia

Good job!

13.3 Conditions Affecting the Intestines

Small Intestine

Duodenum
The first segment of the small intestine, connecting the stomach to the jejunum.

The inferior aspect of the pyloric sphincter is the **duodenum**, the first segment of the small intestine. The duodenum curves around like the letter "C," with the pancreas tucked in the center. The hepatopancreatic sphincter, also called the *sphincter of Oddi*, is the connection point between the duodenum, the pancreatic duct, and the common bile duct that comes from the gallbladder and the liver.

> **EXAMPLES**
>
> K29.80   Duodenitis without bleeding
>
> K31.5   Obstruction of duodenum

As the duodenum trails into that last portion, at the bottom of the "C," it curves around and becomes the **jejunum**, the segment of the small intestine that twists and turns throughout the abdomen (see Figure 13-4). The **mesentery** is a membrane that connects to the jejunum like a spider web filled with blood vessels, nerves, and lymphatic vessels to provide nourishment to the intestine. On the anterior side of the abdominal cavity, coming from the greater curvature of the stomach down to the anterior of the jejunum like a protective curtain, is a double fold of the peritoneum called the *greater omentum*.

The last segment of the small intestine is the **ileum**. The ileum connects to the **cecum**, the bridge to the large intestine via the ileocecal sphincter. This sphincter controls the passage of material from the small intestine into the large intestine.

Gastrojejunal Ulcer

A lesion that develops in the small intestine can be quite problematic because it may interfere with the absorption of nutrients in the digestive process. As you review documentation for a diagnosis of a gastrojejunal ulcer, you will need to abstract some key details:

1. **Is the ulcer identified as acute or chronic?**

    K28.0–K28.3   Acute gastrojejunal ulcer . . .

    K28.4–K28.7   Chronic gastrojejunal ulcer . . .

2. **Is the ulcer hemorrhaging?**

    K28.0   Acute gastrojejunal ulcer with hemorrhage

    K28.4   Chronic or unspecified gastrojejunal ulcer with hemorrhage

> **CODING BITES**
>
> Be careful to not confuse il*e*um (with an *e*), the end of the small intestine, with il*i*um (with an *i*), the widest portion of the pelvic bones.
>
> - il*e*um is the end of the small intestine. Connect *ileum* with *end*.
> - il*i*um is a portion of the hip bone. Think of the *i* in *hip*.

Jejunum
The segment of the small intestine that connects the duodenum to the ileum.

Mesentery
A fold of a membrane that carries blood to the small intestine and connects it to the posterior wall of the abdominal cavity.

Ileum
The last segment of the small intestine.

Cecum
A pouchlike organ that connects the ileum with the large intestine; the point of connection for the vermiform appendix.

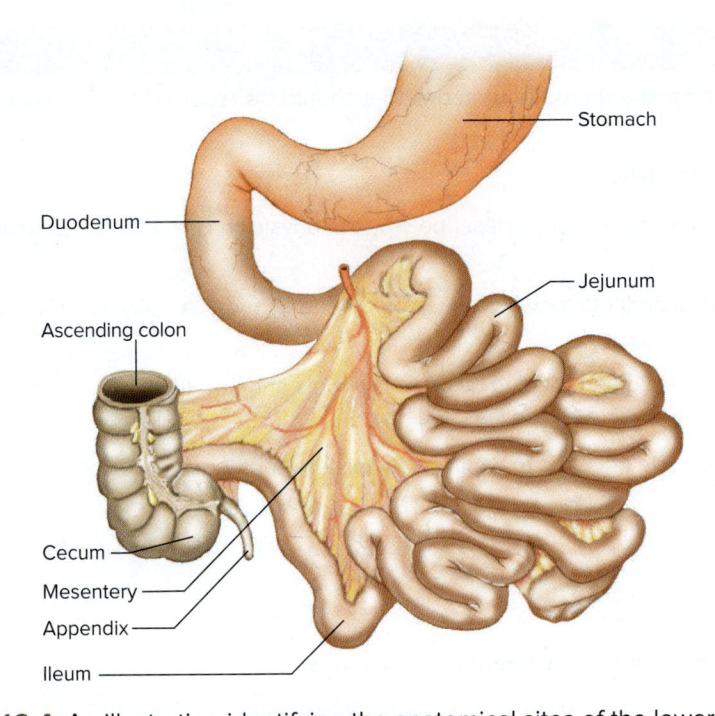

FIGURE 13-4 An illustration identifying the anatomical sites of the lower alimentary canal from the stomach to the cecum   David Shier et al., *HOLE'S HUMAN ANATOMY & PHYSIOLOGY*, 12/e. ©2010 McGraw-Hill Education. Figure 17.31, p. 680. Used with permission.

3. **Has the ulcer perforated the wall of the small intestine?**

   K28.1   Acute gastrojejunal ulcer with perforation
   K28.5   Chronic or unspecified gastrojejunal ulcer with perforation

4. **Are hemorrhage and perforation both documented?**

   K28.2   Acute gastrojejunal ulcer with both hemorrhage and perforation
   K28.6   Chronic or unspecified gastrojejunal ulcer with both hemorrhage and perforation

5. **Has either hemorrhage or perforation been documented individually? If not . . .**

   K28.3   Acute gastrojejunal ulcer without hemorrhage or perforation
   K28.7   Chronic or unspecified gastrojejunal ulcer without hemorrhage or perforation

Of course, be certain to read the notations at the top of this code category:

Use additional code to identify alcohol abuse and dependence (F10.-)

EXCLUDES1 *primary ulcer of small intestine (K63.3)*

Read the documentation carefully, again, to determine if the physician noted whether the patient suffers with alcohol abuse or alcohol dependence. If so, you will need to code this, as well.

The jejunum is one specific part of the small intestine. The small intestine includes the duodenum, jejunum, mesentery, ileum, and cecum.

YOU CODE IT! CASE STUDY

Bernadette Bowers, a 29-year-old female, came to see Dr. Grandem with symptoms of persistent diarrhea and ongoing right lower quadrant (RLQ) abdominal pain. Lab work showed an increased white blood cell count and erythrocyte sedimentation rate. A barium enema showed string sign. A biopsy confirmed a diagnosis of Crohn's disease of the jejunum.

You Code It!

Go through the steps of coding, and determine the code or codes that should be reported for this encounter between Dr. Grandem and Bernadette.

Step #1: Read the case carefully and completely.

Step #2: Abstract the scenario. Which key words or terms describe why the physician cared for the patient during this encounter?

Step #3: Are there any details missing or incomplete for which you would need to query the physician? [If so, ask your instructor.]

Step #4: Check for any relevant guidance, including reading all of the symbols and notations in the Tabular List and the appropriate sections of the Official Guidelines.

Step #5: Determine the correct diagnosis code or codes to explain why this encounter was medically necessary.

Step #6: Double-check your work.

Answer:

Did you determine this to be the correct code?

     K50.00   **Crohn's disease of the small intestine without complications**

Good job!

Large Intestine

The colon is also known as the large intestine. As you look at the illustration (see Figure 13-5), you might wonder why it is considered large when the small intestine seems to be so much longer. This distinction has nothing to do with length; the large intestine has a larger diameter.

You may notice that the two terms *colon* and *large intestine* are used almost interchangeably. In reality, they are technically not the same thing. The large intestine consists of the cecum, the vermiform appendix, the colon, the rectum, and the anus. The colon represents the majority of the large intestine. Let's take a look at the parts of the large intestine.

Starting at the cecum, the colon frames the abdomen almost like the beltway around Washington, D.C., and is referred to in four segments.

The ileum of the small intestine connects to the **ascending colon** on the right side of the large intestine at the cecum. The **vermiform appendix**, a rounded tubular appendage, protrudes from the end of the cecum. The ascending colon stretches upward from the cecum to just below the liver in the superior aspect of the abdomen. At this point, this tubular structure makes a sharp left turn, known as the *hepatic flexure* (named

Ascending Colon
The portion of the large intestine that connects the cecum to the hepatic flexure.

Vermiform Appendix
A long, narrow mass of tissue attached to the cecum; also called *appendix*.

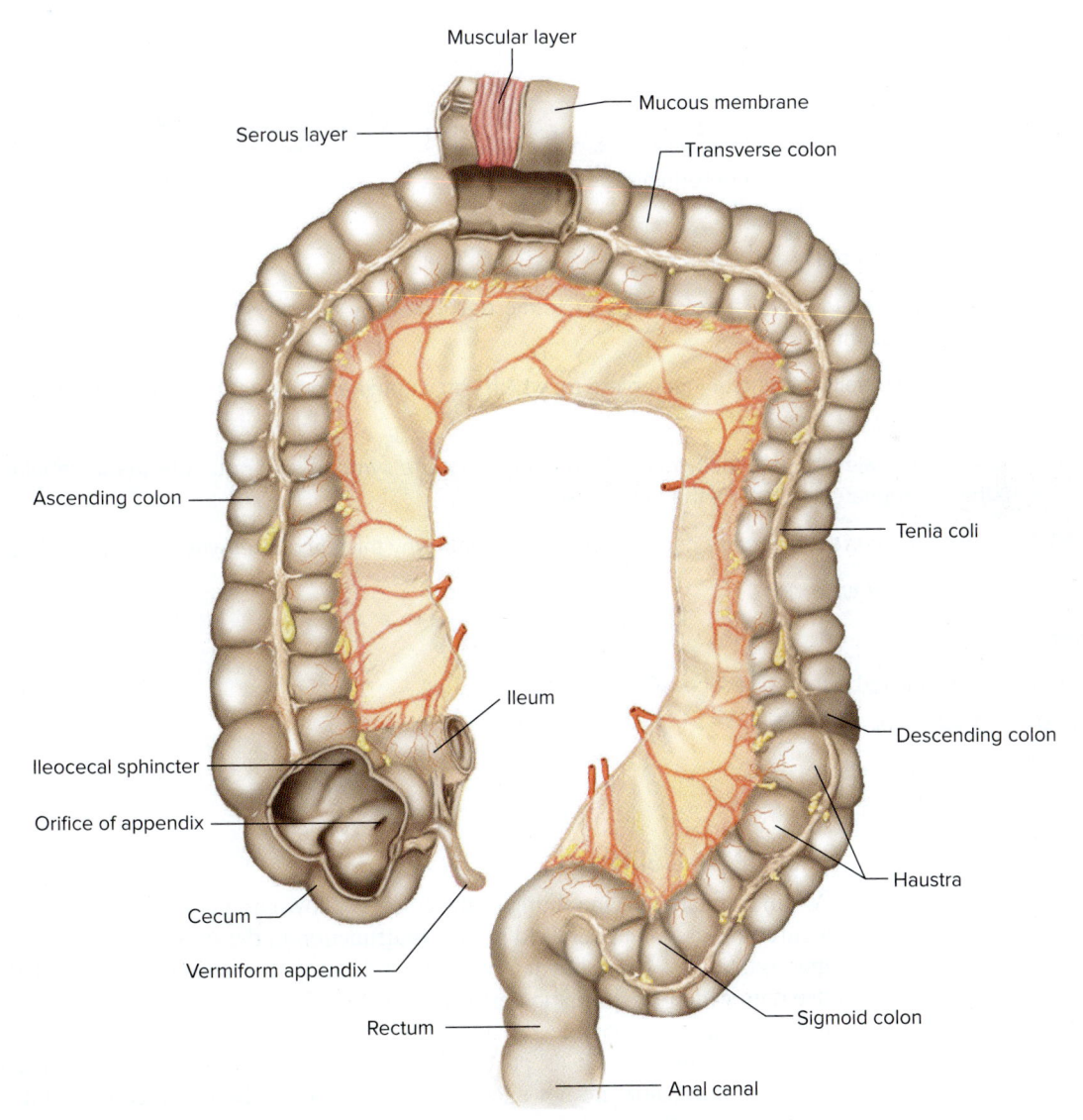

FIGURE 13-5 An illustration identifying the anatomical sites of the large intestine David Shier et al., *HOLE'S HUMAN ANATOMY & PHYSIOLOGY*, 12/e. ©2010 McGraw-Hill Education. Figure 17.43, p. 687. Used with permission.

Transverse Colon
The portion of the large intestine that connects the hepatic flexure to the splenic flexure.

Descending Colon
The segment of the large intestine that connects the splenic flexure to the sigmoid colon.

Sigmoid Colon
The dual-curved segment of the colon that connects the descending colon to the rectum; also referred to as the *sigmoid flexure*.

because of the proximity to the liver) and runs across to the left side. This section is known as the **transverse colon** because it traverses across the abdomen (*transverse* = across). On the left side, the colon turns downward at a curve known as the *splenic flexure* (named because of the proximity to the spleen), becoming the **descending colon**. It continues down until it slightly curves, just above the pelvis, and becomes the **sigmoid colon**.

The large intestine turns again, downward. This area is called the **rectum** (rectal vault), and it leads directly into the anal canal. At the distal end of the anal canal, the *internal and external anal sphincters* form the **anus**—the opening to the outside.

> **EXAMPLES**
> K51.20   Ulcerative (chronic) proctitis without complications
> K56.41   Fecal impaction of the intestine
> K35.3   Acute appendicitis with localized peritonitis

YOU CODE IT! CASE STUDY

Gerald Candahar, a 51-year-old male, was brought into the procedure room so Dr. Avalino could remove his anal polyps.

You Code It!

Go through the steps of coding, and determine the code or codes that should be reported for this encounter between Dr. Avalino and Gerald.

Step #1: Read the case carefully and completely.

Step #2: Abstract the scenario. Which key words or terms describe why the physician cared for the patient during this encounter?

Step #3: Are there any details missing or incomplete for which you would need to query the physician? [If so, ask your instructor.]

Step #4: Check for any relevant guidance, including reading all of the symbols and notations in the Tabular List and the appropriate sections of the Official Guidelines.

Step #5: Determine the correct diagnosis code or codes to explain why this encounter was medically necessary.

Step #6: Double-check your work.

Answer:

Did you determine this to be the correct code?

   K62.0   Anal polyp

Good job!

Rectum
The last segment of the large intestine, connecting the sigmoid colon to the anus.

Anus
The portion of the large intestine that leads outside the body.

Ulcerative Colitis

An inflammation of the lining of the colon is known as ulcerative colitis. This is often a chronic illness and believed to be a malfunction in the immune response within the mucosa. Studies have shown a familial tendency. Signs and symptoms include bloody diarrhea with asymptomatic periods of time between attacks. Abdominal pain, irritability, weight loss, weakness, nausea, and vomiting are also indicators.

Manifestations, such as pancolitis, proctitis, rectosigmoiditis, and inflammatory polyps in the colon are not uncommon. In addition, the presence of rectal bleeding, obstruction within the intestinal tract, fistulae, and abscesses must be included in the code or codes, as documented.

The terms you need to abstract from the documentation will lead you to the correct fourth character to identify the manifestations:

- ☑5 K51.0   Ulcerative (chronic) pancolitis
- ☑5 K51.2   Ulcerative (chronic) proctitis
- ☑5 K51.3   Ulcerative (chronic) rectosigmoiditis
- ☑5 K51.4   Inflammatory polyps of colon
- ☑5 K51.5   Left sided colitis
- ☑5 K51.8   Other ulcerative colitis

Then, fifth and sixth characters will identify the presence of rectal bleeding, intestinal obstruction, fistula, abscess, or other complication.

Diverticular Disease of the Intestine

Since the first page of this book, you have learned that you must read carefully and completely, and this habit will be especially important when determining the code for a patient diagnosed with diverticular disease. There are two conditions, which are very different, reported from code category ☑4 K57 Diverticular disease of intestine:

- *Diverticulosis:* small pouches develop and protrude outward through the intestine
- *Diverticulitis:* when these pouches become inflamed or infected

While abstracting the documentation, you will also need to determine:

1. Is the small intestine, the large intestine, or both affected?
2. Is there mention of perforation, abscess, or bleeding?

YOU CODE IT! CASE STUDY

Lisa Begas, a 63-year-old female, came in complaining of a low-grade fever with chills for 3 days, nausea and vomiting, and cramps. Dr. Allendale did a CT scan of her abdomen and pelvis, and determined that she had diverticulitis without perforation or bleeding of the colon.

You Code It!

Read the scenario of Dr. Allendale's encounter with Lisa, and determine the accurate diagnosis code or codes.

Step #1: Read the case carefully and completely.

Step #2: Abstract the scenario. Which main words or terms describe why the physician cared for the patient during this encounter?

Step #3: Are there any details missing or incomplete for which you would need to query the physician? [If so, ask your instructor.]

Step #4: Check for any relevant guidance, including reading all of the symbols and notations in the Tabular List and the appropriate sections of the Official Guidelines.

Step #5: Determine the correct diagnosis code or codes to explain why this encounter was medically necessary.

Step #6: Double-check your work.

Answer:

Did you determine this to be the code?

K57.32   Diverticulitis of large intestine without perforation or abscess without bleeding

13.4 Dysfunction of the Digestive Accessory Organs and Malabsorption

The digestive **accessory organs** play a role in the way the body processes food and water so that each tissue and organ system has the fuel to function. These organs secrete enzymes, alkalis, and other substances that are required for the process of digestion, and they include the gallbladder, liver, and pancreas. The accessory organs connect to the alimentary canal and support it, but they are not a part of it.

Gallbladder

In the top left corner of Figure 13-6, the pear-shaped pouch is the **gallbladder**. This sac is a storage tank for bile, a yellow-green liquid created by the liver and used by the body to assist in the digestive process. When required, the gallbladder contracts to release bile into the duodenum via the **common bile duct** and the hepatopancreatic ampulla. The common bile duct is the juncture where the *hepatic duct* (which comes from the liver) meets the *cystic duct* (which comes from the gallbladder). At the *hepatopancreatic sphincter,* both the common bile duct and the pancreatic duct meet to continue into the duodenum.

> **EXAMPLES**
>
> K81.0   Acute cholecystitis
>
> K82.3   Fistula of gallbladder

Accessory Organs
Organs that assist the digestive process and are adjacent to the alimentary canal: the gallbladder, liver, and pancreas.

Gallbladder
A pear-shaped organ that stores bile until it is required to aid the digestive process.

Common Bile Duct
The juncture of the cystic duct of the gallbladder and the hepatic duct from the liver.

CODING BITES

Due to the interactive nature of the anatomical organs in this small area of the body, you may notice long, complex medical terms used in diagnostic statements. Don't be intimidated; just use your knowledge from medical terminology class and parse the terms. For example: choledocholithiasis: *chole* = bile + *docho* = common bile duct + *lith* = calculus + *iasis* = pathologic condition.

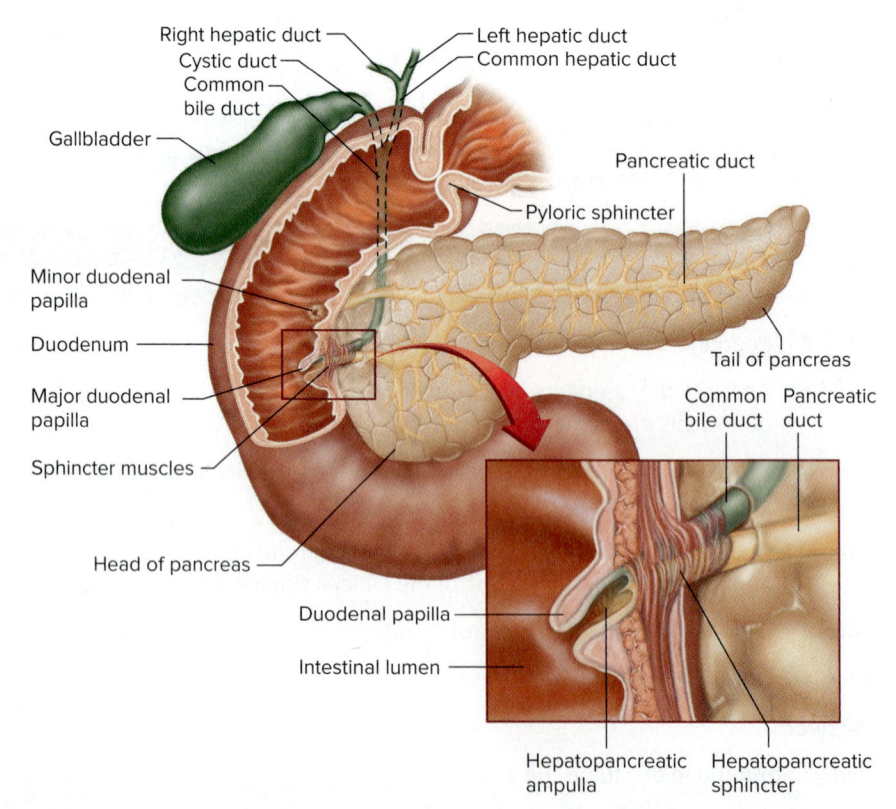

FIGURE 13-6 An illustration identifying the anatomical sites within the accessory organs   David Shier et al., HOLE'S HUMAN ANATOMY & PHYSIOLOGY, 12/e. ©2010 McGraw-Hill Education. Figure 17.23, p. 672. Used with permission.

Cholecystitis

Cholecystitis is the medical term for inflammation of the gallbladder (*chole* = bile + *cyst* = fluid-filled sac + *-itis* = inflammation). In cases where the disease affects the bile duct rather than the gallbladder, the diagnosis is cholangitis.

Calculi can accumulate in this area and harden into small rocks (stones) that may block the flow of bile from the gallbladder. This condition is known as **cholelithiasis**. This may occur with or without cholecystitis, changing the code used to report the condition.

Cholelithiasis
Gallstones.

> **EXAMPLES**
>
> K80.70   Calculus of gallbladder and bile duct without cholecystitis without obstruction
> K81.1   Chronic cholecystitis

Pancreas

Situated posterior to the stomach, tucked inside a curve of the duodenum, is the **pancreas**. The section of the pancreas adjacent to the duodenum, called the *head of the pancreas,* extends to the center section (the body of the pancreas), which extends to the tail of the pancreas, which forms almost a fingerlike shape. The **pancreatic islets** (the islets of Langerhans) create glucagon and insulin, as well as other hormones, and secrete them into the bloodstream. Similar to the gallbladder, the pancreas manufactures certain digestive enzymes that pass into the duodenum via the pancreatic duct (see Figure 13-6).

Malfunction of the pancreas may lead to various health problems, including pancreatic cancer, pancreatitis, cystic fibrosis, and diabetes mellitus. One of the most dangerous concerns about the impact on the body of conditions of the pancreas is that signs and symptoms are few and nonspecific, making diagnosis difficult. For example, there is actually a treatment for pancreatic cancer. However, due to lack of signs and symptoms that typically promote early identification and treatment, diagnosis is not often realized until the malignancy has metastasized to other organs and cannot be halted.

Pancreas
A gland that secretes insulin and other hormones from the islet cells into the bloodstream and manufactures digestive enzymes that are secreted into the duodenum.

Pancreatic Islets
Cells within the pancreas that secrete insulin and other hormones into the bloodstream.

Liver
The organ, located in the upper right area of the abdominal cavity, that is responsible for regulating blood sugar levels; secreting bile for the gallbladder; metabolizing fats, proteins, and carbohydrates; manufacturing some blood proteins; and removing toxins from the blood.

Pancreatitis

Acute pancreatitis occurs suddenly and usually goes away in a few days with treatment. However, when you are determining the correct code for this diagnosis, you must abstract the underlying cause of the pancreatitis:

K85.0-   Idiopathic acute pancreatitis
K85.1-   Biliary acute pancreatitis
K85.2-   Alcohol-induced acute pancreatitis
K85.3-   Drug-induced acute pancreatitis

Note that alcohol-induced acute pancreatitis and alcohol-induced chronic pancreatitis are reported from different code categories.

K86.0   Alcohol-induced chronic pancreatitis

Liver

The **liver** is an almost triangular-shaped organ (see Figure 13-7) located in the right upper quadrant (RUQ) of the abdominal cavity, beneath the diaphragm, anterior to the stomach and pancreas. As the largest gland in the body, it performs many functions, including regulating blood sugar levels and aiding the digestive process by secreting bile to the gallbladder. The liver cleans the blood of toxins; metabolizes proteins, fats, and carbohydrates; and manufactures some blood proteins.

> **CODING BITES**
>
> The medical root *hepa-* or *hepat-* is used in most diagnoses and other descriptive terms to refer to the liver as the anatomical site involved. For example, the term *hepatic failure* identifies a condition that has rendered the liver ineffective.

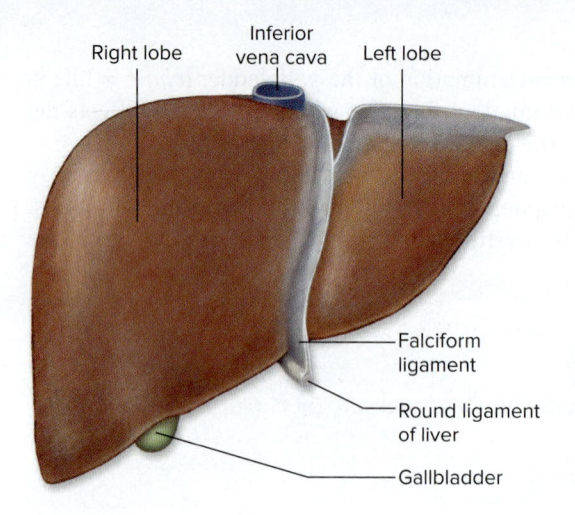

FIGURE 13-7 An illustration identifying the anatomical sites of the liver (anterior view) Michael McKinley and Valerie O'Loughlin, HUMAN ANATOMY, 1/e. ©2006 McGraw-Hill Education. Figure 26.19, p. 815. Used with permission.

CODING BITES

You will need to determine from the documentation if the use (abuse) of alcohol has contributed to the diagnosis because this may affect the determination of the correct code or the need for an additional code. At code category K70, Alcoholic liver disease, is a notation to remind you:

Use additional code **to identify alcohol abuse and dependence (F10.-)**

Hepatitis

Hepatitis (*hepa-* = liver + *-itis* = inflammation or disease) is a swelling of the liver that causes a reduction in function. Most often, hepatitis is caused by a virus, resulting in a diagnosis that includes the specific type of inflammation, such as hepatitis A, hepatitis B, and so on. (For more details on this condition, see the chapter *Coding Infectious Diseases*).

There are cases when drugs and alcohol can lead to this same diagnosis. Identified as acute or chronic nonviral hepatitis, most patients will exhibit signs and symptoms very similar to viral hepatitis, including nausea, vomiting, and jaundice (yellowing of the skin). Take a look at the *Use additional code* notation beneath code category:

K70   **Alcoholic liver disease**

Use additional code to identify: alcohol abuse and dependence (F10.-)

EXAMPLES

B18.2	Chronic viral hepatitis C
K70.10	Alcoholic hepatitis without ascites
K76.4	Peliosis hepatis

Cirrhosis

After a person suffers with chronic hepatic disease, fibrotic tissue may form on hepatic cells causing scarring, known as *cirrhosis of the liver*. This condition may be caused by injury as well. The scar tissue impairs the normal function of the liver and can result in easy bruising or bleeding, abdominal swelling, lower extremity edema, and possibly kidney failure. There is evidence that approximately 5% of patients suffering with cirrhosis will develop liver cancer.

EXAMPLES

K74.3	Primary biliary cirrhosis
K74.69	Other cirrhosis of liver

YOU CODE IT! CASE STUDY

After struggling to deal with a sharp pain that went from his stomach area straight through to his back, Saul Braverman went to see Dr. Spiegel. After a full examination and an ultrasound, Dr. Spiegel confirmed Saul's cholelithiasis and they discussed plans for surgery.

> **You Code It!**
>
> Abstract this documentation about the encounter between Dr. Spiegel and Saul.
>
> Step #1: Read the case carefully and completely.
>
> Step #2: Abstract the scenario. Which main words or terms describe why the physician cared for the patient during this encounter?
>
> Step #3: Are there any details missing or incomplete for which you would need to query the physician? [If so, ask your instructor.]
>
> Step #4: Check for any relevant guidance, including reading all of the symbols and notations in the Tabular List and the appropriate sections of the Official Guidelines.
>
> Step #5: Determine the correct diagnosis code or codes to explain why this encounter was medically necessary.
>
> Step #6: Double-check your work.
>
> **Answer:**
>
> Did you determine this to be the code?
>
> K80.20   Calculus of gallbladder without cholecystitis without obstruction

Celiac Disease

While you may see a great deal in the news and advertisements about gluten-free products, the facts support that celiac disease, also known as gluten enteropathy, is uncommon. This condition is suffered by twice as many women than men, and has been seen to be familial (common in families).

Recurrent attacks of diarrhea, abdominal distention due to flatulence, stomach cramps, and weakness are some of the most frequently experienced signs and symptoms. When diagnosed in adults, celiac disease may be the underlying cause of multiple ulcers forming within the lining of the small intestine. Biopsies from the small bowel, identifying histologic changes, would confirm this diagnosis.

> **EXAMPLE**
>
> K90.0 Celiac disease
> *Use additional code* for associated disorders including:
>   dermatitis herpetiformis (L13.0)
>   gluten ataxia (G32.81)
> **Code also** exocrine pancreatic insufficiency (K86.81)

13.5 Reporting the Involvement of Alcohol in Digestive Disorders

Alcohol abuse can increase the risk of developing several serious disorders of the digestive system. When the documentation includes a connection of alcohol abuse in the diagnosis, you will need to report this with an additional code.

When reading the documentation for digestive system disorders, be aware of these diagnoses which are known to be connected to alcohol abuse. If there is any indication, you might need to query the physician.

- *Mouth cancer and gum disease:* Alcohol abuse increases the risk, second only to tobacco abuse.

> **CODING BITES**
>
> In some cases, throughout the ICD-10-CM Tabular List will remind you that the involvement of alcohol abuse must also be reported:
>
> ✓4 **K05** Gingivitis and periodontal diseases
>
> *Use additional code* to identify:
>   alcohol abuse and dependence (F10.-)

- *GERD and gastritis:* Excessive use of alcohol can damage the sphincter between the esophagus and the stomach, permitting stomachs acids to backwash into the esophagus. The lining of the stomach can also become irritated.
- *Malabsorption and malnutrition:* The consistent and excessive intake of alcohol can interfere with the body's ability to absorb nutrients.
- *Pancreatitis:* Alcohol abuse can cause inflammation in the pancreas and interfere with the proper function of the digestive process.
- *Alcoholic liver disease:* Alcohol abuse can cause this condition, a precursor to cirrhosis.

YOU CODE IT! CASE STUDY

Noel Cooper, a 43-year-old male, came to see Dr. Briscow with complaints of epigastric discomfort, nausea, and indigestion, over the last several days. He admits to drinking alcohol at lunch and dinner daily. He states he often has a couple in the evening as well. A gastroscopy was performed, and Dr. Briscow confirmed a diagnosis of acute gastritis due to alcohol abuse.

You Code It!

Review the details of this encounter between Dr. Briscow and Noel Cooper.

Step #1: Read the case carefully and completely.

Step #2: Abstract the scenario. Which main words or terms describe why the physician cared for the patient during this encounter?

Step #3: Are there any details missing or incomplete for which you would need to query the physician? [If so, ask your instructor.]

Step #4: Check for any relevant guidance, including reading all of the symbols and notations in the Tabular List and the appropriate sections of the Official Guidelines.

Step #5: Determine the correct diagnosis code or codes to explain why this encounter was medically necessary.

Step #6: Double-check your work.

Answer:

Did you determine these to be the codes?

K29.00	Acute gastritis without bleeding
F10.188	Alcohol abuse with other alcohol-induced disorder

Good job!!

Chapter Summary

The organs included in the digestive system run from the head to the bottom of the torso. Therefore, several different health care specialists may be involved in caring for patients with digestive disorders, depending upon where the abnormality is located. Health care issues within the digestive system can occur as the result of a congenital anomaly, a traumatic event, or dietary influence. This means that there may be times when an external cause code is required to be included so that you can tell the whole story about the reasons why (the medical necessity) this patient was cared for.

CODING BITES

Health Conditions Connected to Poor Oral Hygiene

Disease of the gums of the mouth, known as *periodontal disease,* has been shown to affect the health of other organs throughout the body. Some examples include:

Cardiovascular system	• Increased risk of stroke • Increased risk of fatal heart attack • Increased risk of cardiovascular disease • Increased risk of clotting disorder
Respiratory system	Bacteria from mouth, dental plaque buildup, and throat can contribute to pneumonia and other lung diseases.
Musculoskeletal system	Increased risk of osteopenia.
Endocrine system	Interference with control of diabetes mellitus.
Reproductive system	• During gestation, mothers with advanced periodontitis are at increased risk for premature and/or underweight neonates. • Microbes from periodontitis can cross through the placenta and expose the fetus to infection.

CHAPTER 13 REVIEW
Coding Digestive System Conditions

Let's Check It! Terminology

Match each key term to the appropriate definition.

Part I

1. LO 13.1 Small, calcified protrusions with roots in the jaw. **K**
2. LO 13.4 Cells within the pancreas that secrete insulin and other hormones into the bloodstream. **H**
3. LO 13.4 A large gland responsible for creating digestive enzymes. **G**
4. LO 13.3 The last segment of the small intestine. **D**
5. LO 13.2 A saclike organ within the alimentary canal designed to contain nourishment during the initial phase of the digestive process. **J**
6. LO 13.3 A long, narrow mass of tissue attached to the cecum; also called *appendix.* **L**
7. LO 13.3 The last segment of the large intestine, connecting the sigmoid colon to the anus. **I**
8. LO 13.2 The tubular organ that connects the pharynx to the stomach for the passage of nourishment. **C**
9. LO 13.4 The organ, located in the upper right area of the abdominal cavity, that is responsible for regulating blood sugar levels; secreting bile for the gallbladder; metabolizing fats, proteins, and carbohydrates; manufacturing some blood proteins; and removing toxins from the blood. **F**

A. Anus
B. Duodenum
C. Esophagus
D. Ileum
E. Jejunum
F. Liver
G. Pancreas
H. Pancreatic Islets
I. Rectum

CHAPTER 13 REVIEW

10. LO 13.3 The portion of the large intestine that leads outside the body. A
11. LO 13.3 The first segment of the small intestine, connecting the stomach to the jejunum. B
12. LO 13.3 The segment of the small intestine that connects the duodenum to the ileum. E

J. Stomach
K. Teeth
L. Vermiform Appendix

Part II

1. LO 13.3 A pouchlike organ that connects the ileum with the large intestine; the point of connection for the vermiform appendix. B
2. LO 13.3 The segment of the large intestine that connects the splenic flexure to the sigmoid colon. D
3. LO 13.3 The portion of the large intestine that connects the hepatic flexure to the splenic flexure. H
4. LO 13.4 The juncture of the cystic duct of the gallbladder and the hepatic duct from the liver. C
5. LO 13.3 The portion of the large intestine that connects the cecum to the hepatic flexure. A
6. LO 13.3 The dual-curved segment of the colon that connects the descending colon to the rectum. G
7. LO 13.1 The opening in the face that begins the alimentary canal and is used for the input of nutrition; also known as the *mouth*. E
8. LO 13.1 Three sets of bilateral exocrine glands that secrete saliva: parotid glands, submaxillary glands, and the sublingual glands. F

A. Ascending Colon
B. Cecum
C. Common Bile Duct
D. Descending Colon
E. Oral Cavity
F. Salivary Glands
G. Sigmoid Colon
H. Transverse Colon

Part III

1. LO 13.2 A blockage or closing. J
2. LO 13.2 An atypical hole in the wall of an organ or anatomical site. K
3. LO 13.4 Organs that assist the digestive process and are adjacent to the alimentary canal: the gallbladder, liver, and pancreas. A
4. LO 13.4 Gallstones. B
5. LO 13.3 A fold of a membrane that carries blood to the small intestine and connects it to the posterior wall of the abdominal cavity. I
6. LO 13.2 A circular muscle that contracts to prevent passage of liquids or solids. L
7. LO 13.4 A pear-shaped organ that stores bile until it is required to aid the digestive process. E
8. LO 13.2 The section of an organ farthest from its opening. D
9. LO 13.1 Absence of teeth. C
10. LO 13.2 A condition in which one anatomical structure pushes through a perforation in the wall of the anatomical site that normally contains that structure. H
11. LO 13.2 Necrotic tissue resulting from a loss of blood supply. F
12. LO 13.2 Excessive or severe bleeding. G

A. Accessory Organs
B. Cholelithiasis
C. Edentulism
D. Fundus
E. Gallbladder
F. Gangrene
G. Hemorrhage
H. Hernia
I. Mesentery
J. Obstruction
K. Perforation
L. Sphincter

Let's Check It! Concepts

Choose the most appropriate answer for each of the following questions.

1. LO 13.2 The correct code for a diaphragmatic hernia with obstruction without gangrene is
   a. K44
   b. K44.0
   c. K44.1
   d. K44.9

2. LO 13.3 The duodenum, jejunum, and ileum are all parts of the
   a. esophagus.   b. liver.   **c.** small intestine.   d. large intestine.
3. LO 13.1 When you are abstracting the documentation regarding acquired loss of teeth: Class _____ establishes the existence of other factors significantly affecting the outcomes of treatment and the need for surgical revision of the supporting structures (gums and bone) to create an opportunity for prosthodontics.
   a. I   b. II   **c.** III   d. IV
4. LO 13.4 Cirrhosis of the liver can be caused by
   a. abuse of alcohol.   b. trauma.   c. disease.   **d.** all of these.
5. LO 13.2 A hiatal hernia occurs at the
   a. esophagus.   b. small intestine.   c. surgical site.   d. groin.
6. LO 13.3 What is the correct code for an acute appendicitis with localized peritonitis?
   a. K35.2   **b.** K35.3   c. K35.8   d. K35.89
7. LO 13.3 The transverse colon lies between the
   a. ascending colon and the hepatic flexure.   **b.** hepatic flexure and the splenic flexure.
   c. splenic flexure and the sigmoid colon.   d. sigmoid colon and the anus.
8. LO 13.4 Cholelithiasis is commonly known as
   a. disease of the liver.   b. disease of the colon.   **c.** gallstones.   d. pancreatic cancer.
9. LO 13.2 Necrotic tissue resulting from a loss of blood supply is known as
   a. obstruction.   b. hemorrhage.   c. perforation.   **d.** gangrene.
10. LO 13.5 All of the following are known be diagnoses that could be connected to alcohol abuse *except*
    a. GERD.   b. pancreatitis.
    c. malabsorption and malnutrition.   **d.** all of these could be connected to alcohol abuse.

Let's Check It! Rules and Regulations

Please answer the following questions from the knowledge you have gained after reading this chapter.

1. LO 13.1 When you are abstracting the documentation regarding acquired loss of teeth, you will need to identify three specified details from the notes. What are the three details?
2. LO 13.2 Explain the condition of GERD.
3. LO 13.3 What are some of the key details you will need to abstract from the documentation when coding a gastrojejunal ulcer?
4. LO 13.4 Which is the largest gland in the body? Where is it located, and what is its function?
5. LO 13.5 Discuss how alcohol abuse can affect the digestive system.

YOU CODE IT! Basics

First, identify the condition in the following diagnoses; then code the diagnosis.

Example: Acute pulpitis
   a. main term: *Pulpitis*   b. diagnosis: *K04.0*

1. Dental caries on pit and fissure surface, penetrating into dentin:
   a. main term: _____   b. diagnosis: _____

2. Acute generalized periodontitis severe:
   a. main term: _____   b. diagnosis: _____

3. Odontogenic cyst:
   a. main term: _____   b. diagnosis: _____

4. Exfoliative cheilitis:
   a. main term: _____   b. diagnosis: _____

CHAPTER 13 | CODING DIGESTIVE SYSTEM CONDITIONS   377

CHAPTER 13 REVIEW

5. Leukoplakia of oral mucosa:
   a. main term: _____   b. diagnosis: _____
6. Hypertrophy of tongue papillae:
   a. main term: _____   b. diagnosis: _____
7. Eosinophilic esophagitis:
   a. main term: _____   b. diagnosis: _____
8. Acute gastric ulcer:
   a. main term: _____   b. diagnosis: _____
9. Alcoholic gastritis:
   a. main term: _____   b. diagnosis: _____
10. Hyperplasia of the appendix:
    a. main term: _____   b. diagnosis: _____
11. Inguinal hernia with gangrene:
    a. main term: _____   b. diagnosis: _____
12. Inflammatory polyps of colon with abscess:
    a. main term: _____   b. diagnosis: _____
13. Chronic ischemic colitis:
    a. main term: _____   b. diagnosis: _____
14. Rectal prolapse:
    a. main term: _____   b. diagnosis: _____
15. Radiation proctitis:
    a. main term: _____   b. diagnosis: _____

YOU CODE IT! Practice

Using the techniques described in this chapter, carefully read through the case studies and determine the most accurate ICD-10-CM code(s) and external cause code(s), if appropriate, for each case study.

1. Dorothea Greig, a 26-year-old female, presents with the complaint of persistent pain in her lower left abdomen, 1 week duration. Dorothea says she has also experienced nausea and vomiting. Dr. Hendrix notes weakness and a temperature of 102.2 F. The decision is made to admit the patient. Following a review of the laboratory tests, liver function tests, and the CT scan, Dorothea is diagnosed with diverticulitis of both the small and large intestines; abscess is noted.

2. Kent Rhodes, a 28-month-old male, is brought in by his parents for a checkup. Dr. Washington notes Kent's deciduous teeth are smaller than normal and widely spaced with notches on the biting surface. Kent is diagnosed with Hutchinson's teeth.

3. Leigh Norman, a 37-year-old female, comes in today with the complaint of shortness of breath. Dr. Schimek notes tachypnea, tachycardia, and cyanosis. Upon auscultation, bowel sounds are heard in the chest area. Leigh is admitted to Weston Hospital. After reviewing the arterial blood gases, laboratory results, and CT scan, Leigh is diagnosed with a diaphragmatic hernia with obstruction. Surgery is scheduled.

4. John Bandings, a 53-year-old male, presents today with fever and jaundice. John admits to drinking alcohol for decades. After reviewing the test results, Dr. Fong diagnoses John with alcoholic cirrhosis of the liver with ascites.

5. Maxine Weber, a 42-year-old female, comes in today with the complaint of severe pain in the right side of her lower abdomen. Maxine also says she has vomited. Dr. Jefferson documents a temperature of 101 F. Maxine is admitted to the hospital, where a CT scan confirms the diagnosis of acute appendicitis with localized peritonitis.

6. Archie Blume, a 41-year-old male, presents with the complaint of swollen tender gums and bleeding after he brushes his teeth. Dr. Day notes Archie uses tobacco. After an examination and x-rays, Archie is diagnosed with acute gingivitis, non-plaque induced.

7. Allen Klebb, a 36-year-old male, comes in today complaining of diarrhea and vomiting. Allen just finished his radiation treatments for his hand malignancy. Dr. Ard diagnoses Allen with gastroenteritis due to radiation.

8. Paula Dent, a 3-year-old female, is diagnosed with a congenital trachea-esophageal fistula with atresia of the esophagus. Paula is admitted to Weston Hospital for surgical repair.

9. Walter Logan, a 59-year-old male, presents today with a yellow brownish tongue. Walter admits to a bad taste in his mouth. Dr. Roche completes an examination, noting hypertrophy of the central dorsal tongue papillae. The biopsy confirms a diagnosis of black hairy tongue.

10. Robert Thomas, an 82-year-old male, presents today with severe epigastric pain. Robert also has been experiencing sharp chest pain that radiated to the left side of the neck and arm. Robert is admitted to the hospital, where an upper GI series confirms the diagnosis of volvulus of the colon with perforation.

11. Michelle Toatley, a 51-year-old female, presents with the complaints of stomach pain and bloating. Michelle admits to vomiting. Dr. Mobley notes patient has a history of heartburn and current alcohol abuse. The EGD confirms a diagnosis of acute gastric ulcer.

12. Harry Wisemann, a 46-year-old male, comes in today with the complaint of long-lasting heartburn and pain under his breastbone. Harry admits to taking aspirin several times a day for many years. Dr. Camut diagnoses Harry with an ulcer of the esophagus due to ingestion of aspirin.

13. C.E. Molyneaux, a 34-year-old male, comes in today with the complaint of a lump in his groin area. Dr. Williams completes a physical examination of the groin region and notes a bulge on the right side when C.E. is standing erect. A CT scan confirms a diagnosis of a femoral hernia, unilateral. C.E. is admitted to the hospital for surgical repair.

14. Carla Jett, a 45-year-old female, presents today with bloody diarrhea and weakness. Carla states this has been going on over the last few weeks. Dr. Edenton completes a thorough examination, noting a small ulcer on Carla's left leg and a temperature of 102.1 F. Carla is admitted to the hospital for a full workup. After reviewing the laboratory tests and the MRI scan, Carla is diagnosed with ulcerative pancolitis with rectal bleeding and pyoderma gangrenosum.

15. Jonathan Stutts, a 41-year-old male, comes in today with the complaint of abdomen pain with some diarrhea and bloating. Dr. Dresdner completes a thorough examination with the appropriate laboratory tests. Jonathan is diagnosed with idiopathic sclerosing mesenteric fibrosis.

YOU CODE IT! Application

The following exercises provide practice in abstracting physicians' notes and learning to work with documentation from our health care facility, Prader, Bracker, & Associates. These case studies are modeled on real patient encounters. Using the techniques described in this chapter, carefully read through the case studies and determine the most accurate ICD-10-CM code(s) and external cause code(s), if appropriate, for each case study.

WESTON HOSPITAL

629 Healthcare Way • SOMEWHERE, FL 32811 • 407-555-6541

PATIENT: UMBRELL, MORGAN

ACCOUNT/EHR #: UMBRMO001

DATE: 09/16/18

Attending Physician: Renee O. Bracker, MD

S: Patient is a 41-year-old female complaining of localized pain in the upper right quadrant radiating to the right scapular tip. Pain usually begins postprandial and is intense for approximately a 5-hour duration and then subsides. Pain is not relieved by emesis, flatus, or position change.

O: H: 5'3", Wt: 146 lb., R: 19, HR: 125, BP: 135/73, T: 102.4 F. Dr. Bracker notes diaphoresis, slight jaundice, as well as hypoactive bowel sound. CT scan confirms a bile duct calculus. Morgan is admitted for surgery.

A: Choledocholithiasis, acute with cholangitis, and obstruction

P: Laparoscopic cholecystectomy

ROB/pw   D: 09/16/18 09:50:16   T: 09/16/18 12:55:01

Determine the most accurate ICD-10-CM code(s).

PRADER, BRACKER, & ASSOCIATES

A Complete Health Care Facility

159 Healthcare Way • SOMEWHERE, FL 32811 • 407-555-6789

PATIENT: SEQUEN, EUGENE

ACCOUNT/EHR #: SEQUEU001

DATE: 09/16/18

Attending Physician: Oscar R. Prader, MD

Patient is a 49-year-old male diagnosed with chronic acid reflux. Barium swallow fluoroscopy, esophageal pH probe, esophageal manometry, and esophagoscopy were completed. He presents today to discuss the results of those tests.

I explain that the test results indicate that he has GERD. The first course of treatment is to adopt a low-fat, high-fiber diet. The second course would be surgical repair. Patient was instructed not to eat at least 2 hours before going to bed, and the head of the bed should be elevated 6 to 8 inches while in supine position.

Patient was informed that surgery may be necessary if diet and positioning do not relieve symptoms.

ORP/pw   D: 09/16/18 09:50:16   T: 09/16/18 12:55:01

Determine the most accurate ICD-10-CM code(s).

PRADER, BRACKER, & ASSOCIATES

A Complete Health Care Facility

159 Healthcare Way • SOMEWHERE, FL 32811 • 407-555-6789

PATIENT: HERMAN, CONNIE

ACCOUNT/EHR #: HERMCO001

DATE: 10/16/18

Attending Physician: Oscar R. Prader, MD

S: This 43-year-old female comes in with complaints of hematemesis and epigastric pain.

O: Esophageal tears are visualized during a fiberoptic endoscopy.

A: Mallory-Weiss syndrome, confirmed.

P: The options of electrocoagulation therapy for hemostasis and surgery to suture the esophageal lacerations if the condition did not resolve itself were discussed.

ORP/pw   D: 10/16/18 09:50:16   T: 10/18/18 12:55:01

Determine the most accurate ICD-10-CM code(s).

PRADER, BRACKER, & ASSOCIATES
A Complete Health Care Facility
159 Healthcare Way • SOMEWHERE, FL 32811 • 407-555-6789

PATIENT: GRAILLE, VAN

ACCOUNT/EHR #: GRAIVA001

DATE: 09/16/18

Attending Physician: Oscar R. Prader, MD

S: Patient is a 27-year-old male complaining of abdominal pain with alternating diarrhea and constipation. Abdominal distention is evident.

O: Complete history is obtained, including psychological profile. Sigmoidoscopy is completed.

A: Irritable bowel syndrome with diarrhea, confirmed.

P: Patient is asked to keep a food diary in order to identify foods that aggravate the condition.

Follow-up appointment 10–14 days

ORP/pw   D: 09/16/18 09:50:16   T: 09/16/18 12:55:01

Determine the most accurate ICD-10-CM code(s).

PRADER, BRACKER, & ASSOCIATES
A Complete Health Care Facility
159 Healthcare Way • SOMEWHERE, FL 32811 • 407-555-6789

PATIENT: ELLISON, THERESA

ACCOUNT/EHR #: ELLITH001

DATE: 09/16/18

Attending Physician: Renee O. Bracker, MD

S: Patient is a 36-year-old female complaining of regular epigastric pain beginning in the umbilical region and radiating toward her spine. Last night the pain was so severe she vomited.

O: Examination reveals crackles in lower lobe at the base of the lung, tachycardia, and a temperature of 102 F. Lab results show increased serum lipase levels and increased polymorphonuclear leukocytes. Ultrasound shows enlarged pancreas.

A: Acute pancreatitis

P: Admit to hospital.

ROB/pw   D: 09/16/18 09:50:16   T: 09/16/18 12:55:01

Determine the most accurate ICD-10-CM code(s).

14 Coding Integumentary Conditions

Key Terms

Blister
Bulla
Carbuncle
Cyst
Decubitus Ulcer
Dermis
Epidermis
Furuncle
Gangrene
Hair
Hair Follicle
Macule
Nevus
Nodule
Papule
Patch
Phalanges
Pressure Ulcer
Pustule
Scale
Skin
Subcutaneous
Ulcer

Skin
The external membranous covering of the body.

Epidermis
The external layer of the skin, the majority of which is squamous cells.

Dermis
The internal layer of the skin; the location of blood vessels, lymph vessels, hair follicles, sweat glands, and sebum.

Subcutaneous
The layer beneath the dermis; also known as the *hypodermis*.

Learning Outcomes

After completing this chapter, the student should be able to:

LO 14.1 Apply the guidelines for reporting conditions of the skin.
LO 14.2 Analyze disorders of the nails, hair, glands, and sensory nerves.
LO 14.3 Determine the specific characteristics of a lesion as they relate to coding.
LO 14.4 Abstract the reasons for preventive care and report them accurately to support medical necessity.

STOP! Remember, you need to follow along in your ICD-10-CM code book for an optimal learning experience.

14.1 Disorders of the Skin

The Skin

The average person has roughly 2 square yards (5,184 inches) of **skin** surface area. As the largest organ in the human body, the skin does so much more than just keep all your internal organs covered. Each of its layers, the **epidermis** and the **dermis**, plays an important role in protecting the body.

The dermis is a sturdy collagenous layer that connects the epidermis to the fatty tissue layer. Blood vessels, nerves, glands, hair follicles, and lymph channels are all located in this stratum of the skin. In Figure 14-1, you can see how all of the components of the integumentary system work together—the skin (epidermis and dermis) along with the accessory structures (hair, nails, glands, and sensory receptors). Notice how the line between the epidermis and the dermis has hills and ridges, known as *dermal papillae*. Fingerprints are formed by these genetically prompted elevations and valleys, which are then altered further during formation as a fetus presses against the wall of the uterus. This explains why no two people have the same fingerprints, not even identical twins.

Fastening the skin to the underlying elements of the anatomy is the fatty tissue, also known as the *hypodermis* (*hypo* = below + *dermis* = dermal) or the **subcutaneous** layer.

Dermatitis

Dermatitis is technically an inflammation of the skin (*derma* = skin + *-itis* = inflammation). However, it is not as simple as this; there are several types of dermatitis.

Atopic dermatitis (category L20) includes Besnier's prurigo, flexural eczema, infantile eczema, and intrinsic (allergic) eczema. Most often, this chronic inflammation

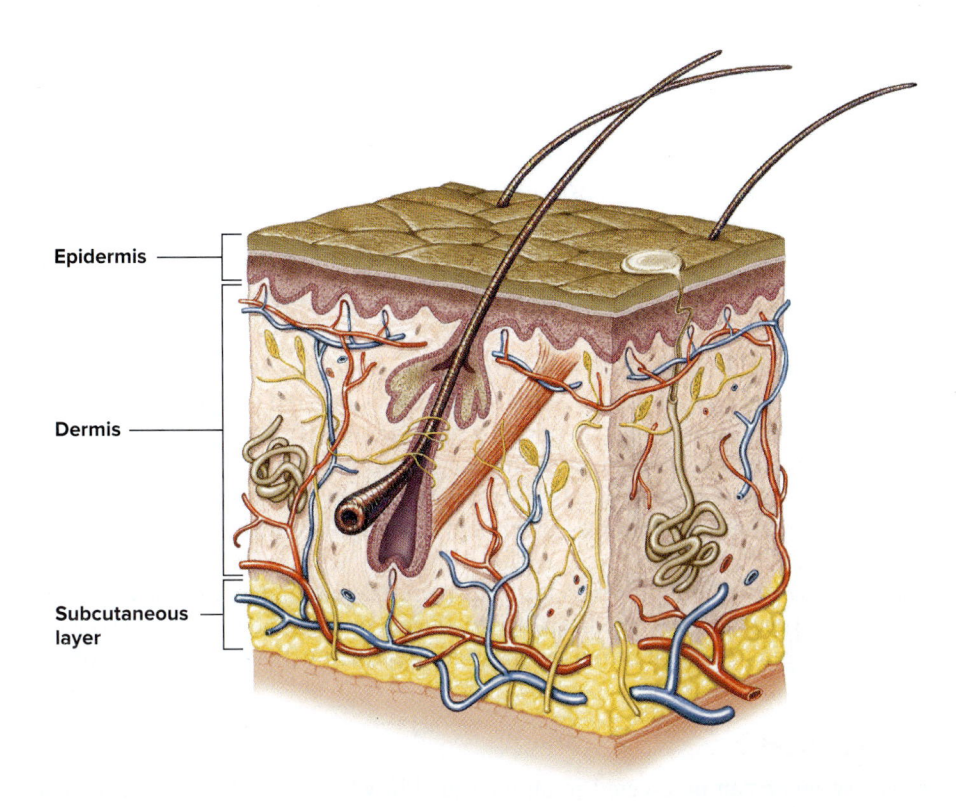

FIGURE 14-1 An illustration identifying the layers of the skin David Shier et al., *Hole's Human Anatomy & Physiology*, 12/e. ©2010 McGraw-Hill Education. Figure 6.2a, p. 172. Used with permission.

affects infants (1 month to 1 year of age) with family histories of atopic conditions such as allergic rhinitis and bronchial asthma. Signs and symptoms include erythematous areas on extremely dry skin, appearing as lesions on the forehead, cheeks, arms, and legs. The pruritus nature of this condition results in scratching that induces scaling and edema.

Seborrheic dermatitis (category L21) includes seborrhea capitis and seborrheic infantile dermatitis, commonly affecting the scalp and face. Symptoms include itching, erythematous areas, and inflammation, characterized by lesions covered with brownish gray or yellow scales in areas in which sebaceous glands are plentiful.

Diaper dermatitis (category L22), commonly referred to as *diaper rash*, is caused by continuously wet skin. Often, this develops when diapers are not changed frequently enough to permit the area to dry out.

Allergic contact dermatitis (category L23) is the result of the skin touching a material or substance to which the patient is sensitive. In addition to erythematous areas, vesicles develop that itch, scale, and may ooze.

Irritant contact dermatitis (category L24) is caused by exposure of the skin to detergents, solvents, acids, or alkalis. Blisters and/or ulcerations may appear in the area that came in contact with the chemical.

Exfoliative dermatitis (category L26) is an acute and chronic inflammation with widespread erythema and scales. The loss of the stratum corneum (the outermost layer of the epidermis) is at the heart of this condition, along with hair loss, fever, and shivering.

Dermatitis due to substances taken internally (category L27) would include an inflammatory eruption of the epidermis in reaction to medications, drugs, ingested food, or other substances. It may be easy to think that this might be limited to a response only to oral medicines, but, technically, a drug injected, infused, or delivered via subcutaneous patch also places the pharmaceutical internally. Keep a watchful eye on the *Use additional code* notations within this code category, which remind you to include an external cause code.

Psoriasis

Identified by epidermal erythematous papules and plaques covered with silvery scales, psoriasis is a chronic illness. Exacerbations (flare-ups) can be treated to relieve the symptoms. Patients can inherit the tendency to develop psoriasis because it is genetically passed from parent to child. Its pruritic nature can sometimes result in pain along with itching in the areas covered with dry, cracked, encrusted lesions appearing on the scalp, chest, elbows, knees, shins, back, and buttocks. The silver scales may flake away easily or create a thickened cover over the lesion. There are several types of psoriasis, including the following:

- *Psoriasis vulgaris*, also known as *nummular psoriasis or plaque psoriasis*, is the most common type of psoriasis. It usually causes dry, red skin lesions (plaques) covered with silvery scales. Reported with code L40.0 Psoriasis vulgaris.
- *Guttate psoriasis* appears more often in young adults (under the age of 30) as well as children. Lesions covered by a fine scale will typically develop as small, teardrop-shaped sores on the scalp, arms, trunk, and legs. Reported with code L40.4 Guttate psoriasis.
- *Psoriatic arthritis mutilans* presents with pain, edema, and/or loss of flexibility in at least one joint. When affecting the fingers or toes, the nails may show pitting or begin to separate from the nail bed. Reported with code L40.52 Psoriatic arthritis mutilans.

Pressure Ulcers

A **pressure ulcer** can be created in an area of skin when tissue breaks down. Also known as a *bedsore, plaster ulcer, pressure sore,* or **decubitus ulcer**, it can occur if the patient is unable to move or shift his or her own weight, such as when an individual is confined to a wheelchair or bed, even for a short period of time. The constant pressure against the skin reduces the blood supply to that particular area, and the affected tissue becomes necrotic (dies). You might have experienced this yourself with a pebble in your shoe or a simple fold of your sock within a tight shoe. The area where the pressure impacted your foot became more and more painful. If you took your shoe right off, you might have noticed a red area. If you waited a length of time before removing your shoe, you found a painful **blister**. The longer the pressure and irritation are maintained, the worse the damage to the skin (see Figure 14-2).

The National Pressure Ulcer Advisory Panel (NPUAP) defines a pressure ulcer as "a localized injury to the skin and/or underlying tissue, usually over a bony prominence, as a result of pressure, or pressure in combination with shear and/or friction."

As a professional coding specialist, you will need to know two factors to determine the correct codes for a diagnosed pressure ulcer:

- Anatomical location (where on the body the ulcer is).
- Depth of the lesion (also known as the *stage of ulcer*).

There are five codeable stages of pressure ulcers (see Figure 14-3):

- *Stage 1* affects the epidermal layer and is recognized by persistent erythema (redness). A stage 1 pressure ulcer is visualized as a reddened area on the skin that, when pressed with the finger, is nonblanchable (does not turn white).
- *Stage 2* is a partial-thickness loss involving both the epidermis and the dermis; sometimes a fluid-filled blister is evident. A stage 2 pressure ulcer shows visible blisters or forms an open sore. The tissue surrounding the sore may be red and irritated like an abrasion, blister, or shallow crater with a red-pink wound bed.
- *Stage 3* pressure ulcer involves skin loss through and including the subcutaneous tissue. A stage 3 pressure ulcer looks like a crater with visible damage to the tissue below the skin. Full-thickness tissue loss may expose subcutaneous fatty tissue but not bone, tendon, or muscle.

Pressure Ulcer
An open wound or sore caused by pressure, infection, or inflammation.

Decubitus Ulcer
A skin lesion caused by continuous pressure on one spot, particularly on a bony prominence.

Blister
A bubble or sac formed on the surface of the skin, typically filled with a watery fluid or serum.

GUIDANCE CONNECTION

Read the ICD-10-CM Official Guidelines for Coding and Reporting, section **I. Conventions, General Coding Guidelines and Chapter Specific Guidelines,** subsection **C. Chapter-Specific Coding Guidelines,** chapter **12. Diseases of the Skin and Subcutaneous Tissue,** subsection **a. Pressure ulcer stage codes.**

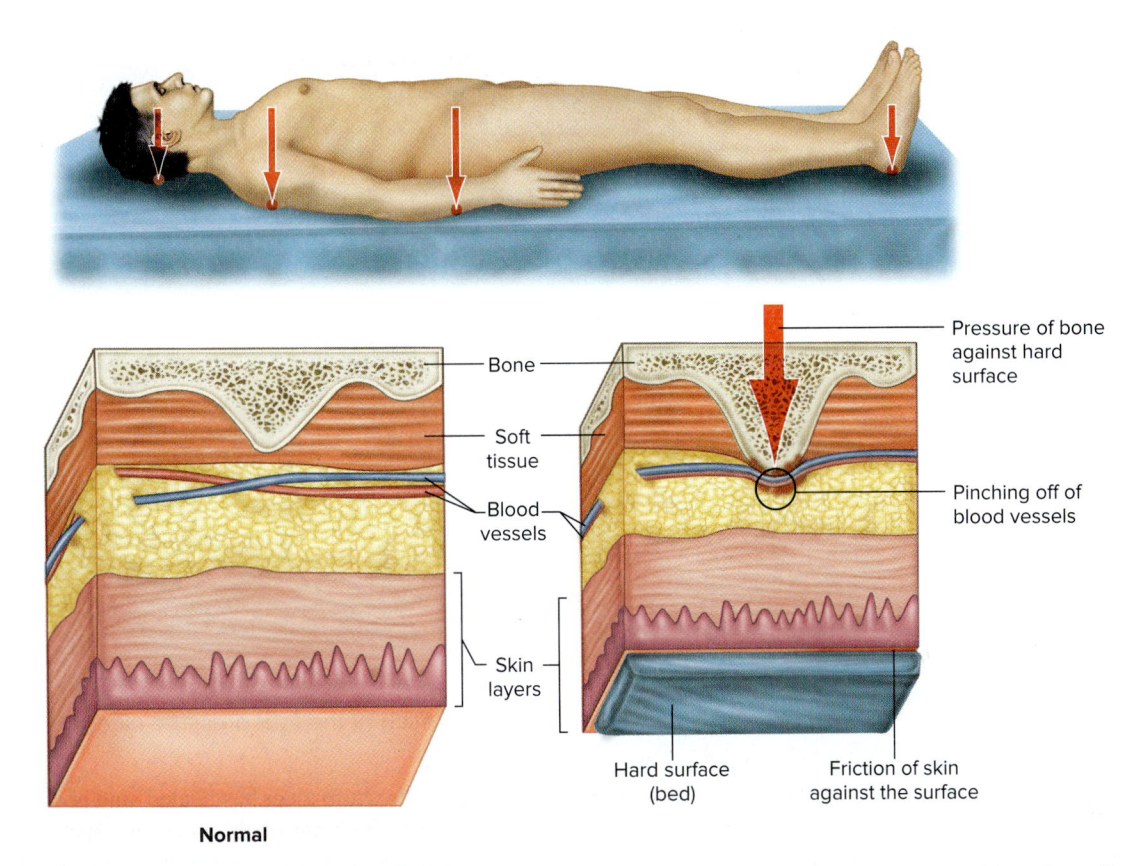

FIGURE 14-2 An illustration identifying the etiology of pressure ulcers including the layers of the skin affected

- *Stage 4* indicates the skin layers are necrotic and the ulcer reaches down into muscle and possibly bone. Stage 4 pressure ulcers have become so deep that there is damage to the muscle and bone, sometimes along with tendon and joint damage. While the depth of the ulcer varies on the basis of the anatomical site, there is full-thickness tissue loss with bone, tendon, or muscle exposed.
- An *unstageable ulcer* is *not* an unspecified stage. There are times when slough and eschar must be removed to reveal the base of the wound before the true depth, or stage, can be accurately determined. The lesion may be inaccessible—because it is covered by a wound dressing that has not been removed or by a sterile blister or because of some other documented reason.

ICD-10-CM has created combination codes, therefore requiring only one code to identify both the anatomical site and the stage of the ulcer.

EXAMPLE

Holder Pronce has a stage 3 pressure ulcer on his left hip.

L89.223   Pressure ulcer of left hip, stage 3

Healing Pressure Ulcers

It is logical that a patient will be attended to by a health care professional during the time the pressure ulcer is healing. Typically, the documentation will identify the original stage and describe the ulcer as "healing." For example, "Harvey Rhoden was seen today by Dr. Steelman to follow up on his stage 2 pressure ulcer. Dr. Steelman documented that the ulcer is healing nicely." In this case, you would continue to code this as a stage 2 pressure ulcer.

> **GUIDANCE CONNECTION**
>
> Read the ICD-10-CM Official Guidelines for Coding and Reporting, section **I. Conventions, General Coding Guidelines and Chapter Specific Guidelines,** subsection **C. Chapter-Specific Coding Guidelines,** chapter **12. Diseases of the Skin and Subcutaneous Tissue,** subsection **a.5) Patients admitted with pressure ulcers documented as healing.**

> **GUIDANCE CONNECTION**
>
> Read the ICD-10-CM Official Guidelines for Coding and Reporting, section **I. Conventions, General Coding Guidelines and Chapter Specific Guidelines,** subsection **C. Chapter-Specific Coding Guidelines,** chapter **12. Diseases of the Skin and Subcutaneous Tissue,** subsection **a.6) Patients admitted with pressure ulcer evolving into another stage during the admission.**

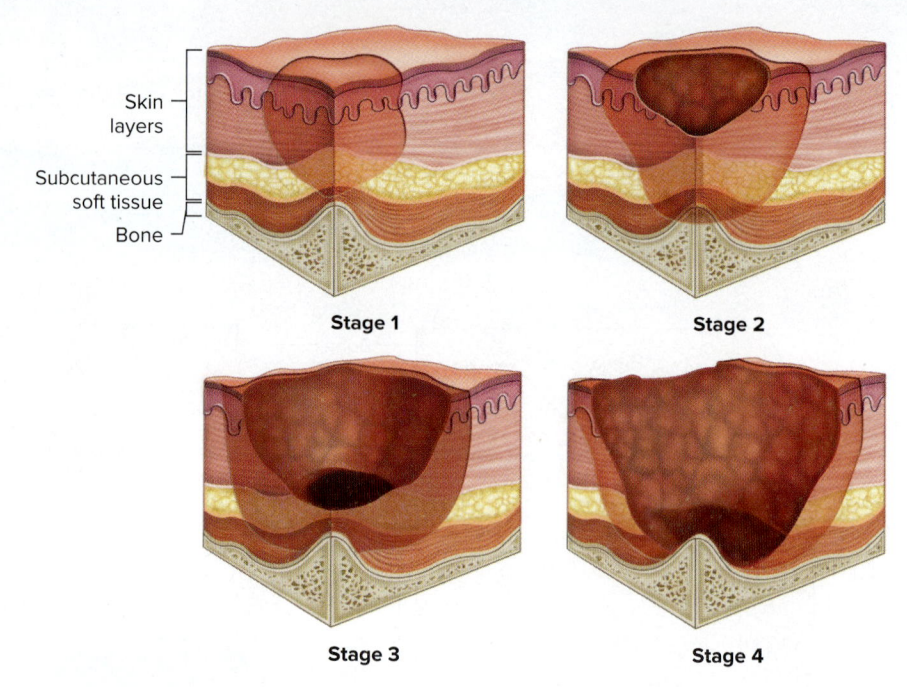

Stage 1   Stage 2   Stage 3   Stage 4

FIGURE 14-3 An illustration showing each of the four pressure ulcer stages

At the time of discharge, if the patient's pressure ulcer has healed, and is documented as healed, you will need to report the stage and site of this ulcer as described in the admissions documentation. This will provide the medical necessity for the treatment of this condition while the patient was in the facility and resulted in the healed outcome.

Evolving Pressure Ulcers

Sadly, there are occasions when a patient is admitted into the hospital with a pressure ulcer that, during his or her stay, gets worse and progresses into a higher stage of ulcer. Should this happen, you will need to report two codes at discharge:

1. Code for the site and stage of the pressure ulcer as documented when the patient was admitted into the hospital.
2. Report an additional code for the site and stage of the ulcer as documented when the patient is discharged.

Presence of Gangrene

Notice the *Code first* notation beneath the code category L89 Pressure ulcer to report the code for any gangrenous condition associated with the ulcer by using code I96 Gangrene, not elsewhere classified (Gangrenous cellulitis). You are directed by this notation to list the gangrene code first, followed by the pressure ulcer code.

Did you notice that the code for gangrene is in the chapter of codes used to report diseases of the circulatory system? This makes sense because **gangrene** is necrosis, cell death, and decay caused by insufficient blood supply to the affected cells. Remember that pressure ulcers are caused by the ongoing compression of the skin, often resulting in the prevention of blood flow into the area. Look again at Figure 14-3.

> **CODING BITES**
>
> Nonpressure ulcers are reported with codes from the **L97** and **L98** code categories. For more details about these skin disorders, see section **Lesions** in this chapter.

Gangrene
Necrotic tissue resulting from a loss of blood supply.

LET'S CODE IT! SCENARIO

After attempting to jump his motorcycle over five barrels and crashing on the other side, Hunter Massler ended up in the hospital for 6 weeks with a left, closed, transverse fractured femur, shaft; a right, closed, oblique fractured *femoral shaft;* and three fractured ribs, left side. He was unable to move without extreme pain, so he lay in bed virtually motionless, except with help from the nurse. After several weeks, while changing the sheets, Nurse Kenesson identified a pressure ulcer on each of his hips. Dr. Weiner staged the ulcers bilaterally as stage 2 and ordered wound care immediately. While there, Dr. Weiner also checked Hunter's progress on the healing of his fractures.

> **Let's Code It!**
>
> Dr. Weiner came in to stage and treat Hunter's pressure ulcers: *bilateral hip pressure ulcers,* both documented as stage 2. Let's turn to the Alphabetic Index and find
>
> **Ulcer, ulcerated, ulcerating, ulceration, ulcerative**
>   **pressure (pressure area) L89.9-**
>   **hip L89.2-**
>
> Perfect! Now let's turn to L89 in the Tabular List and read completely.
>
> ☑4 **L89**   **Pressure Ulcer**
>
> Read the INCLUDES, *Code first*, and EXCLUDES2 notations. There is nothing here to direct you elsewhere, so continue reading and review *all* of the required fourth-character choices to determine the one that matches the physician's notes:
>
> ☑5 **L89.2**   **Pressure ulcer of hip**
>
> This matches the notes, so you know you are in the right place. Next, you must determine the required fifth character for this ulcer code. Check the documentation; is the pressure ulcer on his right hip or left hip? Both, actually, so you will need two codes, one for each hip:
>
> ☑6 **L89.21**   **Pressure ulcer of right hip**
> ☑6 **L89.22**   **Pressure ulcer of left hip**
>
> To identify the sixth characters, you will need to abstract from the documentation regarding the stage of each ulcer. The documentation states stage 2 for both.
>
> **L89.212**   **Pressure ulcer of right hip, stage 2**
> **L89.222**   **Pressure ulcer of left hip, stage 2**
>
> These pressure ulcer codes will be reported first because the ulcers are the principal reason Dr. Weiner came to see Hunter for this encounter. Then follow these steps with the codes to report Hunter's fractures, and you will have the diagnosis codes to report this encounter:
>
> **L89.212**   **Pressure ulcer of right hip, stage 2**
> **L89.222**   **Pressure ulcer of left hip, stage 2**
> **S72.325D**   **Nondisplaced transverse fracture of shaft of left femur, subsequent encounter for closed fracture with routine healing**
> **S72.334D**   **Nondisplaced oblique fracture of shaft of right femur, subsequent encounter for closed fracture with routine healing**
> **S22.42xD**   **Multiple fractures of ribs, left side, subsequent encounter for closed fracture with routine healing**
>
> Good work!

14.2 Disorders of the Nails, Hair, Glands, and Sensory Nerves

Nails

As you can see in Figure 14-4, there are several components of nails—those hard, protective layers at the ends of your **phalanges** (fingers and toes). The most well-known part

Phalanges
Fingers and toes [singular: phalange or phalanx].

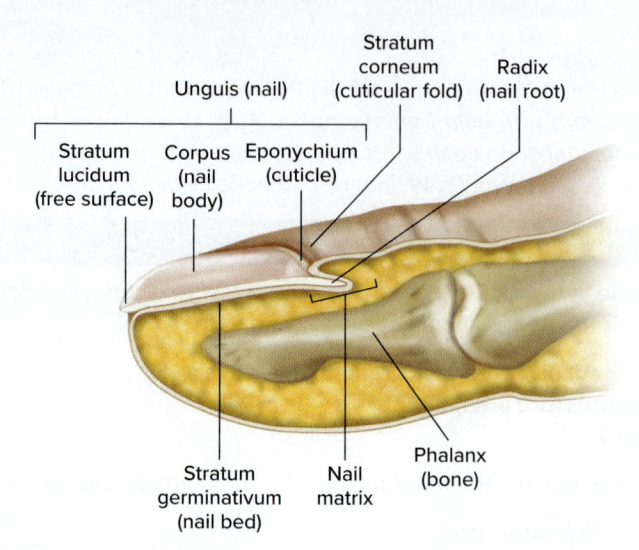

FIGURE 14-4 An illustration identifying the anatomical sites of the basic parts of a human nail: nail plate, lunula, root, sinus, matrix, nail bed, hyponychium, free edge Booth et al., *Medical Assisting*, 5e. Copyright ©2013 by McGraw-Hill Education. Figure 23-4, p. 501. Used with permission.

of the nail is the *nail plate,* the main part of the nail, which lies upon a layer of skin (nail bed). At the point where the nail plate goes beneath the skin [*eponychium* = nail fold + cuticle (lunula)] of the finger (or toe) is the *lunula,* a white area shaped like a crescent moon (therefore, the term *lunula,* from *luna,* meaning moon). As the nail grows over the tip of the phalange, the area of epidermis beneath is called the *hyponychium.*

Nail Disorders

The human body has 20 nails—10 fingernails and 10 toenails—and as with any other anatomical site, things can go wrong.

- *Onycholysis:* This is a detachment of the nail from the bed of the nail. Onset occurs at either the distal or lateral attachment. Patients previously diagnosed with psoriasis or thyrotoxicosis are most often seen with this condition. Reported with code L60.1 Onycholysis.
- *Beau's lines:* These are deeply grooved, horizontal lines (from side to side) on either a fingernail or a toenail. Previous infection, injury, or other disruption to the nail fold, the location of nail formation, may be the cause. Reported with code L60.4 Beau's lines.
- *Yellow nail syndrome:* A thickened nail that has become yellowed is typically seen in patients previously diagnosed with a systemic disease, such as lymphedema or bronchiectasis. This is reported with code L60.5 Yellow nail syndrome.

You have learned, with many diseases in various body systems, that a disease in one location of the body may negatively impact another part of the body. This can happen with the nails as well, so ICD-10-CM provides a specific code to report this:

L62 Nail disorders in diseases classified elsewhere
Code first underlying disease, such as: pachydermoperiostosis (M89.4-)

LET'S CODE IT! SCENARIO

Priscilla Ablerts, an 83-year-old female, was brought in with toenails that had grown out of normal shape. It had gotten to the point that she could no longer wear closed shoes, and her daughter was concerned. After examination, Dr. Terranzo diagnosed Priscilla with onychogryphosis.

> **Let's Code It!**
>
> Dr. Terranzo diagnosed Priscilla with *onychogryphosis*. Turn in the ICD-10-CM Alphabetic Index to find
>
> **Onychogryphosis, onychogryposis L60.2**
>
> Let's turn in the Tabular List to the code category:
>
> ☑4 **L60**   **Nail disorders**
> EXCLUDES2   clubbing of nails (R68.3)
>   onychia and paronychia (L03.0-)
>
> Neither of these conditions applies to Priscilla's reason for seeing Dr. Terranzo for this encounter, so keep reading down to evaluate all of the fourth-character options. Which is the most accurate?
>
> **L60.2**   **Onychogryphosis**
>
> This matches Dr. Terranzo's documentation. However, you know that before you can report this code, you need to check the EXCLUDES1 note for this subsection (right above L60). This does not relate to this case. Now, check the EXCLUDES2 note at the very beginning of this chapter in the ICD-10-CM Tabular List. Last stop at the Official Guidelines, section 1.c.12. There seem to be no guidelines here that relate to Dr. Terranzo's care for Priscilla, so you can now report this code with confidence:
>
> **L60.2**   **Onychogryphosis**
>
> Good job!

Hair

Hair is a pigmented (colored), hard keratin that grows from the **hair follicle**—the location of the hair root. As you can see in Figure 14-5, the follicle is embedded in the dermis and fatty tissue of the skin layers. As you probably know from your own body, hair may grow externally, such as on your scalp, as well as internally, such as inside the nasal or ear cavity. The hairs in the nose help to prevent certain particles from entering the respiratory system.

Disorders of the Hair

For some patients, a bad hair day can be much more serious than a cowlick or frizz.

- *Alopecia mucinosa:* This skin disorder may first be identified by erythematous plaqueing of the skin without any hair growth. The flat patches of hairlessness may occur on the scalp, face, or legs. Reported with code L65.2 Alopecia mucinosa.
- *Trichorrhexis nodosa:* Evidenced by a hair shaft defect that causes weak spots, this disorder results in hair that easily breaks. Most often, this condition is caused by environmental factors such as blow drying, permanent waves, or excessive chemical exposure. Reported with code L67.0 Trichorrhexis nodosa.
- *Hirsutism:* Women with this condition have excessive hair growth on anatomical sites where hair does not typically occur, such as the chest or chin. It is believed to be caused by an abnormal hormonal level, particularly male hormones such as testosterone. Reported with code L68.0 Hirsutism.

Glands

Three different types of glands are located within the skin:

- *Sebaceous glands* produce an oil-rich element, known as *sebum,* that lies on the outer surface of the epidermis and along the hair. The substance has a waterproofing effect. Individuals with oily skin may have overly active sebaceous glands.

Hair
A pigmented, cylindrical filament that grows out from the hair follicle within the epidermis.

Hair Follicle
A saclike bulb containing the hair root.

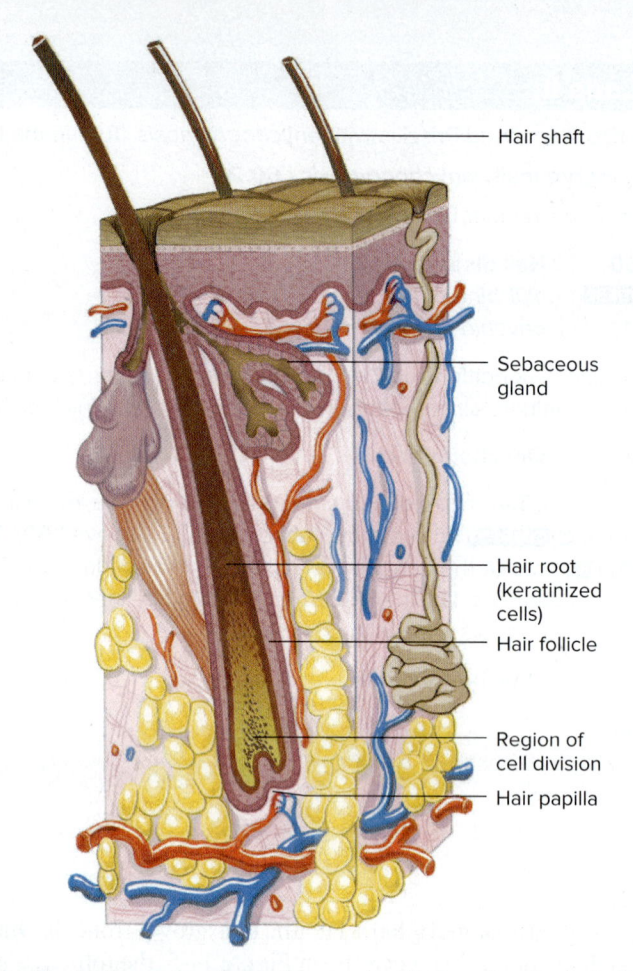

FIGURE 14-5 An illustration identifying the anatomical parts of a hair; from papilla to shaft   David Shier et al., *Hole's Human Anatomy & Physiology*, 12/e. ©2010 McGraw-Hill Education. Figure 6.7a, p. 178. Used with permission.

- *Eccrine glands* are sweat glands that are responsible for maintaining proper body temperature by excreting sweat (water, salt, and wastes) via the pores in the skin. Production of more sweat is the reaction to cool an overheated body (see Figure 14-6).
- *Apocrine glands* release a discharge that is high in protein. Located in the axilla (armpits), anal, and genital areas, bacteria interact with the protein and create an odor.

Eccrine Sweat Disorders

As with any other anatomical site, the eccrine sweat glands can malfunction. One condition is known as *focal hyperhidrosis* (excessive sweating). This is reported with a specific character to identify the region of the body affected (i.e., axillae, face, palms, or soles). Primary hyperhidrosis is an idiopathic condition (no known etiology), whereas secondary focal hyperhidrosis (also known as *Frey's syndrome*) is often caused by damage to the parotid glands, resulting in excessive salivation. Hypohidrosis (code L74.4), also known as *anhidrosis,* is a condition in which the glands do not produce enough perspiration. This may lead to hyperthermia, heat stroke, or heat exhaustion.

You can see that the ICD-10-CM code descriptions use the term *miliaria,* which is the medical term for a skin disorder—the appearance of red bumps or blisters—caused by blocked sweat ducts and trapped sweat beneath the skin. Laypeople call this *heat rash.*

L74.0	Miliaria rubra
L74.1	Miliaria crystallina
L74.2	Miliaria profunda
L74.4	Anhidrosis (Hypohidrosis)

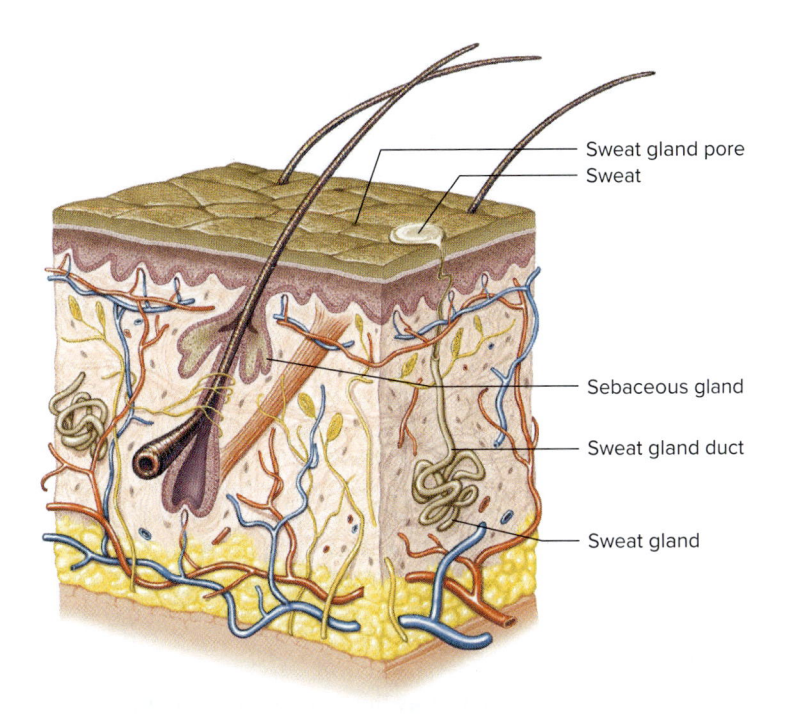

FIGURE 14-6 An illustration identifying the anatomical sites of sweat glands Booth et al., *Medical Assisting*, 5e. Copyright ©2013 by McGraw-Hill Education. Figure 23-1, p. 497. Used with permission.

Apocrine Sweat Disorders

One of the challenges in dealing with an apocrine sweat disorder is the potential for embarrassment due to the increase in body odor. Natural odors can be a natural attraction between humans; however, when body odor is out of balance, this can cause both physiological and psychological problems. Bromhidrosis (foul-smelling perspiration, code L75.0) or chromhidrosis (pigmented perspiration, code L75.1) can be publicly humiliating to any adult.

L75.0	Bromhidrosis
L75.1	Chromhidrosis
L75.2	Apocrine miliaria (Fox-Fordyce disease)
L75.8	Other apocrine sweat disorders

YOU CODE IT! CASE STUDY

Ellyn Pacard, a 41-year-old female, presents to Dr. Grall with what she believes to be nonscarring male-pattern alopecia. Examination reveals small patches of scalp, with some limited mild erythema. "Exclamation point" hairs are located on the periphery with some indication of new patches and regrowth. Explained to patient that complete regrowth is possible in this diagnosis.

Diagnosis: alopecia capitis

Treatment plan: intralesional corticosteroid injections followed by minoxidil applications.

You Code It!

Read Dr. Grall's notes on his encounter with Ellyn carefully, and code the visit.

Step #1: Read the case carefully and completely.

Step #2: Abstract the scenario. Which main words or terms describe why the physician cared for the patient during this encounter?

(continued)

> Step #3: Are there any details missing or incomplete for which you would need to query the physician? [If so, ask your instructor.]
>
> Step #4: Check for any relevant guidance, including reading all of the symbols and notations in the Tabular List and the appropriate sections of the Official Guidelines.
>
> Step #5: Determine the correct diagnosis code or codes to explain why this encounter was medically necessary.
>
> Step #6: Double-check your work.
>
> **Answer:**
>
> Did you determine this to be the correct code?
>
> **L63.0   Alopecia (capitis) totalis**
>
> Good work!

Sensory Nerves

In a part of the nervous system known as the *somatic* (relating to the body) *sensory system*, sensory nerve endings are located in the layers of the skin to provide sensory feedback—the sense of touch. These nerves enable you to feel pressure, pain, temperature (hot and cold), textures (rough and smooth), and more.

There is more about the nervous system in this book's chapter titled *Coding Mental, Behavioral, and Neurological Disorders*.

LET'S CODE IT! SCENARIO

Serena Brynner is a 19-year-old female who came in to see Dr. Trenton with thickened, hardened skin and subcutaneous tissue on her forearms, bilaterally. Examination shows Addison's keloid present. She is given a referral to a plastic surgeon.

Let's Code It!

Dr. Trenton diagnosed Serena with *Addison's keloid* on both of her forearms. Let's begin by finding this key term in the Alphabetic Index:

Keloid, cheloid L91.0
   Addison's L94.0

Let's find this code category in the Tabular List:

☑4 **L94   Other localized connective tissue disorders**

The terms here don't match exactly. Let's check a medical encyclopedia to find out exactly what an Addison's keloid is:

Addison's keloid is a skin disease consisting of patches of yellowish or ivory-colored hard, dry, smooth skin. It is more common in females. Also known as morphea or circumscribed scleroderma.

This helps a great deal. Read the complete code descriptions in this code category. Did you connect to this code?

L94.0   Localized scleroderma [morphea] (Circumscribed scleroderma)

Fantastic!

14.3 Lesions

Many people believe a lesion is a sore on the epidermis; however, lesions might also occur internally. Skin lesions are categorized as primary or secondary and are pathologically determined to be benign or malignant. Even though the majority of lesions are external, reporting them is not confined to the codes in the L00–L99 section, *Diseases of the Skin and Subcutaneous Tissue*. Essentially, lesion codes are located throughout the code set; they are most often found in the section related to the anatomical location or by a specific term. Many skin lesions (see Figure 14-7) are identified by name or type, including

- **Cyst**: a fluid-filled or gas-filled bubble in the skin.
- **Furuncle**: a staphylococcal infection in the subcutaneous tissue; commonly known as a *boil*.
- **Papule**: a raised lesion with a diameter of less than 5 mm.
- **Nodule**: a tissue mass or papule larger than 5 mm.
- **Macule**: a flat lesion with a different pigmentation (color) when compared with the surrounding skin. An *ephelidis* (freckle) is a small macule.
- **Nevus**: an abnormally pigmented area of skin. A birthmark is an example.
- **Patch**: a flat, small area of differently colored or textured skin; a large macule.
- **Bulla**: a large vesicle that is filled with fluid.
- **Pustule**: a swollen area of skin; a vesicle filled with pus.
- **Scale**: flaky exfoliated epidermis; a flake of skin.
- **Ulcer**: an erosion or loss of the full thickness of the epidermis.

EXAMPLE

L02.32   Furuncle of buttock

Let's turn to the Alphabetic Index and find the key term *lesion*. Review the terms shown in the indented list that follows, providing additional description for the type of lesion documented. For the most part, these lesions are directly described by their anatomical location, with no additional clinical terminology.

EXAMPLES

Lesion, aortic (valve) I35.9 (an internal lesion)
Lesion, lip K13.0 (an external lesion)
Lesion, basal ganglion G25.9 (an internal lesion)
Lesion, eyelid H00.03- (an external lesion)

Often, a skin lesion is diagnosed with a specific name or by type. Therefore, the most effective way to find the codes in the Alphabetic Index is to look up the exact term that the physician used in the diagnostic statement first, before trying to generalize by interpreting *lesion* and using that term. For example, **carbuncles** and furuncles, also known as *boils* (a type of pustule caused by an infection), are listed by the terms *carbuncle* and *furuncle,* rather than under the main term of *lesion,* with the fourth character identifying the anatomical location of the skin condition.

EXAMPLES

Carbuncle, chin L02.03
Carbuncle, hand L02.53-
Carbuncle, scalp L02.831

Cyst
A fluid-filled or gas-filled bubble in the skin.

Furuncle
A staphylococcal infection in the subcutaneous tissue; commonly known as a *boil*.

Papule
A raised lesion with a diameter of less than 5 mm.

Nodule
A tissue mass or papule larger than 5 mm.

Macule
A flat lesion with a different pigmentation (color) when compared with the surrounding skin.

Nevus
An abnormally pigmented area of skin. A birthmark is an example.

Patch
A flat, small area of differently colored or textured skin; a large macule.

Bulla
A large vesicle that is filled with fluid.

Pustule
A swollen area of skin; a vesicle filled with pus.

Scale
Flaky exfoliated epidermis; a flake of skin.

Ulcer
An erosion or loss of the full thickness of the epidermis.

Carbuncle
A painful, pus-filled boil due to infection of the epidermis and underlying tissues, often caused by staphylococcus.

PRIMARY LESIONS

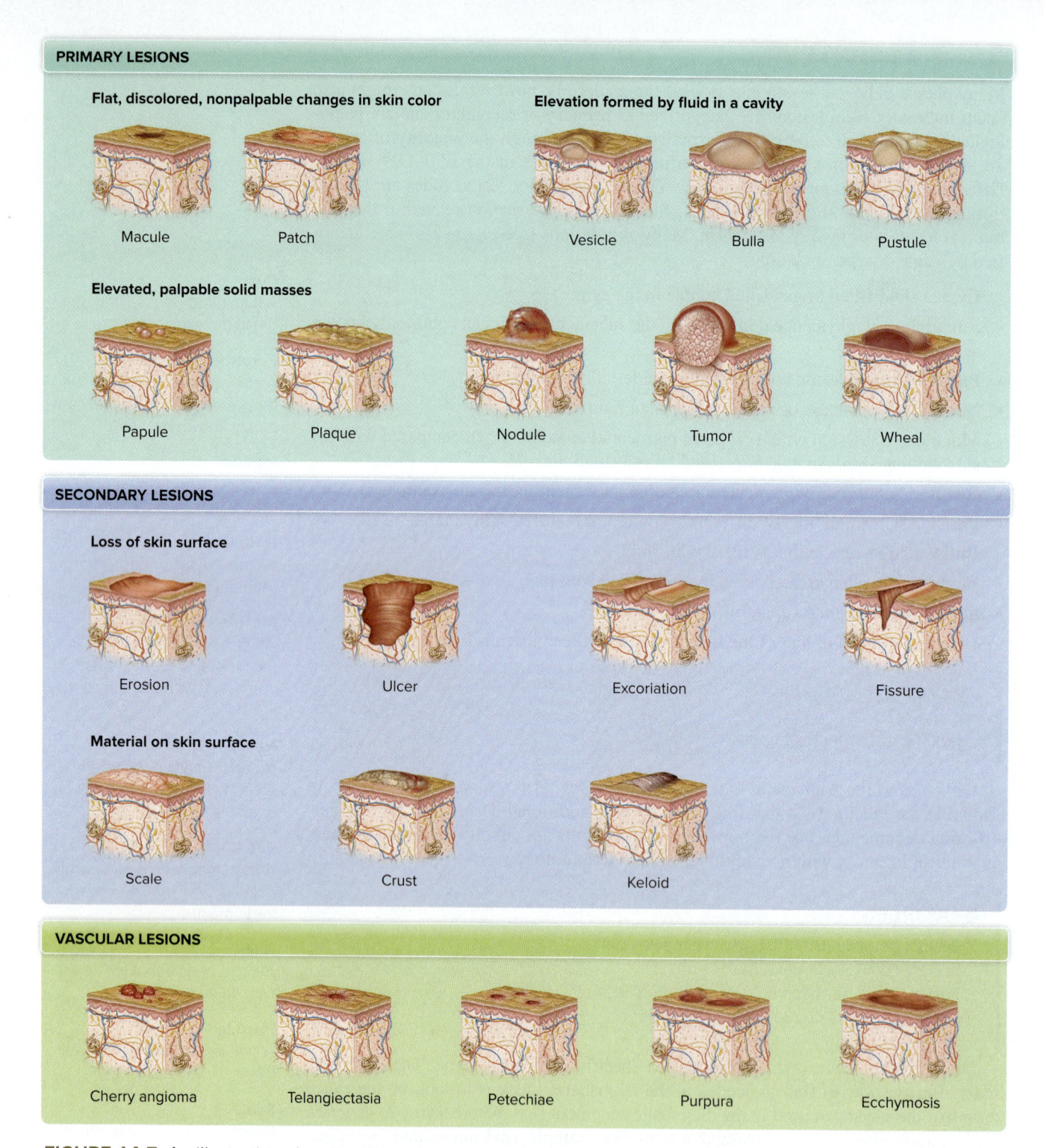

Flat, discolored, nonpalpable changes in skin color: Macule, Patch

Elevation formed by fluid in a cavity: Vesicle, Bulla, Pustule

Elevated, palpable solid masses: Papule, Plaque, Nodule, Tumor, Wheal

SECONDARY LESIONS

Loss of skin surface: Erosion, Ulcer, Excoriation, Fissure

Material on skin surface: Scale, Crust, Keloid

VASCULAR LESIONS

Cherry angioma, Telangiectasia, Petechiae, Purpura, Ecchymosis

FIGURE 14-7 An illustration showing the various types of skin lesions   Booth et al., *Medical Assisting*, 5e. Copyright ©2013 by McGraw-Hill Education. Figure 23-2, p. 498. Used with permission.

Malignant Lesions

The majority of skin lesions diagnosed are benign. However, there are certain skin lesions that are pathologically identified as malignant.

Malignant melanoma is the most deadly type of skin malignancy, causing 80% of all skin malignancy fatalities. The most frequently identified sites of melanoma metastases are the lymph nodes, liver, lung, and brain. The ABCDE method is used most often to evaluate a possible site, then confirmed by a biopsy. Confirmed diagnoses will be reported with a code from the category C43.- Malignant melanoma of skin, with an additional character or characters based on the specific anatomical site.

Merkel cell carcinoma (also known as *neuroendocrine carcinoma*) is a rare diagnosis. Most often found on the face and neck, it can be recognized by a bluish-red or flesh-colored nodule. This malignancy grows quickly and will metastasize quickly, meaning that early diagnosis and treatment are an essential component of a positive outcome. Report this confirmed diagnosis with a code from category C4A.- Merkel cell carcinoma with an additional character or characters based on the specific anatomical site.

Squamous cell carcinoma is often pink and scaly with notched or irregular borders. It has the potential to become erythematous (reddened) or ulcerated with easy bleeding. Metastasis is common, making early detection and treatment very important. Report this confirmed diagnosis with a code from category C44.- Other and unspecified malignant melanoma of skin with an additional character or characters based on the specific anatomical site.

Basal cell carcinoma is the most frequently seen skin malignancy, with patients aged 80 or older at highest risk. Report this confirmed diagnosis with a code from category C44.- Other and unspecified malignant melanoma of skin with an additional character or characters based on the specific anatomical site.

> **CODING BITES**
>
> For more information on malignant neoplasms, refer to the chapter titled **Coding Neoplasms** in this text.

YOU CODE IT! CASE STUDY

Carlos Monteverde, a 63-year-old male, comes in to see Dr. Harris, complaining of an extremely painful spot on his thigh. He states he has been very tired lately, especially since he noticed this bump. Patient history reveals a preexistent furunculosis.

Examination shows deep follicular abscess of several follicles with several draining points. CBC shows an elevated white blood cell count. Wound culture identifies Staphylococcus aureus.

Area is cleaned thoroughly. Instructions given to patient to apply warm, wet compresses at home.

A: Carbuncle of the thigh, left

P: Rx for erythromycin, q8h and mupirocin ointment

You Code It!

Read Dr. Harris's notes on his encounter with Carlos carefully, and code the visit.

Step #1: Read the case carefully and completely.

Step #2: Abstract the scenario. Which main words or terms describe why the physician cared for the patient during this encounter?

Step #3: Are there any details missing or incomplete for which you would need to query the physician? [If so, ask your instructor.]

Step #4: Check for any relevant guidance, including reading all of the symbols and notations in the Tabular List and the appropriate sections of the Official Guidelines.

Step #5: Determine the correct diagnosis code or codes to explain why this encounter was medically necessary.

Step #6: Double-check your work.

Answer:

Did you determine these to be the correct codes?

L02.436	Carbuncle of left lower limb
B95.61	Methicillin susceptible Staphylococcus aureus infection as the cause of diseases classified elsewhere

Good job!

14.4 Prevention and Screenings

The most frequently diagnosed malignancy in the United States is skin cancer. While some individuals have a higher risk of developing this type of malignant neoplasm, the truth is that anyone can find himself or herself with this diagnosis.

The best way to prevent skin lesions is to avoid known causes. Of course, some suggest staying out of the sun altogether, but this could decrease a patient's exercise and outdoor activities, which are also good for one's health. Therefore, protective clothing and use of sunscreen with a sun protection factor (SPF) of 15 or higher is strongly recommended prior to going out into the sun. Tanning beds also may cause an increased risk.

The Centers for Disease Control and Prevention (CDC) suggests ways to protect yourself from UV rays that can cause harm:

- Stay in the shade as much as possible, especially during the hours of 10 a.m. through 4 p.m.
- Keep your extremities (arms and legs) covered with clothing.
- Use a wide-brimmed hat to shade and protect your head, face, neck, and ears.
- Wear sunglasses to protect your eyes (and reduce your risk for cataracts).
- Apply sunscreen with an SPF of 15 or higher.
- Avoid the use of any indoor tanning beds or booths including sunlamps.

Physicians are encouraged by the CDC to perform an annual exam of all patients, especially those who are older and higher at risk. The scalp, ears, nasolabial folds, and wrinkles are key points.

EXAMPLES

There can be other reasons for a healthy patient to see a physician about skin-related issues:

Z12.83	Encounter for screening for malignant neoplasm of skin
Z20.7	Contact with and (suspected) exposure to pediculosis, acariasis and other infestations
Z52.11	Skin donor, autologous
Z52.19	Skin donor, other
Z84.0	Family history of diseases of the skin and subcutaneous tissue
Z86.31	Personal history of diabetic foot ulcer
Z87.2	Personal history of disease of the skin and subcutaneous tissue
Z94.5	Skin transplant status
Z96.81	Presence of artificial skin

YOU CODE IT! CASE STUDY

PATIENT NAME: Christopher Flemming

SUBJECTIVE: The patient is a 54-year-old male who presents for his annual preventive screening of moles. He has no particular lesions he is concerned about, although he states his wife has told him that he has a lot of moles on his back. He does not think any of them are changing. He did have an atypical nevus removed from one of the toes on his left foot about 3 years ago. He did not require re-excision after the biopsy. He was told to have annual skin exams and he just has not followed through with it. His other complaint is acne on his chest and back.

PAST MEDICAL HISTORY: Negative for skin cancer.

MEDICATIONS: None.

ALLERGIES: NKDA.

FAMILY HISTORY: Negative for melanoma.

SOCIAL HISTORY: Moderate sun exposure. He does use sunscreen, when he remembers.

OBJECTIVE: Alert and oriented x3. Normal mood. Normal body habitus. Examined his face, neck, chest, abdomen, back, upper extremities and lower extremities, hands and feet bilaterally. There were no lesions anywhere worrisome for cutaneous malignancy; however, he does have an above-average number of pigmented macular nevi. These range from 2–6 mm in diameter. The lesions appear similar to each other and are widely distributed on his chest, abdomen, and back; few on his upper and lower extremities and face. On his upper back, there are scattered 2.5 mm inflammatory papules and pustules.

ASSESSMENT:

1. Mild truncal acne.
2. Multiple nevi.
3. History of solitary atypical nevus.

PLAN:

1. Reviewed ABCDs of pigmented lesions, sun protection. Discussed self-exam. Advised he return for skin examination annually as the mole pattern he has does put him at a higher lifetime risk of development of melanoma.
2. He was given erythromycin solution to use b.i.d. for acne.
3. Follow-up is scheduled in 1 year.

You Code It!

Review this documentation from Dr. Stirpe's evaluation of Christopher, and determine the correct code or codes to report the medical necessity for this encounter.

Step #1: Read the case carefully and completely.

Step #2: Abstract the scenario. Which main words or terms describe why the physician cared for the patient during this encounter?

Step #3: Are there any details missing or incomplete for which you would need to query the physician? [If so, ask your instructor.]

Step #4: Check for any relevant guidance, including reading all of the symbols and notations in the Tabular List and the appropriate sections of the Official Guidelines.

Step #5: Determine the correct diagnosis code or codes to explain why this encounter was medically necessary.

Step #6: Double-check your work.

Answer:

Did you determine these to be the correct codes?

Z12.83	Encounter for screening for malignant neoplasm of skin
D22.5	Melanocytic nevi of trunk
L70.8	Other acne

Chapter Summary

With all the advertising about lotions to preserve youthful skin, shampoos and conditioners for soft hair, and manicures and pedicures for nails, you may forget that the elements of the integumentary system (skin, hair, nails) are not just cosmetic or decorative elements of our bodies. In addition, the glands embedded in the skin support the ongoing proper function of the body.

> **CODING BITES**
>
> Early detection is the best, most effective way to deal with any malignancy, including skin cancer. This means that a regular habit of self-examination is wise. The CDC developed a five-point checklist to help you check yourself for melanoma.
>
> "A" stands for Asymmetrical. Does the mole or spot have an irregular shape with two parts that look very different?
>
> "B" stands for Border. Is the border irregular or jagged?
>
> "C" is for Color. Is the color uneven? Do you see variations of brown, black, blue, or white?
>
> "D" is for Diameter. Is the mole or spot larger than the size of a pea (6 mm)?
>
> "E" is for Evolving. Has the mole or spot changed during the past few weeks or months?
>
> If the answer to any of these steps is Yes, the patient should contact a dermatologist for a complete screening.

CHAPTER 14 REVIEW
Coding Integumentary Conditions

Enhance your learning by completing these exercises and more at connect.mheducation.com!

Let's Check It! Terminology

Match each key term to the appropriate definition.

Part I

1. **LO 14.1** A bubble or sac formed on the surface of the skin, typically filled with a watery fluid or serum.
2. **LO 14.1** An open wound or sore caused by pressure, infection, or inflammation.
3. **LO 14.2** Death and decay of tissue due to inadequate blood supply.
4. **LO 14.1** The layer beneath the dermis; also known as the *hypodermis*.
5. **LO 14.3** A painful, pus-filled boil due to infection of the epidermis and underlying tissues, often caused by staphylococcus.
6. **LO 14.1** A skin lesion caused by continuous pressure on one spot, particularly on a bony prominence.
7. **LO 14.2** A saclike bulb containing the hair root.
8. **LO 14.2** Fingers and toes.
9. **LO 14.2** A pigmented, cylindrical filament that grows out from the hair follicle within the epidermis.
10. **LO 14.1** The external layer of the skin, the majority of which is squamous cells.
11. **LO 14.1** The internal layer of the skin; the location of blood vessels, lymph vessels, hair follicles, sweat glands, and sebum.
12. **LO 14.1** The external membranous covering of the body.

A. Blister
B. Carbuncle
C. Decubitus Ulcer
D. Dermis
E. Epidermis
F. Gangrene
G. Hair
H. Hair Follicle
I. Phalanges
J. Skin
K. Subcutaneous
L. Pressure Ulcer

Part II

1. LO 14.3 An erosion or loss of the full thickness of the epidermis.
2. LO 14.3 A large macule.
3. LO 14.3 A raised lesion with a diameter of less than 5 mm.
4. LO 14.3 An abnormally pigmented area of skin. A birthmark is an example.
5. LO 14.3 A flat lesion with a different pigmentation (color) when compared with the surrounding skin.
6. LO 14.3 A papule larger than 5 mm.
7. LO 14.3 A fluid-filled or gas-filled bubble in the skin.
8. LO 14.3 A boil.
9. LO 14.3 Flaky exfoliated epidermis.
10. LO 14.3 A large vesicle that is filled with fluid.
11. LO 14.3 A vesicle filled with pus.

A. Bulla
B. Cyst
C. Furuncle
D. Macule
E. Nevus
F. Nodule
G. Papule
H. Patch
I. Pustule
J. Scale
K. Ulcer

Let's Check It! Concepts

Choose the most appropriate answer for each of the following questions.

1. LO 14.1 The _____ is a sturdy collagenous layer that connects the _____ to the fatty tissue layer.
   a. epidermis, dermis
   b. dermis, epidermis
   c. fatty tissue, dermis
   d. subcutaneous, epidermis

2. LO 14.1 Seborrheic dermatitis is coded from category _____.
   a. L20
   b. L21
   c. L22
   d. L23

3. LO 14.3 Latoya Gregson was diagnosed with a left hand nevus. The correct code would be
   a. D22.6
   b. D22.60
   c. D22.61
   d. D22.62

4. LO 14.2 Women with this condition have excessive hair growth on anatomical sites where hair does not typically occur, such as the chest or chin. This condition is known as
   a. trichotillomania.
   b. hirsutism.
   c. alopecia.
   d. cilia.

5. LO 14.1 Kathy Harrington, a 17-year-old female, comes in today complaining of red, tender skin and having chills. Kathy admits to sun bathing all day yesterday. After an examination, Dr. Dills diagnoses Kathy with a 2nd degree sunburn. What is the correct code?
   a. L55.9
   b. L55.0
   c. L55.1
   d. L55.2

6. LO 14.2 _____ are sweat glands that are responsible for maintaining proper body temperature by excreting sweat (water, salt, and wastes) via the pores in the skin.
   a. Sebaceous glands
   b. Eccrine glands
   c. Apocrine glands
   d. Holocrine glands

7. LO 14.3 _____ is recognized by a bluish-red or flesh-colored nodule.
   a. Basal cell carcinoma
   b. Malignant melanoma
   c. Merkel cell carcinoma
   d. Squamous cell carcinoma

CHAPTER 14 REVIEW

8. LO 14.1 When skin layers are lost through and including the subcutaneous tissue, this is a _____ pressure ulcer.
   a. stage 1
   b. stage 2
   c. stage 3 ✓
   d. stage 4

9. LO 14.1 _____ presents with pain, edema, and/or loss of flexibility in at least one joint. When affecting the fingers or toes, the nails may show pitting or begin to separate from the nail bed.
   a. Psoriatic arthritis mutilans ✓
   b. Psoriasis vulgaris
   c. Guttate psoriasis
   d. Plaque psoriasis

10. LO 14.4 All of the following are ways to protect yourself from UV rays that can cause harm *except*
    a. keep your extremities covered with clothing.
    b. use indoor tanning beds regularly.
    c. use a wide-brimmed hat to shade and protect your head, face, neck, and ears.
    d. wear sunglasses to protect your eyes (and reduce your risk for cataracts).

Let's Check It! Guidelines

Refer to the Official Guidelines and fill in the blanks according to the Chapter 12, Diseases of the Skin and Subcutaneous Tissue, Chapter-Specific Coding Guidelines.

all	site	clinical	documentation	no
completely	highest	progresses	ulcer	admitted
terms	L89	healing	stage	two

1. Codes from category L89, Pressure _____, identify the _____ of the pressure ulcer as well as the stage of the ulcer.
2. Assign as many codes from category _____ as needed to identify _____ the pressure ulcers the patient has, if applicable.
3. When there is _____ documentation regarding the _____ of the pressure ulcer, assign the appropriate code for unspecified stage (L89.--9).
4. Assignment of the pressure ulcer stage code should be guided by _____ documentation of the stage or documentation of the _____ found in the Alphabetic Index.
5. No code is assigned if the documentation states that the pressure ulcer is _____ healed.
6. Pressure ulcers described as _____ should be assigned the appropriate pressure ulcer stage code based on the _____ in the medical record.
7. If a patient is _____ with a pressure ulcer at one stage and it _____ to a higher stage, _____ separate codes should be assigned: one code for the site and stage of the ulcer on admission and a second code for the same ulcer site and the _____ stage reported during the stay.

Let's Check It! Rules and Regulations

Please answer the following questions from the knowledge you have gained after reading this chapter.

1. LO 14.1 What are two factors a professional coding specialist needs to know to determine the correct code(s) for a diagnosed pressure ulcer?
2. LO 14.1 List the stages of pressure ulcers, and explain how you differentiate among the stages.
3. LO 14.1 Read the ICD-10-CM Official Guidelines for Coding and Reporting, section I. Conventions, General Coding Guidelines and Chapter Specific Guidelines, subsection C. Chapter-Specific Coding Guidelines, chapter 12. Diseases of the Skin and Subcutaneous Tissue, subsection a.2) Unstageable pressure ulcers. Explain the guideline, including instructions concerning clinical documentation.

4. **LO 14.2** Explain the different types of glands that are located within the skin. What is the function of each?
5. **LO 14.3** List two types of malignant lesions; describe each one, including the category code.

YOU CODE IT! Basics

First, identify the condition in the following diagnoses; then code the diagnosis.

Example: Bullous impetigo

    a. main term: *impetigo*   b. diagnosis: *L01.03*

1. Carbuncle of perineum:
   a. main term _____   b. diagnosis: _____
2. Acute lymphangitis:
   a. main term _____   b. diagnosis: _____
3. Coccygeal fistula with abscess:
   a. main term _____   b. diagnosis: _____
4. Pemphigus vulgaris:
   a. main term _____   b. diagnosis: _____
5. Flexural eczema:
   a. main term _____   b. diagnosis: _____
6. Seborrhea capitis:
   a. main term _____   b. diagnosis: _____
7. Irritant contact dermatitis due to cosmetics:
   a. main term _____   b. diagnosis: _____
8. Psoriasis vulgaris:
   a. main term _____   b. diagnosis: _____
9. Psoriatic arthritis mutilans:
   a. main term _____   b. diagnosis: _____
10. Lichen nitidus:
    a. main term _____   b. diagnosis: _____
11. Telogen effluvium:
    a. main term _____   b. diagnosis: _____
12. Alopecia universalis:
    a. main term _____   b. diagnosis: _____
13. Acne conglobata:
    a. main term _____   b. diagnosis: _____
14. Pilar cyst:
    a. main term _____   b. diagnosis: _____
15. Livedoid vasculitis:
    a. main term _____   b. diagnosis: _____

YOU CODE IT! Practice

Using the techniques described in this chapter, carefully read through the case studies and determine the most accurate ICD-10-CM code(s) and external cause code(s), if appropriate, for each case study.

1. Angie Ullman, a 7-year-old female, is brought into the ER by her parents due to a painful rash on her legs. The ER physician documents a temperature of 101 F and admits Angie to the hospital with the diagnosis of severe poison ivy. Angie's mother admitted she was walking their dog at the local park this morning and must have come in contact with the poison ivy there.
2. Anna Morris, a 22-year-old female, presents today with a blister on her left elbow. Her elbow is painful and warm to the touch. After an examination, Dr. Lane diagnoses Anna with a pressure ulcer of the elbow, stage 2.
3. A.G. Harrison, a 62-year-old male, complains of a deep sore on his right heel. After an examination, Dr. Miles notes that the subcutaneous tissue is visible with necrosis and admits A.G. to the hospital. Dr. Miles diagnoses A.G. with a decubitus ulcer of the heel, stage 3.
4. George Bowden, a 34-year-old male, presents today with a painful pus-filled lump on the nape of his neck. After an examination, Dr. Harris diagnoses George with a neck carbuncle.
5. Maechearda McConico, a 23-year-old female, presents with a bleeding mole on her left eyebrow. After a thorough examination and the appropriate tests, Dr. Ardis diagnoses Maechearda with a malignant melanoma in situ.

CHAPTER 14 REVIEW

6. Matt Kicklighter, an 18-year-old male, presents today with fluid-filled blisters on his back. Matt states that the blisters are easily broken. After an examination and testing, Dr. Gardener diagnoses Matt with staphylococcal scalded skin syndrome with 14% exfoliation due to erythematosis.

7. Judy Shirer, a 48-year-old female, comes in today with swollen, red, and painful skin on her face. Judy says she also feels nauseous. Dr. Lee notes red streaking around the cheeks and eyes and a temperature of 103 F. After examining Judy, Dr. Lee admits her to the hospital, where further laboratory test results confirm the diagnosis of facial cellulitis, MRSA.

8. Aaron Ragin, a 17-year-old male, presents today with a painful red lump on his chest. Dr. Godwin completes an examination and the appropriate laboratory tests. Aaron is diagnosed with a furuncle due to staphylococcus.

9. Harriett Mooney, a 6-year-old female, is brought in by her parents. Harriett has dry scaly skin. Dr. Lebrun completes an examination and a patch test, which confirms the diagnosis of infantile eczema.

10. Kathy Neal, a 56-year-old female, presents today with an itchy purple-colored lower lip. Dr. Grimsley notes flat-topped papules intermingled with lacy white lines. Kathy is diagnosed with bullous lichen planus.

11. Brenda Mets, a 32-year-old female, was diagnosed with basal cell carcinoma on her nose 10 days ago. Brenda is admitted to the hospital today for electrodesiccation and curettage by Dr. Dease.

12. Donald Ross, a 33-year-old male, presents today with raised bumps on his back. Dr. Margroff notes pustules. Don admits to skin tenderness. Dr. Margroff completes an examination and diagnoses Donald with generalized pustular psoriasis.

13. Beth Whitman, an 81-year-old female, presents with a sore on the medial side of her right calf. After examining the area and documenting edema and ulceration, Dr. Sanoski decides to admit Beth to the hospital. After a workup, Beth is diagnosed with a venous stasis ulcer with muscle necrosis, right calf. A possible skin graft is discussed with the patient.

14. Eugene Sanford, a 49-year-old male, comes in today with the complaint of a small red prickly rash under his scrotum. Dr. Kimrey completes an examination and the appropriate tests. Eugene is diagnosed with apocrine miliaria.

15. Gary Sanders, a 78-year-old male, comes in today with the complaint that the mole on his right ankle has begun to rapidly change in shape and color. Dr. Jones completes an examination noting ABCD - asymmetry, elevation above skin surface with an irregular border, blue-grey in color, firm to the touch, and a diameter of 8 mm and thickness of 1.63 mm. Gary is admitted to Weston Hospital. Skin and lymph node biopsies were ordered as well as imaging studies and blood tests. After reviewing the results of the pathology report and other tests, Gary is diagnosed with a malignant nodular melanoma. Excision of lesion is scheduled.

YOU CODE IT! Application

The following exercises provide practice in abstracting physicians' notes and learning to work with documentation from our health care facility, Prader, Bracker, & Associates. These case studies are modeled on real patient encounters. Using the techniques described in this chapter, carefully read through the case studies and determine the most accurate ICD-10-CM code(s) and external cause code(s), if appropriate, for each case study.

PRADER, BRACKER, & ASSOCIATES

A Complete Health Care Facility

159 Healthcare Way • SOMEWHERE, FL 32811 • 407-555-6789

PATIENT: CHILDERS, AARON

ACCOUNT/EHR #: CHILAA001

DATE: 09/16/18

Attending Physician: Oscar R. Prader, MD

This 59-year-old male presents today with a rash on the bottom of his feet. Patient admits he is also having trouble with his vision and has dysuria.

VS normal; on visual foot examination, rash has a cobblestone appearance. After a thorough examination and testing, patient is diagnosed with acquired keratoderma due to reactive arthritis of the foot joint (Reiter's disease).

Patient is given 5 mg IM, methotrexate

Rx: Methotrexate, 2.5 mg tab, PO, once a day, x 10 days

P: Return PRN

ORP/pw   D: 09/16/18 09:50:16   T: 09/16/18 12:55:01

Determine the most accurate ICD-10-CM code(s).

PRADER, BRACKER, & ASSOCIATES
A Complete Health Care Facility
159 Healthcare Way • SOMEWHERE, FL 32811 • 407-555-6789

PATIENT: STEEVANG, BRANDON

ACCOUNT/EHR #: STEEBR001

DATE: 10/16/18

Attending Physician: Oscar R. Prader, MD

S: This is a 39-year-old male with advanced human immunodeficiency virus infection who has presented to the emergency department with severe itching with a duration of approximately 10 days. On a scale of 1 to 10, he rates the itching as 10 of 10 in severity. Patient states he has been compliant with his antiretroviral therapy. He has been drinking excessively and taking diphenhydramine every 4 hours for the last several days.

O: H: 6'1", Wt: 176, T: 98.9, R: 19, P: 66, BP: 132/76. On examination, he is constantly scratching his skin. There are spots of blood on his clothing. Xerosis is noted as well as several brown patches on his extremities. The scrotum appears leathery and thickened. A skin scraping for scabies mite is performed and sent to the lab for analysis.

A: Scabies, HIV

Rx: Permethrin, 5% cream, apply to all skin surfaces. Leave on for at least 9 hours, then wash off with warm water.

P: Follow-up appointment with PCP

ORP/pw   D: 10/16/18 09:50:16   T: 10/18/18 12:55:01

Determine the most accurate ICD-10-CM code(s).

CHAPTER 14 REVIEW

PRADER, BRACKER, & ASSOCIATES

A Complete Health Care Facility

159 Healthcare Way • SOMEWHERE, FL 32811 • 407-555-6789

PATIENT: CHARLES, RICHARD

ACCOUNT/EHR #: CHARRI001

DATE: 09/16/18

Attending Physician: Renee O. Bracker, MD

S: This 35-year-old male came in after experiencing a severe episode with a prodrome of tingling of his lip before the appearance of lesions. He has been diagnosed with recurrent herpes simplex labialis. These episodes typically last between 1 and 2 weeks. He has no other medical problems and would like some easy-to-follow recommendations to manage this chronic illness.

O: VS normal. On visual examination, a small blister/sore on the lower lip is documented.

A: Recurrent herpes simplex labialis

Rx: Valacyclovir 2g, PO, followed by 2g in 12 hours

P: Return PRN

ROB/pw   D: 09/16/18 09:50:16   T: 09/16/18 12:55:01

Determine the most accurate ICD-10-CM code(s).

WESTON HOSPITAL

629 Healthcare Way • SOMEWHERE, FL 32811 • 407-555-6541

PATIENT: MEDINA, LEAH

ACCOUNT/EHR #: MEDILE001

DATE: 09/16/18

Attending Physician: Renee O. Bracker, MD

S: Leah Medina, a 6-year-old female, was at home helping her father clean out the attic when she was bitten by a black spider. Her father, Jacob, thought quickly and captured the spider in an old jar. Leah began to run a fever and vomited several hours later, so her father rushed her to the ED.

O: H: 50.5", Wt: 58.0 lbs., T: 102 F, R: 22, P: 90, BP: 127/88. Leah says she feels really tired and hurts all over. She has constantly scratched the bite area since arriving at the ED. She appears lethargic; rash is noted over body; heart is regular with no gallops or murmurs; lungs are clear; a dark blue/purple wound is noted on the right thigh. PMH and FH are both noncontributory. Dr. Bracker was able to identify the spider as a black widow spider and admits Leah to the hospital.

A: Black widow spider bite

P: Anitvenom 6000 units IV in 50 mL of normal saline over 15 minutes

ROB/pw   D: 09/16/18 09:50:16   T: 09/16/18 12:55:01

Determine the most accurate ICD-10-CM code(s).

WESTON HOSPITAL

629 Healthcare Way • SOMEWHERE, FL 32811 • 407-555-6541

PATIENT: CHABANNI, LORI

ACCOUNT/EHR #: CHABLO001

DATE: 09/16/18

Attending Physician: Renee O. Bracker, MD

S: This 46-year-old female with a 3-month history of ulcerations and abscesses involving both breasts was admitted today. Patient states the ulcerations began to appear after breast reduction surgery, approximately 2 weeks postop. The patient had no history of ulcerations before the breast reduction surgery. She also states that her muscles and joints ache.

O: VS: T: 102 F, all other VS are within normal range; patient is in obvious distress. PMH: remarkable for hypertension and quiescent ulcerative colitis. FH: Noncontributory. Deep ulcers under breast, bilaterally, are noted with well-defined borders. Ulcer edges are worn and surrounding skin is red. Coloration of ulcers is violet to blue. Incision and drainage of breast abscesses is scheduled.

A: Pyoderma gangrenosum.

P: Pulse IV methylprednisolone, 500 mg daily for 3 consecutive days

ROB/pw   D: 09/16/18 09:50:16   T: 09/16/18 12:55:01

Determine the most accurate ICD-10-CM code(s).

15 Coding Muscular and Skeletal Conditions

Key Terms

Arthropathy
Articulation
Chondropathy
Dorsopathy
Intervertebral Disc
Laterality
Myopathy
Site
Spondylopathy
Vertebra

Learning Outcomes

After completing this chapter, the student should be able to:

LO 15.1 Code accurately arthropathic conditions of the muscles.
LO 15.2 Determine the proper way to report dorsopathies and spondylopathies.
LO 15.3 Interpret the details required to report soft tissue disorders.
LO 15.4 Identify the specifics of diseases that affect the musculoskeletal system reported from other areas of ICD-10-CM.
LO 15.5 Report diagnoses related to pathological fractures accurately.

STOP! Remember, you need to follow along in your ICD-10-CM code book for an optimal learning experience.

15.1 Arthropathies

As you can see in Figure 15-1, the entire skeleton appears to be wrapped with muscles from top to bottom and all the way around. Each muscle has a specific function.

Injuries are not the only concern that can affect an individual's musculoskeletal health. Diseases, infections, and other problems can occur. There are pathogens (bacteria, viruses, and fungi) that directly attack the muscles of the body. The physician's notes might identify the patient's condition as **myopathy**, **arthropathy**, **chondropathy**, **dorsopathy**, or **spondylopathy**. Some of these conditions are described in this list:

CODING BITES

Myopathy: *myo* = muscle + *-pathy* = disease.
Arthropathy: *arthro* = joint + *-pathy* = disease.
Chondropathy: *chondro* = cartilage + *-pathy* = disease.
Dorsopathy: *dorso* = back + *-pathy* = disease.
Spondylopathy: *spondylo* = vertebra + *-pathy* = disease.

Myopathy
Disease of a muscle [plural: myopathies].

Arthropathy
Disease or dysfunction of a joint [plural: arthropathies].

Chondropathy
Disease affecting the cartilage [plural: chondropathies].

Dorsopathy
Disease affecting the back of the torso [plural: dorsopathies].

Spondylopathy
Disease affecting the vertebrae [plural: spondylopathies].

Rheumatoid arthritis (RA) is an autoimmune systemic inflammatory disease that affects joints as well as the surrounding muscles, tendons, and ligaments. Report a code from category M05 Rheumatoid arthritis with rheumatoid factor or M06 Other rheumatoid arthritis. To determine the complete valid code, you will need to identify, from the documentation, the specific anatomical site. Be alert because more than one anatomical site may be involved, and ICD-10-CM provides you with combination codes to report the complete story of this patient's condition.

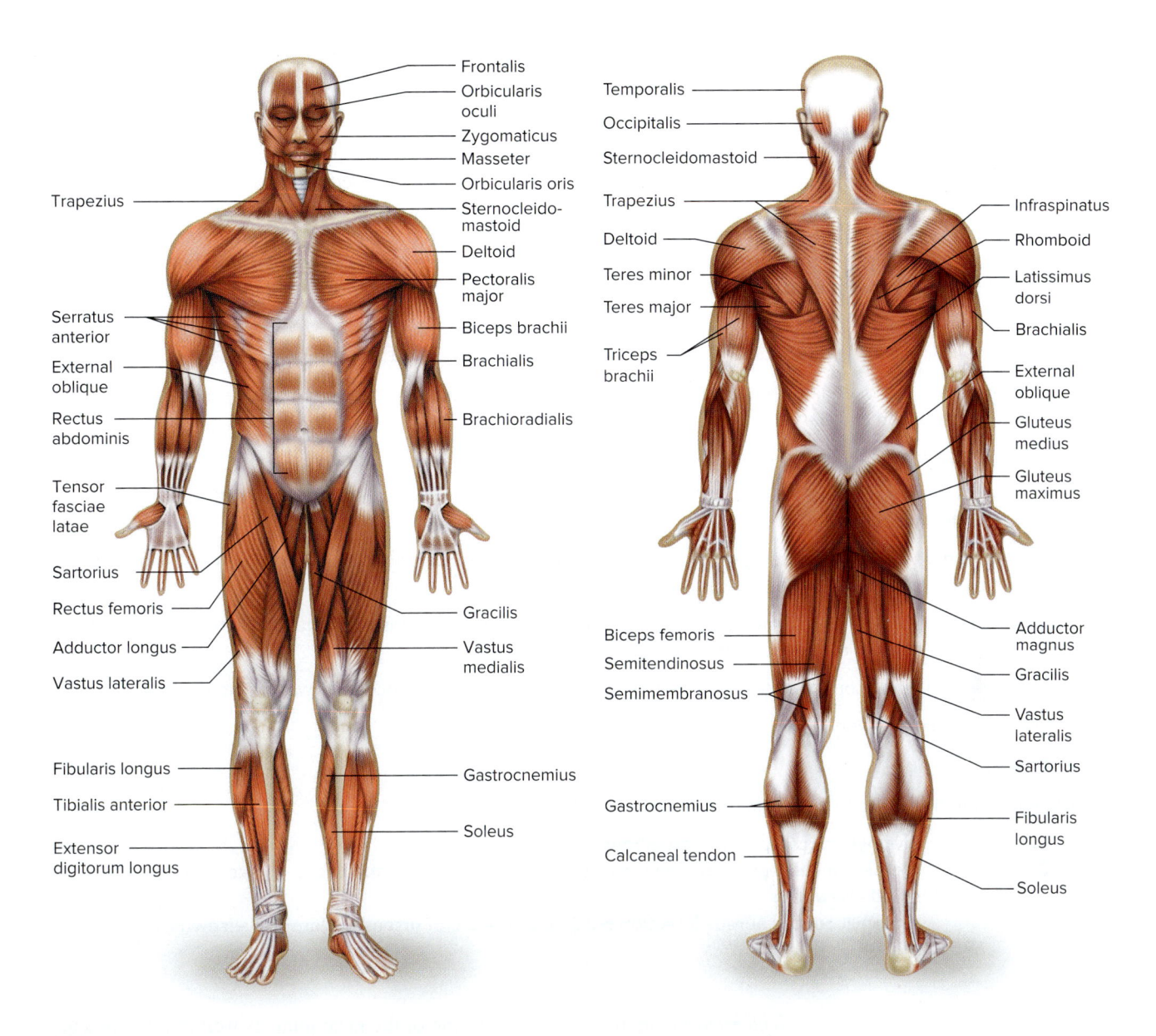

FIGURE 15-1 An illustration identifying the muscles of the body: anterior and posterior David Shier et al., *Hole's Human Anatomy & Physiology*, 12/e. ©2010 McGraw-Hill Education. Figure 9.23 and 9.24, p. 305–306. Used with permission.

CODING BITES

Many people confuse RA (rheumatoid arthritis) with OA (osteoarthritis). RA is a condition that affects the muscles, joints, and/or connective tissue, whereas OA is the deterioration of cartilage within joints as well as spinal vertebrae.

EXAMPLES

M05.151	Rheumatoid lung disease with rheumatoid arthritis of right hip
M05.242	Rheumatoid vasculitis with rheumatoid arthritis of the left hand
M05.361	Rheumatoid heart disease with rheumatoid arthritis of right knee
M06.022	Rheumatoid arthritis without rheumatoid factor, left elbow
M06.071	Rheumatoid arthritis without rheumatoid factor, right ankle and foot

Rheumatoid factor (RF) is a test that quantifies the amount of the RF antibodies in the blood. A positive RF is the abnormal result indicating a higher number of antibodies have been detected—confirmation of the autoimmune response mechanism. You would find the data on the pathology report.

CHAPTER 15 | CODING MUSCULAR AND SKELETAL CONDITIONS

> # YOU CODE IT! CASE STUDY
>
> Gary Simmons, a 19-year-old male, came in with complaints of intense pain and swelling of his left elbow. Vital signs evidence a low-grade fever. Gary states that he injured his forearm in hockey practice and it got infected, but he was too busy with classes and practice to go to the medical clinic on campus. Now, all of a sudden, he has pain in his elbow that he cannot ignore. Dr. Lannahan applied a local anesthetic and used fine needle aspiration to extract some synovial fluid. Analysis shows gross pus and testing shows a high white blood cell count. The synovial fluid glucose is 55 mg/dL. This confirmed a diagnosis of acute septic arthritis, due to gram-positive Staphylococcus aureus.
>
> ## You Code It!
>
> Go through the steps of coding, and determine the code or codes that should be reported for this encounter between Dr. Lannahan and Gary.
>
> Step #1: Read the case carefully and completely.
>
> Step #2: Abstract the scenario. Which main words or terms describe why the physician cared for the patient during this encounter?
>
> Step #3: Are there any details missing or incomplete for which you would need to query the physician? [If so, ask your instructor.]
>
> Step #4: Check for any relevant guidance, including reading all of the symbols and notations in the Tabular List and the appropriate sections of the Official Guidelines.
>
> Step #5: Determine the correct diagnosis code or codes to explain why this encounter was medically necessary.
>
> Step #6: Double-check your work.
>
> **Answer:**
>
> Did you determine these to be the correct codes?
>
> | | |
> |---|---|
> | M00.022 | Staphylococcal arthritis, left elbow |
> | B95.61 | Methicillin susceptible Staphylococcus aureus infection as the cause of diseases classified elsewhere |
> | | (Staphylococcus aureus infection NOS as the cause of diseases classified elsewhere) |

Genu recurvatum, the backward curving of the knee joint, as well as other bowing of the long bones of the leg, may be treated with braces, casting, and/or orthotics. Congenital genu recurvatum is reported with code Q68.2 Congenital deformity of knee. When this condition is the sequela (late effect) of rickets, it is reported with M21.26- Flexion deformity, knee, followed by code E64.3 Sequela of rickets.

Gout, also known as *gouty arthritis,* is the result of the buildup of uric acid in the body; caused by either a malfunction that produces too much uric acid or an anomaly that makes it difficult for the body to get rid of uric acid. The specific underlying cause may be idiopathic or secondary, as a manifestation of renal impairment, adverse reaction to a drug, or a toxic effect. Gout presents in the joints, most often a toe, knee, or ankle, and begins with a throbbing or extreme pain in the middle of the night. The joint will be tender, warm to the touch, and erythematous (red). The most common treatment is a prescription for NSAIDs (nonsteroidal anti-inflammatory drugs). In ICD-10-CM, gout is reported from code category M10- Gout or from code category M1A- Chronic Gout, with additional characters required to report the underlying cause (i.e., drug-induced, idiopathic, etc.) as well as the specific anatomical location (i.e., ankle, elbow, foot, etc.).

Osteoarthritis is a chronic degeneration of the articular cartilage simultaneous with the formation of bone spurs on the underlying bone within a joint. The cause of the osteoarthritis might be an idiomatic condition (such as code M17.11 Unilateral primary osteoarthritis, right knee); secondary to another underlying condition (such as code M18.52 Other unilateral secondary osteoarthritis of first carpometacarpal joint, left hand); or post-traumatic (such as code M19.172 Post-traumatic osteoarthritis, left ankle and foot). Treatments typically begin with NSAIDs and/or corticosteroid injections. In some cases, a brace or crutches may be helpful.

> ### LET'S CODE IT! SCENARIO
>
> *Timothy Metrosky, a 55-year-old male, came to see Dr. Weingard with complaints of acute pain in his left hip. He had been diagnosed with stage 1 chronic kidney disease about 1 year ago, but it has been under control with medication. Dr. Weingard aspirated synovial fluid from his hip, and the pathology report confirmed that Timothy had developed secondary gout in his hip.*
>
> #### Let's Code It!
>
> Dr. Weingard diagnosed Timothy with gout in his left hip, secondary to his renal impairment. Turn to the Alphabetic Index, look up *Gout,* and read down the list. Hmmm.
>
> **Gout, gouty (acute) (attack) (flare)** (*see also* **Gout, chronic) M10.9**
>
> Was Timothy diagnosed with chronic gout? Check the notes. No. So, look down the indented list to find "secondary," or something similar . . .
>
> **Gout, gouty**
>   **in (due to) renal impairment M10.30**
>   **hip M10.35-**
>
> Great! The terms "*due to*" and "*secondary*" both indicate the condition [gout] was caused by another condition [kidney disease]. Now turn to the Tabular List and confirm the code.
>   Start reading at the code category
>
> ☑4 **M10**   **Gout**
>
> Read the *Use additional code* notation carefully to see if it applies. None are applicable. Now check the **EXCLUDES2** note. You have already confirmed that the patient does not have chronic gout; therefore, this does not apply either.
>   Continue reading to find the accurate fourth character:
>
> ☑5 **M10.3**   **Gout due to renal impairment**
>
> There is a *Code first* notation that states you need to report Timothy's renal impairment as the first code, followed by this code for the gout. But, as long as you are here, keep reading down the column to review the fifth-character and sixth-character options and determine which matches Dr. Weingard's documentation:
>
>   **M10.352**   **Gout due to renal impairment, left hip**
>
> Very good! Now go back to the Alphabetic Index and find
>
>   **Disease, kidney, chronic, stage 1 N18.1**
>
> Double-check this code in the Tabular List.
>
> ☑4 **N18**   **Chronic kidney disease (CKD)**
>
> Read the *Code first* and *Use additional code* notations carefully. Do they apply to this case? No. So, continue down to find the accurate fourth character.
>
>   **N18.1**   **Chronic kidney disease, stage 1**
>
> You have the two codes required to report Dr. Weingard's diagnosis for Timothy. And remember that the *Code first* notation directed you to the correct sequencing of these two codes.
>
>   **N18.1**   **Chronic kidney disease, stage 1**
>   **M10.352**   **Gout due to renal impairment, left hip**
>
> *(continued)*

Make certain to check the top of both subsections and the head of both chapters in ICD-10-CM. There are notations at the beginning: an INCLUDES notation, a *Code first* notation, a *Use additional code* notation, **NOTE**s at the head of both chapters, and EXCLUDES2 notations. Read carefully. Do any relate to Dr. Weingard's diagnosis of Timothy? No. Turn to the Official Guidelines and read Section 1.c.13 (for the musculoskeletal system) and 1.c.14 (for the renal disease). There is nothing specifically applicable here, either. Now you can report N18.1, M10.352 for Timothy's diagnosis with confidence. Good coding!

Systemic lupus erythematosus (SLE) is an autoimmune disease affecting the joints, kidneys, brain, skin, and other organs. Interestingly, ICD-10-CM places this code category within the musculoskeletal system chapter. SLE may be an adverse effect of certain drugs. When this is documented, you will code M32.0 Drug-induced systemic lupus erythematosus, as well as an additional external cause code to identify the specific drug involved. If the etiology of the SLE is unknown, you will need to abstract from the physician's notes if any organ or organ system is specifically affected. When this is documented, use a combination code from subcategory M32.1- Systemic lupus erythematosus with organ or system involvement, with the fifth character naming that system or issue, such as

M32.11   Endocarditis in systemic lupus erythematosus
M32.13   Lung involvement in systemic lupus erythematosus

LET'S CODE IT! SCENARIO

Manuel Daniels, a 43-year-old male, came to see Dr. Biehl complaining of pain and stiffness in his lower jaw. Upon examination, Dr. Biehl noted swelling and erythema at the temporomandibular joint. Dr. Biehl diagnosed Manuel with *arthralgia of temporomandibular joint, right side*.

Let's Code It!

Dr. Biehl diagnosed Manuel with *arthralgia of temporomandibular joint*. In the Alphabetic Index, find

Arthralgia –
    Temporomandibular M26.62

Let's turn to the Tabular List and locate the beginning of the code category:

☑4 **M26**   Dentofacial anomalies (including malocclusion)

Beginning at the code category was a good idea. There is an EXCLUDES1 notation. Read it carefully and determine whether any of this guidance is applicable to this specific encounter. There is nothing here that relates to Manuel's condition, so review all of the choices for the fourth character to determine what matches Dr. Biehl's documentation about Manuel's diagnosis:

☑5 **M26.6**   Temporomandibular joint disorders

There is an EXCLUDES2 notation with two temporomandibular conditions listed. Again, read it carefully and determine whether any of this guidance is applicable to this specific encounter. There is nothing here that relates to Manuel's condition, so review all of the choices for the fifth character to determine what matches Dr. Biehl's documentation about Manuel's diagnosis. This part of the coding process is very important to determining the correct code to report.

Review the list of fifth characters. The documentation will bring you to this code:

M26.62   Arthralgia of temporomandibular joint

Very good. Now, a sixth character is required to report the laterality. Check the documentation, which side of Manuel's jaw was affected? The right side. Read through all of the sixth character options and determine the correct code to report:

M26.621   Arthralgia of right temporomanibular joint

Good job!

15.2 Dorsopathies and Spondylopathies (Conditions Affecting the Joints of the Spine)

Components of the Spine

From the neck, where the *atlas* (C1—the first cervical vertebra) articulates with the skull, and all the way down the column to the *coccyx*, the spine is a long stack of individual bones called **vertebrae**, separated by **intervertebral discs**.

Vertebrae

An individual vertebra is more than just a bone—it is actually a complex segment of the anatomical structure. In each of the sections of the vertebral column, the size and shape of the vertebrae change. The cervical, thoracic, and lumbar vertebrae are shaped slightly differently as the bones reconfigure on the basis of their position in the column and the support that is necessary. The cervical vertebrae are the smallest of all, and the lumbar vertebrae are the largest. The various aspects of all the vertebrae, however, are the same. As you can see in Figure 15-2, the vertebral body protects the spinal cord anteriorly, while the spinous process and pedicle protect it posteriorly.

Vertebrae are identified by their location and position in each section of the spinal column (see Figure 15-3):

- *Cervical vertebrae:* There are seven cervical vertebrae—beginning with the atlas (the first cervical vertebra) followed by the axis (the second cervical vertebra)—that run down the posterior (back) of the neck to the top of the shoulder area. These vertebrae are identified as C1, C2, C3, C4, C5, C6, and C7.
- *Thoracic vertebrae:* There are 12 thoracic vertebrae that run along the posterior segment of the torso (the thoracic cavity). The rib cage connects at these points. These vertebrae are identified as T1, T2, T3, T4, T5, T6, T7, T8, T9, T10, T11, and T12.
- *Lumbar vertebrae:* The five lumbar vertebrae are located at approximately the waist/hips area and are identified as L1, L2, L3, L4, and L5.

> **Vertebra**
> A bone that is a part of the construction of the spinal column [plural: vertebrae].
>
> **Intervertebral Disc**
> A fibrocartilage segment that lies between vertebrae of the spinal column and provides cushioning and support.

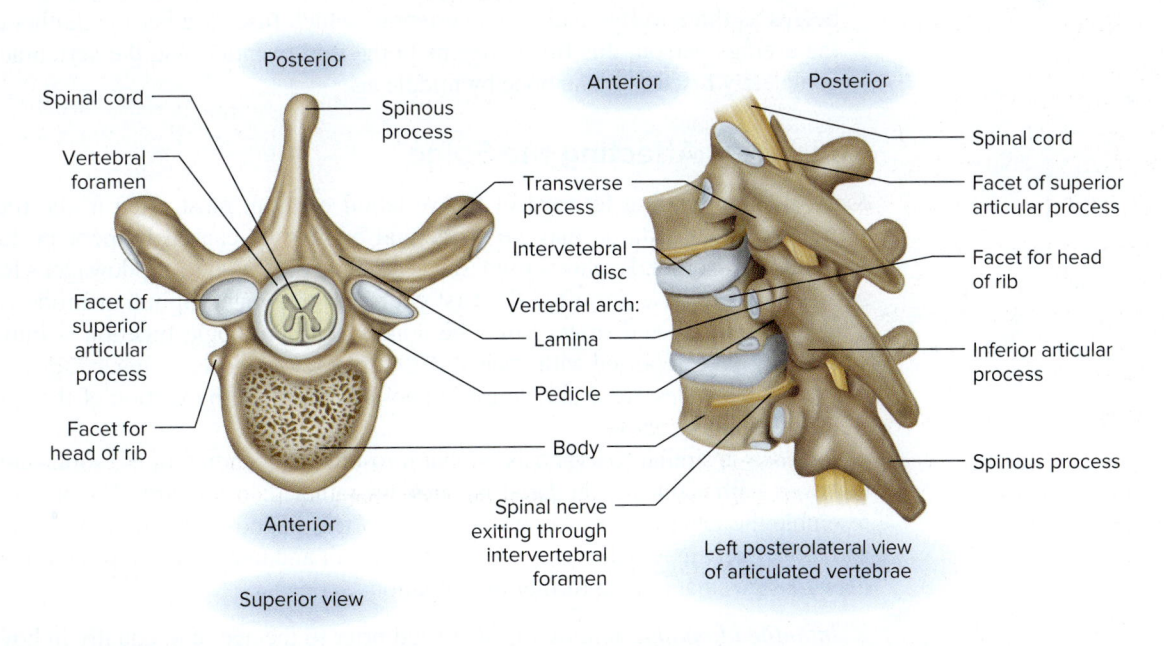

FIGURE 15-2 An illustration identifying the aspects of the vertebrae: anterior and posterior

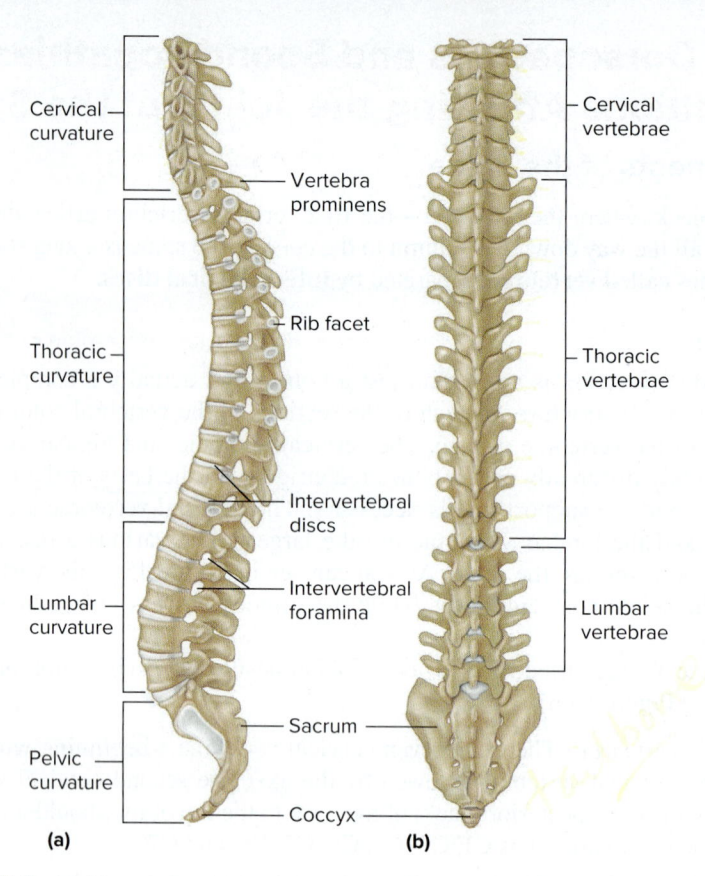

FIGURE 15-3 An illustration identifying the anatomical sites of the spinal column
Source: David Shier et al., *Hole's Human Anatomy & Physiology,* 12/e. ©2010 McGraw-Hill Education. Figure 7.32, p. 219. Used with permission.

- *Sacrum:* This is a triangular-shaped bone that begins as five individual vertebrae, which fuse together by the time the average person is in his or her mid-twenties. The sacrum vertebrae may be identified as S1, S2, S3, S4, and S5.
- *Coccyx:* Also known as the *tailbone,* this bottommost tip of the spinal column begins as three to five individual vertebrae, which fuse together in adulthood. For the average person, this fusion begins in the mid-twenties, and the vertebrae have completely fused into one bone by middle age.

Conditions Affecting the Spine

Kyphosis is a bending forward of the vertebral column, most often at the thoracic vertebrae. This condition may be congenital or may be caused by poor posture or other spinal disorder. Kyphosis used to be commonly referred to as "dowager's hump." A brace and exercise are often the first course of treatment. Spinal arthrodesis may relieve symptoms, and surgery may be done when neurologic function is impaired. This condition is reported with code M40.04 Postural kyphosis, thoracic region. However, multiple codes are available for kyphosis determined by section of the spine as well as underlying cause.

Scoliosis is similar to kyphosis, in that it results in a bending of the spinal column; however, with scoliosis, the bend is sideways rather than forward. The spine might resemble the letter S or C. Scoliosis is most often diagnosed in children aged 0–18, and more likely in females than males. Uneven gait and unbalanced hips and/or shoulders are signs that initiate further investigation.

Infantile idiopathic scoliosis is identified prior to the age of 4, equally in boys and girls, and more than 90% of these cases resolve without medical treatment.

Juvenile idiopathic scoliosis is diagnosed in children between the ages of 4 and 10, and is found more frequently in males than females. The curve in these children is often left-sided.

Adolescent idiopathic scoliosis is seen in patients aged 10–18 and may be evidenced in as high as 4% of this portion of the population. Researchers believe there may be a genetic connection; however, this has not yet been proven.

EXAMPLE

In all scoliosis diagnoses, you will need to abstract the specific region of the spine affected.

M41.02	Infantile idiopathic scoliosis, cervical region
M41.115	Juvenile idiopathic scoliosis, thoracolumbar region
M41.127	Adolescent idiopathic scoliosis, lumbosacral region

YOU CODE IT! CASE STUDY

Marci Wakefield started having pain in her back, after completing a full course of radiation treatments for a malignant tumor. Dr. Diaz diagnosed her with scoliosis of the thoracic region as a result of the radiation.

You Code It!

Go through the steps of coding, and determine the code or codes that should be reported for this encounter between Dr. Diaz and Marci.

Step #1: Read the case carefully and completely.

Step #2: Abstract the scenario. Which key words or terms describe why the physician cared for the patient during this encounter?

Step #3: Are there any details missing or incomplete for which you would need to query the physician? [If so, ask your instructor.]

Step #4: Check for any relevant guidance, including reading all of the symbols and notations in the Tabular List and the appropriate sections of the Official Guidelines.

Step #5: Determine the correct diagnosis code or codes to explain why this encounter was medically necessary.

Step #6: Double-check your work.

Answer:

Did you determine these to be the correct codes?

M41.54	Other secondary scoliosis, thoracic region
Y84.2	Radiological procedure and radiotherapy as the cause of abnormal reaction of the patient, or of later complication, without mention of misadventure at the time of the procedure

Spinal ankylosis is the fusion within a vertebral joint caused by disease. This is not a procedure where the physician may fuse a joint. Code subcategory M43.2 Fusion of spine requires a fifth character to report the specific region affected.

Ankylosing spondylitis (AS) is actually a type of inflammation within the vertebral joint (arthritis). This may also be seen in the joints between the spine and the pelvic girdle. AS affects men more than women. Code category M45 Ankylosing spondylitis is used to report AS, with a fourth character to specify the region affected.

Intervertebral disc infection is caused by a pathogen and is different from the inflammation of arthritis because it is suppurative (produces pus). Code subcategory

CODING BITES

Why is Marci's condition coded as *secondary scoliosis* and not . . .

M41.24   **Other idiopathic scoliosis, thoracic region**

Idiopathic means with no known cause. But the notes *do* state a cause of her scoliosis—the radiation. So this cannot be correct.

What about this code:

Q67.5   **Congenital deformity of spine (Congenital scoliosis)**

Congenital means present at birth. But Marci was not born with scoliosis—it developed as a result of her having radiation treatments.

Secondary means that something else (other than nature or something unknown) caused this condition. In this case, the radiation caused the scoliosis. The radiation came first, and the scoliosis came second.

M46.3 Infection of intervertebral disc (pyogenic) requires a fifth character to identify the specific region where the infection is located, as well as an additional code from B95–B97 to identify the pathogen.

LET'S CODE IT! SCENARIO

George Cornelius came to see Dr. Rymer with complaints of sudden-onset, severe low back pain. He states that the pain is in the left side of his buttocks, his left leg, and sometimes his left foot. At times, he states that his leg seems weak as well. Dr. Rymer takes a complete patient history, including specific times and actions that intensify the pain. Then x-rays, followed by an MRI, are taken of George's spine, showing a herniated (intervertebral) disc at L3–L4.

Let's Code It!

Dr. Rymer diagnosed George with a *herniated (intervertebral) disc.* Turn to the Alphabetic Index, look up *herniated,* and read down the list to find *disc.* Hmmm. It is not there. Try looking for *intervertebral.* Look down and see

Hernia, hernial (acquired) (recurrent) K46.9
    intervertebral cartilage or disc — see Displacement, intervertebral disc

OK, let's turn to that in the Alphabetic Index:

Displacement, displaced
    intervertebral disc NEC
        lumbar region M51.26

You might ask, How do we know that it is the lumbar region? Look back at Dr. Rymer's notes. He wrote that the herniated disk is at L3–L4. The "L" means the lumbar vertebrae, and the notation L3–L4 indicates that the affected intervertebral disc is between the third and fourth lumbar vertebrae. Now turn to the Tabular List and confirm the code.

Start reading at

✓4 **M51**   **Thoracic, thoracolumbar, and lumbosacral intervertebral disc disorders**

There is an EXCLUDES2 note that mentions disorders of the cervical and sacral discs. However, George's lumbar disc is what is dislocated, so you can keep reading down the column to review the fourth-character and fifth-character options and determine which matches Dr. Rymer's documentation:

✓5 **M51.2**   **Other thoracic, thoracolumbar, and lumbosacral intervertebral disc displacement**
     M51.26   **Other intervertebral disc displacement, lumbar region**

> Go back to Dr. Rymer's notes and see that while this doesn't match exactly, it does tell the story of why Dr. Rymer cared for George. Terrific!
>
> This code tells the whole story about George's specific injury. Now ask yourself, Do I need to find the external cause code(s) to explain how George's injury happened? No. A herniated disc is not necessarily the result of a traumatic event. Therefore, there is no need to report any external cause.
>
> Good work!

15.3 Soft Tissue Disorders

Fibromyalgia, also known as myofibrositis, or fibromyositis, causes the patient to experience tenderness on his or her extremities, as well as his or her neck and shoulders, back, and hips. In addition, the patient will suffer headaches, trouble sleeping, and sometimes forgetfulness and difficulties thinking. Code M79.7 Fibromyalgia.

Myositis identifies the inflammation of a muscle caused by a muscle strain. When a diagnosis of infective myositis is documented, you will need to report a code from subcategory M60.0 Infective myositis, with a fifth character to identify the specific anatomical site (shoulder, upper arm, hand, thigh, etc.) and a sixth character to report laterality. In addition to the M60.0-- code, you will need *an additional code* from B95–B97 to report the specific pathogen.

Polymyositis is a systemic rheumatic disorder evidenced by inflammatory and degenerative changes in the muscles. The signs and symptoms of muscle weakness, discomfort, and tenderness appear suddenly, most often in the proximal muscles. These symptoms interrupt the patient's ability to perform activities of daily living (ADL). To report this diagnosis accurately, you will need to abstract from the documentation the involvement of the respiratory system (M33.21), myopathy (M33.22), or other specific organs being hampered by this condition (M33.29).

Dermatopolymyositis is a systemic rheumatic disorder characterized by inflammatory and degenerative changes in the skin and muscles. The first sign is often an erythematous rash that appears on the face, neck, torso (front and back), and upper extremities. In addition, there may be a heliotropic rash on the eyelids along with periorbital edema. To report this diagnosis accurately, you will need to abstract from the documentation the involvement of the respiratory system (M33.11), myopathy (M33.12), or other specific organs being hampered by this condition (M33.19).

Juvenile dermatomyositis (JDM) is a systemic, autoimmune, inflammatory muscle condition that often appears with vasculopathy in children 18 years of age or younger. To report this diagnosis accurately, you will need to abstract from the documentation the involvement of the respiratory system (M33.01), myopathy (M33.02), or other specific organs being hampered by this condition (M33.09).

Bursitis is a painful inflammation of a bursa, most often the result of recurring trauma. Once you make your way to code category M71 Other bursopathies, you will need to abstract from the physician's notes the type of problem: Is there an abscess or infection? If so, in addition to identifying the specific anatomical site (shoulder, elbow, hand, etc.) and laterality, you will need to find the confirmation of the pathogen, so you can accurately add a second code from B95.- or B96.- to report this detail as well.

Epicondylitis is an inflammation of the elbow joint that typically begins as a small tear in the muscle and then is aggravated by activities. *Lateral epicondylitis* is commonly known as "tennis elbow," while *medial epicondylitis* is commonly known as "golfer's elbow," reported by codes M77.1 Lateral epicondylitis and M77.0 Medial epicondylitis, respectively. Both codes require a fifth character to identify the right or left elbow.

Achilles tendon contracture is a shortening of the tendocalcaneus (heel cord), which is caused by chronic poor posture, continual wearing of high-heeled shoes, or landing on the ball of the foot rather than the heel while jogging or is a manifestation of cerebral palsy or poliomyelitis. Use code M67.0 Short Achilles tendon (acquired), with a fifth character to identify the right or left ankle, or Q66.89 Other specified congenital deformities of feet.

Torticollis is a condition in which the sternocleidomastoid muscle becomes spasmed (shortened), causing the head to bend to one side and the chin to the opposite side. This condition may be acquired, reported with code M43.6 Torticollis, unless the documentation states Q68.0 Congenital deformity of sternocleidomastoid muscle, F45.8 Other somatoform disorders, G24.3 Spasmodic torticollis, or other diagnosis shown in the notation beneath M43.6.

Muscle spasms, commonly known as *muscle cramps,* are involuntary twitches and are often caused by myositis or fibromyositis. Sometimes these spasms are caused by metabolic or mineral imbalances. Abstract the documentation to identify the anatomical site. Use code M62.830 Muscle spasm of back, M62.831 Muscle spasm of calf (Charley-horse), M62.838 Other muscle spasm, or R25.2 Cramp and spasm.

Type III traumatic spondylolisthesis of the axis (C2) is a displacement of the vertebra anteriorly over the vertebra below it. An open reduction of the C2 vertebra followed by a posterior spinal fusion with a pedicle lag screw is used to repair the injury. Report this with code M43.12 Spondylolisthesis, cervical region.

LET'S CODE IT! SCENARIO

Elliott Carlyle, a 17-year-old male, is believed to be an up-and-coming star on the golf course. He explains to Dr. Carole that the pain in his left elbow has become severe and his ability to grasp the club is weakened. Physical exam included flexion and pronation, confirming medial epicondylitis.

Let's Code It!

Dr. Carole diagnosed Elliott with *medial epicondylitis*. In the ICD-10-CM Alphabetic Index, let's turn to find the documented term. . . . Find

Epicondylitis (elbow)

There are only two items on the indented list:

Epicondylitis (elbow)
　lateral M77.1-
　medial M77.0-

Check the scenario to confirm which diagnosis was documented. Let's go to the Tabular List to check this code category. Find

　☑4 **M77**　　Other enthesopathies

Check the diagnoses shown in the **EXCLUDES1** and **EXCLUDES2** notations. Do either of them relate to Elliott's diagnosis? No, good. Now, read down and review all of the fourth-character options. Which matches the documentation?

　☑5 **M77.0**　　Medial epicondylitis
　　　M77.01　　Medial epicondylitis, right elbow
　　　M77.02　　Medial epicondylitis, left elbow

Therefore, the most accurate code is

　M77.02　　Medial epicondylitis, left elbow

Check the top of this subsection and the head of this chapter in ICD-10-CM. Both a **NOTE** and an **EXCLUDES2** notation appear at the beginning of this ICD-10-CM chapter. Read carefully. Do any relate to Dr. Carole's diagnosis of Elliott? No. Turn to the Official Guidelines and read Section 1.c.13. There is nothing specifically applicable here, either.

　Now you can report M77.02 for Elliott's diagnosis with confidence.
　Good coding! Good work!

Osteochondrosis, also known as *osteochondropathy* or *Osgood-Schlatter disease,* is a painful separation of the epiphysis of the tibial tubercle from the tibial shaft. This condition most often affects preteen and early teenage boys after a traumatic event. Treatments include immobilization of the knee and rest. In severe cases, surgical repair may be required. One code example is M93.1 Kienbock's disease of adults (adult osteochondrosis of carpal lunates).

Osteitis deformans, also known as *Paget's disease,* may cause severe and chronic pain as well as impaired movement due to abnormal bone growth on the spinal cord. The preferred first phase of treatment is pharmaceutical. Report this from code category M88 Osteitis deformans (Paget's disease of bone), with additional characters to report the specific bone affected as well as laterality.

Osteoporosis is a disease that is believed to be the manifestation of slowing bone formation that occurs simultaneously with an increase in the body's reabsorption of bone. One exception is *post-traumatic osteoporosis,* also known as *Sudeck's atrophy.* The existence of osteoporosis increases the patient's susceptibility to fractures. The presence of a pathologic fracture will change the code determination in ICD-10-CM. Code category M80 reports osteoporosis *with* a current pathologic fracture, while code category M81 reports osteoporosis *without* a current pathologic fracture.

> **GUIDANCE CONNECTION**
>
> Read the ICD-10-CM Official Guidelines for Coding and Reporting, section **I. Conventions, General Coding Guidelines and Chapter Specific Guidelines,** subsection **C. Chapter-Specific Coding Guidelines,** chapter **13. Diseases of the Musculoskeletal System and Connective Tissue,** subsection **d. Osteoporosis.**

LET'S CODE IT! SCENARIO

Everett Rotarine, a 43-year-old male, was having pain in his left thigh, which his orthopedist, Dr. Nixon, identified as excessive bone resorption, the osteoclastic phase of Paget's disease. X-rays and a urinalysis showing elevated levels of hydroxyproline confirmed the osteoclastic hyperactivity. Everett comes in today to discuss the test findings and treatment options.

Let's Code It!

Dr. Nixon diagnosed Everett with *Paget's disease.* You may remember that this is an eponym and will be shown in the ICD-10-CM Alphabetic Index, so let's turn to find the suggested code. Find

Paget's disease

Notice the long list of additional descriptors of this condition indented beneath this listing. Look at the scenario again.

Paget's disease
    bone M88.9
        femur M88.85-

Let's go to the Tabular List to check this code category. Find

   ☑4 **M88**   **Osteitis deformans (Paget's disease of bone)**

Let's keep reading:

   ☑5 **M88.8**   **Osteitis deformans of other bones**
   ☑6 **M88.85**   **Osteitis deformans of thigh**
        M88.852   **Osteitis deformans of left thigh**

Therefore, the most accurate code is

   M88.852   **Osteitis deformans of left thigh**

Good work!

15.4 Musculoskeletal Disorders from Other Body Systems

Acquired Conditions

Muscle tumors do not occur frequently and can often be malignant. Use code categories C49 Malignant neoplasm of other connective and soft tissue, C79.89 Secondary malignant neoplasms of other specified sites, or D21 Other benign neoplasms of connective and other soft tissue.

Duchenne's muscular dystrophy (DMD) is caused by a mutation of the DMD gene within the X chromosome, resulting in the body's inability to create the dystrophin protein within the muscles. Due to this, males are more likely to contract the condition because females have an additional X chromosome that may counteract the mutated gene, as long as the second X chromosome is not damaged as well. Initial signs and symptoms of DMD include leg muscle weakness followed by weakness of the shoulder muscles. DMD is most often diagnosed in early childhood and may be terminal by age 21 should the weakness spread to either heart or respiratory muscles. New trials using gene therapy are hopeful. Use code G71.0 Muscular dystrophy.

Myasthenia gravis is a chronic autoimmune condition that causes muscle weakness, primarily in the face and neck, due to the immune system incorrectly attacking the muscle cells in the body. It may progress and involve additional weakness in the muscles of the extremities (arms and legs). Use code G70.00 Myasthenia gravis without (acute) exacerbation or G70.01 Myasthenia gravis with (acute) exacerbation.

Paralytic syndromes are conditions in which muscle control is reduced or nonexistent. Cerebral palsy (code category G80), hemiplegia and hemiparesis (code category G81), and paraplegia (paraparesis) and quadriplegia (quadriparesis) (code category G82) are some of the conditions that may interfere with the activities of daily living.

Congenital Disorders

Congenital myopathies include minicore disease, nemaline myopathy, and fiber-type disproportion. One code, G71.2, reports several muscle abnormalities diagnosed in a neonate or infant. Most often, the infant will not meet normal developmental milestones, particularly those involving muscular actions, such as sitting up or rolling over. Such babies may also have problems feeding.

Developmental dysplasia of the hip (DDH), also known as *congenital hip dysplasia*, is most common in a baby born breech, a large neonate, or a multiparity baby. DDH is a condition in which the head of the femur is displaced from the acetabulum. Use code Q65.89 Other specified congenital deformities of hip (congenital acetabular dysplasia).

Ectromelia or *hemimelia* can occur in either the upper or lower limb. Ectromelia is the congenital absence or imperfection of one or more limbs. Hemimelia is a congenital abnormality affecting only the distal segment of either the upper or lower limb. This condition is reported with code Q73.8 Other reduction defects of unspecified limb (ectromelia of limb NOS) (hemimelia of limb NOS).

Klippel-Feil syndrome is a condition characterized by the development of a short, wide neck due to either an abnormal number of cervical vertebrae or fused hemivertebrae (the incomplete development of one side of a vertebra). Use code Q76.1 Klippel-Feil syndrome (cervical fusion syndrome).

Spina bifida is a condition in which the bony encasement of the spinal cord fails to close. Surgical repair is done as soon as possible in an effort to reduce serious handicaps. There have been some successful cases of in utero surgical repair. This condition is reported from code category Q05- Spina bifida, with an additional character to identify the specific area of the spine that is affected.

> **CODING BITES**
>
> NOTICE that these conditions—*congenital myopathies, muscular dystrophy, myasthenia gravis,* and *paralytic syndromes*—are reported with codes from the ***Diseases of the Nervous System*** chapter of ICD-10-CM. Remember that the nerves signal the muscles to function. Therefore, paralysis is actually a dysfunction of the nerves that communicate with the affected specific muscles.

YOU CODE IT! CASE STUDY

Theda Granddura, a 37-year-old female, came to see Dr. Lyndon complaining of weakness in her arms and hands. She stated that sometimes, she is unsteady on her feet, and her right eyelid was droopy. Two days ago, she tried to pick up a glass and could not get her fingers to "work right." An EMG was performed in the office, confirming a diagnosis of myasthenia gravis.

You Code It!

Review the details in Dr. Lyndon's documentation of this encounter with Theda to determine the accurate ICD-10-CM code or codes to report her diagnosis.

Step #1: Read the case carefully and completely.

Step #2: Abstract the scenario. Which main words or terms describe why the physician cared for the patient during this encounter?

Step #3: Are there any details missing or incomplete for which you would need to query the physician? [If so, ask your instructor.]

Step #4: Check for any relevant guidance, including reading all of the symbols and notations in the Tabular List and the appropriate sections of the Official Guidelines.

Step #5: Determine the correct diagnosis code or codes to explain why this encounter was medically necessary.

Step #6: Double-check your work.

Answer:

Did you determine this to be the correct code?

G70.00   Myasthenia gravis without (acute) exacerbation

15.5 Pathological Fractures

The skeleton of the human body (see Figure 15-4) provides the structure for both form and function. The 206 bones in the adult body comprise a framework hinged together at the **articulations** (joints) that is stabilized by muscles and connective tissues.

In your job as a professional coding specialist, it is important to abstract from the documentation details regarding the **site** of the disease or injury (the specific bone) as well as the **laterality** (right side or left side), when applicable.

Some conditions may affect any part of the skeletal system and therefore require that the specific anatomical location be documented. For instance, when a long bone, such as an ulna or femur, is affected, you might find that knowing the name of the bone is insufficient; you will also need to know the part of the bone, such as the shaft. When the segment of the bone that is diseased leads into, and participates in, the formation of a joint (articulation), read the documentation carefully. Even if the part of the bone affected is *at the joint,* you must report the bone as the diseased anatomical site.

Diseases and other conditions can create problems with the bones and may be caused by a congenital malformation, pathology, or a traumatic event. As always, these are important details for coders to know.

The bones are, typically, the strongest parts of our bodies. However, in some cases, disease can deteriorate the structure of a bone so much that it breaks under the slightest pressure. Even normal activity can result in the weakened part of the bone breaking (fracture). When this happens, it is known as a pathological fracture.

The most common underlying cause of a pathological fracture is osteoporosis. However, other health conditions, such as a bone cyst, an infection, genetic disorders, and malignancy, may do just as much harm.

Articulation
A joint.

GUIDANCE CONNECTION

Read the ICD-10-CM Official Guidelines for Coding and Reporting, section **I. Conventions, General Coding Guidelines and Chapter Specific Guidelines,** subsection **C. Chapter-Specific Coding Guidelines,** chapter **13. Diseases of the Musculoskeletal System and Connective Tissue,** subsection **a. Site and laterality.**

Site
The specific anatomical location of the disease or injury.

Laterality
The right or left side of anatomical sites that have locations on both sides of the body; e.g., right arm or left arm; *unilateral* means one side and *bilateral* means both sides.

> **GUIDANCE CONNECTION**
>
> Read the ICD-10-CM Official Guidelines for Coding and Reporting, section **I. Conventions, General Coding Guidelines and Chapter Specific Guidelines,** subsection **C. Chapter-Specific Coding Guidelines,** chapter **13. Diseases of the Musculoskeletal System and Connective Tissue,** subsection **a.1) Bone versus joint.**

> **GUIDANCE CONNECTION**
>
> Read the ICD-10-CM Official Guidelines for Coding and Reporting, section **I. Conventions, General Coding Guidelines and Chapter Specific Guidelines,** subsection **C. Chapter-Specific Coding Guidelines,** chapter **13. Diseases of the Musculoskeletal System and Connective Tissue,** subsection **c. Coding of Pathologic Fractures.**

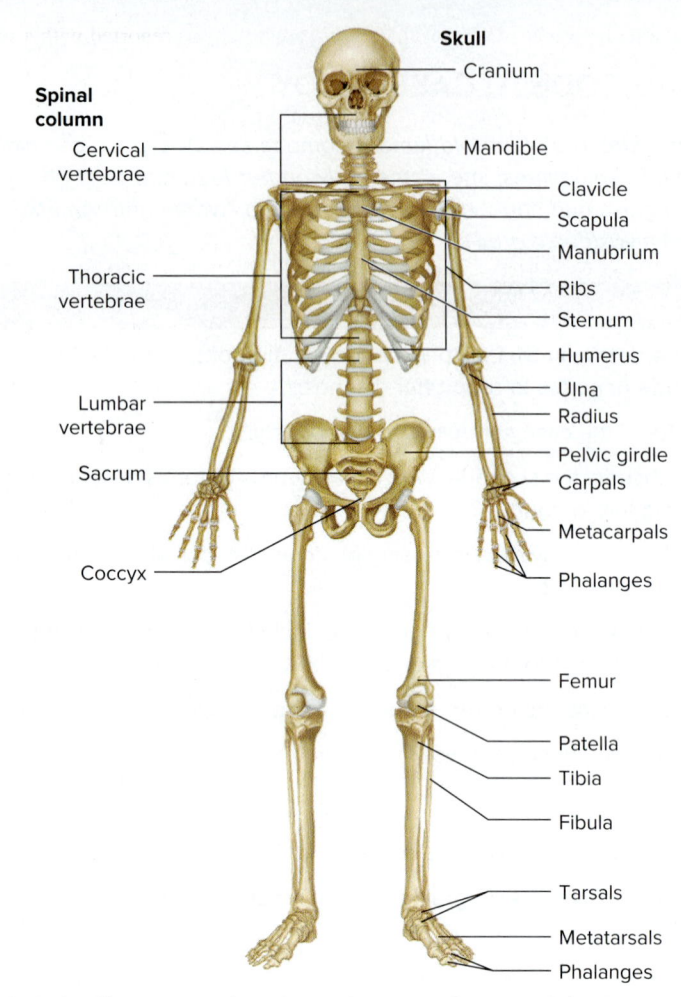

FIGURE 15-4 An illustration identifying the major bones of the human skeleton

Treatment for pathological fractures may be similar to that for a traumatic fracture. However, not always. In virtually all cases, the underlying condition is treated as well.

> **EXAMPLES**
>
> Pathological fractures are reported from these code subcategories:
>
> | | |
> |---|---|
> | M84.4- | Pathological fracture, not elsewhere classified |
> | M84.5- | Pathological fracture in neoplastic disease |
> | M84.6- | Pathological fracture in other diseases |

When reporting a code for a pathologic fracture, you will need to assign a seventh character to identify the point in the treatment for this condition.

A   Use the seventh character A for the entire scope of time that the patient is receiving active treatment for this fracture. This seventh character reports the status of "active treatment," not the relationship between physician and patient (new patient).

D   Once the patient has completed active treatment, this character should be reported to identify follow-up for routine healing.

G   The seventh character G would be reported for subsequent care for a pathological fracture with delayed healing.

K   Subsequent care provided for a nonunion would be identified with a seventh character of K.

P   When a malunion occurs, the subsequent care would be reported with a seventh character of P.

S   Care for any sequela (late effect) of the original pathological fracture is identified with a seventh character of S.

> **GUIDANCE CONNECTION**
>
> Read the ICD-10-CM Official Guidelines for Coding and Reporting, section **I. Conventions, General Coding Guidelines and Chapter Specific Guidelines**, subsection **C. Chapter-Specific Coding Guidelines**, chapter **13. Diseases of the Musculoskeletal System and Connective Tissue**, subsection **c. Coding of Pathologic Fractures**, and chapter **2. Neoplasms**, subsection **I.6) Pathologic fracture due to a neoplasm**.

YOU CODE IT! CASE STUDY

Deliah Livingston, a 49-year-old female, was diagnosed with breast cancer a year ago. She had a double mastectomy 6 months ago. She came to see Dr. Wells for a checkup and he discovered that Deliah's malignancy had metastasized to the proximal portion of her right femur. Dr. Wells suggested surgery to insert a metal rod to support the bone. She told him she would think about it. Yesterday, she was walking down her driveway and all of a sudden her thighbone splintered and she fell. In the Emergency Department, Dr. Travers diagnosed Deliah with a pathological fracture of the proximal femur, just below the hip joint, due to metastatic malignancy.

You Code It!

Abstract the documentation about this ED encounter between Deliah and Dr. Travers and determine how to report the reasons for this visit.

*HINT: You will need some of what you learned from the **Coding Neoplasms** chapter here.*

Step #1: Read the case carefully and completely.

Step #2: Abstract the scenario. Which main words or terms describe why the physician cared for the patient during this encounter?

Step #3: Are there any details missing or incomplete for which you would need to query the physician? [If so, ask your instructor.]

Step #4: Check for any relevant guidance, including reading all of the symbols and notations in the Tabular List and the appropriate sections of the Official Guidelines.

Step #5: Determine the correct diagnosis code or codes to explain why this encounter was medically necessary.

Step #6: Double-check your work.

Answer:

Did you determine these to be the correct codes?

M84.551A	Pathological fracture in neoplastic disease, right femur, initial encounter for fracture
C79.51	Secondary malignant neoplasm of bone
Z85.3	Personal history of malignant neoplasm of breast

Chapter Summary

The entire body is wrapped from head to toe and all the way around by muscles: voluntary muscles that assist movement of the skeleton and involuntary muscles that are controlled by the nervous system. Each muscle has its specific function and they are all susceptible to injury, inflammation, and disease.

The 206 bones of the adult human skeleton provide the foundational structure for the components of the body. These bones protect internal organs as well as enable certain functions. Each bone is categorized by its shape: long bones, flat bones, short bones, irregularly shaped bones, and sesamoid bones. Any of these bones can be afflicted by malformation during gestation (congenital conditions), disease (pathologic conditions), or injury (traumatic conditions).

> **CODING BITES**
>
> *Interesting Facts about Human Muscles*
> Longest muscle = Sartorious (thigh) muscle
> Smallest muscle = Stapedius (in the ear)
> Largest muscle = Gluteus maximus (buttocks)
> Strongest muscle = Masseter (chewing)
> Busiest muscles = Eye muscles
> Goosebump muscles = Tiny muscles in the hair root
> Smiling requires 17 facial muscles.
> Frowns require 42 facial muscles.

CHAPTER 15 REVIEW
Coding Muscular and Skeletal Conditions

Let's Check It! Terminology

Match each key term to the appropriate definition.

1. **LO 15.2** A fibrocartilage segment that lies between vertebrae of the spinal column and provides cushioning and support.
2. **LO 15.5** A joint.
3. **LO 15.5** The specific anatomical location of the disease or injury.
4. **LO 15.2** A bone that is a part of the construction of the spinal column.
5. **LO 15.5** The right or left side of anatomical sites that have locations on both sides of the body.

A. Articulation
B. Intervertebral Disc
C. Laterality
D. Site
E. Vertebra

Let's Check It! Concepts

Choose the most appropriate answer for each of the following questions.

1. **LO 15.2** Jane Timmerman was diagnosed with lower back strain, subsequent encounter. What is the correct code?
   a. S39.002A
   b. S39.012D
   c. S39.022D
   d. S39.092S

2. **LO 15.1** _____ is an autoimmune systemic inflammatory disease that affects joints as well as the surrounding muscles, tendons, and ligaments.
   a. Duchenne's muscular dystrophy
   b. Nemaline myopathy
   c. Rheumatoid arthritis
   d. Myasthenia gravis

3. **LO 15.1** A chronic degeneration of the articular cartilage simultaneous with the formation of bone spurs on the underlying bone within a joint is known as
   a. rheumatoid arthritis.
   b. gout.
   c. genu recurvatum.
   d. osteoarthritis.

4. LO 15.3 ____ is a condition in which the sternocleidomastoid muscles become spasmed (shortened), causing the head to bend to one side and the chin to the opposite side.
   a. Bursitis
   b. Epicondylitis
   c. Achilles tendon contracture
   d. Torticollis

5. LO 15.2 Sammie Blane was diagnosed with cervicothoracic postural kyphosis. How is this coded?
   a. M40.209
   b. M40.202
   c. M40.03
   d. M40.12

6. LO 15.3 A systemic rheumatic disorder characterized by inflammatory and degenerative changes in the skin and muscles is known as
   a. myositis.
   b. juvenile dermatomyositis.
   c. osteochondrosis.
   d. dermatopolymyositis.

7. LO 15.4 Myotonic muscular dystrophy is coded
   a. G71.11
   b. G71.0
   c. G71.12
   d. G71.13

8. LO 15.4 ____ is a chronic autoimmune condition that causes muscle weakness, primarily in the face and neck, due to the immune system incorrectly attacking the muscle cells in the body.
   a. Duchenne's muscular dystrophy
   b. Myasthenia gravis
   c. Ectromelia
   d. Paralytic syndromes

9. LO 5.5 Ben Watson is diagnosed with a malunion. It will be reported with which seventh character?
   a. A
   b. G
   c. P
   d. K

10. LO 15.5 When disease deteriorates the structure of a bone so much that it breaks under the slightest pressure, this is known as a ____ fracture.
    a. malformation
    b. traumatic
    c. congenital
    d. pathologic

Let's Check It! Guidelines

Refer to the Official Guidelines and fill in the blanks according to the Chapter 13, Diseases of the Musculoskeletal System and Connective Tissue, Chapter-Specific Coding Guidelines.

no	laterality	joint	Z87.310	without
systemic	history	active	A	multiple
healed	not	site	bone	time
fracture	affected	current	known	musculoskeletal
represents	traumatic	one		

1. Most of the codes within Chapter 13 have ____ and ____ designations. The site ____ the bone, joint or the muscle involved.

2. For categories where ____ multiple site code is provided and more than ____ bone, joint or muscle is involved, ____ codes should be used to indicate the different sites involved.

3. For certain conditions, the bone may be affected at the upper or lower end (e.g., avascular necrosis of bone, M87, Osteoporosis, M80, M81). Though the portion of the bone ____ may be at the ____, the site designation will be the ____, not the joint.

4. Bone, joint, or muscle conditions that are the result of a ____ injury are usually found in Chapter 13.

5. 7th character ____ is for use as long as the patient is receiving ____ treatment for the fracture.

CHAPTER 15 REVIEW

6. Osteoporosis is a ____ condition, meaning that all bones of the ____ system are affected.
7. Category M81, Osteoporosis ____ current pathological fracture, is for use for patients with osteoporosis who do ____ currently have a pathologic fracture due to the osteoporosis, even if they have had a ____ in the past.
8. For patients with a ____ of osteoporosis fractures, status code ____, Personal history of (healed) osteoporosis fracture, should follow the code from M81.
9. Category M80, Osteoporosis with ____ pathological fracture, is for patients who have a current pathologic fracture at the ____ of an encounter.
10. A code from category M80, not a ____ fracture code, should be used for any patient with ____ osteoporosis who suffers a fracture, even if the patient had a minor fall or trauma, if that fall or trauma would not usually break a normal, healthy bone.

Let's Check It! Rules and Regulations

Please answer the following questions from the knowledge you have gained after reading this chapter.

1. LO 15.1 What is arthropathy? Include ways that the physician might identify the patient's condition; also include an example of an arthropathic condition.
2. LO 15.2 List two conditions that affect the spine and explain each one.
3. LO 15.3 Explain the difference between osteochondrosis and osteoporosis.
4. LO 15.4 List an acquired musculoskeletal disorder and a congenital disorder and discuss each.
5. LO 15.5 Explain the difference between a traumatic fracture and a pathologic fracture. Why is it important to know the difference?

YOU CODE IT! Basics

First, identify the condition in the following diagnoses; then code the diagnosis.

Example: Trigger thumb, right:
   a. main term: *Trigger*   b. diagnosis: *M65.311*

1. Infective myositis, left foot:
   a. main term: ____   b. diagnosis: ____
2. Pyogenic arthritis, left knee:
   a. main term: ____   b. diagnosis: ____
3. Foreign body granuloma of soft tissue, right thigh:
   a. main term: ____   b. diagnosis: ____
4. Juxtaphalangeal distal osteoarthritis:
   a. main term: ____   b. diagnosis: ____
5. Nontraumatic rupture of muscle, left shoulder:
   a. main term: ____   b. diagnosis: ____
6. Hallux valgus, left foot:
   a. main term: ____   b. diagnosis: ____
7. Ischemic infarction of muscle, left hand:
   a. main term: ____   b. diagnosis: ____
8. Osteomyelitis neonatal jaw:
   a. main term: ____   b. diagnosis: ____
9. Infantile idiopathic scoliosis, lumbosacral:
   a. main term: ____   b. diagnosis: ____
10. Contracture of right ankle:
    a. main term: ____   b. diagnosis: ____
11. Atrophy of left lower leg:
    a. main term: ____   b. diagnosis: ____
12. Ankylosis of right wrist:
    a. main term: ____   b. diagnosis: ____
13. Abscess of tendon sheath, right forearm:
    a. main term: ____   b. diagnosis: ____
14. Spinal stenosis, cervicothoracic region:
    a. main term: ____   b. diagnosis: ____
15. Calcific tendinitis, left pelvic region:
    a. main term: ____   b. diagnosis: ____

YOU CODE IT! Practice

Using the techniques described in this chapter, carefully read through the case studies and determine the most accurate ICD-10-CM code(s) and external cause code(s), if appropriate, for each case study.

1. Nancy Nottingham, a 52-year-old female, presents today with a severe burning pain and swelling in her upper right arm and fingers. Dr. Olden notes edema and allodynia. After a thorough examination, Nancy is diagnosed with reflex sympathetic dystrophy (RSD).

2. Arturo Garwood, a 57-year-old male, comes in today with left shoulder pain and weakness. Arturo admits that he struggles to raise his left arm above his head. Dr. Dow completes an examination and orders an MRI scan. The MRI results confirm the diagnosis of incomplete rotator cuff tear.

3. Sharron Webster, a 3-year-old female, was brought in by her parents to see her pediatrician, Dr. Surrant, 4 days ago. Sharron had a boil on her left thigh that Dr. Surrant incised and drained. Sharron is now running a fever of 102 F. Dr. Surrant decides to admit Sharron to Weston Hospital. The MRI scan revealed abscess of the vastus intermedius muscle. A wound culture grew *Staphylococcus aureus*. Sharron is diagnosed with pyomyositis.

4. Tamara Gibbons, a 37-year-old female, presents today with pain on the inside of her right knee. Dr. Booker completes a history and physical examination. After reviewing the MRI results, Tamara is diagnosed with Plica syndrome.

5. Jay Lawson, a 13-year-old male, is brought in by his parents to see Dr. Bouknight, his pediatrician. Jay is complaining of left hip pain and stiffness. Dr. Bouknight completes a physical examination and notes limited left hip motion as well as soft tissue swelling. Jay is admitted to Weston Hospital. Aspiration of synovial fluid reveals an elevated cell count of 136 cells/mL with 52% being polymorphonuclear leukocytes. Jay is diagnosed with intermittent hydrarthrosis.

6. Terrell Meddy, a 58-year-old male, comes in today to see Dr. McNair with the complaint his left elbow is stiff, painful and feels warm. Terrell doesn't remember hitting his elbow on anything. After an examination, Dr. McNair diagnosed Terrell with olecranon bursitis of the elbow.

7. Shirley Moody, an 11-year-old female, is brought in by her mother. Mrs. Moody states that Shirley is experiencing severe muscle weakness. Dr. Bernstein completes a physical examination and notes heart arrhythmias, aphasia, and dyspnea. Shirley says that the weakness seems to last about 4 hours and comes and goes. Dr. Bernstein admits Shirley into the hospital and orders an electromyographic (EMG) test. The results of the ECG, EMG, and muscle biopsy confirm the diagnosis of hypokalemic periodic paralysis.

8. Angie Dawson, a 4-year-old female, is brought in by her parents. Angie is having difficulty chewing her food as well as having some speech problems. Dr. Hunt notes misalignment between the teeth of the dental arches as Angie's jaw closes. Dr. Hunt completes a thorough examination and the appropriate tests. Angie is diagnosed with malocclusion, Angle's class II.

9. Ned Taylor, a 33-year-old male, presents today with severe weakness in his left hip. Dr. Louthan notes enlarged neck lymph node, a rash, and high fever. Ned admits to some eye and chest pain with general lethargy. After a thorough examination, Dr. Louthan decides to admit Ned to the hospital. The laboratory test and MRI confirmed the diagnosis of arthritis of the hip due to O'nyong-nyong fever.

10. Rykia Huffman, a 21-year-old female, presents today with the complaint of uneven hips and leg length. Dr. Gamble completes a physical examination and orders a weight-bearing, full-length spine x-ray, AP, which confirms the diagnosis of idiopathic scoliosis, lumbosacral region.

11. Kendall Everett, a 41-year-old female, comes in today with the complaint her right hand aches and itches. Kendall also admits it has become harder to hold objects in her right hand. Dr. Inabinet completes an examination and a table top test, which was positive for Dupuytren's disease.

12. Jason Okoro, a 46-year-old male, presents with pain in his right foot. Jason admits it hurts to walk. Dr. Denka completes an examination and after reviewing the results of the MRI, Jason is diagnosed with a synovial cyst rupture between the second and third metatarsal bones.

CHAPTER 15 REVIEW

13. Valerie Halsey, a 51-year-old female, complains of lower back pain and numbness. Valerie also admits it is sometimes difficult to control her left leg. Dr. Spratt completes a physical examination and history of the symptoms. Dr. Spratt has Valerie perform the straight leg raise test, which was positive for Lasegue's sign. Valerie is diagnosed with wallet sciatica, left side.

14. James Ard, a 31-year-old male, comes in today to see Dr. Smyth. Jim complains his head is tilting and he can't control it. He also admits to neck spasms and it seems to him that it is worse after he has taken his afternoon run. After a thorough examination and testing, Dr. Smyth diagnoses Jim with spasmodic torticollis.

15. Marygrace Fuller, a 16-year-old female, participated in rhythmic gymnastics yesterday at the local gym. She woke up this morning and her left ankle was stiff and aches. After an examination, Dr. Jefferson diagnosed Marygrace with Achilles tendinitis.

YOU CODE IT! Application

The following exercises provide practice in abstracting physicians' notes and learning to work with documentation from our health care facility, Prader, Bracker, & Associates. These case studies are modeled on real patient encounters. Using the techniques described in this chapter, carefully read through the case studies and determine the most accurate ICD-10-CM code(s) and external cause code(s), if appropriate, for each case study.

PRADER, BRACKER, & ASSOCIATES

A Complete Health Care Facility

159 Healthcare Way • SOMEWHERE, FL 32811 • 407-555-6789

PATIENT: LOPEZ, JUANA

ACCOUNT/EHR #: LOPEJU001

DATE: 07/16/18

Attending Physician: Oscar R. Prader, MD

S: Patient is a 15-year-old female with complaints of dysphagia and occasional problems speaking. She complains of dyspnea and finds it painful to raise her arms over her head. In the last couple of days, she states that climbing stairs and even getting up from a chair are painful and challenging.

O: ROM indicates weakness in the proximal muscles, specifically shoulders and hips. Both MRI and electromyography indicate polymyositis with myopathy. This was confirmed by autoimmune antibody testing.

A: Polymyositis with myopathy

P: Rx: Prednisone

   Rx: Methotrexate

ORP/pw   D: 07/16/18 09:50:16   T: 07/17/18 12:55:01

Determine the most accurate ICD-10-CM code(s).

PRADER, BRACKER, & ASSOCIATES

A Complete Health Care Facility

159 Healthcare Way • SOMEWHERE, FL 32811 • 407-555-6789

PATIENT: MARCHEON, GABRIELLA

ACCOUNT/EHR #: MARCGA001

DATE: 07/16/18

Attending Physician: Renee O. Bracker, MD

Assessment: Derangement of anterior horn medial meniscus due to old tear, right knee.

Order for physical therapy:

    Moist heat, cryotherapy, muscle stimulation, whirlpool, massage

    ROM: active, active assistive, passive

    Exercise: isometric, isotonic ambulation training, as tolerated

    3 a week for 6 weeks.

Session # 3/6: Pain Level: 4/10

Pt states pain shooting down right medial lower leg and numbness in toes.

    Total time: 35 minutes

    10 min. Cold pack/right knee

    25 min. Therapeutic exercise . . . to increase strength and ROM

Symptoms began to return in right lower leg toward the end of the exercise. No new exercises added.

Donata R. Chen, MPT

DRC/pw D: 07/16/18 09:50:16 T: 07/17/18 12:55:01

Determine the most accurate ICD-10-CM code(s).

PRADER, BRACKER, & ASSOCIATES

A Complete Health Care Facility

159 Healthcare Way • SOMEWHERE, FL 32811 • 407-555-6789

PATIENT: STRICK, JOSEPH

ACCOUNT/EHR #: STRIJO001

DATE: 09/16/18

Attending Physician: Oscar R. Prader, MD

On Sept. 10, the patient's daughter noticed him walking on his toes, in obvious pain, and having trouble moving his left foot. She insisted on him coming here to have me check, because she was worried.

PE: Patient states sharp pain is experienced during dorsiflexion of the left foot. ROM is limited. Circulation good.

DX: Achilles tendon contracture, left

PLAN: Referral for physical therapy

      Rx for specialized series of shoes

ORP/mg D: 9/16/18 09:50:16 T: 9/18/18 12:55:01

Determine the most accurate ICD-10-CM code(s).

CHAPTER 15 REVIEW

PRADER, BRACKER, & ASSOCIATES

A Complete Health Care Facility

159 Healthcare Way • SOMEWHERE, FL 32811 • 407-555-6789

PATIENT: LAO, HANNAH

ACCOUNT/EHR #: LAOHAN001

DATE: 09/16/18

Attending Physician: Oscar R. Prader, MD

Hannah Lao, a 59-year-old female, came to see Dr. Prader with pain, swelling, and erythema in her left foot and ankle. She stated that she was diagnosed with open-angle glaucoma and prescribed acetazolamide (a diuretic) by Dr. Carson, her ophthalmologist. She stated she never mentioned she was using a topical lotion of urea (a diuretic) prescribed by her dermatologist to hydrate her dry skin. Hannah stated she didn't think a lotion would count when asked about current medications.

Dr. Prader realized the combination of the two diuretics lowered her serum uric acid too quickly, causing drug-induced gout.

ORP/pw   D: 9/16/18 09:50:16   T: 9/18/18 12:55:01

Determine the most accurate ICD-10-CM code(s).

PRADER, BRACKER, & ASSOCIATES

A Complete Health Care Facility

159 Healthcare Way • SOMEWHERE, FL 32811 • 407-555-6789

PATIENT: BRACKSLEY, NATASHA

ACCOUNT/EHR #: BRACNA001

DATE: 09/16/18

Attending Physician: Renee O. Bracker, MD

It has been 8 months since I saw this 67-year-old female. She states experiencing terrible "knee pain" in both legs. Patient states taking extra-strength Tylenol around the clock (two tablets every 4 hours) with little or no relief.

PE: She has Heberden's and Bouchard's nodes and deformity of the knee joints with decreased range of motion. On the basis of the patient's history and this examination, osteoarthritis is suspected. Patient is taken to x-ray. AP, 2 views, x-rays of each knee confirm diagnosis of osteoarthritis. There are no other findings.

DX: Osteoarthritis, bilateral

Rx: Tripod cane

Patient is advised to begin taking OTC glucosamine plus chondroitin sulfate. Patient to return prn

ROB/pw   D: 9/16/18 09:50:16   T: 9/18/18 12:55:01

Determine the most accurate ICD-10-CM code(s).

Coding Injury, Poisoning, and External Causes

16

Learning Outcomes

After completing this chapter, the student should be able to:

LO 16.1 Analyze the documentation to determine when external cause codes are required.

LO 16.2 Apply guidelines for coding traumatic injuries.

LO 16.3 Determine seventh characters for injury codes accurately.

LO 16.4 Identify a suggested code from the Table of Drugs and Chemicals.

LO 16.5 Distinguish between poisonings and adverse effects.

LO 16.6 Abstract documentation to accurately report burns.

LO 16.7 Demonstrate coding protocols for reporting abuse and neglect.

LO 16.8 Evaluate documented complications of care to report them accurately.

Key Terms

Abuse
Avulsion
Burn
Corrosion
Dislocation
Extent
First-Degree Burn
Fracture
Laceration
Malunion
Myalgia
Nonunion
Physicians' Desk Reference (PDR)
Rule of Nines
Second-Degree Burn
Severity
Site
Third-Degree Burn

STOP! Remember, you need to follow along in your ICD-10-CM code book for an optimal learning experience.

16.1 Reporting External Causes of Injuries

When a patient has been injured traumatically, the first code or codes you need to report will explain the specific injury, such as a fractured arm or a burned foot. We will discuss those details as you move through this chapter. There are more codes required for these circumstances to tell the whole story. This means that you also need to report codes that explain the:

- *Cause of the injury,* such as a car accident or a fall off a ladder.
- *Place of the occurrence,* such as the park or the kitchen.
- *Activity during the occurrence,* such as playing basketball or gardening.
- *Patient's status,* such as paid employment, on-duty military, or leisure activity.

That's a lot of information. However, think of how important these details are to the reimbursement process as well as to research studies. When you report that the patient's status was "civilian activity done for income or pay," it will be clear that this is a workers' compensation case and not a claim to be sent to the patient's health insurance carrier. If the cause of the injury was "driver of pickup truck or van injured in collision with heavy transport vehicle or bus in nontraffic accident," this information may direct the claim to the auto insurance company (not the health insurance carrier), and there may be the possibility that the information can support any legal action. Including a code to report a "fall into swimming pool" may help with getting improved fencing and saving others.

> **CODING BITES**
>
> An external cause code can *never* be a first-listed code, and it can *never* be the only code reported. External cause codes are reported secondary to the codes that report the injury itself.

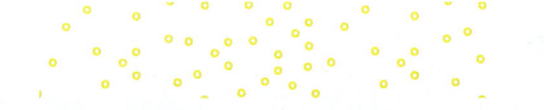

429

> **GUIDANCE CONNECTION**
>
> Read the ICD-10-CM Official Guidelines for Coding and Reporting, section **I. Conventions, General Coding Guidelines and Chapter Specific Guidelines,** subsection **C. Chapter-Specific Coding Guidelines,** chapter **20. External Causes of Morbidity,** subsection **a. General External Cause Coding Guidelines.**

Dislocation
The movement of a muscle away from its normal position.

> **GUIDANCE CONNECTION**
>
> Read the ICD-10-CM Official Guidelines for Coding and Reporting, section **I. Conventions, General Coding Guidelines and Chapter Specific Guidelines,** subsection **C. Chapter-Specific Coding Guidelines,** chapter **20. External Causes of Morbidity,** subsection **b. Place of Occurrence Guideline.**

> **GUIDANCE CONNECTION**
>
> Read the ICD-10-CM Official Guidelines for Coding and Reporting, section **I. Conventions, General Coding Guidelines and Chapter Specific Guidelines,** subsection **C. Chapter-Specific Coding Guidelines,** chapter **20. External Causes of Morbidity,** subsection **c. Activity Code.**

To begin the process of determining the appropriate external cause codes for a specific encounter, you will start in the Alphabetic Index. However, these codes have a separate index. You will not use the *Alphabetic Index to Diseases,* which you have been using in previous chapters and cases. Instead, you will use the *Alphabetic Index to External Causes,* often located after the *Alphabetic Index to Diseases,* after the *Table of Drugs and Chemicals,* and before the *Tabular List.*

Cause of the Injury Code

When a part of the body meets with an external object and the result is injury, you must explain what that external object or force was, along with the code or codes for the injury itself. The cause may be anything from being stepped on by a cow (W55.29x-) to falling from scaffolding (W12.xxx-) to the forced landing of a (hot air) balloon injuring the occupant (V96.02x-). Domestic violence, child abuse, and elder abuse are considered assault and may be the cause of a physical injury (code category Y07). Whatever it may have been, you need to determine from the documentation what it was that caused the fracture, **dislocation**, sprain, or strain and report it with the appropriate code or codes.

Place of the Occurrence Code

Where was the patient when he or she was injured? Code category Y92 Place of occurrence of the external cause provides you with many options so you can report, for example, that the swimming pool at which the patient slipped and tore his deltoid muscle was at a single-family (private) house, a mobile home, a boarding house, a nursing home, or another noninstitutional or institutional location. The codes are quite specific, so you need to ensure that your physicians understand the need to be equally specific in their documentation.

Activity Code

Code category Y93 Activity codes provides you with many activities from which to choose to identify what exactly the patient was doing when he or she became injured. Dancing, yoga, gymnastics, trampolining, cheerleading . . . each has its own code, and this is just one subcategory!

Patient's Status

This sounds a bit obscure, certainly. What was the patient's status at the time the injury occurred? There are four options within code category Y99 External cause status:

- *Civilian activity done for income or pay*—in other words, on the job for pay or other compensation, excluding on-duty military or volunteers.
- *Military activity,* excluding off-duty status at the time.
- *Volunteer activity.*
- *Other external cause status,* which includes leisure activities, student activities, and working on a hobby.

As we discussed earlier in this section, this detail is important to the entire process, including reimbursement as well as continuity of care.

> **GUIDANCE CONNECTION**
>
> Read the ICD-10-CM Official Guidelines for Coding and Reporting, section **I. Conventions, General Coding Guidelines and Chapter Specific Guidelines,** subsection **C. Chapter-Specific Coding Guidelines,** chapter **20. External Causes of Morbidity,** subsection **k. External cause status.**

LET'S CODE IT! SCENARIO

Phyllis Bush, a 27-year-old female, was learning to rock climb at her gym. As she was scaling the wall, her foot slipped and Phyllis grabbed on with her right hand, pulling something in her shoulder. The severe pain caused her to stop by her physician's office on her way home. Dr. Dellin took x-rays and determined that she had an inferior dislocation of the humerus, right side. Dr. Dellin put Phyllis's arm into a sling and gave her a prescription for a pain reliever.

Let's Code It!

Dr. Dellin diagnosed Phyllis with an *inferior dislocation of the humerus, right side*. Turn to the Alphabetic Index and look up *dislocation, humerus*. Read down the list and see

Dislocation, humerus, proximal end — *see* **Dislocation, shoulder**

Even though Dr. Dellin's notes didn't specify proximal, that was necessary to get to inferior—anatomically:

Dislocation, shoulder
    humerus S43.00-
        inferior S43.03-

Perfect! Now, turn to the Tabular List and confirm the code. Start reading at

✓4 **S43**   **Dislocation and sprain of joints and ligaments of shoulder girdle**

There is a **Code also** note reminding you to also report a code for any associated open wound. Phyllis does not have an open wound, so this does not apply. There is also an **EXCLUDES2** note that mentions a strain of muscle, fascia, and tendon of the shoulder and upper arm (S46.-). However, Phyllis dislocated her humerus, so you can keep reading down the column to review the fourth-character and fifth-character options and determine which matches Dr. Dellin's documentation:

✓5 **S43.0**   **Subluxation and dislocation of shoulder joint**
    ✓6 **S43.03**   **Inferior subluxation and dislocation of humerus**

Go back to Dr. Dellin's notes and see that this matches exactly. Terrific! Now a sixth character is required. Review the options, check the documentation again, and determine

✓7 **S43.034-**   **Inferior dislocation of right humerus**

Fantastic! A seventh character is required to explain where in the treatment path this encounter is. You can see the options directly under the code category S43. This is the first time that Dr. Dellin is treating Phyllis's dislocation. Great! This leads you to the complete, most accurate code to report Phyllis's injury:

S43.034A   **Inferior dislocation of right humerus, initial encounter**

This code tells the whole story about Phyllis's specific injury.

Now you need to find the external cause code(s) to explain how Phyllis's injury happened. Turn to the *External Cause Code* Alphabetic Index. *Climb*—no; *exercise*—no; *fall*—possibly. None of these listings really describes how Phyllis got hurt. Actually, she was involved in an "activity," so let's take a look:

Activity (involving) (of victim at time of event) Y93.9

Keep reading down the long indented list below until you get to

    climbing NEC Y93.39
        mountain Y93.31
        rock Y93.31
        wall climbing Y93.31

Perfect! That is exactly what she was doing. Let's take a look in the Tabular List:

(continued)

> ☑4 **Y93**   **Activity codes**
>   ☑5 **Y93.3**   **Activities involving climbing, rappelling, and jumping off**
>
> The EXCLUDES1 note lists activities not related to Phyllis's injury, so keep reading down the list:
>
>   **Y93.31**   **Activity, mountain climbing, rock climbing and wall climbing**
>
> A code is needed to report the place of occurrence. Where was Phyllis when she got injured? At her gym.
>
> ☑4 **Y92**   **Place of occurrence of the external cause**
> **Y92.39**   **Other specific sports and athletic area as the place of occurrence of the external cause (Gymnasium)**
>
> One more thing: What was Phyllis's status, which you can describe using the codes within **Y99 External cause status**? The wall climbing was a leisure activity for Phyllis, so you will report
>
>   **Y99.8**   **Other external cause status (hobby not done for income)**
>
> Now you have all of the codes you need to tell the *whole story* about Phyllis's injury and why Dr. Dellin treated her:
>
>   **S43.034A**   Inferior dislocation of right humerus, initial encounter
>   **Y93.31**   Activity, mountain climbing, rock climbing and wall climbing
>   **Y92.39**   Other specific sports and athletic area as the place of occurrence of the external cause (Gymnasium)
>   **Y99.8**   Other external cause status (hobby not done for income)
>
> Good work!

16.2 Traumatic Injuries

The term *injury* refers to traumatic damage to some aspect of the body, virtually always caused by a fall, crash, weapon, or some other external cause. The damage may be minor (superficial) or it may be life-threatening. It may occur during time at work or while playing. It may be the result of an automobile accident or a fight. Or it may occur during an indoor or outdoor activity.

Traumatic Fractures

Fracture
Broken cartilage or bone.

Both bone and cartilage can break—that is, become fractured. **Fractures** can be the result of trauma, such as a fall or car accident, or they can be the result of a pathologic condition (underlying disease), such as osteoporosis, that causes the bone to weaken so much that it breaks. This is important information for you to abstract from the physician's documentation because traumatic fractures and pathologic fractures are coded differently. Actually, they have separate listings in the Alphabetic Index: Fracture, pathological, and Fracture, traumatic.

When a fracture of a bone occurs, the coder must identify the segment of the bone that was affected. For example: The sternal end of the clavicle is called this because it is the end that connects to the sternum (ICD-10-CM code S42.011 Anterior displaced fracture of sternal end of right clavicle). The acromial or lateral end of the clavicle connects to the acromioclavicular joint (ICD-10-CM code S42.031 Displaced fracture of lateral end of right clavicle).

Types of Fractures

One of the first factors needed for accurate coding of a fracture is whether the fracture is *open* or *closed* (see Figure 16-1).

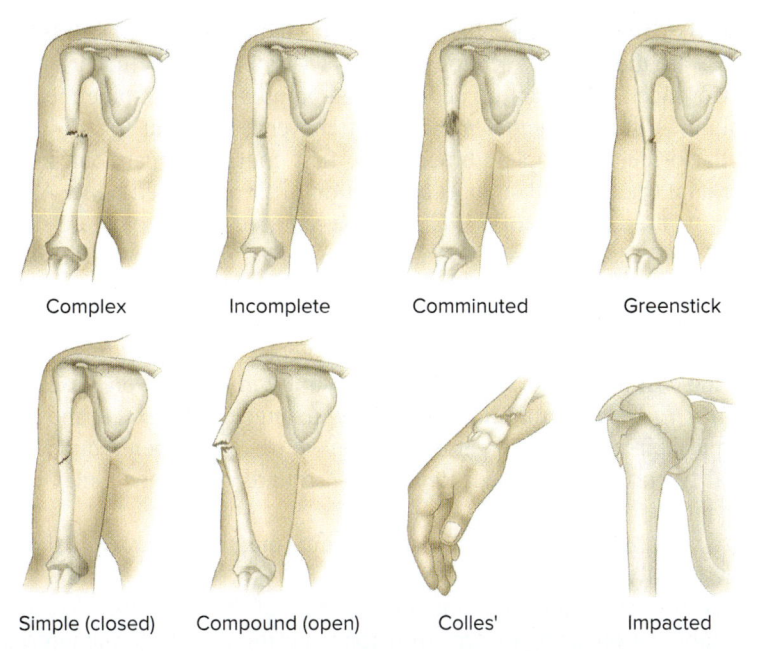

FIGURE 16-1 Illustrations of several different types of fractures

An open fractured bone is found in conjunction with an open wound through which the bone may or may not extend. A closed, or simple, fracture has no accompanying wound and remains within the confines of the body. Some types of fractures are explained in the following paragraphs.

Avulsion fractures happen when a tiny bone piece breaks off at the point where a ligament or tendon attaches to the bone. This is an occurrence of a piece of bone that has broken away at a tubercle. When the fracture is not displaced, treatment is similar to that for a soft tissue injury. In severe cases, surgery may be required to realign and stabilize an affected growth plate.

Burst fractures occur when a vertebra has been crushed in all directions. This fracture may be described as stable or unstable. Imaging (x-rays, CT scan, or MRI), as well as physical and neurologic exams, typically will support a diagnosis. Stable burst fractures may be treated with a molded turtle shell brace or a body cast. If neurologic damage is identified, then the fracture is considered unstable and will require surgery. An anterior or posterior approach may be used to insert internal fixation, a bone graft, and/or fusion. The specific bone affected will determine the code.

Comminuted fracture identifies the breaking of the bone into several pieces. A closed reduction may be required prior to immobilization by cast or splint. Internal fixation may be necessary to correct an impacted fracture with an open reduction.

Depressed fracture indicates that the bone has been displaced inward.

Fatigue fractures occur most often in the second or third metatarsal shaft and are typically the result of continuous weight-bearing activities such as long-distance running, ballet dancing, or sports. An example is M48.4- Fatigue fracture of vertebra. Additional names for this type of fracture include march fracture, Deutschlander's disease, and stress fracture—reported from subcategory M84.3- Stress fracture (fatigue fracture) (march fracture).

Fissured (linear) fracture is a break that runs along the length of a long bone.

Greenstick fracture is one in which the fracture exists on one side of the bone while the other side is not broken but bent. Example: S42.311A Greenstick fracture of shaft of humerus, right arm, initial encounter for closed fracture.

Impacted fracture occurs when a fragment from the broken bone embeds itself into the body of another.

Infected fracture documents that there is presence of an infection at the fracture site. This often will require additional codes to report the underlying bacterium or virus, as well as the infection itself.

CODING BITES

Open fractures may also be documented as infected, missile, puncture, compound, or with a foreign body.

Closed fractures may also be documented as comminuted, depressed, elevated, fissured, greenstick, impacted, linear, simple, slipped epiphysis, or spiral.

Lateral mass fracture of the atlas (C1), as the name implies, involves the lateral masses. These are the sturdiest sections of the C1 vertebra and include a superior facet and an inferior facet. This fracture occurs at the point where the spine meets the base of the cranium. A stable fracture means the transverse ligament is still intact, and a cervical collar or cervicothoracic brace is the first course of treatment. For unstable fractures, cranial traction will support a reduction of the displaced bone. After time, a halo vest can be used. Fusion of C1–C3 may be required for more severe subluxation. Use code S12.040 Displaced lateral mass fracture of first cervical vertebra or S12.041 Non-displaced lateral mass fracture of first cervical vertebra.

Maisonneuve's fracture is a spiral fracture of the proximal portion of the fibula. This type of fracture includes a disruption of ligaments. Stable fractures can be treated with a long leg cast. Internal fixation may be required in more severe cases.

Oblique fracture is a fracture line that runs at an angle to the axis of the bone. Casting is the typical first course of treatment. In severe cases, an open reduction and possibly internal fixation will be used. Repair to surrounding ligaments may be required as well.

Periosteal fractures occur below the periosteum (membrane covering the bone surface) and are usually not displaced.

Pilon fracture is an oblique, comminuted fracture of the distal tibia. Treatment may begin with stabilization, using external traction to permit the soft tissue injuries to heal prior to surgical intervention. Open reduction with internal fixation, as well as external fixation and percutaneous plating, may be used once the soft tissue has recovered.

Puncture fracture can identify that a puncture from outside the body penetrated to cause the fracture or that the broken bone has punctured the skin after the fracture occurred. Example: S91.231A Puncture wound without foreign body of right great toe with damage to nail, initial encounter.

Segmental fracture is similar to the comminuted fracture; however, the broken pieces of the bone separate. Internal fixation with open reduction is used to prevent misalignment of the bone fragments. In some cases, bone cement is included in the repair. Some surgical procedures also include attachment of external fixation.

Salter-Harris physeal fracture is a fracture of the epiphyseal plate (a thin layer of bone; a growth plate, an area near the end of a long bone that contains growing tissue, also known as the *physis*), and it is commonly found in children. ICD-10-CM separately codes four of the nine types of Salter-Harris fracture: Salter-Harris type I is a transverse fracture of the growth plate; type II is a fracture of the growth plate and the metaphysis; type III is a fracture of the growth plate and the epiphysis; and type IV is a fracture line that travels through all three: the growth plate, metaphysis, and epiphysis. Closed reductions and traction can be used for less severe cases. Types III and IV more often will require surgical intervention using open reduction and internal fixation. For example: S79.011A Salter-Harris type I physeal fracture of upper end of right femur, initial encounter for closed fracture.

Spiral fracture happens when a twisting force causes the bone to break around a long bone in a spiral direction. Example: S52.244A Nondisplaced spiral fracture of shaft of ulna, right arm, initial encounter for closed fracture.

Torus fracture is also known as a *buckle fracture;* it is a compression of one side of a bone's protrusion, also known as the *torus,* while the other side is bent. This fracture is typically nondisplaced and, therefore, is correctable with a cast or splint.

Transverse fracture is a fracture line that runs across the bone; it may be an open or closed fracture. An open reduction with internal fixation may be required if the bone has separated. A closed reduction might alternatively be employed. Casting is typical.

Transcondylar fracture is a fracture that runs through a condyle (a rounded knoblike prominence at the end of a bone). Such fractures are categorized as flexion or extension fractures. Treatment can begin with immobilization for nondisplaced injury. However, treatment for this type of fracture can be difficult due to the break's location and the lack of bone available for successful union. Example: S42.431A Displaced fracture (avulsion) of lateral epicondyle of right humerus, initial encounter for closed fracture.

> **GUIDANCE CONNECTION**
>
> Read the ICD-10-CM Official Guidelines for Coding and Reporting, section **I. Conventions, General Coding Guidelines and Chapter Specific Guidelines,** subsection **C. Chapter-Specific Guidelines,** chapter **19. Injury, poisoning, and certain other consequences of external causes,** subsection **c. Coding of Traumatic Fractures.**

Wedge compression fracture occurs when only the anterior portion of a vertebra is crushed, which causes the vertebra to take on a wedge shape. Vertebroplasty will stabilize the fracture and prevent further damage. Example: A wedge compression fracture of L3 would be reported with code S32.030A Wedge compression fracture of third lumbar vertebra, initial encounter for closed fracture.

Skull Fracture

A skull fracture will first be qualified by the area injured, such as the vault of the skull (frontal or parietal bone—code S02.0xxA) or the base of the skull (sphenoid or temporal bone—code S02.19xA). *Note:* A second code would report any intracranial injury, if applicable.

Fractures of the skull are characterized differently than others throughout the body and include the following:

- *Basal skull fracture* is a break in the floor of the skull.
- *Blowout fracture* indicates a break in the floor of the orbit that is typically caused by a severe blow to the eye.
- *Depressed skull fracture* identifies an inward displacement of one of the bones of the skull.
- *Stellate fracture* is one with a clear central point of the fracture and with break lines radiating from this central spot.

Maxillary Fracture

Facial trauma might result in a LeFort fracture, which is a bilateral maxillary fracture with involvement of the surrounding bone, including the zygomatic bones. Such fractures are identified by type: A LeFort I fracture (code S02.411-) is a downward horizontal facial fracture and typically involves the maxillary alveolar rim and inferior nasal aperture. A LeFort II fracture (code S02.412-) is more triangular, involving the inferior orbital rim, the nasal bridge, and the frontal processes of the maxilla. A LeFort III fracture (code S02.413-) is a transverse fracture, sometimes referred to as a *craniofacial dissociation*. This fracture involves the zygomatic arch, the nasal bridge, and the upper maxilla and extends along the orbit floor (posteriorly).

EXAMPLES

S02.402A   Zygomatic fracture, unspecified side, initial encounter for closed fracture
S02.413D   LeFort III fracture, subsequent encounter for fracture with routine healing

Sequelae (Late Effects) of Fractures

Once a bone has been given the opportunity to heal, it may not heal properly. The most common types of late effects of fractures are **malunion** and **nonunion**. A malunion (*mal* = bad + *union* = together) of a fractured bone means that the pieces of the bone healed back together but not in an effective way. Unfortunately, the most common treatment for a malunion is for the physician to rebreak the bone and set it again, hoping that it will heal properly the second time. When the parts of a broken bone do not heal back together at all, despite the proper treatment and time allotment, this is known as a nonunion (*non* = not + *union* = together).

In ICD-10-CM's Alphabetic Index, when you look up *Fracture, malunion,* you will see the notation "*See* Fracture, by site." When you look up *Fracture, nonunion,* you will see the notation "*See* Nonunion, fracture." At *Nonunion, fracture,* the notation states, "*See* Fracture, by site."

CODING BITES

The Tabular List categorizes the codes used to report injuries first by anatomical site (the location of the injury) and then by the specific injury (contusion, insect bite, etc.).

Malunion
A fractured bone that did not heal correctly; healing of bone that was not in proper position or alignment.

Nonunion
A fractured bone that did not heal back together; no mending or joining together of the broken segments.

Laceration
Damage to the epidermal and dermal layers of the skin made by a sharp object.

> **GUIDANCE CONNECTION**
>
> Review the ICD-10-CM Official Guidelines for Coding and Reporting, section **I. Conventions, General Coding Guidelines and Chapter Specific Guidelines,** subsection **C. Chapter-Specific Coding Guidelines,** chapter **13. Diseases of the Musculoskeletal System and Connective Tissue,** subsection **b, Acute traumatic versus chronic or recurrent musculoskeletal conditions,** in addition to chapter **19. Injury, poisoning, and certain other consequences of external causes,** subsection **b. Coding of Injuries.**

Traumatic Wounds

Lacerations (Superficial Wounds)

Each one of us has had a laceration at some time or another. Perhaps it was a paper cut or a cut from a knife while chopping vegetables. This smooth slit or opening in the epidermal layer is typically superficial and does not bleed. A **laceration** caused by a sharp object is generally a ragged wound (see Figure 16-2). Unlike a superficial cut, a laceration is deeper, damaging the dermal layer of the skin. It penetrates the blood vessels, resulting in bleeding. These more severe injuries may also be vulnerable to infection and pain. Depending upon the specific object or event that caused the laceration, the physician may order an x-ray to determine whether any foreign bodies, such as shards of glass or splinters from wood, are lodged within the wound.

Contusions and Hematomas

A *contusion,* commonly known as a *bruise* or "black-and-blue mark," is an injury to the body that typically does not break the skin but that does damage to the underlying blood vessels. The bleeding in the dermal layer is seen only through the epidermis as a dark color. As the contusion heals, the colors change until the collected blood is dissipated and everything has healed. When the bleeding coagulates into a blood clot, this is called a *hematoma.* The seriousness of these injuries largely depends on the anatomical site where the bleeding and/or clot is located. A contusion or hematoma on the leg or arm is typically a minor event that rarely requires a physician's skill, whereas a contusion to the brain or a subdural hematoma could be life-threatening.

Puncture Wounds

When a pointed, narrow object enters deeply into the visceral (inside) aspects of the body, the injury is known as a *puncture wound* (see Figure 16-2). A carpenter's nail, a knife, scissors, and a fishhook are just a few items that can cause an injury of this nature. Due to the characteristics of this type of wound, infection and internal damage

Contusion   Incision   Laceration

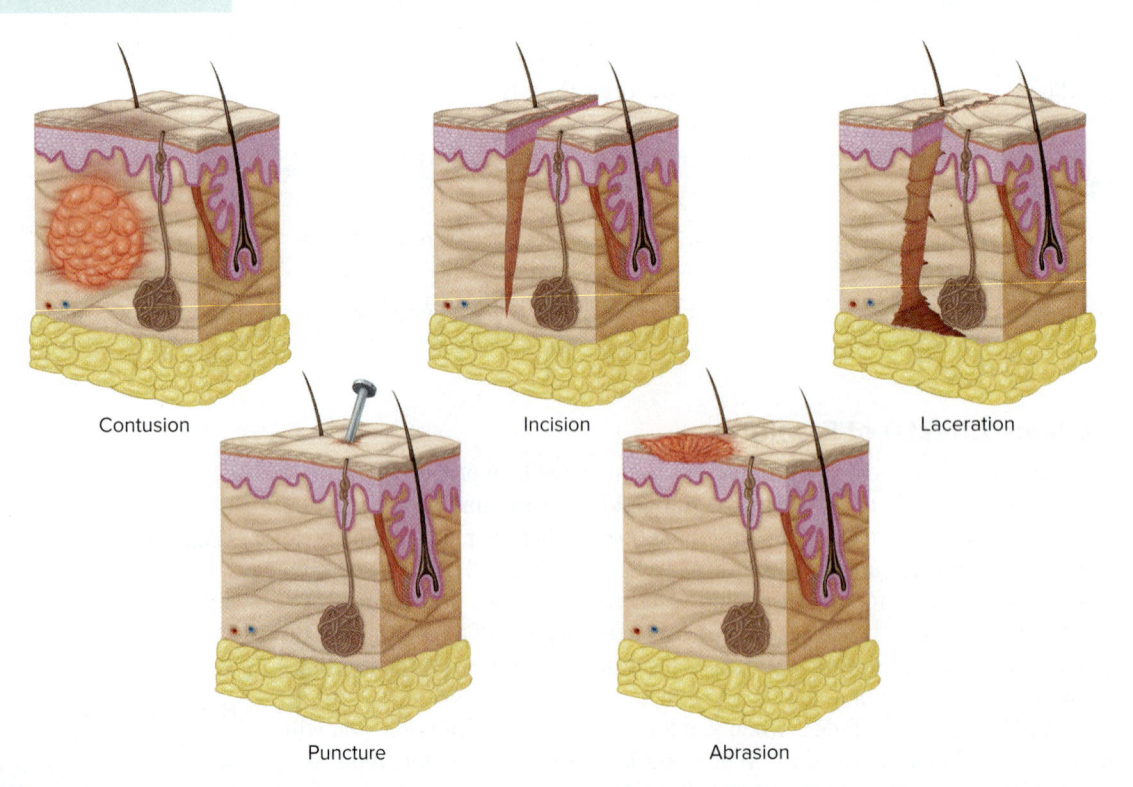

Puncture   Abrasion

FIGURE 16-2 Illustrations of different types of wounds, including lacerations and puncture wounds Booth et al., *Medical Assisting,* 5e. Copyright ©2013 by McGraw-Hill Education. Figure 57-7, p. 1191. Used with permission.

are possible. The physician may check for dirt, debris, or foreign objects within the wound. He or she may also order blood tests to check for a pathogen that might cause an infection. Stitches and possible surgery may be required, depending upon the specific depth and location of the injury.

Avulsions

The medical term **avulsion** describes a situation in which all layers of the skin (epidermis and dermis) are forcibly torn away from the body, typically a surface trauma. Due to the pulling off of the dermal layers, the underlying structures, including adipose tissue, muscles, tendons, and bone, become open to the outside. Rock climbers may suffer "flappers," an avulsion of the fingertip pad. When this occurs to a fingernail or toenail, it is known as a *nail avulsion*—the nail plate is torn off the nail bed. Unlike the case with avulsions at other anatomical sites, in nail avulsions the nail is not reattached. Instead, the fingertip and nail bed are covered to protect the area until the keratin has formed a new nail.

Avulsion
Injury in which layers of skin are traumatically torn away from the body.

Animal, Insect, or Human Bites

Animal bites and human bites can be a particular concern due to the potential spread of bacteria and viruses via saliva transference. Insects may transmit their own fluids and sometimes venom.

LET'S CODE IT! SCENARIO

Nathan Kirchner, an 8-year-old male, was hiking in a public park with his Boy Scout troop when they came to a clearing and he saw a foal and its mother looking over the fence in a corral in the northeast edge of the park. He reached out his left hand to pet the foal, and the mother horse bit his thumb. His scout leader took him to the emergency room. After examination and some tests, Dr. Clifton cleaned the wound, applied a sterile dressing, and gave Nathan an antibiotic.

Let's Code It!

Dr. Clifton's notes state that Nathan had been bitten on the thumb by a horse. When you turn to the Alphabetic Index, you see

> **Bite(s) (animal)(human)**
> **thumb S61.05**

Remember the Coding Tip from the beginning of this chapter? These codes are first categorized by the anatomical site and then by the specific injury.
When you turn to the Tabular List, you confirm

> ✓4 **S61**   Open wound of wrist, hand and fingers

Before you continue reading, be certain to pay attention to the notations here. There is a *Code also* if a wound infection is documented; there is an EXCLUDES1 notation with two diagnoses that do not relate to Nathan's case; and there are options for the required seventh character. You will need to come back to this after you determine the correct code. So keep reading to determine the correct fourth character:

> ✓5 **S61.0**   Open wound of thumb without damage to nail

There is another EXCLUDES1 notation. Has Dr. Clifton documented that the nail was also damaged? No. So continue reading to determine the correct fifth character:

> ✓6 **S61.05**   Open bite of thumb without damage to nail

There is another detail you need to abstract from the documentation: Nathan's right or left thumb?

> **S61.052-**   Open bite of left thumb without damage to nail

Now you need to determine the correct seventh character. Go back to the beginning of this code category and review your choices.

(continued)

CHAPTER 16 | CODING INJURY, POISONING, AND EXTERNAL CAUSES

> **S61.052A**   Open bite of left thumb without damage to nail, initial encounter
>
> Perfect! Yet you have not explained the whole story about why Dr. Clifton cared for Nathan. This code states he was bitten on the left thumb, but not by whom or what. To report how Nathan got bitten and by what, you will need external cause codes. Turn to the Alphabetic Index to External Causes and look up
>
>   **Bite**
>   horse W55.11
>
> Turn in the Tabular List to
>
>   ☑4 **W55**   **Contact with other mammals**
>
> Of course, you are going to read this code's **EXCLUDES1** notation carefully. None of the exclusions apply to this case. And there are your options for the seventh character. But, first, read down to determine the correct fourth, fifth, and sixth characters:
>
>   ☑5 **W55.1**   **Contact with horse**
>   **W55.11x-**   **Bitten by horse**
>
> And now, go back up for the seventh character:
>
>   **W55.11xA**   **Bitten by horse, initial encounter**
>
> Terrific! You will also need to determine the codes to report the place of occurrence, activity, and the external cause status. Try this on your own. Did you determine that these are the codes?
>
>   **Y92.830**   Public park as the place of occurrence of the external cause
>   **Y93.01**   Activity, walking, marching and hiking
>   **Y99.8**   Other external cause status
>
> You are really getting to be a great coder!

Myalgia
Pain in a muscle.

CODING BITES

Remember that whenever you are reporting an injury, you will also need to report external cause codes to explain how the patient got injured and identify the place of occurrence. To learn more, see the section *Reporting External Causes of Injuries* in this chapter. Also, many of the codes from ICD-10-CM code book's *Chapter 19, Injury, poisoning, and certain other consequences of external causes* require seventh characters for reporting the type of encounter.

Traumatic Injury to the Muscles

A muscle injury is most often the result of some type of trauma or overexertion during exercise or sports. Traumatic injuries to muscles may be described in a number of ways:

- *Strain* is a tearing of the fibers of the muscle involved, most often the result of overstretching the muscle during movement.
- *Sprain* is a partially torn or overstretched ligament.
- *Contusion* is usually the result of a minor trauma to a muscle, causing a bruise.
- *Tear* (muscle tear) is a separation within the muscle fibers. A bowstring tear, also known as a *bucket-handle tear,* occurs longitudinally in the meniscus.
- **Myalgia** is the medical term for muscle pain.
- *Rupture* is the tear in an organ or tissue.

EXAMPLES

S53.21xA	Traumatic rupture of right radial collateral ligament, initial encounter
S76.122A	Laceration of left quadriceps muscle, fascia, and tendon, initial encounter
S83.211A	Bucket-handle tear of medial meniscus, current injury, right knee, initial encounter

PART II | REPORTING DIAGNOSES

> **YOU CODE IT! CASE STUDY**
>
> Theresa Flores experienced her first parachute jump with her boyfriend 3 months ago. She loved it and is now working on her certification for parachute jumping. On her last jump, she sprained the lateral collateral ligament of her left knee after landing the wrong way. Dr. Hadden confirmed the injury and treated it.
>
> ### You Code It!
>
> Go through the steps of coding, and determine the code or codes that should be reported for this encounter between Dr. Hadden and Theresa.
>
> Step #1: Read the case carefully and completely.
>
> Step #2: Abstract the scenario. Which main words or terms describe why the physician cared for the patient during this encounter?
>
> Step #3: Are there any details missing or incomplete for which you would need to query the physician? [If so, ask your instructor.]
>
> Step #4: Check for any relevant guidance, including reading all of the symbols and notations in the Tabular List and the appropriate sections of the Official Guidelines.
>
> Step #5: Determine the correct diagnosis code or codes to explain why this encounter was medically necessary.
>
> Step #6: Double-check your work.
>
> **Answer:**
>
> Did you determine these to be the correct codes?
>
> | | |
> |---|---|
> | S83.422A | Sprain of lateral collateral ligament of left knee, initial encounter |
> | V97.22xA | Parachutist injured on landing, initial encounter |
> | Y99.8 | Other external cause status (leisure activity) |

16.3 Using Seventh Characters to Report Status of Care

Throughout the long list of codes available to report traumatic injury, you will see that a majority require seventh (7th) characters. These characters report where the patient is, at this encounter, in the treatment plan.

Character	Description	Meaning
A	Initial encounter	Patient is receiving active treatment including evaluation and continuing treatment by any physician.
D	Subsequent encounter	Patient has completed active treatment and is receiving routine care for the condition during the healing process or the recovery phase.
S	Sequela	Late effects, also known as residual effects, of another condition, such as scar formation after a burn.

> **CODING BITES**
>
> When reporting an encounter for *sequela* care, the principal (first-listed) code is the one identifying the specific sequela (i.e., scar, malunion of fractured bone, etc.), followed by the code that reports the original injury or poisoning with a 7th character of S.

Seventh Characters for Fracture Care

When reporting a code identifying that the patient has a fracture (more about this in *16.2 Traumatic Injuries* in this chapter), the definitions of the seventh characters change a bit to provide more details about the specific fracture.

> **GUIDANCE CONNECTION**
>
> Read the ICD-10-CM Official Guidelines for Coding and Reporting, section **I. Conventions, General Coding Guidelines and Chapter Specific Guidelines,** subsection **C. Chapter-Specific Coding Guidelines,** chapter **19. Injury, poisoning, and certain other consequences of external causes,** subsection **a. Application of 7th Characters in Chapter 19.**

Skeletal Fractures

Character	Description
A	Initial encounter for closed fracture
B	Initial encounter for open fracture
D	Subsequent encounter for fracture with routine healing
G	Subsequent encounter for fracture with delayed healing
K	Subsequent encounter for fracture with nonunion
P	Subsequent encounter for fracture with malunion
S	Sequela

> **CODING BITES**
>
> Example of a *subsequent encounter* for fracture care might include a cast change, removal of a cast, x-ray to evaluate healing of a fracture, or adjusting a patient's medication.

> **GUIDANCE CONNECTION**
>
> Read the ICD-10-CM Official Guidelines for Coding and Reporting, section **I. Conventions, General Coding Guidelines and Chapter Specific Guidelines,** subsection **C. Chapter-Specific Coding Guidelines,** chapter **19. Injury, poisoning, and certain other consequences of external causes,** subsection **c.1) Initial vs. Subsequent Encounter for Fractures.**

Fracture of Forearm, Femur, and Lower Leg (Including Ankle)

Character	Description
A	Initial encounter for closed fracture
B	Initial encounter for open fracture type I or II (or NOS)
C	Initial encounter for open fracture type IIIA, IIIB, or IIIC
D	Subsequent encounter for closed fracture with routine healing
E	Subsequent encounter for open fracture type I or II with routine healing
F	Subsequent encounter for open fracture type IIIA, IIIB, or IIIC with routine healing
G	Subsequent encounter for closed fracture with delayed healing
H	Subsequent encounter for open fracture type I or II with delayed healing
J	Subsequent encounter for open fracture type IIIA, IIIB, or IIIC with delayed healing
K	Subsequent encounter for closed fracture with nonunion
M	Subsequent encounter for open fracture type I or II with nonunion
N	Subsequent encounter for open fracture type IIIA, IIIB, or IIIC wtih nonunion
P	Subsequent encounter for closed fracture with malunion
Q	Subsequent encounter for open fracture type I or II with malunion
R	Subsequent encounter for open fracture type IIIA, IIIB, or IIIC with malunion
S	Sequela

> **CODING BITES**
>
> Aftercare codes from ICD-10-CM's Chapter 21 (Z codes) should *NOT* be reported when the injury or poisoning code uses a 7th character.

16.4 Using the Table of Drugs and Chemicals

Often located directly after the alphabetical listing is the Table of Drugs and Chemicals (see Figure 16-3). (*Note:* Different published versions of the ICD-10-CM book may place sections in a different order.) The Table of Drugs and Chemicals is used when a drug or chemical caused an adverse reaction, poisoned the patient, or caused a toxic effect. Similar to the Neoplasm Table, the Table of Drugs and Chemicals is organized in columns.

Substance	Poisoning, Accidental (unintentional)	Poisoning, Intentional self-harm	Poisoning, Assault	Poisoning, Undetermined	Adverse Effect	Underdosing
		#			–	–
1-propanol	T51.3X1	T51.3X2	T51.3X3	T51.3X4	–	–
2-propanol	T51.2X1	T51.2X2	T51.2X3	T51.2X4	–	–
2,4-D (dichlorophen-oxyacetic acid)	T60.3X1	T60.3X2	T60.3X3	T60.3X4	–	–
2,4-toluene diisocyanate	T65.0X1	T65.0X2	T65.0X3	T65.0X4	–	–
2,4,5-T (trichloro-phenoxyacetic acid)	T60.1X1	T60.1X2	T60.1X3	T60.1X4	–	–
14-hydroxydihyrdo-morphinone	T40.2X1	T40.2X2	T40.2X3	T40.2X4	T40.2X5	T40.2X6
		A				
ABOB	T37.5X1	T37.5X2	T37.5X3	T37.5X4	T37.5X5	T37.5X6
Abrine	T62.2X1	T62.2X2	T62.2X3	T62.2X4	–	–
Abrus(seed)	T62.2X1	T62.2X2	T62.2X3	T62.2X4	–	–
Absinthe	T51.0X1	T51.0X2	T51.0X3	T51.0X4	–	–
- beverage	T51.0X1	T51.0X2	T51.0X3	T51.0X4	–	–
Acaricide	T60.8X1	T60.8X2	T60.8X3	T60.8X4	–	–
Acebutolol	T44.7X1	T44.7X2	T44.7X3	T44.7X4	T44.7X5	T44.7X6
Acecarbromal	T42.6X1	T42.6X2	T42.6X3	T42.6X4	T42.6X5	T42.6X6
Aceclidine	T44.1X1	T44.1X2	T44.1X3	T44.1X4	T44.1X5	T44.1X6
Acedapsone	T37.0X1	T37.0X2	T37.0X3	T37.0X4	T37.0X5	T37.0X6
Acetylline piperazine	T48.6X1	T48.6X2	T48.6X3	T48.6X4	T48.6X5	T48.6X6
Acemorphan	T40.2X1	T40.2X2	T40.2X3	T40.2X4	T40.2X5	T40.2X6
Acenocoumarin	T45.511	T45.512	T45.513	T45.514	T45.515	T45.516
Acenocoumarol	T45.511	T45.512	T45.513	T45.514	T45.515	T45.516
Acepifylline	T48.6X1	T48.6X2	T48.6X3	T48.6X4	T48.6X5	T48.6X6
Acepromazine	T43.3X1	T43.3X2	T43.3X3	T43.3X4	T43.3X5	T43.3X6
Acesulfamethoxypyrida-zine	T37.0X1	T37.0X2	T37.0X3	T37.0X4	T37.0X5	T37.0X6
Acetal	T52.8X1	T52.8X2	T52.8X3	T52.8X4	–	–
Acetaldehyde (vapor)	T52.8X1	T52.8X2	T52.8X3	T52.8X4	–	–
- liquid	T65.891	T65.892	T65.893	T65.894	–	–
P-Acetamidophenol	T39.1X1	T39.1X2	T39.1X3	T39.1X4	T39.1X5	T39.1X6
Acetominaphen	T39.1X1	T39.1X2	T39.1X3	T39.1X4	T39.1X5	T39.1X6
Acetalminosalol	T39.1X1	T39.1X2	T39.1X3	T39.1X4	T39.1X5	T39.1X6
Acetanilide	T39.1X1	T39.1X2	T39.1X3	T39.1X4	T39.1X5	T39.1X6
Acetarsol	T37.3X1	T37.3X2	T37.3X3	T37.3X4	T37.3X5	T37.3X6
Acetazolamide	T50.2X1	T50.2X2	T50.2X3	T50.2X4	T50.2X5	T50.2X6
Acetiamine	T45.2X1	T45.2X2	T45.2X3	T45.2X4	T45.2X5	T45.2X6
Acetic						
- acid	T54.2X1	T54.2X2	T54.2X3	T54.2X4	–	–

(continued)

Substance	Poisoning, Accidental (unintentional)	Poisoning, Intentional self-harm	Poisoning, Assault	Poisoning, Undetermined	Adverse Effect	Underdosing
-- with sodium acetate (ointment)	T49.3X1	T49.3X2	T49.3X3	T49.3X4	T49.3X5	T49.3X6
-- ester (solvent) (vapor)	T52.8X1	T52.8X2	T52.8X3	T52.8X4	–	–
-- irrigating solution	T50.3X1	T50.3X2	T50.3X3	T50.3X4	T50.3X5	T50.3X6
-- medicinal (lotion)	T49.2X1	T49.2X2	T49.2X3	T49.2X4	T49.2X5	T49.2X6
- anhydride	T65.891	T65.892	T65.893	T65.894	–	–

FIGURE 16-3 ICD-10-CM Table of Drugs and Chemicals, in part, from 1-propanol through acetic anhydride *Source: ICD-10-CM Official Guidelines for Coding and Reporting* The Centers for Medicare and Medicaid Services (CMS) and the National Center for Health Statistics (NCHS)

> **GUIDANCE CONNECTION**
>
> Read the ICD-10-CM Official Guidelines for Coding and Reporting, section **I. Conventions, General Coding Guidelines and Chapter Specific Guidelines**, subsection **C. Chapter-Specific Coding Guidelines**, chapter **19. Injury, poisoning, and certain other consequences of external causes**, subsections **e. Adverse Effects, Poisoning, Underdosing and Toxic Effects** and **e.1) Do not code directly from the Table of Drugs.**

Physicians' Desk Reference (PDR)
A series of reference books identifying all aspects of prescription and over-the-counter medications, as well as herbal remedies.

Drug and Chemical Names

The first column of the table lists the names of drugs and chemicals, in alphabetic order. The list includes prescription medications, over-the-counter medications, household and industrial chemicals, and many other items with a chemical basis. Aspirin, indigestion relief medication, drugstore-brand allergy relievers, alcohol (for drinking or sterilization), window cleaner, battery acid, and lots of other similar substances are included, as well as medications prescribed by a physician.

Sometimes, it is easy to find what you're looking for. For example, Giselle had a bad reaction to Nytol. Even though *Nytol* is the brand name of an over-the-counter sleep medication, you will find it easily in the list of substances in the first column of the Table of Drugs and Chemicals.

Other times, it may not be this easy, and the name—whether brand name, generic name, or chemical name—that is documented in the physician's notes may not be in the table. If you don't find it, you may have to do some research. Some of the drugs and chemicals are listed by their brand or common names, such as Metamucil or Nytol. Others are listed by their chemical or generic names, such as barbiturates (sedatives). If you are not certain, consult a *Physicians' Desk Reference* **(PDR)**, a group of books that list all the approved drugs, herbal remedies, and over-the-counter medications by brand name, chemical name, generic name, and drug category.

> **EXAMPLE**
>
> Vesicare—the brand name.
> Solifenacin succinate—the generic or chemical name.
> Muscarinic receptor antagonist—the drug category.
> Anticholinergic—the general drug category.

In our example, you can see Vesicare is shown as the trade or brand name. The generic or chemical name is solifenacin succinate. If a physician prescribed it for a patient, who then had an adverse reaction or took an overdose, you would most likely see one or the other of those names in the notes. However, you will find neither of them listed in the Table of Drugs and Chemicals. The next piece of information given to you by the PDR is found in the description of the drug: muscarinic receptor antagonist. Unfortunately, there is nothing in the table under *muscarinic* either. Because the patient either had an adverse reaction or had taken an overdose, take a look at the following paragraphs from the PDR:

ADVERSE REACTIONS
. . . Expected side effects of antimuscarinic agents . . .
OVERDOSAGE
. . . Overdosage with Vesicare can potentially result in severe *anticholinergic* effects . . .

The two paragraphs provide us with two new descriptors for the drug: *antimuscarinic* and *anticholinergic*. Both of them are shown in the Table of Drugs and Chemicals and, interestingly, lead you to the same codes.

LET'S CODE IT! SCENARIO

Kurt Hershey found an unmarked barrel in the back of the warehouse where he works. He opened the top and leaned over to see what was inside. Vapors from the benzene solvent being stored in that barrel overcame Kurt. He had difficulty breathing because he accidentally inhaled the chemical. He was taken to the doctor immediately. Dr. Blanchard diagnosed Kurt with respiratory distress syndrome, a toxic effect from inhaling the benzene.

Let's Code It!

Kurt had *a toxic effect from inhaling the benzene*. The notes also state that Kurt had *respiratory distress*. You learned that you need at least two codes: toxic effect + external cause code.

The first code identifies the chemical or substance and intent. In Kurt's case, the substance was the vapor from a barrel of benzene solvent. Turn to the Alphabetic Index's Table of Drugs and Chemicals. Look down the first column and find *benzene:*

Benzene
  homologues (acetyl) (dimethyl) (methyl) (solvent)

You know from the documentation that this was an accidental poisoning, so look across the line to the first column titled "Poisoning, Accidental (Unintentional)":

Benzene   T52.1x1
  homologues (acetyl) (dimethyl) (methyl) (solvent)   T52.2x1

Hmm. It can be difficult to know what was in that barrel. You can get more information from the Tabular List and see if that helps. Start at the three-character number and be certain to check any notations or directives:

☑4 **T52**   **Toxic effect of organic solvents**

Be sure to read the **EXCLUDES1** notation. Does it relate to Kurt's diagnosis? No. Good! There are the seventh-character options for later, but first you must determine the rest of the code, so keep reading down the column:

☑5 **T52.1**   **Toxic effects of benzene**
☑5 **T52.2**   **Toxic effects of homologues of benzene**

Homologues are not mentioned in the documentation, so review the options for fifth and sixth characters under T52.1:

☑7 **T52.1x1**   **Toxic effects of benzene, accidental (unintentional)**

Remember, you need to include the seventh character.

T52.1x1A   **Toxic effects of benzene, accidental (unintentional), initial encounter**

Great! You now have the first-listed code for Kurt's encounter.
  The next code reports the *effect* that the benzene vapors had on Kurt.
  The notes state he had respiratory distress. In the main section of the Alphabetic Index, find

Distress
  respiratory (adult) (child) **R06.03**

Look up the code in the Tabular List

R06.03   **Acute respiratory distress**

(continued)

This matches!

Two more codes—remember, you also need external cause codes to report where the accident occurred and Kurt's status (why he was doing this). In the Index to External Causes, turn to "Place of occurrence." The notes state that Kurt was in a warehouse when this accident happened, so read down the list, and you will see

> **Place of occurrence**
> **warehouse Y92.59**

Go to the Tabular List, beginning with the code category:

> ☑4 **Y92**   **Place of occurrence of the external cause**

Read down the column to review your choices for the required fourth and fifth characters.

> **Y92.59**   Other trade areas as the place of occurrence of the external cause (warehouse as the place of occurrence of the external cause)

Your last code will report Kurt's status. You know he was at work, so you will use this code:

> **Y99.0**   **Civilian activity done for income or pay**

This completes the report.

> **T52.1x1A**   Toxic effects of benzene, accidental (unintentional), initial encounter
> **R06.03**   Acute respiratory distress
> **Y92.59**   Other trade areas as the place of occurrence of the external cause (warehouse as the place of occurrence of the external cause)
> **Y99.0**   Civilian activity done for income or pay

You are really becoming a great coder!

16.5 Adverse Effects, Poisoning, Underdosing, and Toxic Effects

When an individual comes in contact with a drug or a chemical that has an unhealthy impact, it must be coded. The person might have had an unusual reaction to a medication prescribed by a health care professional or might have been exposed to something noxious.

The first step is for you to determine whether the patient was poisoned, suffering an adverse effect (or reaction), or experiencing a toxic effect.

Adverse Reaction

When health care providers determine that a pharmaceutical substance may improve an individual's health status, they will typically prescribe that medication for therapeutic use. A patient is diagnosed with an adverse effect, or reaction, when *all* of the following occur and the patient has a negative outcome anyway:

- A health care professional correctly *prescribes* a drug for a patient.
- The correct patient receives the correct *drug*.
- The correct dosage is given to the patient (or taken by the patient). [The correct dosage includes the correct *amount* in the correct *frequency*.]
- The correct *route* of administration is used.

> **GUIDANCE CONNECTION**
>
> Read the ICD-10-CM Official Guidelines for Coding and Reporting, section **I. Conventions, General Coding Guidelines and Chapter Specific Guidelines,** subsection **C. Chapter-Specific Coding Guidelines,** chapter **19, Injury, poisoning, and certain other consequences of external causes,** subsection e. **Adverse Effects, Poisoning, Underdosing and Toxic Effects.**

> **EXAMPLE**
> Dr. Levinson prescribed 10 mg of Lexapro, bid, po, for Terence Romulles for anxiety.
>
> Lexapro is the brand name of an anti-anxiety medication.
> 10 mg is the quantity (amount) of the dosage.
> bid is the abbreviation meaning twice per day—the frequency.
> po is the abbreviation meaning "by mouth"—the route of administration.

CODING BITES

You might need more than one code to report the negative effect of this medication on this patient. Remember, you need to tell the whole story in codes.

The patient then has an unexpected bad reaction to that drug. There may have been no way to know the patient was allergic to this medication because he had never taken it before. Unpredictable reactions to drugs can be prompted by genetic factors, other conditions or diseases, allergies, or other issues.

When an adverse reaction has occurred, you will need a minimum of two codes.

First, code for the effect. The code or codes will report exactly what the reaction was, such as a rash, vomiting, or unconsciousness. When you abstract the physician's documentation, you may find this is a confirmed diagnosis, or signs and symptoms experienced by the patient as a result of taking the medication.

Second, code for the external cause. The external cause code will explain that the patient took the drug for therapeutic use. You can find this code in the Table of Drugs and Chemicals by first locating the name of the drug (either the brand name or the generic name) in the first column and then reading across that row to the column under the heading "Adverse Effect."

CODING BITES

Think P.E. for Poison

P = poison code is reported first [the code suggested by the appropriate column of the Table of Drugs and Chemicals]

E = effect of the poisoning is reported next [the bad reaction the patient had to the substance, such as a rash, vomiting, or unconsciousness]

The effect of the poisoning might be a confirmed diagnosis or documentation of signs and/or symptoms. You may need more than one code to tell the whole story about how this poisoning has affected the patient.

> **EXAMPLE**
> Giana Roman took her prescription for amoxicillin exactly as the doctor and the pharmacist instructed. She broke out in a rash because it turned out she was allergic to this antibiotic and no one knew.
>
> The "effect" is the rash "dermatitis due to drugs taken internally" = **L27.0 Generalized skin eruption due to drugs and medicaments taken internally**
>
> +
>
> The external cause code explains "therapeutic use of amoxicillin" = **T36.0x5A Adverse effect of penicillins, initial encounter**

Poisoning

Most people think of poisoning as something from a great detective novel or movie; however, a poisoning can happen under many different circumstances. In reality, when a person comes in contact with a drug (not prescribed by a physician or not taken as prescribed) or a chemical and a health problem results, it is called a poisoning.

The drug or substance might have been ingested, inhaled, absorbed through the skin, injected, or taken by some other method. Remember that this may be a drug, or it may be a chemical, such as cleaning supplies, gasoline, or other type of poison or toxic substance. Your first step is to abstract the name of the substance that poisoned the patient so you can look it up on the Table of Drugs and Chemicals.

Next, you will need to discover the circumstances under which this patient came to be poisoned. Was it . . .

- *An accident (unintentional).* Things happen, such as a child finding a bottle of medication and thinking it's candy or finding cleaning spray and thinking it would be fun to wash his face with it. A patient mistakenly took the wrong amount of a medication or the clinician mistakenly administered the wrong quantity to the

GUIDANCE CONNECTION

The ICD-10-CM guidelines reduce the number of codes you will need to report some conditions. Codes in categories T36–T65 are combination codes that include the substances related to adverse effects, poisonings, toxic effects, and underdosing, as well as the external cause.

> **GUIDANCE CONNECTION**
>
> Read the ICD-10-CM Official Guidelines for Coding and Reporting, section **I. Conventions, General Coding Guidelines and Chapter Specific Guidelines,** subsection **C. Chapter-Specific Coding Guidelines,** chapter **19. Injury, poisoning, and certain other consequences of external causes,** subsection **e.5)(b) Poisoning.**

wrong patient (if this was a drug). Two substances could also be taken that contradicted each other.

- *A suicide attempt (intentional self-harm).* Sadly, a person might take an overdose while trying to harm himself or herself, intentionally.
- *An assault.* This occurs when someone tries to cause intentional harm to someone else. It sounds like a scene from that detective movie, but it does happen in real life.
- *Underdosing.* Most often, this occurs when the patient cannot afford the medication, so he or she takes less each time so one prescription will last longer. Or, this may occur because a label is misread or an implanted medication pump malfunctions. In any of these situations, the patient is not receiving the quantity necessary for therapeutic value and thus does not improve as expected due to the medication's ineffectiveness.

Underdosing and Patient Noncompliance

Sometimes, a patient has an adverse effect because he or she did not take the medication as ordered by the physician or didn't take the drugs at all. Some patients forget, some are resistant to needing a drug, and some cannot afford the required number of pills. When taking too little of the quantity prescribed (underdosing) is the patient's action, rather than an error on the part of a health care professional, this is considered noncompliance and is reported with an additional code to explain:

Z91.120	Patient's intentional underdosing of medication regimen due to financial hardship
Z91.128	Patient's intentional underdosing of medication regimen for other reason
Z91.130	Patient's unintentional underdosing of medication regimen due to age-related debility
Z91.138	Patient's unintentional underdosing of medication regimen for other reason
Z91.14	Patient's other noncompliance with medication regimen

> **CODING BITES**
>
> Code subcategories Z91.12- and Z91.13- both have a *Code first* notation, so you don't have to wonder about proper sequencing.

> **CODING BITES**
>
> The difference between a poisoning and a toxic effect is the substance. A poisoning or adverse effect is a reaction to a natural or medicinal substance, whereas a toxic effect is a reaction to a harmful substance.

Toxic Effects

A toxic effect, such as irritation or carcinogenicity, may result from a part of the human body interacting with a chemical or other nonmedicinal substance. When an individual comes in contact with a toxic substance, whether ingested (such as liquid window cleaner), inhaled (such as asbestos), or touched (such as acid), you will report this using the same coding process as reporting a poisoning. The external cause code will come from a different range of codes, that's all.

T51-T65 Toxic effects of substances chiefly nonmedicinal as to source

---

LET'S CODE IT! SCENARIO

Dr. Barry, a pediatrician, was called in to see Abigail Scanter, a 3-year-old female, brought in by her mother after she discovered Abigail on the floor with part of a detergent pod in her mouth, half empty. Abigail was having difficulty breathing; she had vomited; and her mouth, throat, and esophagus were erythmatous, swollen, and irritated. Dr. Barry ordered blood tests and immediately began to pump Abigail's stomach based on his diagnosis of a toxic effect of the accidental ingestion of detergent.

Let's Code It!

Dr. Barry confirmed that Abigail was ill due to the toxic effects of ingesting the detergent.

Turn to the Table of Drugs and Chemicals to find "detergent" in the first column, "**Substance**":

> **Detergent**
>   external medication
>   local
>   medicinal
>   nonmedicinal
>   specified NEC
>
> Were you surprised to see so many different options? I was. Which fits this diagnosis? Let's think this through:
>
> **Detergent**
>   external medication — *the problem here was not external*
>   local — *she swallowed the detergent, so it was not local*
>   medicinal — *definitely not*
>   nonmedicinal — *this fits!*
>   specified NEC — *possibly*
>
> Look across the row where *nonmedicinal* is listed to the first column to the right, the column "**Poisoning, Accidental (unintentional)**" . . . you will see code T55.1x1 suggested. This is the same code suggested on the next row for "*specified NEC*" so that will save some time.
>   Turn in the ICD-10-CM Tabular List to the code category
>
> ☑4 **T55**   **Toxic effect of soaps and detergents**
>
> The fourth character requires you to determine if Abigail was affected by soap or detergent, leading you to
>
> ☑5 **T55.1**   **Toxic effect of detergents**
> ☑6 **T55.1x**   **Toxic effect of detergents**
>   ☑7 **T55.1x1**   **Toxic effect of detergents, accidental (unintentional)**
>
> You will find the seventh-character options in the box immediately below the code category. You can tell this is the first time Dr. Barry is caring for Abigail for this reason, and this is the first time Abigail is receiving care for this event, leading you to confirm this code:
>
> **T55.1x1A**   **Toxic effect of detergents, accidental (unintentional), initial encounter**
>
> Good job!

Substance Interactions

When the cause of the poisoning or toxic effect is the interaction between two substances (e.g., drugs and alcohol), then you will need to report both substances involved. You will need one poisoning code for each substance causing the reaction, as well as one or more codes to accurately report the effect of the interaction.

   Interactions can occur between two or more drugs, drugs and alcohol or other drinks, drugs and food, or many other combinations. For example, you might notice a warning "*Don't take this drug with milk or other dairy products.*" This is a warning provided to prevent an interaction—the mixture of two or more substances that changes the effect of any of the individual substances.

> ### 🛑 LET'S CODE IT! SCENARIO
>
> *Meryl Brighton was prescribed Zyprexa (olanzapine), a psychotropic, by her psychiatrist, Dr. Cauldwell, for treatment of her bipolar disorder. Meryl mentioned that her family doctor, Dr. Wall, had her on Norvasc (amlodipine), an antihypertensive, for her high blood pressure. Dr. Cauldwell told Meryl to stop taking the Norvasc while on the Zyprexa. Meryl forgot and took both medicines at the same time. Meryl suffered a dangerous case of severe hypotension and was rushed to the ED by ambulance.*
>
> *(continued)*

Let's Code It!

Meryl was diagnosed with severe hypotension as a result of taking both Zyprexa and Norvasc. She was told not to take both medications, but she forgot and took them both anyway. This means that this was an accidental drug interaction.

First, you will need to determine the codes for the substances and intent. Open your ICD-10-CM code book to the Table of Drugs and Chemicals and look for

Zyprexa

Move across the row to find the suggested code in the first column for Poisoning, Accidental (Unintentional) . . . T43.591

Turn in the Tabular List to code category

☑4 **T43**   **Poisoning by, adverse effect of and underdosing of psychotropic drugs, not elsewhere classified**

Carefully read the EXCLUDES1 and EXCLUDES2 notes. Do they have any connection to Meryl's diagnosis? Not this time, so read down and review all of the fourth-character options.

☑5 **T43.5**   **Poisoning by, adverse effect of and underdosing of other and unspecified antipsychotics and neuroleptics**

Carefully read the EXCLUDES1 note. Meryl did not become poisoned by rauwolfia, so continue reading to find the appropriate fifth character.

☑6 **T43.59**   **Poisoning by, adverse effect of and underdosing of other antipsychotics and neuroleptics**

Next, find the appropriate sixth character for Meryl's accidental ingestion of Zyprexa.

T43.591   **Poisoning by, adverse effect of and underdosing of other antipsychotics and neuroleptics, accidental (unintentional)**

Almost done; find the appropriate seventh character. You will find the box with the options at the top of this subsection, right under the T43 code.

T43.591A   **Poisoning by, adverse effect of and underdosing of other antipsychotics and neuroleptics, accidental (unintentional), initial encounter**

Good job! Now, you need to go back to the Table of Drugs and Chemicals, and look for

Norvasc

It is not listed. So, use a PDR (*Physicians' Desk Reference*) or the website [www.pdr.net] and learn that the generic name for Norvasc is amlodipine besylate and it is an antihypertensive.

Antihypertensive drug NEC

Move across the row to find the suggested code in the first column for Poisoning, Accidental (Unintentional) . . . T46.5x1

Turn in the Tabular List to code category

☑4 **T46**   **Poisoning by, adverse effect of and underdosing of agents primarily affecting the cardiovascular system**

Carefully read the EXCLUDES1 note. Meryl did not become poisoned by metaraminol, so continue reading to find the appropriate fourth character.

☑5 **T46.5**   **Poisoning by, adverse effect of and underdosing of other antihypertensive drugs**

Carefully read the EXCLUDES2 notes. Meryl did not become poisoned by any of these, so continue reading to find the appropriate fifth character.

☑6 **T46.5x**   **Poisoning by, adverse effect of and underdosing of other antihypertensive drugs**

Next, find the appropriate sixth character for Meryl's accidental ingestion of Norvasc.

> **T46.5x1** Poisoning by, adverse effect of and underdosing of other antihypertensive drugs accidental (unintentional)

Almost done, find the appropriate seventh character. You will find the box with the options at the top of this subsection, right under the T46 code.

> **T46.5x1A** Poisoning by, adverse effect of and underdosing of other antihypertensive drugs accidental (unintentional), initial encounter

Good job! One more code to go. You need to report the effect that this interaction had on Meryl. Turn to the Alphabetic Index and find:

> **Hypotention (arterial) (constitutional) I95.9**

with a list indented beneath. Stop and review the scenario again. What exactly caused Meryl's hypotension? The interaction of the two drugs. Therefore, it was drug-induced. Read down and find

> **Hypotention (arterial) (constitutional) I95.9**
>   drug-induced I95.2

Turn to the Tabular List, and begin at the code category . . .

> ☑4 **I95** Hypotension

Carefully read the **EXCLUDES1** note. None of these apply to this encounter with Meryl, so continue reading to find the appropriate fourth character.

> **I95.2** Hypotension due to drugs
>   *Use additional code* for adverse effect, if applicable, to identify drug (T36-T50 with fifth or sixth character 5)

Does this turn your sequencing upside down? No. Read this carefully. In this case, for Meryl's current issue, she did not have an adverse effect. It was a poisoning. Great!

Now you can report, with confidence . . .

> **T43.591A** Poisoning by, adverse effect of and underdosing of other antipsychotics and neuroleptics, accidental (unintentional), initial encounter
> **T46.5x1A** Poisoning by, adverse effect of and underdosing of other antihypertensive drugs accidental (unintentional), initial encounter
> **I95.2** Hypotension due to drugs

Good coding!

YOU INTERPRET IT!

Identify if this is an accidental poisoning, an adverse effect, a suicide attempt, or an assault.

1. The EMTs brought Katherine into the ER. Her roommate found her unconscious with an empty pill bottle by her side, along with a suicide note. _____

2. Harrison rushed his 3-year-old son into the ER. He had found him sitting on the bathroom floor with his bottle of Synthroid, half empty. _____

3. Roger picked up his new prescription at the drug store. Within 30 minutes of taking the first tablet, he began to break out in a rash. _____

4. Ellen was brought into the Urgent Care late one night by her friends. They were out at a club and she suddenly lost consciousness. The blood tests showed that someone at the club had put something in her drink. _____

16.6 Reporting Burns

A patient can sustain a **burn** or **corrosion** to any part of the body in many different ways. It can be the result of the skin coming near to or in actual contact with a flame, such as a candle or the flame on a gas stove. A burn can happen when contact is made with a hot object, such as a hot plate or curling iron. Chemicals, such as lye or acid, can cause a corrosion upon contact with a person's skin. As a professional coding specialist, you may need to code the diagnosis of a burn or corrosion.

When a patient has suffered a burn, virtually every case will require multiple codes to tell the whole story. So, we came up with a memory tip to help you remember the details you need, the minimum number of codes you need, and the sequencing of (the order in which to report) the codes. To report these diagnoses correctly, you have to *S/S.E.E.* the burn. You need at least three codes to properly report the diagnosis of a burn:

First-listed code(s): S/S = *s*ite and *s*everity (from categories T20–T25)
Next-listed code: E = *e*xtent (from code category T31)
Last-listed code(s): E = *e*xternal cause code(s)

Let's look at these components and what they mean.

Site and Severity

Site

Your first-listed code or codes will be combination codes that report both the **site** and **severity** of the injury. *Site* refers to the anatomical site that is affected by the burn. When you look at the descriptions for the codes in range T20–T28, you see that each code category is first defined by a general part or section of the human body:

T20	Burn and corrosion of head, face, and neck
T21	Burn and corrosion of trunk
T22	Burn and corrosion of shoulder and upper limb, except wrist and hand
T23	Burn and corrosion of wrist and hand
T24	Burn and corrosion of lower limb, except ankle and foot
T25	Burn and corrosion of ankle and foot
T26	Burn and corrosion confined to eye and adnexa
T27	Burn and corrosion of respiratory tract
T28	Burn and corrosion of other internal organs

EXAMPLE

Hope Rockfield suffered a burn to her left knee. Lower limb is the general anatomical site, and knee is the specific site of the burn.

Severity

The fourth character for each category (except categories T26–T28) identifies the severity. Using the layers of the skin, the severity of a burn is identified by degree (see Figure 16-4):

- **First-degree burns** are evident by erythema (redness of the epidural layer).
- **Second-degree burns** are identified by fluid-filled blisters in addition to the erythema.
- **Third-degree burns** have damage evident in the epidermis, dermis, and fatty tissue layers and can involve the muscles and nerves below.
- *Deep third-degree burned* skin will show necrosis (death of the tissue) and at times may result in the loss (amputation) of a body part.

The fourth characters available in this section give you the ability to report the documented severity of the burn or corrosion:

CODING BITES

A burn is caused by fire or heat, while a corrosion is caused by a chemical.

GUIDANCE CONNECTION

Read the ICD-10-CM Official Guidelines for Coding and Reporting, section **I. Conventions, General Coding Guidelines and Chapter Specific Guidelines,** subsection **C. Chapter-Specific Coding Guidelines,** chapter **19. Injury, poisoning, and certain other consequences of external causes,** subsection **d. Coding of Burns and Corrosions.**

GUIDANCE CONNECTION

Read the ICD-10-CM Official Guidelines for Coding and Reporting, section **I. Conventions, General Coding Guidelines and Chapter Specific Guidelines,** subsection **C. Chapter-Specific Coding Guidelines,** chapter **19. Injury, poisoning, and certain other consequences of external causes,** subsections **d.2) Burns of the same local site** and **d.5) Assign separate codes for each burn site.**

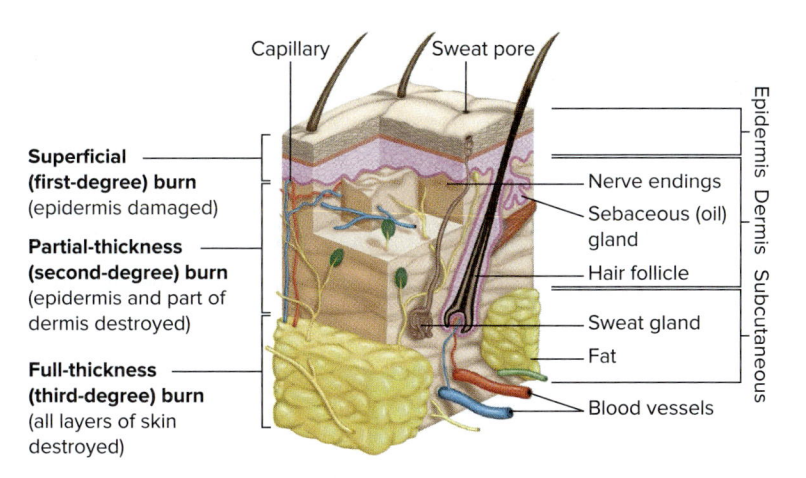

FIGURE 16-4 An illustration identifying the impact on the layers of skin for the different degrees of burns

.0	Unspecified degree
.1	Erythema (first degree)
.2	Blisters, epidermal loss (second degree)
.3	Full-thickness skin loss (third degree NOS)
.4	Corrosion of unspecified degree
.5	Corrosion of first degree
.6	Corrosion of second degree
.7	Corrosion of the third degree

Specific Site

The fifth character gives you the opportunity to report additional details regarding the anatomical site of the burn. Of course, these details will change in accordance with the anatomical region of the code category. Let's take a look at samples from code category T23 Burn and corrosion of wrist and hand:

T23.-1	Burn . . . of thumb (nail)
T23.-2	Burn . . . of single finger (nail) except thumb
T23.-3	Burn . . . of multiple fingers (nail), not including thumb
T23.-4	Burn . . . of multiple fingers (nail), including thumb
T23.-5	Burn . . . of palm
T23.-6	Burn . . . of back of hand
T23.-7	Burn . . . of wrist
T23.-9	Burn . . . of multiple sites of wrist and hand

> **EXAMPLE**
>
> Troy was talking to his buddy and stepped back, hitting the back of his right calf on the hot tailpipe of his motorcycle. The doctor at the emergency room documented second-degree burns.
>
> The first three characters = **T24 Burn and corrosion of lower limb, except ankle and foot.**
> The fourth character = **T24.2 Burn of second degree of lower limb, except ankle and foot.**
> The fifth character = **T24.23 Burn of second degree of lower leg.**
> The sixth character = **T24.231 Burn of second degree of right lower leg.**
> The seventh character = **T24.231A Burn of second degree of right lower leg, initial encounter.**
>
> And there you have the complete code to report Troy's injury. Of course, as you remember, you will also need to report an external cause code to explain how Troy's leg became burned.

Burn
Injury by heat or fire.

Corrosion
A burn caused by a chemical; chemical destruction of the skin.

Site
The specific anatomical location of the disease or injury.

Severity
The level of seriousness.

First-Degree Burn
Redness of the epidermis (skin).

Second-Degree Burn
Blisters on the skin; involvement of the epidermis and the dermis layers.

Third-Degree Burn
Destruction of all layers of the skin, with possible involvement of the subcutaneous fat, muscle, and bone.

> **CODING BITES**
>
> The code descriptions in this section all include both the medical terms (such as *blisters*) and the degree (such as *second degree*), so you can match either to the documentation.

> **CODING BITES**
>
> The description of the fifth character 0 (zero) states "unspecified site." Use this character *very, very* rarely. Think about it: How can a physician diagnose and treat a burn and not know exactly where it is?

LET'S CODE IT! SCENARIO

Anthony, a 15-year-old male, was working on a school project in the basement and accidentally released the hot glue gun onto the palm of his left hand. Dr. Clermont treated him for third-degree burns of the palm of his hand.

Let's Code It!

Anthony was diagnosed with *third-degree burns of the palm*. Let's turn to the Alphabetic Index and look up *burns*:

> **Burn**
> palm(s) T23.059

Turn to the Tabular List, and read

> ☑4 **T23** **Burn and corrosion of wrist and hand**

Notice the available seventh-character options listed directly beneath this code. You will need that information later. First, you need to determine the other characters, so read through your choices for the fourth character:

> ☑5 **T23.3** **Burn of third degree of wrist and hand**

That is much more specific and accurate. Now you have to review the fifth-character choices for code T23.3. Did you notice that there is a character to specify that the burn was on his palm?

> ☑6 **T23.35** **Burn of third degree of palm**

The choices for the sixth character clearly identify which palm:

> ☑7 **T23.352** **Burn of third degree of left palm**

One more character—remember, the options for the seventh character for this code are shown directly beneath the three-character code category. Is this the first time Dr. Clermont is seeing Anthony for this burn? Yes.

> **T23.352A** **Burn of third degree of left palm, initial encounter**

This code tells the complete story, doesn't it? Of course, you will need to also report the external cause code.

Multiple Sites Fall into the Same Code Category

When various sites fall into the same code category (the first three characters of the code), you will report all of these sites with just one code. If the burns are of different severity, use the fourth character that reports the most severe burn (determined by severity), the highest degree.

Then identify that more than one specific site has been burned by using the fifth character that reports "multiple sites," such as T25.19- Burn of first degree of multiple sites of ankle and foot.

LET'S CODE IT! SCENARIO

Damien Connell opened the cover of the bar-b-que to see how the coals were doing. He decided to add some lighter fluid to hurry it along, and the flames roared up into his face. Gina, his wife, rushed him to the emergency department. After an exam, Dr. Hawks diagnosed Damien with a third-degree burn on his chin and second-degree burns on his nose and cheek.

Let's Code It!

Let's begin by abstracting Damien's condition. He has

> Third degree burn on his chin
> Second degree burn on his nose
> Second degree burn on his cheek

In the Alphabetic Index, turn to the term *burn*. You will notice that the long, long list of terms indented beneath this main term all identify anatomical sites, the location on the body that has been burned. Find the suggested codes for all three of Damien's burns:

Burn, chin, third-degree T20.33
Burn, nose, second-degree T20.24
Burn, cheek, second-degree T20.26

Notice that the code category T20 is the same for all three sites: chin, nose, and cheek. Therefore, you use only one code to report these burn sites. Turn to code T20 in the Tabular List:

✓4 **T20**   **Burn and corrosion of head, face, and neck**

Read carefully the EXCLUDES2 listed diagnoses. None of them apply to Damien's condition. Remember that your seventh-character options are listed here as well, for later.

Go ahead and read down the column to review all of the choices for the required fourth character. Now you need to determine which fourth character to use. The burn on his chin is a third-degree burn (fourth character 3), but the burns on his nose and cheek are only second-degree burns (fourth character 2). Should you report both? The guidelines direct you to report only one code, with the fourth character that reports the *most severe* of all the burns, so you need to use the fourth character of 3:

✓5 **T20.3**   **Burn of third degree of head, face, and neck**

Notice that the *Use additional external cause code* notation is here to remind you that you need to do this next, after you determine all of the appropriate codes to report the injury itself.

Review the fifth-character options in this subcategory:

The fifth character 3 reports his chin was burned.
The fifth character 4 reports his nose was burned.
The fifth character 6 reports his cheek was burned.

Again, the guidelines tell you that you must combine all of these into one accurate code. Take a look at the fifth character 9, which reports multiple sites of face, head, and neck. Perfect!

Put it all together and get the most accurate code that tells the whole story:

✓6 **T20.39-**   **Burn of third degree of multiple sites of head, face, and neck**

Look back up to the beginning of the code category to review your options for the seventh character. This is the first time Dr. Hawks is caring for Damien's burns. Now you have the complete code to report:

T20.39xA   **Burn of third degree of multiple sites of head, face, and neck, initial encounter**

Excellent!

Extent

The next code you have to report indicates the **extent**, or percentage, of the body involved. The three-character category for reporting the extent of a burn is T31 and the extent of a corrosion is T32. Either of these codes requires a total of five characters to be valid, no matter what the extent of the burn or corrosion.

T31   **Burns classified according to extent of body surface involved**
T32   **Corrosions classified according to extent of body surface involved**

Turn to code T31 in the Tabular List. The required fourth character will identify the percentage of the patient's *entire body* that is affected by any and all burns, of all degrees (severity). The code descriptions refer to this as *percentage of body surface*, also known as *total body surface area (TBSA)*.

The physician may specify the percentages directly in his or her notes. A statement like "third-degree burns over 10% of the body" or "7% of the body burned" will give

> **Extent**
> The percentage of the body that has been affected by the burn or corrosion.

> **GUIDANCE CONNECTION**
>
> Read the ICD-10-CM Official Guidelines for Coding and Reporting, section **I. Conventions, General Coding Guidelines and Chapter Specific Guidelines,** subsection **C. Chapter-Specific Coding Guidelines,** chapter **19. Injury, poisoning, and certain other consequences of external causes,** subsection **d.6) Burns and Corrosions Classified According to Extent of Body Surface Involved.**

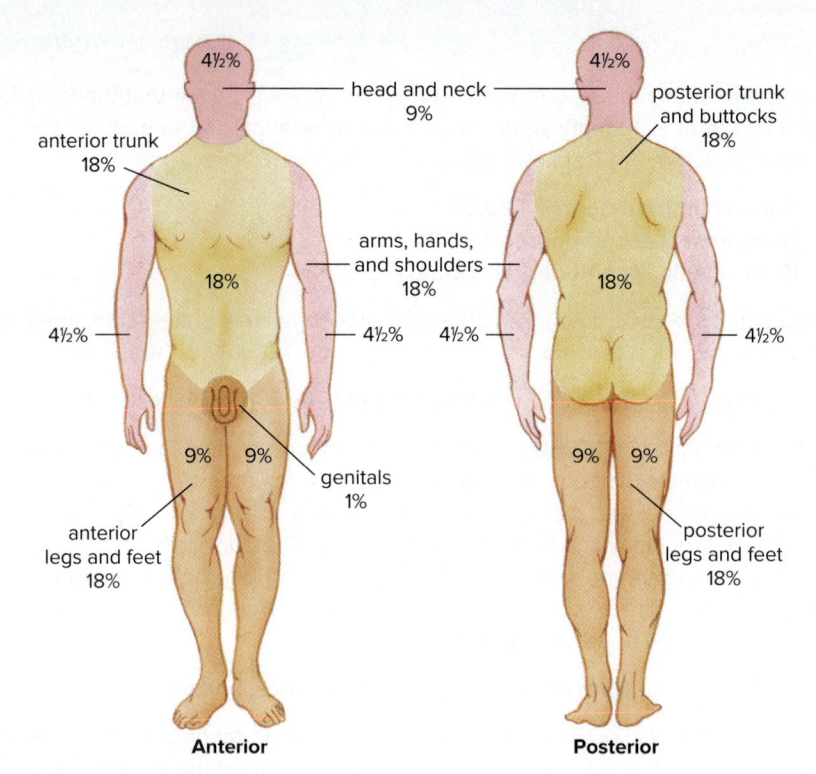

FIGURE 16-5 An illustration identifying the rule of nines, which can be used to estimate the extent of burns

Rule of Nines
A general division of the whole body into sections that each represents 9%; used for estimating the extent of a burn.

> **GUIDANCE CONNECTION**
>
> Read the ICD-10-CM Official Guidelines for Coding and Reporting, section **I. Conventions, General Coding Guidelines and Chapter Specific Guidelines,** subsection **C. Chapter-Specific Coding Guidelines,** chapter **19. Injury, poisoning, and certain other consequences of external causes,** subsection **d.1) Sequencing of burn and related condition codes.**

you the information you need to find the correct fourth character for code T31 or T32. However, other times, the physician may not use a number, and you will have to calculate the percentage yourself. To calculate, you can use the **rule of nines**.

The rule of nines is used to estimate the total body surface area that has been affected by the burns. The body is divided into sections, each section representing 9% of the human body (see Figure 16-5):

Head and neck 9%

Arm, right 9%

Arm, left 9%

Chest 9%

Abdomen 9%

Upper back 9%

Lower back 9%

Leg, right, anterior (front) 9%

Leg, right, posterior (back) 9%

Leg, left, anterior (front) 9%

Leg, left, posterior (back) 9%

Genitalia 1%

As you read through the physician's notes, be aware of the anatomical site, not only for your site code but also for your calculation of the extent of the body involved in the burns.

Next, you must determine the most accurate fifth character for this code. The fifth character identifies the percentage of the patient's body that is *suffering with third-degree burns* only. You can also use the rule of nines to calculate the percentage of area affected by third-degree burns to find the best fifth character.

Of course, these percentages are general—to be used for estimation purposes. As you look at the code descriptions for the fourth and the fifth characters, you will see that the choices for codes T31 and T32 all have descriptors that require you to know the percentage of the body involved only within a 10% range. Therefore, you don't have to worry too much about narrowing down the number.

When you are determining the fourth and fifth characters for code T31 or T32, you may have to add the percentages for several anatomical sites together.

While everyone knows that the rule of nines provides an estimate and is not expected to be precise, it is a professional coder's job to be as specific as possible. Therefore, you want to adjust the percentage as appropriate.

> **EXAMPLE**
>
> Celia suffered third-degree burns on her lower back and the back of her left leg and second-degree burns on her anterior forearm, wrist, and hand:
>
> Lower back (9%) + left leg, back (9%) + anterior forearm (2%) + wrist and hand (1%) = total body surface (21%)
>
> ☑5 T31.2   Burns involving 20%–29% of body surface
>
> Only her back and leg had *third*-degree burns:
>
> Lower back (9%) + left leg, back (9%) = 18%
>
> T31.21   Burns involving 20%–29% of body surface with 10–19% third-degree burns

LET'S CODE IT! SCENARIO

Eli Glosyck, a 28-year-old male, was trying to start a campfire when the flames flared and burned him on the back of his right hand, right forearm, and right elbow. He was rushed to the emergency room, where Dr. Compton determined that he had third-degree burns on his hand and forearm and second-degree burns on his elbow.

Let's Code It!

Dr. Compton diagnosed Eli with *third-degree burns on his hand and forearm* and *second-degree burns on his elbow*. Go to the Alphabetic Index and look up *burn, hand*. Find that listing and the others:

Burn, hand, third-degree T23.309
Burn, forearm, third-degree T22.319
Burn, elbow, second-degree T22.229

Does the Tabular List confirm the codes? Let's check each one:

☑4 **T23**   **Burn and corrosion of wrist and hand**

You can see that a fourth character is required, so read down the column to

☑5 **T23.3**   **Burn of third degree of wrist and hand**

The burns on Eli's hand were documented as third-degree, so that is correct. Now you need to determine the required fifth and sixth characters. Read all of the choices and determine which is the most accurate.

☑6 **T23.36**   **Burn of third degree of back of hand**
☑7 **T23.361-**   **Burn of third degree of back of right hand**

Don't forget the seventh character. The options are at the beginning of this code category.

(continued)

T23.361A   Burn of third degree of back of right hand, initial encounter

This code tells the whole story about the burn to Eli's hand. Now look at the other codes suggested by the Alphabetic Index:

Burn, forearm, third degree T22.319
Burn, elbow, second-degree T22.229

Did you notice that both of these burns are reported using the same three-character code category, T22?

✓4 T22   Burn and corrosion of shoulder and upper limb, except wrist and hand

You have two codes with the same three-character code category. The guidelines state that you must combine these into one code, T22, but which fourth character should you use? Remember, the guidelines also direct you to use the character that reports the greatest severity (the highest degree) of the burn. Third degree is more severe than second degree, so you will use

✓5 T22.3   Burn of third-degree of shoulder and upper limb, except wrist and hand

Read the fifth-character choices for this code category. Which one code can report the burn to both Eli's forearm and his elbow?

✓6 T22.39   Burn of third-degree of multiple sites of shoulder and upper limb, except wrist and hand

The sixth character will report which forearm and elbow were burned:

✓7 T22.391   Burn of third-degree of multiple sites of right shoulder and upper limb, except wrist and hand

And the seventh character will report which encounter this is:

T22.391A   Burn of third-degree of multiple sites of right shoulder and upper limb, except wrist and hand, initial encounter

Good! Next, you need a code to report the extent of the burns. Eli was burned on the following sites:

Hand (part of the arm), 9%
Forearm (part of the same arm), 9%
Elbow (also part of the same arm), 9%

The rule of nines states that one arm represents 9%. Eli had burns on his hand, forearm, and elbow of the same arm. You can see that it would not make sense to add 9% for each of these injuries, as it is still only one arm, so you get a TBSA of 9%. Of this 9%, you must note that only an estimated 4% of his body (his hand and forearm) suffered third-degree burns. Therefore, the next code on Eli's chart will be:

T31.0   Burns involving less than 10% of body surface

The codes you have for Eli's burns are T23.361A, T22.391A, and T31.10 (plus the external cause codes, of course!). Good work!

GUIDANCE CONNECTION

Read the ICD-10-CM Official Guidelines for Coding and Reporting, section **I. C. 19. Injury, poisoning, and certain other consequences of external causes,** subsection **d.4) Infected Burn.**

Infection in the Burn Site

If not treated properly, a burn site can become infected. This can happen because the inner layers of the tissue are exposed, and it might be difficult to keep the wound clean and sterile. If an infection occurs, you should add a code for the specific pathogen. Sequence the infection code after the burn code but before the T31 or T32 code.

Solar and Radiation Burns

When a patient has been burned not by fire or chemicals but by some kind of radiation, the injuries are not reported with codes from the T20–T28 range.

Even with all the ads promoting sunblock lotions and ointments to protect the skin, individuals still manage to get sunburns. These burns are also identified in three degrees to report damage to the skin as a result of overexposure to the natural sun, and each degree has its own code:

L55.0	Sunburn of first degree
L55.1	Sunburn of second degree
L55.2	Sunburn of third degree

Some individuals have a hypersensitivity to the sun, similar to an allergic reaction. Actually, this can be diagnosed as a photoallergic or a phototoxic response to the sun. This type of severe reaction can be determined to be an effect of solar radiation and is reported with one of the following codes:

L56.0	Drug phototoxic response
L56.1	Drug photoallergic response
L56.2	Photocontact dermatitis (berloque dermatitis)
L56.3	Solar urticaria

In addition to physiological sensitivity to the sun, certain medications can cause a patient to develop a sensitivity to the sun. When this is the case, you will need to add an external cause code to report the specific drug that caused this situation.

Sequelae (Late Effects) of Burns and Corrosions

Often, a scar or contracture develops at the site of a healed burn or corrosion. There are times when this lasting condition requires treatment or a procedure. In these cases, you will report the original burn or corrosion code using the seventh character "S," for sequela, to identify that the care and treatment are directed at the late effect of the burn or corrosion.

16.7 Abuse, Neglect, and Maltreatment

Some people treat other people terribly. Such treatment may be physical or sexual **abuse**, neglect, or abandonment. Often, people consider unacceptable behavior as being directed toward a child, yet adults also are abused, neglected, and maltreated. As our elder population increases, these adults are also vulnerable and need health care professionals to watch out for them and protect them.

T74-	Adult and child abuse, neglect, and other maltreatment, confirmed
T76-	Adult and child abuse, neglect, and other maltreatment, suspected
O9A.3-	Physical abuse complicating pregnancy, childbirth and the puerperium
O9A.4-	Sexual abuse complicating pregnancy, childbirth and the puerperium
O9A.5-	Psychological abuse complicating pregnancy, childbirth and the puerperium
Z04.4-	Encounter for examination and observation following alleged rape
Z04.7-	Encounter for examination and observation following alleged physical abuse

The difference between categories T74 and T76 is important and is determined by the documentation: category T74 reports that the physician knows (confirms) this situation; category T76 records a suspicion. You know that suspected conditions are generally not coded and reported. However, most states require health care

---

> **GUIDANCE CONNECTION**
>
> Read the ICD-10-CM Official Guidelines for Coding and Reporting, section **I. Conventions, General Coding Guidelines and Chapter Specific Guidelines**, subsection **C. Chapter-Specific Coding Guidelines**, chapter **19. Injury, poisoning, and certain other consequences of external causes**, subsections **d.7) Encounters for treatment of late effects of burns** and **d.8) Sequelae with a late effect code and current burn**.

Abuse
This term is used in different manners: (a) extreme use of a drug or chemical; (b) violent and/or inappropriate treatment of another person (child, adult, elder).

> **GUIDANCE CONNECTION**
>
> Read the ICD-10-CM Official Guidelines for Coding and Reporting, section **I. Conventions, General Coding Guidelines and Chapter Specific Guidelines**, subsection **C. Chapter-Specific Coding Guidelines**, chapter **19. Injury, poisoning, and certain other consequences of external causes**, subsection **f. Adult and child abuse, neglect and other maltreatment**, and chapter **20. External Causes of Morbidity**, subsection **g. Child and Adult Abuse Guidelines**.

professionals to report any instances of abuse or neglect, even if it is just a suspicion at this point.

When applicable, the code from T74 or T76 should be the first-listed or principal diagnosis, followed by the injury code and/or mental health code. For cases in which the circumstances have been confirmed, a code to report the specific cause of the injury should be included, most often from code range X92–Y08. In any case of abuse, neglect, or maltreatment, if the perpetrator is known, an additional code from category Y07 should be included.

YOU CODE IT! CASE STUDY

Judah Messner, a 5-month-old male, was brought into the ED with third-degree burns on all five fingers of his left hand and both second-degree and third-degree burns on the back of his left hand. His aunt brought him in after visiting the home and seeing her sister's boyfriend stick the baby's hand into a pot of boiling water on the stove. She states she quickly grabbed the baby from this man and rushed him here. She stated that she did not want to risk staying on the premises awaiting the ambulance. When asked about the baby's mother, the aunt stated she just stood there, crying, and did not come with the child. The child was taken into treatment and the police were notified.

You Code It!

Read this scenario, and determine the correct codes to report Judah's injuries.

Step #1: Read the case carefully and completely.

Step #2: Abstract the scenario. Which main words or terms describe why the physician cared for the patient during this encounter?

Step #3: Are there any details missing or incomplete for which you would need to query the physician? [If so, ask your instructor.]

Step #4: Check for any relevant guidance, including reading all of the symbols and notations in the Tabular List and the appropriate sections of the Official Guidelines.

Step #5: Determine the correct diagnosis code or codes to explain why this encounter was medically necessary.

Step #6: Double-check your work.

Answer:

Did you determine these to be the codes?

T23.342A	Burn of third degree of multiple left fingers (nail), including thumb, initial encounter
T23.362A	Burn of third degree of back of left hand, initial encounter
T74.12xA	Child physical abuse, confirmed, initial encounter
X12.xxxA	Contact with other hot fluids, initial encounter

16.8 Complications of Care

Even though medical procedures and the standards of care are heavily researched and tested, things can go wrong. Complications can occur for any number of reasons. Before a condition can be coded as a "complication of care," the documentation must specifically identify the cause-and-effect relationship between the health care procedure, service, or treatment and the current condition that is noted as a complication.

Pain caused by medical devices and grafts previously implanted is reported with a code from categories T80–T88 (such as T82.847A Pain from cardiac prosthetic devices, implants and grafts, initial encounter), along with either code G89.18 Other acute postprocedural pain or G89.28 Other chronic postprocedural pain, as appropriate.

As you might imagine, transplanting an organ from one individual to another is a complex surgical accomplishment and saves thousands of lives. When a complication of the transplantation has been documented, a code from category T86 Complications of transplanted organs and tissue should be reported, followed by a second code to specify the complication itself.

Not all intraprocedural or postprocedural complications are reported from code categories T80–T88. They may be reported with codes from any chapter of the code set. The Alphabetic Index will guide you.

> **GUIDANCE CONNECTION**
>
> Read the ICD-10-CM Official Guidelines for Coding and Reporting, section **I. Conventions, General Coding Guidelines and Chapter Specific Guidelines,** subsection **B.16. Documentation of Complications of Care,** as well as subsection **C. Chapter-Specific Coding Guidelines,** chapter **19. Injury, poisoning, and certain other consequences of external causes,** subsection **g. Complications of care.**

EXAMPLES

J95.2	Acute pulmonary insufficiency following non-thoracic surgery
K91.840	Postprocedural hemorrhage of a digestive system organ or structure following a digestive system procedure

YOU CODE IT! CASE STUDY

Dr. Prentiss ordered 1 pint of A+ to be transfused into Sami Yariz in the postoperative area. The nurse was in a hurry and did not read carefully when she grabbed the blood and hung it on the IV pole. A few hours later, the patient began to complain of feeling very hot (temperature of 103 F) and pain in his back. At that time, one of the assistants noticed that the patient was given AB+ blood. The patient was treated immediately for ABO incompatibility. Hemolytic transfusion reaction was confirmed.

You Code It!

Review this scenario, and determine the correct ICD-10-CM code or codes to report.

Step #1: Read the case carefully and completely.

Step #2: Abstract the scenario. Which main words or terms describe why the physician cared for the patient during this encounter?

Step #3: Are there any details missing or incomplete for which you would need to query the physician? [If so, ask your instructor.]

Step #4: Check for any relevant guidance, including reading all of the symbols and notations in the Tabular List and the appropriate sections of the Official Guidelines.

Step #5: Determine the correct diagnosis code or codes to explain why this encounter was medically necessary.

Step #6: Double-check your work.

Answer:

Did you determine this to be the correct code?

T80.310A	ABO incompatibility with acute hemolytic transfusion reaction, initial encounter

Chapter Summary

People injure themselves in many different ways under many different circumstances, or others may harm someone—by accident or on purpose. Some patients may try to hurt themselves. Whether a fractured bone, a third-degree burn, a pulled muscle, or an adverse effect of a medication, when something like this happens, those of us working in health care help them.

As professional coding specialists, you must remember that, in these situations, you not only need to determine the code or codes to explain *why* the patient needs health care services, you also must explain how the patient got hurt and where the injury occurred.

> **CODING BITES**
>
> External cause codes explain
>
> - *Cause of the injury,* such as a car accident or a fall off a ladder.
> - *Place of the occurrence,* such as the park or the kitchen.
> - *Activity during the occurrence,* such as playing basketball or gardening.
> - *Patient's status,* such as paid employment, on-duty military, or leisure activity.

You Interpret It! Answers

1. Attempted suicide, **2.** Accidental poisoning, **3.** Adverse effect, **4.** Assault

CHAPTER 16 REVIEW
Coding Injury, Poisoning, and External Causes

Enhance your learning by completing these exercises and more at connect.mheducation.com!

Let's Check It! Terminology

Match each key term to the appropriate definition.

Part I

1. **LO 16.2** Layers of skin traumatically torn away from the body.
2. **LO 16.5** Redness of the epidermis (skin).
3. **LO 16.5** A burn caused by a chemical; chemical destruction of the skin.
4. **LO 16.5** Destruction of all layers of the skin, with possible involvement of the subcutaneous fat, muscle, and bone.
5. **LO 16.5** Injury by heat or fire.
6. **LO 16.5** The level of seriousness.
7. **LO 16.5** Blisters on the skin; involvement of the epidermis and the dermis layers.
8. **LO 16.5** A general division of the whole body portioned out to each represent 9%; used for estimating the extent of a burn.
9. **LO 16.2** Damage to the epidermal and dermal layers of the skin made by a sharp object.
10. **LO 16.5** The location on or in the human body; the anatomical part of the body.

A. Avulsion
B. Burn
C. Corrosion
D. First-Degree Burn
E. Laceration
F. Rule of Nines
G. Second-Degree Burn
H. Severity
I. Site
J. Third-Degree Burn

Part II

1. **LO 16.6** This term is used in different manners: (a) extreme use of a drug or chemical; (b) violent and/or inappropriate treatment of another person.
2. **LO 16.5** The percentage of the body that has been affected by the burn or corrosion.
3. **LO 16.2** A fractured bone that did not heal correctly; healing of bone that was not in proper position or alignment.
4. **LO 16.1** The displacement of a limb, bone, or organ from its customary position.
5. **LO 16.2** Broken cartilage or bone.
6. **LO 16.2** Pain in a muscle.
7. **LO 16.3** A series of reference books identifying all aspects of prescription and over-the-counter medications, as well as herbal remedies.
8. **LO 16.2** A fractured bone that did not heal back together; no mending or joining together of the broken segments.

A. Abuse
B. Dislocation
C. Extent
D. Fracture
E. Malunion
F. Myalgia
G. Nonunion
H. *Physicians' Desk Reference* (PDR)

Let's Check It! Concepts

Choose the most appropriate answer for each of the following questions.

1. **LO 16.1** Karen Graysen, a 31-year-old female, lives in a mobile home. This morning she was working in her garden and was injured. What is the correct external cause code for the place of occurrence?
   a. Y92.015   b. Y92.046   c. Y92.027   d. Y92.096

2. **LO 16.2** _____ fracture identifies the breaking of the bone into several pieces.
   a. Burst   b. Depressed   c. Comminuted   d. Fatigue

3. **LO 16.2** A bruise or black and blue mark is known as a(n)
   a. contusion.   b. avulsion.   c. puncture.   d. bite.

4. **LO 16.2** How would you code an avulsion of the left eye, initial encounter?
   a. S05.02XA   b. S05.72XA   c. S05.52XA   d. S05.92XA

5. **LO 16.3** Drugs and chemicals are listed in the *Table of Drugs and Chemicals* in all of these manners except
   a. the brand name.
   b. the chemical name.
   c. the drug category.
   d. the size of the dose.

6. **LO 16.3** The *Table of Drugs and Chemicals* does not include a specific listing for
   a. adhesives.
   b. lettuce opium.
   c. marsh gas.
   d. vodka.

7. **LO 16.4** The columns in the ICD-10-CM *Table of Drugs and Chemicals* include
   a. Intentional Self-Harm.
   b. Malignant.
   c. Toxin.
   d. Ca in situ.

8. **LO 16.5** An example of a late effect of a burn is
   a. malunion.
   b. contracture.
   c. infection.
   d. epidermal loss.

9. **LO 16.5** A third-degree burn of the chin, subsequent encounter, would be coded
   a. T20.33XD
   b. S01.411A
   c. S00.83XD
   d. T20.33XS

10. **LO 16.6** Jennie James, a 28-year-old female, is pregnant and in her third trimester. Jennie presents today with the complaint that her right forearm hurts. Upon examination, bruises are noted. When asked how she got the bruises, Jennie stated that her husband came home upset and twisted her arm because dinner was not ready. What is the correct code for the physical abuse complicating the pregnancy?

   a. O9A.311   b. O9A.312   c. O9A.313   d. O9A.319

Let's Check It! Guidelines
Part I
Refer to the Official Guidelines and fill in the blanks according to the Chapter 19, Injury, poisoning, and certain other consequences of external causes, Chapter-Specific Coding Guidelines.

aftercare	highest	active	local
extent	Superficial	separate	first
primary	acute	7th	T31
degree	minor	external	severity
Z	initial	late	subsequent
	T31	"S"	

1. Most categories in chapter 19 have a _____ character requirement for each applicable code.
2. The aftercare _____ codes should not be used for _____ for conditions such as injuries or poisonings, where 7th characters are provided to identify _____ care.
3. _____ injuries such as abrasions or contusions are not coded when associated with more severe injuries of the same site.
4. When a primary injury results in _____ damage to peripheral nerves or blood vessels, the _____ injury is sequenced _____ with additional code(s) for injuries to nerves and spinal cord (such as category S04), and/or injury to blood vessels (such as category S15).
5. Traumatic fractures are coded using the appropriate 7th character for _____ encounter (A, B, C) for each encounter where the patient is receiving _____ treatment for the fracture.
6. Multiple fractures are sequenced in accordance with the _____ of the fracture.
7. When the reason for the admission or encounter is for treatment of _____ multiple burns, sequence first the code that reflects the burn of the _____ degree.
8. Classify burns of the same _____ site (three-character category level, T20-T28) but of different _____ to the subcategory identifying the highest degree recorded in the diagnosis.
9. Non-healing burns are coded as _____ burns.
10. When coding burns, assign _____ codes for each burn site.
11. Assign codes from category _____, Burns classified according to extent of body surface involved, or _____, Corrosions classified according to _____ of body surface involved, when the site of the burn is not specified or when there is a need for additional data.
12. Encounters for the treatment of the _____ effects of burns or corrosions (i.e., scars or joint contractures) should be coded with a burn or corrosion code with the 7th character _____ for sequela.

Part II
Refer to the Official Guidelines and fill in the blanks according to the Chapter 19, Injury, poisoning, and certain other consequences of external causes, Chapter-Specific Coding Guidelines.

external	adverse	many	assault	properly	sequelae
improper	toxic	current	Underdosing	Z04.71	complication
confirmed	correctly	individually	suspected	source	T36-T50

1. When appropriate, both a code for a _____ burn or corrosion with 7th character "A" or "D" and a burn or corrosion code with 7th character "S" may be assigned on the same record (when both a current burn and _____ of an old burn exist).
2. An _____ cause code should be used with burns and corrosions to identify the _____ and intent of the burn, as well as the place where it occurred.
3. Use as _____ codes as necessary to describe completely all drugs, medicinal or biological substances.
4. If two or more drugs, medicinal or biological substances are reported, code each _____ unless a combination code is listed in the Table of Drugs and Chemicals.
5. When coding an _____ effect of a drug that has been _____ prescribed and _____ administered, assign the appropriate code for the nature of the adverse effect followed by the appropriate code for the adverse effect of the drug (T36-T50).
6. When coding a poisoning or reaction to the _____ use of a medication (e.g., overdose, wrong substance given or taken in error, wrong route of administration), first assign the appropriate code from categories _____.
7. _____ refers to taking less of a medication than is prescribed by a provider or a manufacturer's instruction.
8. When a harmful substance is ingested or comes in contact with a person, this is classified as a _____ effect.
9. For cases of _____ abuse or neglect an external cause code from the _____ section (X92-Y09) should be added to identify the cause of any physical injuries.
10. If a _____ case of abuse, neglect, or mistreatment is ruled out during an encounter code _____, Encounter for examination and observation following alleged physical adult abuse, ruled out, or code Z04.72, Encounter for examination and observation following alleged child physical abuse, ruled out, should be used, not a code from T76.
11. Intraoperative and postprocedural _____ codes are found within the body system chapters with codes specific to the organs and structures of that body system.

Part III

Refer to the Official Guidelines and fill in the blanks according to the Chapter 20, External Causes of Morbidity, Chapter-Specific Coding Guidelines.

A00.0-T88.9	never	Y92	encounter
secondary	assault	data	Y38.9
Y93	"S"	full	initial
completely	Y99	once	status

1. External cause codes are intended to provide _____ for injury research and evaluation of injury prevention strategies.
2. An external cause code may be used with any code in the range of _____, Z00-Z99, classification that is a health condition due to an external cause.
3. Assign the external cause code, with the appropriate 7th character (initial encounter, subsequent encounter or sequela) for each _____ for which the injury or condition is being treated.
4. Use the _____ range of external cause codes to _____ describe the cause, the intent, the place of occurrence, and if applicable, the activity of the patient at the time of the event, and the patient's status, for all injuries, and other health conditions due to an external cause.
5. An external cause code can _____ be a principal (first-listed) diagnosis.
6. Codes from category _____, Place of occurrence of the external cause, are secondary codes for use after other external cause codes to identify the location of the patient at the time of injury or other condition.
7. Generally, a place of occurrence code is assigned only _____, at the _____ encounter for treatment.
8. Assign a code from category _____, Activity code, to describe the activity of the patient at the time the injury or other health condition occurred.

9. Adult and child abuse, neglect, and maltreatment are classified as _____.
10. Sequela are reported using the external cause code with the 7th character _____ for sequela.
11. Assign code _____, Terrorism, _____ effects, for conditions occurring subsequent to the terrorist event.
12. Assign a code from category _____, External cause status, to indicate the work _____ of the person at the time the event occurred.

Let's Check It! Rules and Regulations

Please answer the following questions from the knowledge you have gained after reading this chapter.

1. LO 16.2 Explain the difference between a traumatic fracture and a pathologic fracture. Why is it important to know the difference?
2. LO 16.5 What does the acronym *S/S.E.E.* mean in relation to a burn? What details does it help you remember?
3. LO 16.5 How do you identify the severity of burns? Include the description of each stage.
4. LO 16.6 Turn to the Official Guidelines for Chapter 19. Injury, poisoning, and certain other consequences of external causes—I.C.19.f. Discuss adult and child abuse, neglect, and other maltreatment as outlined in the Chapter 19 guidelines; include reference to *Abuse in a pregnant patient*.
5. LO 16.4 Explain patient noncompliance and the different codes that represent noncompliance.

YOU CODE IT! Basics

First, identify the condition in the following diagnoses; then code the diagnosis.

Example: Abrasion of scalp, initial encounter:

a. main term: <u>Abrasion</u>   b. diagnosis: <u>S00.01XA</u>

1. Underdosing of succinimides, initial encounter:
   a. main term: _____   b. diagnosis: _____
2. External constriction of left eyelid, initial encounter:
   a. main term: _____   b. diagnosis: _____
3. Laceration without foreign body of nose, initial encounter
   a. main term: _____   b. diagnosis: _____
4. Open bite of left cheek, subsequent encounter:
   a. main term: _____   b. diagnosis: _____
5. Corrosion of trachea, sequela:
   a. main term: _____   b. diagnosis: _____
6. Toxic effect of ethanol, assault, subsequent encounter:
   a. main term: _____   b. diagnosis: _____
7. Puncture wound with foreign body of scalp, initial encounter:
   a. main term: _____   b. diagnosis: _____
8. Second degree burn of the right axilla, initial encounter:
   a. main term: _____   b. diagnosis: _____
9. Displaced shaft fracture of the left clavicle (traumatic), subsequent encounter for fracture with malunion:
   a. main term: _____   b. diagnosis: _____
10. Concussion with loss of consciousness of 35 minutes, initial encounter:
    a. main term: _____   b. diagnosis: _____
11. Contusion of left ear, subsequent encounter:
    a. main term: _____   b. diagnosis: _____
12. Crushing injury of larynx:
    a. main term: _____   b. diagnosis: _____
13. Corrosion of third degree of left shoulder, initial encounter:
    a. main term: _____   b. diagnosis: _____
14. Adverse effect of antimycobacterial drugs, combination:
    a. main term: _____   b. diagnosis: _____
15. Pathological fracture of right tibia due to neoplastic disease, delayed healing:
    a. main term: _____   b. diagnosis: _____

YOU CODE IT! Practice

Using the techniques described in this chapter, carefully read through the case studies and determine the most accurate ICD-10-CM code(s) and external cause code(s), if appropriate, for each case study.

1. Richard Pittmon, a 22-year-old male, was playing baseball with some friends at the local park and as he was crossing home plate, he was struck on his right leg by the baseball. The ED physician, Dr. Bonneville, took a history of the injury and completed an examination and the appropriate tests. Richard is diagnosed with an open shaft fracture type I, oblique, of the tibia.

2. Jamie McIntyre, a 43-year-old female, presents today with a painful blister on her right hand. Jamie is trying to get in shape and has begun to play handball. Dr. Brown completes an examination and diagnoses Jamie with a superficial blister on the palm of her hand between the third and fourth metacarpals.

3. Billy Ugro, a 7-year-old male, was brought in by his mother. Billy was playing this afternoon in his backyard on the sliding board and fell, scraping his left cheek. Dr. Tucker, his pediatrician, examines the area and cleans and dresses the wound. Billy is diagnosed with a second-degree abrasion.

4. Janie Walters, a 27-year-old female, presents today with burns on her left hand. Over the weekend, Janie was at a campout and while toasting marshmallows over a bonfire, got too close to the flame, burning her left fingers. Dr. Platzs thoroughly examines Janie's hand and fingers, noting redness with blisters on the second, third, and fourth phalanges. Janie is diagnosed with second-degree burns of the fingers, multiple sites.

5. Jerry Ard, a 31-year-old male, presents today with a cut to his thigh. Jerry was dressing a piece of venison when the knife slipped and cut his left thigh accidentally. Dr. Phillips examines the incised wound and cleans the area, then closes with sutures. Jerry is diagnosed with a laceration to the thigh.

6. Grace Fuller, a 16-year-old female, was brought into the ED by her parents. They found Grace extremely drowsy. Dr. Rowell, the ED physician, notes slow heart rate and breathing. Dr. Rowell also notes constricted pupils. Grace's parents state she has been diagnosed with bipolar depression and has been taking cyclazocine. Grace is drowsy; however, she will not respond to Dr. Rowell. Dr. Rowell completes a thorough examination with the appropriate laboratory tests, which confirm an overdose of cyclazocine. Grace is admitted to Weston Hospital for a full workup.

7. Patricia Neil, a 34-year-old female, presents today with a painful left foot. Patricia accidentally hit her foot on a desk this morning and is concerned she might have broken it. Dr. Dickerson examines Patricia's foot and notes swelling and discoloration. Dr. Dickerson orders an x-ray, which confirms no fractures. Patricia is diagnosed with a contusion, bruise harm score 1.

8. Michael George, a 28-year-old male, presents today with a wound to his lower right leg. Michael stated this morning at home he accidentally stepped on his cat's tail and the cat bit him. The cat has been vaccinated for rabies. Dr. Coleman examines, cleans, and dresses the area and prescribes a round of antibiotics as a precaution.

9. Kim Horton, a 4-year-old female, is brought in today by her father. Kim was playing with her father's pocket change and swallowed a nickel. Dr. Grebner, her pediatrician, notes labored breathing and orders an x-ray, which shows the nickel is lodged in the oropharynx. Dr. Grebner is able to remove the nickel without difficulty.

10. Dean Williams, a 5-year-old male, is brought into the ED by ambulance. Dean's grandmother stated he was playing in the yard where she has ornamental plants. One plant has mezereon berries and the birds were eating them, so Dean ate one too. Dean began to have a choking sensation. Dr. Adams completes a thorough examination and the laboratory results confirmed the diagnosis of accidental poisoning.

11. Annie Froster, an 8-year-old female, was brought in by her mother to see her pediatrician, Dr. Benton. Annie has been having difficulty swallowing. After an examination and the appropriate tests, Dr. Lukenson diagnoses Annie with a lye stricture of the esophagus. Annie admitted that her stepfather forced her to drink lye, confirmed by local police.

12. Carolina Tanner, an 18-year-old female, came into the emergency department with a wrist sprain where a baseball had hit her. She is on her school baseball team and was at a practice game being played on the school

baseball field and got hit by the ball. She was in obvious pain, and the wrist was swollen and too painful upon attempts to flex. After Dr. Rodgers reviewed the x-ray Carolina is diagnosed with a Salter-Harris, type II fracture of the distal radius, left.

13. Tricia Thornwell, a 68-year-old female, was going walking when she fell down the icy front steps of her house; now she can't bear weight on her right leg. She is brought into the ER by ambulance. After the ER physician completed a thorough exam and reviewed the x-ray, he diagnosed her with a femoral neck base fracture, nondisplaced.

14. Paula Caine, a 41-year-old female, was deep-frying fish and the kettle fell over and burned her right thigh. Paula was rushed to the ER by her husband, where the ER physician, Dr. Dinkins, diagnosed her with a second degree burn on her right thigh. Dr. Dinkins dressed the wounds and sent her to the burn unit.

15. Helen Carrizo, an 18-year-old female, presents to the ED with a painful left ankle. Helen is accompanied by her mother. Helen had been rollerblading and tripped, falling on the sidewalk. Helen is unable to flex her ankle, which has begun to swell. Dr. Webber gathered a brief history of the incident that caused the injury, as well as any history relating to her legs and feet. He then performed a limited examination of her left leg, ankle, and foot. The imaging confirmed a sprained calcaneofibular ligament and a sprained anterior tibiofibular ligament.

YOU CODE IT! Application

The following exercises provide practice in abstracting physicians' notes and learning to work with documentation from our health care facility, Prader, Bracker, & Associates. These case studies are modeled on real patient encounters. Using the techniques described in this chapter, carefully read through the case studies and determine the most accurate ICD-10-CM code(s) and external cause code(s), if appropriate, for each case study.

WESTON HOSPITAL

629 Healthcare Way • SOMEWHERE, FL 32811 • 407-555-6541

PATIENT: TRUMAN, HERBERT

ACCOUNT/EHR #: TRUMHE001

DATE: 07/16/18

Attending Physician: Oscar R. Prader, MD

S: Pt is a 47-year-old male brought in by ambulance accompanied by his wife. Wife states he has been confused, dizzy, and vomiting all morning.

O: Ht. 5′11″, Wt. 187 lb., R 16. During the physical examination, the patient has a dramatic drop in vital sign measurements and suffers cardiac arrest. The crash team takes over and patient is successfully resuscitated. Blood work reveals overdose of digoxin. After Pt is stabilized, he states he was rushing to get to work this morning and couldn't remember if he had taken his medication, so he took it again.

A: Cardiac arrest due to overdose of digoxin, accidental

P: Admit for stabilization

   Oxygenation

   Hydration IV fluids

   Monitor electrolyte balance

ORP/pw   D: 07/16/18 09:50:16   T: 07/17/18 12:55:01

Determine the most accurate ICD-10-CM code(s).

PRADER, BRACKER, & ASSOCIATES

A Complete Health Care Facility

159 Healthcare Way • SOMEWHERE, FL 32811 • 407-555-6789

PATIENT: JANKOWSKI, HILDA

ACCOUNT/EHR #: JANKHI001

DATE: 07/16/18

Attending Physician: Renee O. Bracker, MD

S: Patient, a 9-year-old female, was brought in by her mother. She had just returned from a school hiking trip when her parents noticed a problem with her right shoulder. The patient states that her shoulder started bothering her early Sunday morning, but by the time she arrived home Sunday evening, it was much worse. Her mother called a nurse hotline and the nurse suggested an anti-inflammatory, so the parents gave her 250 mg of Tylenol.

The patient is right-handed and noticed, upon waking this morning, that she could not move her arm without a great deal of pain and that her hand was tingling, particularly her fingers. She denies any fall or accident during the trip.

O: Exam revealed some muscle wasting, observed around the right scapula. Movements of the elbow and wrist were both within normal range. However, abduction of her right arm was difficult. She denies being able to extend the arm without support, and she required movement of her entire upper arm to accomplish abduction of this arm.

Additional specific history about activities during the trip revealed that throughout the weekend, she carried a heavy backpack. The left strap had broken, so the entire weight was supported by her right shoulder and arm, creating a traction-countertraction force centered on the axilla and neck area, which produced a stretching force. She stated that each day she carried this on her right shoulder for as long as 10 or 12 hours.

A: Dislocation of the inferior acromioclavicular joint

P: Sling

   Rest and Ice packs

   Rx: Nonsteroidal anti-inflammatory

ROB/pw   D: 07/16/18 09:50:16   T: 07/17/18 12:55:01

Determine the most accurate ICD-10-CM code(s).

PRADER, BRACKER, & ASSOCIATES

A Complete Health Care Facility

159 Healthcare Way • SOMEWHERE, FL 32811 • 407-555-6789

PATIENT: ZIMMER, CYRUS

ACCOUNT/EHR #: ZIMMCY001

DATE: 09/16/18

Attending Physician: Oscar R. Prader, MD

S: This new Pt is a 56-year-old male who was involved in an accident when the motorcycle he was driving was struck by a car on a street near his house. Cyrus admits to riding motorcycles for recreation. He is complaining about some neck pain. He has tingling into his hand and feet. He states that his left arm hurts when he tries to pull it overhead. PMH is remarkable for kidney trouble. Past bronchoscopy, laparoscopy, and kidney stone surgery, otherwise noncontributory as per the medical history form completed by the patient and reviewed this encounter.

O: Ht. 5′9″, Wt. 181 lb., R 18. On exam, the left shoulder demonstrates full passive motion. He has normal strength testing. He has no deformity. He has some tenderness over the trapezial area. The reflexes are brisk and symmetric. X-rays of his chest 2 views and C spine AP/LAT are relatively benign, as are complete x-rays of the shoulder.

A: Anterior displaced type II dens fracture of the second cervical vertebra, and an anterior dislocation of the proximal end of the left humerus.

P: 1. Rx Naprosyn

2. Referral to PT

3. Referral to orthopedist

ORP/mg   D: 9/16/18 09:50:16   T: 9/18/18 12:55:01

Determine the most accurate ICD-10-CM code(s).

PRADER, BRACKER, & ASSOCIATES

A Complete Health Care Facility

159 Healthcare Way • SOMEWHERE, FL 32811 • 407-555-6789

PATIENT: KIM, LINDA

ACCOUNT/EHR #: KIMLI001

DATE: 09/16/18

Attending Physician: Oscar R. Prader, MD

S: This new Pt is a 29-year-old female who presents with splatter burns on the back of her right hand and her right cheek. She stated that she was deep-frying shrimp for a dinner party at her home in the kitchen and the grease splattered unexpectedly.

O: Ht. 5′6″, Wt. 152 lb., R 20. Skin is red and blistered on both sites. There is some epidermal loss. Area was cleansed with antiseptic, and ointment was applied before a clean gauze bandage was put on the hand. The facial area was also cleansed and bandaged.

A: Second-degree burns to back of hand and face.

P: 1. Rx: Aspirin for pain, prn

2. Return in 1 week for dressing change.

ORP/pw   D: 9/16/18 09:50:16   T: 9/18/18 12:55:01

Determine the most accurate ICD-10-CM code(s).

WESTON HOSPITAL

629 Healthcare Way • SOMEWHERE, FL 32811 • 407-555-6541

PATIENT: O'MALLEY, REGINA

ACCOUNT/EHR #: OMALRE001

DATE: 09/16/18

Attending Physician: Renee O. Bracker, MD

S: Pt is a 6-year-old female seen in our emergency facility. She was brought in by ambulance, accompanied by her mother. Mother states that they were baking cookies when the phone rang; she turned to answered it and when she returned, the child was unconscious on the kitchen (apartment) floor, a bottle of wintergreen oil found empty next to the patient.

O: Pt is listless and unresponsive. Respiration labored, BP 80/65, P slow and erratic. Skin is pale and moist. Stomach pumped. Pt responding to treatment.

A: Poisoning by overdose of wintergreen oil, accidental

P: Admit to pediatric unit.

ROB/pw   D: 9/16/18 09:50:16   T: 9/18/18 12:55:01

Determine the most accurate ICD-10-CM code(s).

17 Coding Genitourinary, Gynecology, Obstetrics, Congenital, and Pediatrics Conditions

Key Terms

Abortion
Anemic
Anomaly
Benign Prostatic Hyperplasia (BPH)
Bladder Cancer
Chronic Kidney Disease (CKD)
Clinically Significant
Congenital
Deformity
Genetic Abnormality
Gestation
Glomerular Filtration Rate (GFR)
Gynecologist (GYN)
Low Birth Weight (LBW)
Malformation
Morbidity
Mortality
Obstetrics (OB)
Perinatal
Prematurity
Prenatal
Prostatitis
Puerperium
Urea
Urinary System
Urinary Tract Infection (UTI)

Learning Outcomes

After completing this chapter, the student should be able to:

LO 17.1 Identify the details required to accurately report renal and urologic malfunctions.
LO 17.2 Explain the conditions affecting the male genital system.
LO 17.3 Abstract the components for reporting sexually transmitted diseases accurately.
LO 17.4 Enumerate the reasons for gynecologic care.
LO 17.5 Apply the guidelines for coding routine obstetrics care.
LO 17.6 Determine the correct codes for reporting complications of pregnancy.
LO 17.7 Utilize the official guidelines for well-baby encounters and congenital anomalies.

STOP! Remember, you need to follow along in your ICD-10-CM code book for an optimal learning experience.

17.1 Renal and Urologic Malfunctions

Components of the Urinary System

The components of the **urinary system** (see Figure 17-1) are the same in both men and women. This organ system is responsible for removing waste products (known as **urea**) that are left behind by protein (food), excessive water, disproportionate amounts of electrolytes, and other nitrogenous compounds from the blood and the body. A failure to eliminate these wastes from the body in a timely fashion may actually result in the body poisoning itself. The organ components of the urinary system include

- *Kidney* (right and left), each leading to a
- *Ureter* (right and left), each leading to the
- *Urinary bladder,* which then passes urine through the
- *Urethra,* to travel outside the body.

Urinary System
The organ system responsible for removing waste products that are left behind in the blood and the body.

Urea
A compound that is excreted in urine.

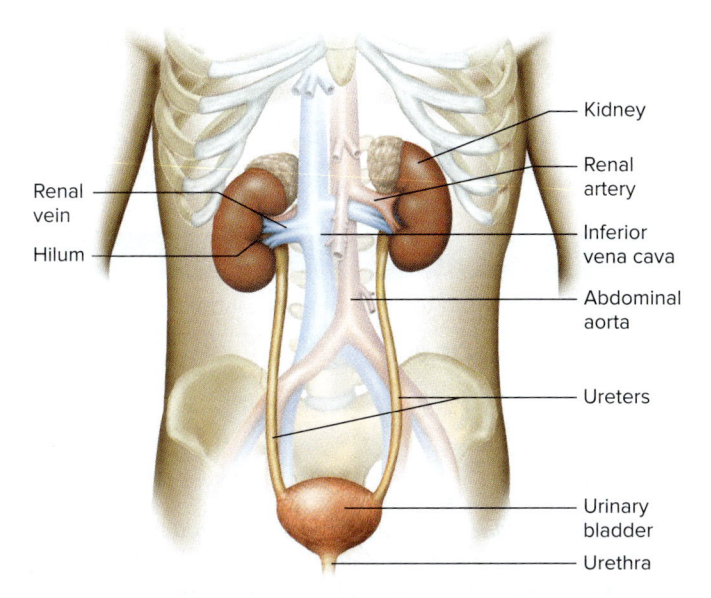

FIGURE 17-1 An illustration identifying the anatomical sites of the urinary system   David Shier et al., *Hole's human anatomy & physiology*, 12/e. ©2010 McGraw-Hill Education. Figure 20.1, p. 776. Used with permission.

As with many body systems, diseases and illnesses, congenital anomalies, medications, and pathogens can cause havoc within the urinary system. These problems may require straightforward treatments, such as using antibiotics for a **urinary tract infection (UTI)**, or more complex treatments, such as dialysis or transplantation.

Renal malfunction affects every organ and body system, so physical examination may alert the physician to a concern in this area. The skin's color and texture can change, periorbital edema can modify vision, or the patient may develop difficulty with muscle function, including gait and posture. Mental status can also be influenced. Electrolyte imbalance can alter hypertension levels, while metabolic acidosis can result in hyperventilation.

Urinary Tract Infection (UTI)
Inflammation of any part of the urinary tract: kidney, ureter, bladder, or urethra.

Diagnostic Tools

A patient history of hypertension, diabetes mellitus, and/or bladder infections may also be indicative of urinary system conditions. Genetic predispositions can be identified with family histories that include glomerulonephritis or polycystic kidney disease. Nephrotoxicity can be caused by the patient's abuse of antibiotics or analgesics.

Blood tests can measure the levels of uric acid, creatinine, and blood urea nitrogen (BUN), providing insight into kidney function. Of course, urinalysis can add data about pH as well as clarity, color, and odor of the specimen. Measurement of urine output may require 24-hour specimen collection. Checking levels of antidiuretic hormone (ADH), produced by the pituitary gland, and/or levels of aldosterone, a hormone produced by the adrenal cortex, may also indicate kidney concerns.

Kidney-ureter-bladder (KUB) radiography can measure the size, shape, and position of these organs, as well as identify any possible areas of calcification.

Ultrasonography, fluoroscopy, computerized tomography (CT) scans, and/or magnetic resonance imaging (MRI) of the urinary system may also be appropriate to support the confirmation of a diagnosis.

An intravenous pyelogram (IVP) records a series of x-ray images, taken rapidly, as contrast material injected intravenously passes through the urinary tract. A retrograde pyelogram also uses contrast material; however, this iodine-based fluid is injected through the ureters to investigate a suspicion of an obstruction, such as kidney stones (calculi).

LET'S CODE IT! SCENARIO

Nila Taglia, a 33-year-old female, just returned from her honeymoon in the islands. She is feeling a burning sensation and some pain on urination, so she came to see Dr. Slater. After exam and urinalysis, Nila was diagnosed with *acute cystitis due to* E. coli.

Let's Code It!

Dr. Slater's notes state that Nila has *acute cystitis.* When you turn to the Alphabetic Index, you see

> Cystitis (exudative) (hemorrhagic) (septic) (suppurative) N30.90
>   acute N30.00

When you turn to the Tabular List, you confirm

> ✓4 **N30**   Cystitis

Take a second to read the **Use additional code** and **EXCLUDES1** notations carefully. Do you know what the infectious agent is so you can code it? Yes, you do. Dr. Slater included this detail *(E. coli)* in his notes. And Nila does not have prostatocystitis. Great! But first, we must determine the code for the cystitis. Did you find

> ✓5 **N30.0**   Acute cystitis

There is an **EXCLUDES1** notation listing two diagnoses. Take a minute to review them and determine whether either one applies to Nila's condition. No, neither of them does, so continue down and review all of the fifth-character choices. Which matches Dr. Slater's notes?

> **N30.00**   Acute cystitis without hematuria

Wait, you are not done yet. You still need to report the infectious agent. The **Use additional code** notation referred you to code range B95–B97. Let's turn to B95 in the Tabular List. Review all of the code descriptions in this subsection. Did you find

> **B96.2**   Escherichia coli [E. coli] as the cause of diseases classified elsewhere

That's good. However, you need more information to determine the accurate fifth character. Did you realize there was more than one type of *E. coli*? Hmm. Even though you have documentation that the infectious agent is *E. coli,* it is not enough information. For this exercise, you will need to report the unspecified version. Once you get on the job, you will need to double-check the pathology report to be more specific.

> **N30.00**   Acute cystitis without hematuria
> **B96.20**   Unspecified Escherichia coli [E. coli] as the cause of diseases classified elsewhere

---

Glomerular Filtration Rate (GFR)
The measurement of kidney function; used to determine the stage of kidney disease. GFR is calculated by the physician using the results of a creatinine test in a formula with the patient's gender, age, race, and other factors; normal GFR is 90 and above.

Chronic Kidney Disease (CKD)
Ongoing malfunction of one or both kidneys.

Chronic Kidney Disease

The kidneys are so important to the extraction of waste within the body. Therefore, when one or both malfunction, toxicity can form and the patient can become very ill. Chronic kidney disease (CKD) can be caused by disease, trauma, or an adverse reaction to medication.

In the section about the kidneys, you learned that glomerular filtration is an important process in removing wastes (creatinine) from the blood as it flows through the kidneys. The **glomerular filtration rate (GFR)** is measured by blood tests to check the creatinine level. When kidney function is not at an optimum level, creatinine continues to amass in the blood because it is not being removed as necessary. The National Kidney Foundation identifies a normal GFR range as 90–120 mL/min. GFR decreases with age, so geriatric patients are likely to have lower levels. Actually, a 90-year-old patient may have kidney function at 50% solely due to age-related changes.

Monthly tests would be performed to identify a chronic condition. **Chronic kidney disease (CKD)** may be indicated by the following lab results:

- *Normal GFR:* Kidney damage may exist even with a normal GFR—CKD stage 1, code N18.1
- *GFR of 60–89:* CKD stage 2 (mild renal disease), code N18.2
- *GFR of 30–59:* CKD stage 3 (moderate renal disease), code N18.3
- *GFR of 15–29:* CKD stage 4 (severe renal disease), code N18.4
- *GFR below 15:* CKD stage 5, code N18.5
- *End-stage renal disease (ESRD):* CKD stage 5 requiring ongoing dialysis or transplantation, code N18.6

> ### YOU CODE IT! CASE STUDY
>
> Shane Moyet, a 41-year-old male, was tested as part of his annual physical. He came in today with his wife to get his test results. Dr. Contreras diagnosed him with moderate chronic kidney disease. She sat and discussed treatment options with Shane and his wife.
>
> #### You Code It!
>
> Go through the steps of coding, and determine the code or codes that should be reported for this encounter between Dr. Contreras and Shane Moyet.
>
> Step #1: Read the case carefully and completely.
>
> Step #2: Abstract the scenario. Which key words or terms describe why the physician cared for the patient during this encounter?
>
> Step #3: Are there any details missing or incomplete for which you would need to query the physician? [If so, ask your instructor.]
>
> Step #4: Check for any relevant guidance, including reading all of the symbols and notations in the Tabular List and the appropriate sections of the Official Guidelines.
>
> Step #5: Determine the correct diagnosis code or codes to explain why this encounter was medically necessary.
>
> Step #6: Double-check your work.
>
> **Answer:**
>
> Did you determine this to be the correct code?
>
> N18.3   Chronic kidney disease, stage 3 (moderate)

CKD with Other Conditions

CKD can be caused by hypertension, diabetic neuropathy (diabetes mellitus), untreated obstruction such as renal calculi (kidney stones), or a congenital anomaly such as polycystic kidneys. CKD progresses slowly; therefore, early diagnosis and treatment provide the best prognosis.

Hypertensive Chronic Kidney Disease

When a patient is documented to have both hypertension and CKD, you are to assume that there is a cause-and-effect relationship between the two conditions. The physician does not have to specifically state that one caused the other in the documentation. Report this with a code from category I12 Hypertensive chronic kidney disease.

Diabetes with Renal Manifestations

A patient who has been diagnosed with diabetes may develop problems with his or her kidneys, such as chronic kidney disease, diabetic nephropathy, or Kimmelstiel-Wilson syndrome. When this is documented, regardless of the specific reason for the encounter, you will report a code from one of the following code categories, depending upon the type of diabetes mellitus:

- E08.2- Diabetes mellitus due to underlying condition with kidney complications
- E09.2- Drug or chemical induced diabetes mellitus with kidney complications
- E10.2- Type 1 diabetes mellitus with kidney complications
- E11.2- Type 2 diabetes mellitus with kidney complications
- E13.2- Other specified diabetes mellitus with kidney complications

In all of these code categories, if the patient's kidney complication is CKD, you will need to report an additional code to identify the stage of the disease. You will see the *Use additional code* notation.

LET'S CODE IT! SCENARIO

Sergio Prisma, a 21-year-old male, was diagnosed with type 1 diabetes mellitus when he was 7 years old. He has been lax about testing his glucose and giving himself his insulin shots because he has been so busy with his courses and activities at Hillgraw University. After a complete HPI and exam, Dr. Allenson performed a glucose test and a urinalysis. The results showed the early signs of type 1 diabetic nephrosis.

Let's Code It!

Dr. Allenson's notes state that Sergio has *type 1 diabetic nephrosis*. When you turn to the Alphabetic Index, you see

Diabetes, diabetic (mellitus) (sugar) E11.9

The word *nephrosis* is not there, but "kidney complications" is shown, suggesting code E11.29. Let's take a look in the Tabular List:

☑4 **E11** Type 2 diabetes mellitus

Oh, wait a minute. This code category is for type 2 diabetes. Dr. Allenson's notes document that Sergio has type 1 diabetes. Turn the pages and review this whole section to see if you can determine a more accurate code category. Did you find this code category:

☑4 **E10** Type 1 diabetes mellitus

There is an INCLUDES note as well as an EXCLUDES1 notation listing several diagnoses. Take a minute to review them and determine whether any apply to Sergio's condition. No, none of them do, so continue down and review all of the fourth-character choices. Which matches Dr. Allenson's notes?

E10.2 Type 1 diabetes mellitus with kidney complications

You remember that *nephrosis* is an abnormal condition of the kidney. Review the three potential fifth-character options. Which do you believe most accurately reports Sergio's condition?

E10.21 Type 1 diabetes mellitus with diabetic nephropathy

Nephropathy (*nephro* = kidney + *-pathy* = disease) means the same as *nephrosis*, so you have found the correct code. Good job!

Anemic
Any of various conditions marked by deficiency in red blood cells or hemoglobin.

Anemia in CKD

The malfunction of the kidneys as they attempt to filter out the impurities in the body may trigger an **anemic** condition in the body. This condition can leave the patient weak, fatigued, and potentially short of breath because there is less oxygen carried through the bloodstream to the cells. When the patient is documented with these two conditions, you will need to

- *Code first* the underlying chronic kidney disease (CKD) (N18.-).
- Follow this with code D63.1 Anemia in chronic kidney disease.

Dialysis

There are two types of dialysis that may be used to treat a patient with renal malfunction: peritoneal dialysis and hemodialysis.

Peritoneal dialysis infuses a dialysate solution into the peritoneal cavity. Subsequently, the solution passes through the peritoneal membrane (which lines the abdominal cavity), collecting waste. The solution is then drained and thereby removes the waste.

Hemodialysis draws blood out of the body via an intravenous tube and passes the blood through a machine that removes waste products and returns clean blood to the body via a second intravenous connection.

When the patient is preparing for the dialysis treatments, you will need to know which type of dialysis the patient will be receiving:

Z49.01 Encounter for fitting and adjustment of extracorporeal dialysis catheter

or

Z49.02 Encounter for fitting and adjustment of peritoneal dialysis catheter

Plus, note the reminder directly beneath the code category:

Code also associated end stage renal disease (N18.6)

Within the first few weeks after beginning the series of dialysis treatments, the physician will want to have the patient come in for an efficiency or adequacy test. The purpose of the test is to measure the exchanges to ensure that the treatments are removing enough urea. The test results enable the health care professionals to adjust the dose, or amount, of the dialysis in each treatment. To report the reason for the encounter, report one of these codes:

Z49.31 Encounter for adequacy testing for hemodialysis

or

Z49.32 Encounter for adequacy testing for peritoneal dialysis

Most patients will need to receive dialysis several times each week, usually until a transplant is available. For each of these encounters, the diagnosis codes to report will include this code:

Z99.2 Dependence on renal dialysis (hemodialysis status) (peritoneal dialysis status) (presence of arteriovenous shunt for dialysis)

Sadly, some patients cannot deal with an ongoing need for treatment and may not come in for their sessions. As you learned, this can have a negative impact on their health, and it must be documented. The diagnosis codes to report will include this:

Z91.15 Patient's noncompliance with renal dialysis

Transplantation

At the point when the kidney is so severely damaged that it cannot be rehabilitated, a transplant may be the only solution to improve the patient's health and possibly save his or her life. A patient receiving a transplant must deal with the challenge of needing lifelong medication as well as follow-up care. However, great success has been

> **GUIDANCE CONNECTION**
>
> Read the ICD-10-CM Official Guidelines for Coding and Reporting, section **I. Conventions, General Coding Guidelines and Chapter Specific Guidelines,** subsection **C. Chapter-Specific Coding Guidelines,** chapter **14. Diseases of Genitourinary System,** subsection **a.2) Chronic kidney disease and kidney transplant status.**

> **CODING BITES**
>
> Code category **T86 Complications of transplanted organs and tissue** has a *Use additional code* notation to remind you to also report any other transplant complications, such as
>
> Graft-versus-host disease (D89.81-)
>
> Malignancy associated with organ transplant (C80.2-)
>
> Post-transplant lymphoproliferative disorders (PTLD) (D47.Z1)

achieved in increasing transplant patients' quality of life. Of course, there is always the possibility that the patient's body might reject the new organ, but the greatest roadblock for these patients is the long wait for a donor:

Z76.82   Awaiting organ transplant status

Of course, a donor is needed. With kidney transplants, the donor may be either a live individual or a cadaver. If the donor is live, the individual will need this diagnosis code to support medical necessity for the preoperative testing, the procedure itself to remove the donated organ, and the postoperative care:

Z52.4   Kidney donor

Organ transplantation is an incredible health care procedural accomplishment, giving thousands of individuals with previously terminal conditions a second chance to live a normal and productive life. Patients who have received an organ transplant will typically need to take antirejection medication and receive regular checkups. Therefore, after the transplant has taken place, the patient's posttransplant status may need to be reported:

Z94.0   Kidney transplant status

Transplanting an organ from one person into another person is not always a perfect cure. There may be several issues that may require additional treatment. In some cases, the transplant does not eliminate all of the kidney disease. One kidney may have a milder case of CKD and not need transplantation, whereas the other kidney does. Therefore, it is acceptable to report both posttransplant status and current CKD in the same patient at the same time when the physician documents both conditions concurrently.

When a transplanted organ begins to show signs of rejection, failure, infection, or other complication, this will need to be treated and, in some cases, the transplanted organ will need to be removed.

T86.11   Kidney transplant rejection
T86.12   Kidney transplant failure
T86.13   Kidney transplant infection
          (use additional code to report specific infection)
T86.19   Other complication of kidney transplant
Z98.85   Transplanted organ removal status

Acute Renal Failure

Acute renal failure (ARF) is a sudden malfunction of the kidney often caused by an obstruction, a circulatory problem, or possible renal parenchymal disease. This condition is often reversible with medical treatment.

The most typical cause of ARF in critically ill patients and the cause of approximately 75% of all cases of ARF is a condition known as *acute tubular necrosis (ATN),* also called *acute tubulointerstitial nephritis (ATIN)*—code N10. Nephrotoxic injury, such as that caused by the ingestion of certain chemicals, can cause ATN but is reversible when diagnosed and treated early. Ischemic ATN may be the result of an injury to the glomerular epithelial cells causing cellular collapse or injury to the vascular endothelium, resulting in cellular swelling and therefore obstruction.

Report this condition with a code from category N17 Acute kidney failure, with an additional character to identify accompanying tubular necrosis, acute cortical necrosis, or medullary necrosis.

Treatment typically includes the provision of diuretics and fluids to flush the system. Electrolyte and fluid balances must be maintained to avoid fluid overload. Some cases require peritoneal dialysis.

> **CODING BITES**
>
> Infections can occur commonly, particularly in an organ system that is open to the outside of the body. Conditions such as a kidney infection, cystitis (bladder infection), or a urinary tract infection (UTI) are certainly not exotic infectious conditions. In these cases, you will need to
>
> *Use additional code* **to identify organism.**
>
> You may have to check the pathology report to determine what the organism is if it is not specified in the physician's notes.

> ## YOU CODE IT! CASE STUDY
>
> Frieda Sacks, an 81-year-old female, has been having problems with her kidneys for a while, with two kidney infections over the last 5 years. Dr. Cannon diagnosed her with acute renal insufficiency.
>
> ### You Code It!
>
> Go through the steps of coding, and determine the code or codes that should be reported for this encounter between Dr. Cannon and Frieda.
>
> Step #1: Read the case carefully and completely.
>
> Step #2: Abstract the scenario. Which key words or terms describe why the physician cared for the patient during this encounter?
>
> Step #3: Are there any details missing or incomplete for which you would need to query the physician? [If so, ask your instructor.]
>
> Step #4: Check for any relevant guidance, including reading all of the symbols and notations in the Tabular List and the appropriate sections of the Official Guidelines.
>
> Step #5: Determine the correct diagnosis code or codes to explain why this encounter was medically necessary.
>
> Step #6: Double-check your work.
>
> **Answer:**
>
> Did you determine this to be the correct code?
>
> N28.9   Disorder of kidney and ureter, unspecified (renal insufficiency (acute))

Urinary Tract Infection

Cystitis and urethritis are both lower urinary tract infections (UTIs), which are often resolved easily with treatment. Ten times more women than men are affected by one of these conditions. In the elderly, a weakening of the bladder muscles may create a foundation for bladder infections (cystitis). Children with a confirmed UTI should be examined for a urinary tract abnormality. This condition would not only predispose them to UTIs but may also present a greater likelihood for renal damage in the future. Report this with a code from category N30 Cystitis, with an additional character to report specifics.

Most UTIs are caused by a Gram-negative enteric bacterium. The pathology report will identify which one. This is important to know because there is a *Use additional code* notation to identify the infectious agent. Additionally, a urinary catheter, a neurogenic (neuromuscular dysfunction) bladder, or a fistula between the intestine and the bladder might cause a UTI. Medicare may consider a UTI caused by a urinary catheter to be a nonreimbursable hospital-acquired condition (HAC).

Urinalysis of a clean-catch midstream void will confirm this diagnosis and will provide the specific name of the pathogen for coding.

Renal Calculi

Renal calculi, commonly known as *kidney stones,* might actually form anywhere within the urinary system; however, formation in the renal pelvis or the calyces of the kidneys is most common. While the precise cause of these uncomfortable formations is not known, decreased urine production, infection, urinary stasis, and metabolic conditions, such as gout, are considered predispositions. Code category N20 Calculus of kidney and ureter, N21 Calculus of lower urinary tract, or N22 Calculus of urinary tract in diseases classified elsewhere would be appropriate for reporting this diagnosis.

When the individual stones are small, hydration is prescribed to enable natural passage of the calculi. Larger stones may need to be removed surgically, most often using a cystoscope or using lithotripsy to break up the larger pieces to permit natural passage.

YOU CODE IT! CASE STUDY

Brandon Markinson, a 51-year-old male, was in so much pain that he was doubled over. He went to the emergency department at the hospital near his house. Dr. Deitz took an x-ray and determined that Brandon had nephrolithiasis. She discussed treatment options with him.

You Code It!

Go through the steps of coding, and determine the code or codes that should be reported for this encounter between Dr. Deitz and Brandon.

Step #1: Read the case carefully and completely.

Step #2: Abstract the scenario. Which key words or terms describe why the physician cared for the patient during this encounter?

Step #3: Are there any details missing or incomplete for which you would need to query the physician? [If so, ask your instructor.]

Step #4: Check for any relevant guidance, including reading all of the symbols and notations in the Tabular List and the appropriate sections of the Official Guidelines.

Step #5: Determine the correct diagnosis code or codes to explain why this encounter was medically necessary.

Step #6: Double-check your work.

Answer:

Did you determine this to be the correct code?

N20.0   Calculus of kidney (Nephrolithiasis)

Malignant Neoplasm of the Bladder

Bladder Cancer
Malignancy of the urinary bladder.

Malignant neoplasm of the bladder, commonly known as **bladder cancer**, is the fourth most frequently diagnosed cancer in men and the eighth most frequent in women. While various types of malignant cells can invade this organ, transitional cell carcinoma is seen most often and develops in the lining of the urinary bladder. This would be reported with a code from category C67 Malignant neoplasm of the bladder, with an additional character to report the specific location of the tumor (trigone, dome, etc.). The definitive test to confirm this condition is a cystoscopy with biopsy.

YOU CODE IT! CASE STUDY

Corneilus St. Augusteine contracted syphilis of his kidney, and now Dr. Acosta determines that an anterior urethral stricture has developed as a result.

> **You Code It!**
>
> Go through the steps of coding, and determine the code or codes that should be reported for this encounter between Dr. Acosta and Corneilus.
>
> Step #1: Read the case carefully and completely.
>
> Step #2: Abstract the scenario. Which key words or terms describe why the physician cared for the patient during this encounter?
>
> Step #3: Are there any details missing or incomplete for which you would need to query the physician? [If so, ask your instructor.]
>
> Step #4: Check for any relevant guidance, including reading all of the symbols and notations in the Tabular List and the appropriate sections of the Official Guidelines.
>
> Step #5: Determine the correct diagnosis code or codes to explain why this encounter was medically necessary.
>
> Step #6: Double-check your work.
>
> **Answer:**
>
> Did you determine these to be the correct codes?
>
> | | |
> |---|---|
> | N35.114 | Post-infective anterior urethral stricture, not elsewhere classified, male |
> | A52.75 | Syphilis of kidney and ureter |

17.2 Diseases of the Male Genital Organs

Due to the proximity of the prostate to the urethra and bladder (see Figure 17-2), the most common underlying condition promoting UTI is **prostatitis**. In men, the prostate is a gland that sits inferior to (below) the urinary bladder. It is shaped like a chestnut and wraps around the urethra as the urethra descends from the bladder to the outside of the body. *E. coli* is the pathogen causing approximately 80% of these cases. A urine

Prostatitis
Inflammation of the prostate.

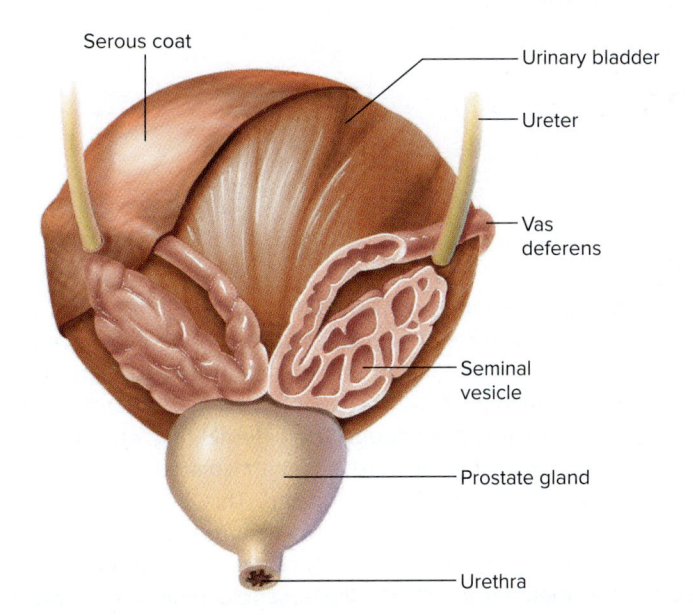

FIGURE 17-2 An illustration identifying the anatomical sites of the prostate Booth et al., *Medical Assisting*, 5e. Copyright ©2013 by McGraw-Hill Education. Figure 31-6 (b), p. 616. Used with permission.

culture of specimens collected using a four-step process known as the *Meares and Stamey technique* provides the best data for a confirmed diagnosis. Antibiotics are the standard-of-care treatment. Code category N41 Inflammatory diseases of the prostate requires a fourth character to identify whether the inflammation is acute, chronic, an abscess, or another issue.

Benign prostatic hyperplasia (BPH), also known as *benign prostatic hypertrophy,* most often diagnosed in men over 50 years of age, is a condition in which the prostate enlarges and results in depressing the urethra. This interferes with the flow of urine from the bladder to the outside. Code category N40 Enlarged prostate with a fourth character would be used to report this condition. BPH can also result in urine retention, severe hematuria (blood in urine), or hydronephrosis.

Hydrocele is a condition that occurs when fluid collects within the tunica vaginalis of the scrotum, the testis, or the spermatic cord. The physician will not only diagnose and treat this condition, but also needs to investigate to determine the underlying cause, especially when associated with pathology that is considered clinically significant. As you abstract the documentation, you will need to identify if the hydrocele is congenital, encysted, infected, or other type, as well as any identified underlying conditions.

Benign Prostatic Hyperplasia (BPH)
Enlarged prostate that results in depressing the urethra.

N43.0	Encysted hydrocele
N43.1	Infected hydrocele
	Use additional code (B95-B97), to identify infectious agent
N43.2	Other hydrocele
P83.5	Congenital hydrocele

YOU CODE IT! CASE STUDY

PATIENT NAME: Walter Primiera

PREOPERATIVE DIAGNOSES:

1. Left hydrocele, possible right.
2. Urethral meatal stenosis.

POSTOPERATIVE DIAGNOSES:

1. Left encysted hydrocele.
2. Urethral meatal stenosis.

OPERATIONS PERFORMED:

1. Left hydrocelectomy.
2. Diagnostic laparoscopy.
3. Urethral meatoplasty.

ANESTHESIA: General and caudal.

DESCRIPTION OF PROCEDURE: After informed consent was acquired, the patient was brought into the surgical suite. The patient was placed on the table in a supine position, and prepped and draped in the usual sterile manner. General anesthesia was accomplished, and a caudal block was administered. A left inguinal skin crease incision was made and the dissection proceeded to expose the external oblique fascia. After placing self-retaining retractors, the external oblique was opened in the direction of its fibers. The external ring was opened. The ilioinguinal nerve was identified and moved away to avoid any injury. The cord was then isolated and a vessel loop placed around it. The fibers of cord were separated and hydrocele sac was identified. This was carefully dissected away from the cord structures, taking care to identify and avoid any injury to the vas or vessels.

Once the sac was completely isolated, bladder was doubly clamped and divided on the proximal aspect as well as up to the internal ring. The sac was then opened, 5 mm laparoscopic trocar sheath was placed under vision into the peritoneum, and a 2-0 silk stitch was secured in order to maintain the pneumoperitoneum. CO_2 was then insufflated to a pressure of 10 mmHg. With the patient in Trendelenburg position, the contralateral internal ring was inspected with a 25 degree lens. The vas and vessels were seen exiting a closed internal ring. Thus, a repair on the right was required. The scope was removed, pneumoperitoneum was released, and the trocar was removed. The hydrocele sac was gathered in the right-angled clamp, twisted, and high ligation was performed with 3-0 Vicryl suture ligature and tied.

Attention was turned to the distal aspect of the sac and the testis was delivered. Tunica vaginalis was opened, redundant tunica was excised, hydrocele fluid drained. A very small testicular appendage was also excised with cautery. The testis was then returned to its normal scrotal location. The floor of the canal was inspected, and there was no evidence of any weakness to suggest a direct hernia. The external oblique was then closed with a running 3-0 Vicryl, taking care to avoid any injury to the nerve. The subcutaneous tissues were closed with interrupted 4-0 chromic, and the skin with running 4-0 Monocryl. Steri-Strip and Tegaderm dressing were placed over the inguinal incision.

Attention was now turned towards the urethral meatus and the tissue in the ventral midline. The meatus was stenotic, so the tissue in the ventral midline was crushed with a mosquito clamp and then opened sharply with Westcott scissors. A 7-0 Vicryl stitch was placed at the apex. Some redundant tissue was crimped and then excised along either the left or right side. To make a normal appearance and help with avoiding interrupting the stream, this tissue was excised. The edge of the urethral mucosa was attached to the glans skin. This was done also with 7-0 Vicryl sutures. Bacitracin ointment was placed over the meatus. The patient was awakened. He was taken to the recovery room in stable condition. All counts were correct. He tolerated the procedure well. There were no complications.

Signed: Stefan Olsen, MD

You Code It!

Review Dr. Olsen's operative notes regarding this procedure performed on Walter. Then, determine the accurate ICD-10-CM code or codes that will explain the medical necessity for this encounter.

Step #1: Read the case carefully and completely.

Step #2: Abstract the scenario. Which main words or terms describe why the physician cared for the patient during this encounter?

Step #3: Are there any details missing or incomplete for which you would need to query the physician? [If so, ask your instructor.]

Step #4: Check for any relevant guidance, including reading all of the symbols and notations in the Tabular List and the appropriate sections of the Official Guidelines.

Step #5: Determine the correct diagnosis code or codes to explain why this encounter was medically necessary.

Step #6: Double-check your work.

Answer:

Did you determine these to be the correct codes?

N43.0	Encysted hydrocele
N35.8	Other urethral stricture

Oligospermia is a type of male infertility, commonly known as a low sperm count. ICD-10-CM code options are combination codes that will include the general type of underlying cause, so you will need to be alert for this when you are abstracting the physician's notes. In most cases, you will also need a second code to provide more specifics about that underlying cause.

N46.11	Organic oligospermia
N46.121	Oligospermia due to drug therapy
N46.122	Oligospermia due to infection
N46.123	Oligospermia due to obstruction of efferent ducts
N46.124	Oligospermia due to radiation
N46.125	Oligospermia due to systemic disease
N46.129	Oligospermia due to other extratesticular causes

Erectile dysfunction is broadcast in television and Internet ads as easily solved by a little blue pill. However, whether or not it is that simple to cure, the reporting of the diagnosis is complex. As you will discover turning to code category N52 Male erectile dysfunction, you will need to determine, from the documentation, the underlying cause because all of these code options are combination codes.

N52.01	Erectile dysfunction due to arterial insufficiency
N52.02	Corporo-venous occlusive erectile dysfunction
N52.03	Combined arterial insufficiency and corporo-venous occlusive erectile dysfunction
N52.1	Erectile dysfunction due to diseases classified elsewhere
	Code first underlying disease
N52.31	Erectile dysfunction following radical prostatectomy
N52.32	Erectile dysfunction following radical cystectomy
N52.33	Erectile dysfunction following urethral surgery
N52.34	Erectile dysfunction following simple prostatectomy
N52.39	Other and unspecified post-surgical erectile dysfunction

17.3 Sexually Transmitted Diseases

Age, employment status, income level, gender, number of sexual encounters . . . nothing except taking proper precautions during sex shields someone from getting a sexually transmitted disease (STD). This is true for all types of sexual encounters in which bodily fluids are exchanged—not just intercourse. The paragraphs below present an overview of the STDs considered the most common by the Centers for Disease Control and Prevention (CDC).

Bacterial Vaginosis

Bacterial vaginosis (BV)—the most common vaginal infection in women 16 to 45 years of age, often affecting pregnant women—is caused by an overgrowth of bacteria. Symptoms include odor, itching, burning, pain, and/or a discharge. Code N76.0 Acute vaginitis would be reported, along with a second code to identify the infectious agent.

Chlamydia

Caused by a bacterium *(Chlamydia trachomatis)*, *chlamydia* can result in infertility or other irreversible damage to a woman's reproductive organs. The symptoms are mild or absent, so most women don't know they have a problem unless their partner is diagnosed. Chlamydia can cause a penile discharge in men. It is the most commonly reported bacterial STD in the United States, according to the CDC. In ICD-10-CM, code A55 Chlamydial lymphogranuloma (venereum) is reported for chlamydia that is transmitted by sexual contact. *Note:* Do not confuse this with A70 Chlamydia psittaci infections, A74.0 Chlamydial conjunctivitis, A74.81 Chlamydial peritonitis, A74.89 Other chlamydial diseases, or A74.9 Chlamydial infection unspecified, all of which are reported when chlamydia causes another disease.

Genital Herpes

Genital herpes is caused by one of the herpes simplex viruses: type 1 (HSV-1) or type 2 (HSV-2). In this STD, one or more blisters may appear on or in the genital or rectal area. Once the blister bursts, it can take several weeks for the ulcer to heal. The virus will remain in the body indefinitely, even though no more breakouts may be experienced, because there is no cure. Treatment can reduce the number of outbreaks and diminish the opportunity of transmission to a partner. To code from category A60 Anogenital herpesviral [herpes simplex] infections, you must know the specific anatomical site, such as penis or cervix, to determine the additional characters required.

Gonorrhea

Gonorrhea, a bacterial STD, can develop in the reproductive organs of men (urethra) and women (cervix, uterus, fallopian tubes, and urethra), in addition to the mouth, throat, eyes, and anus. Symptoms in men include a burning sensation during urination, a penile discharge (white, yellow, or green), and/or swelling or pain in the testes. Women typically do not experience any symptoms. You will report this diagnosis from ICD-10-CM code category A54 Gonococcal infection, which requires identification of the specific anatomical site of the infection to determine additional characters.

Human Immunodeficiency Virus

Both types of *human immunodeficiency virus (HIV)*—HIV-1 and HIV-2—destroy cells within the body that are responsible for helping fight disease (those that are part of the immune system). Soon after the initial infection, some individuals may suffer flu-like symptoms, while others will have no symptoms at all and feel fine. Current medications can help individuals continue to feel well and decrease their ability to transmit the disease. HIV, especially untreated HIV, has known manifestations, including cardiovascular, renal, and liver disease. In the late stages of the disease, when the patient's immune system is quite damaged, acquired immune deficiency syndrome (AIDS) may develop. Currently, there is no cure for HIV or AIDS. You will report a confirmed diagnosis of HIV with code B20 Human Immunodeficiency Virus [HIV] disease when the patient has, or has had, manifestations or code Z21 Asymptomatic human immunodeficiency virus [HIV] infection status when the patient is asymptomatic.

Human Papillomavirus

There are over 40 different types of *human papillomavirus (HPV)* that can infect the genital regions, mouth, and/or throat of both men and women. This infection will not cause any signs or symptoms; however, it is known to contribute to the development of genital warts as well as cervical cancer (in women). A connection has also been made between HPV and malignancies in the penis, anus, vulva, vagina, and oropharynx. A patient getting a test to screen for HPV will be reported with code Z11.51 Encounter for screening for human papillomavirus (HPV). Reporting for a female patient with a positive test result will come from subcategory R87.8 Other abnormal findings in specimens from female genital organs. Additional characters are required based on the anatomical location (cervix or vagina) and on whether the patient is identified as high risk or low risk. Male and female patients would both be reported with a code from subcategory R85.8 Other abnormal findings in specimens from digestive organs and abdominal cavity for HPV-positive results in the anus. A confirmed diagnosis for either a male or female patient would be reported with A63.0 Anogenital (venereal) warts [due to (human) papillomavirus (HPV)].

Pelvic Inflammatory Disease

Pelvic inflammatory disease (PID) is often a complication of previous chlamydial, gonococceal, or other STD infection, occurring when the bacterium moves from the vagina into a woman's uterus or fallopian tubes. It causes lower abdominal pain. Serious consequences of untreated PID include chronic pelvic pain, formation of abscesses, ectopic pregnancy, and possible infertility. Use code A56.11 Chlamydial female pelvic inflammatory disease or A54.24 Gonococcal female pelvic inflammatory disease, or use a code from category N73 Other female pelvic inflammatory diseases or code N74 Female pelvic inflammatory disorders in diseases classified elsewhere.

Syphilis

In its early stages, *syphilis*, caused by a bacterium *(Treponema pallidum)*, is easy to cure. Signs and symptoms include a rash, particularly on the palmar and plantar surfaces, as well as a small, round, painless sore on the genitals, anus, or mouth. However, these symptoms mimic many other diseases, often resulting in delayed diagnosis. Code category A50 Congenital syphilis, A51 Early syphilis, A52 Late syphilis, or A53 Other and unspecified syphilis would be reported when this condition is sexually transmitted.

Trichomoniasis

Trichomoniasis (trich), a protozoan parasitic *(Trichomonas vaginalis)* STD, is more common in older women than in men. Most individuals do not know they are infected because only approximately 30% develop any symptoms, such as a genital discharge. While the condition is curable, a person who has trich and goes without treatment increases his or her risk of getting human immunodeficiency virus (HIV). Trich, when present in a pregnant woman, can cause premature delivery of low-birth-weight neonates. Code category A59 Trichomoniasis requires additional characters to identify the specific anatomical site of the infection.

YOU CODE IT! CASE STUDY

PATIENT: AMELIA MADISON

DATE OF OPERATION: 05/22/2018

PREOPERATIVE DIAGNOSES:

1. Severe pelvic pain.
2. History of pelvic inflammatory disease and pelvic adhesion.
3. Probable left hydrosalpinx.

POSTOPERATIVE DIAGNOSES:

1. Chronic pelvic inflammatory disease.
2. Extensive pelvic adhesion and left hydrosalpinx.

PROCEDURES PERFORMED:

1. Pelvic examination under anesthesia.
2. Total abdominal hysterectomy.
3. Bilateral salpingo-oophorectomy.
4. Lysis of adhesions.

SURGEON: Gabriel Underwood, MD

ANESTHESIA: General.

ESTIMATED BLOOD LOSS: 100 mL.

COMPLICATIONS: None.

DESCRIPTION OF OPERATION: The patient was taken to the operating room, where general anesthesia was administered without complication. The patient was placed in the dorsal lithotomy position, and examination under anesthesia revealed a normal-appearing vagina and cervix. Bimanual exam reveals a normal-sized uterus with no right adnexal pathology noted. There was an adnexal mass in the left adnexa of approximately 4–5 cm. The patient was placed in the supine position. She was prepped and draped in the usual fashion.

A Pfannenstiel skin incision was performed and carried down to the fascial layer. The fascia was transected. The rectus muscles were retracted laterally, and the peritoneum was entered under direct visualization. The pelvic cavity was inspected, and there were extensive pelvic adhesions noted. The bowel was packed into the upper abdomen using moist laps. There was a large left hydrosalpinx present with bilateral tubal-ovarian adhesions. The left hydrosalpinx was first freed up using careful sharp dissection. The tube and ovary on the right side were likewise mobilized with sharp dissection. The right round ligament was doubly clamped, cut, and tied with 0 Vicryl suture. The visceroperitoneum was dissected free to the midline. The left round ligament was likewise doubly clamped, cut, and tied and the visceroperitoneum was dissected free to the midline. The bladder was carefully dissected off the lower uterine segment. The right infundibulopelvic ligament was clamped, cut, and doubly tied with 0 Vicryl suture. The left infundibulopelvic ligament was likewise doubly clamped, cut, and doubly tied with 0 Vicryl suture. The right uterine vessels and cardinal ligament were doubly clamped, cut, and doubly tied with 0 Vicryl suture. The left uterine vessels and cardinal ligament were likewise clamped, cut, and doubly tied with 0 Vicryl suture. The bladder was retracted inferiorly. The right uterosacral ligament was clamped, cut, and tied with 0 Vicryl suture. This step was repeated until the specimen was mobilized on the right side. The left uterosacral ligament was likewise clamped, cut, and tied with 0 Vicryl suture. Again, the step was repeated until the specimen was mobilized on the left side.

The anterior aspect of the vagina was entered with a scalpel and heavy curved scissors were used to remove the uterus, tubes, and ovaries, which were sent to pathology for microscopic examination. Angled sutures were placed on either side of the vaginal cuff using 0 Vicryl suture. The vaginal cuff was closed with interrupted figure-of-eight sutures of 0 Vicryl. A thorough search was made to ensure that there was complete hemostasis. The pelvic peritoneum was reapproximated with 0 Vicryl suture. The instruments were removed from the abdomen. The sponge, needle, and instrument counts were all correct. The parietal peritoneum was reapproximated with 2-0 Vicryl suture. The rectus muscles were reapproximated with interrupted 0 Vicryl suture. The fascia was closed with 0 PDS suture. The subcutaneous tissue was reapproximated with 3-0 Vicryl suture. The skin was closed with staples. A dry sterile dressing was placed over the incision. The patient was then awoken in the operating room and transferred to the recovery room in good condition.

DISPOSITION: The patient was taken to the recovery room in good condition at the end of the procedure.

You Code It!

Read these operative notes, written by Dr. Underwood, about Amelia's procedure, and determine the correct ICD-10-CM code or codes to explain the reason *why* the procedures were medically necessary.

Step #1: Read the case carefully and completely.

Step #2: Abstract the scenario. Which main words or terms describe why the physician cared for the patient during this encounter?

Step #3: Are there any details missing or incomplete for which you would need to query the physician? [If so, ask your instructor.]

Step #4: Check for any relevant guidance, including reading all of the symbols and notations in the Tabular List and the appropriate sections of the Official Guidelines.

Step #5: Determine the correct diagnosis code or codes to explain why this encounter was medically necessary.

Step #6: Double-check your work.

Answer:

Did you determine these to be the codes?

N73.1	Chronic parametritis and pelvic cellulities
N73.6	Female pelvic peritoneal adhesions (post-infective)
N70.11	Chronic salpingitis

Good job!

17.4 Gynecologic Care

Females of all ages may go to the **gynecologist (GYN)** for specialized health care. Sometimes, the physician is referred to as an *OB/GYN*, an abbreviation for the dual

Gynecologist (GYN)
A physician specializing in the care of the female genital tract.

Obstetrics (OB)
A health care specialty focusing on the care of women during pregnancy and the puerperium.

Puerperium
The time period from the end of labor until the uterus returns to normal size, typically 3 to 6 weeks.

specialization of **obstetrics (OB)**, which focuses on care during pregnancy and the **puerperium**, and gynecology. Concerns and disorders relating to other aspects of the female anatomy are not always related to pregnancy. Let's investigate some of the most common reasons a woman would seek the care of a gynecologist and how to report them.

Routine Encounters

Most women understand the importance of getting their annual well-woman examination. It may take place at the office of a specialized OB/GYN or be performed by a family or general practitioner. Typically, the visit includes a routine physical exam, pelvic exam, and breast exam. Often, the visit also includes a Papanicolaou *cervical* smear, better known as a *Pap smear*. The encounter is coded

Z01.411 Encounter for routine gynecological examination (general) (routine) with abnormal findings

or

Z01.419 Encounter for routine gynecological examination (general) (routine) without abnormal findings

These codes include a *cervical* Pap smear. However, when a *vaginal* Pap smear (which is different from a *cervical* Pap smear and must be specified in the documentation) is included in the visit, add a second code:

Z12.72 Encounter for screening for malignant neoplasm of vagina (vaginal pap smear)

Endometriosis

Endometriosis (code category N80) is an inflammation or swelling of the tissue that lines the uterus. The condition is estimated to affect 2% to 10% of women of childbearing age in the United States. Although the disorder is identified as being within the uterus, endometriosis can be observed in a woman's ovary, cul-de-sac, uterosacral ligaments, broad ligaments, fallopian tube, uterovesical fold, round ligament, vermiform appendix, vagina, and/or rectovaginal septum. This means that a diagnosis of endometriosis is not sufficient to determine the most accurate code. You have to know the specific site of the condition.

Uterine Fibroids

Also known as *uterine leiomyoma* or *uterine fibromyoma*, *uterine fibroids* (code category D25 Leiomyoma of uterus) are tumors located in the female reproductive system. Only about one-third of women with these tumors are actually diagnosed. Uterine fibroids are not related to cancer, do not increase the patient's risk of developing cancer later, and are found to be benign 99% of the time.

Pelvic Pain

Female pelvic and perineal pain (code R10.2) may be related to a specific genital organ or an area around a genital organ or may be psychological in nature. The physician may be able to diagnose a particular cause, such as sexual intercourse or menstruation, or the source of the pain may remain unknown.

YOU CODE IT! CASE STUDY

Clarisse Battle, a 31-year-old female, came to see Dr. Legg with complaints of feeling bloated. She stated that she has felt this way for over a month and cannot connect it to anything she has been eating. After taking a complete history, doing an exam, and performing an ultrasound, Dr. Legg explained that Clarisse had a simple cyst on her right ovary.

> **You Code It!**
>
> Go through the steps of coding, and determine the code or codes that should be reported for this encounter between Dr. Legg and Clarisse.
>
> Step #1: Read the case carefully and completely.
>
> Step #2: Abstract the scenario. Which key words or terms describe why the physician cared for the patient during this encounter?
>
> Step #3: Are there any details missing or incomplete for which you would need to query the physician? [If so, ask your instructor.]
>
> Step #4: Check for any relevant guidance, including reading all of the symbols and notations in the Tabular List and the appropriate sections of the Official Guidelines.
>
> Step #5: Determine the correct diagnosis code or codes to explain why this encounter was medically necessary.
>
> Step #6: Double-check your work.
>
> **Answer:**
>
> Did you determine this to be the correct code?
>
>   **N83.291**   Other ovarian cysts (simple cyst of ovary), right
>
> You are really getting to be a great coder!

Procreative Management

A woman may want to see her doctor regarding her desire to have children now or in the future. Code category Z31 Encounter for procreative management is used only for testing conducted with anticipation of procreation (having children). Code subcategory Z31.6 Encounter for general counseling and advice on procreation will provide you with a few fifth-character options to include additional details.

Perhaps a patient comes in for a test to determine whether or not she is a carrier of a genetic disease before getting pregnant. Most often, such a woman wants to be aware of the possibilities of passing inherited diseases, such as sickle cell anemia or Tay-Sachs, to her baby. The code or codes to report her encounter would be code(s):

    Z31.430   Encounter of female for testing for genetic diseases carrier status for procreative management

and/or

    Z31.438   Encounter for other genetic testing of female for procreative management

Code Z31.5 Encounter for genetic counseling would be used after a genetic test has been done and shown positive results.

With good news so far, our female patient may come in next time for fertility testing or, perhaps, a pregnancy test:

    Z31.41   Encounter for fertility testing
    Z32.00   Encounter for pregnancy test, result unknown
    Z32.01   Encounter for pregnancy test, result positive
    Z32.02   Encounter for pregnancy test, result negative

> ### LET'S CODE IT! SCENARIO
>
> Priscilla Sharp, a 25-year-old female, came to see Dr. Trenton to have an intrauterine device (IUD) inserted. She and her husband, Eli, want to wait a while before having children.
>
> #### Let's Code It!
>
> Priscilla came to get an *IUD*. The purpose of this visit is to prevent Priscilla from getting pregnant, also termed *contraception*. Let's go to the Alphabetic Index and look up *contraception*. Look down the list indented under *contraception* and you see *device*. However, none of the terms indented under *device* seems to really match Dr. Trenton's notes. This is the first encounter relating to contraception, so perhaps "initial prescription" would be a place to begin.
>
> **Contraception, contraceptive**
> **device (intrauterine) (in situ) Z97.5**
>   **initial prescription Z30.014**
>
> Turn to the Tabular List and confirm that this is the best, most accurate code:
>
> ☑4 **Z30**   **Encounter for contraceptive management**
>
> There are no notations or directives, so continue reading down the column to determine the most accurate required fourth and fifth characters:
>
> **Z30.014**   **Encounter for initial prescription of intrauterine contraceptive device**
>
> Be sure to read further down the column to determine whether any other code descriptions may be more accurate than this description. Sometimes, the Alphabetic Index gets us to only the best subsection of the Tabular List.
>
> **Z30.430**   **Encounter for insertion of intrauterine contraceptive device**
>
> There it is! Good job!

17.5 Routine Obstetrics Care

Fertilization and Gestation

When a sperm fertilizes an oocyte, a zygote is created. This will typically occur while the egg is still in the last portion of the fallopian tube. Each oocyte (egg) has 23 chromosomes, and each sperm contains 23 chromosomes (in the nucleus in the head of the sperm). When they combine during fertilization, the zygote then has the complete set of 46 chromosomes. This may be confirmed by a pregnancy test; the medical necessity for this visit is reported with a code such as Z32.01 Encounter for pregnancy tests, result positive.

The *embryonic period*, from weeks 2 through 8 after fertilization, is the time during which external structures and internal organs begin to form. Additionally, the placenta, umbilical cord, amnion, yolk sac, and chorion are established during this time. At week 8, the embryo, about 1 inch in length, is considered a fetus, and all organ systems are in place.

Gestation, the length of the pregnancy, is measured in trimesters, beginning on the first day of the last menstrual period (LMP). For coding purposes, ICD-10-CM provides the following definitions:

- *First trimester:* from the first day of the last menstrual period (LMP) to less than 14 weeks 0 days.
- *Second trimester:* 14 weeks 0 days to less than 28 weeks 0 days.

Gestation
The length of time for the complete development of a baby from conception to birth; on average, 40 weeks.

- *Third trimester:* 28 weeks 0 days until delivery.
- *Preterm (premature) neonate:* one with a gestation of 28 completed weeks or more but less than 37 completed weeks (between 196 and 258 completed days).
- *Postterm neonate:* one with over 40 completed weeks up to 42 completed weeks of gestation.
- *Prolonged gestation of a neonate:* a gestational period that has lasted over 42 completed weeks (294 days or more).

Weeks of Gestation

Cases in which a complication has been identified require additional specificity, beyond the current trimester of the pregnancy, and you will need to report the specific number of weeks of gestation. Code category Z3A Weeks of gestation provides you with codes that specify the individual week, from 8 weeks to 42 weeks gestation. In addition, codes are available for less than 8 weeks and greater than 42 weeks.

When a pregnant patient is admitted and stays in the hospital for more than 1 week, you should use the date of admission to determine the weeks of gestation.

> ### EXAMPLE
> Amy went into labor and ultimately delivered the baby. She and her husband were very concerned because the baby was only at 33 weeks:
>
> | O60.14X0 | Preterm labor third trimester with preterm delivery third trimester, single gestation |
> |---|---|
> | Z3A.33 | 33 weeks gestation of pregnancy |

Prenatal Visits

A woman often has three items noted in her chart: *gravida (G)* reports how many times the woman has been pregnant; *para*, or *parity (P)*, reports how many babies this woman has given birth to (after 20 weeks of gestation); and *abortus (A)* identifies how many pregnancies did not come to term or make it past the 20th week. Gravida and para may be noted using an abbreviation, such as G2 P1.

> ### EXAMPLE
> | G1 P1 | tells you that the woman has been pregnant once and given birth once. |
> |---|---|
> | G1 P2 | tells you that the woman has been pregnant once and given birth twice—twins! |
> | G2 P1 | tells you that the woman has been pregnant twice and given birth once. If she is pregnant now, this is her second pregnancy; if she is not pregnant now, she may have had a miscarriage in the past. |

Normal Pregnancy

Routine outpatient **prenatal** checkups are very important to the health and well-being of both the mother and the baby. For a healthy pregnant woman, the visits are typically scheduled at specific points throughout the pregnancy, as determined by the number of weeks of gestation.

When coding routine visits, with the patient having no complications, you will choose from the available Z codes. Remember that you will use a Z code when the

---

GUIDANCE CONNECTION

Read the ICD-10-CM Official Guidelines for Coding and Reporting, section **I. Conventions, General Coding Guidelines and Chapter Specific Guidelines,** subsection **C. Chapter-Specific Coding Guidelines,** chapter **15. Pregnancy, Childbirth, and the Puerperium,** subsections **a.3) Final character for trimester, a.4) Selection of trimester for inpatient admissions that encompass more than one trimester, a.5) Unspecified trimester,** and **b.3) Episodes when no delivery occurs.**

CODING BITES

Code category Z3A codes are not reported in cases of

- Pregnancies with abortive outcomes
- Elective termination of pregnancy
- Postpartum conditions

Prenatal
Prior to birth; also referred to as *antenatal*.

> **GUIDANCE CONNECTION**
>
> Read the ICD-10-CM Official Guidelines for Coding and Reporting, section **I. Conventions, General Coding Guidelines and Chapter Specific Guidelines,** subsection **C. Chapter-Specific Coding Guidelines,** chapter **15. Pregnancy, Childbirth, and the Puerperium,** subsection **b.1) Routine outpatient prenatal visits.**

patient is not encountering the health care provider because of any current illness or injury. A healthy, pregnant woman has neither a current illness nor a current injury.

Z34.01 Encounter for supervision of normal first pregnancy, first trimester
Z34.82 Encounter for supervision of other normal pregnancy, second trimester

As you can see, you will need to determine which code to use on the basis of the physician's notes on the woman's gravida.

High-Risk Pregnancy

In cases where the pregnancy is considered to be medically high risk, you will use a code from category O09 Supervision of high-risk pregnancy for the routine visit.

You will determine the fourth digit for the O09 code according to the reason stated in the physician's notes that the pregnancy is considered high risk. The reason might be a history of infertility (O09.0-), a very young mother (O09.61-), an older mother (O09.51-), or another issue.

The fifth or sixth character is used to report which trimester the patient is in at the encounter.

> **EXAMPLES**
>
> O09.211 Supervision of pregnancy with history of pre-term labor, first trimester
> O09.32 Supervision of pregnancy with insufficient antenatal care, second trimester

Incidental Pregnant State

You may be in an office when a pregnant woman comes in for services or treatment from a physician for a reason that has nothing to do with her pregnancy at all. Even though the actual treatment or service is not related to her pregnancy, the fact that she is pregnant will affect the way the doctor treats her condition. Therefore, you must always include code Z33.1 Pregnant state, incidental, to indicate the pregnancy. It will never be a first-listed code.

> **GUIDANCE CONNECTION**
>
> Read the ICD-10-CM Official Guidelines for Coding and Reporting, section **I. Conventions, General Coding Guidelines and Chapter Specific Guidelines,** subsection **C. Chapter-Specific Coding Guidelines,** chapter **15. Pregnancy, Childbirth, and the Puerperium,** subsection **b.2) Supervision of High-Risk Pregnancy.**

> **EXAMPLE**
>
> Wendy Weingarter is 15 weeks pregnant and works at a bank. As she was walking to her car, she slipped and fractured her toe. Dr. Stewart prescribed one pain medication rather than another because Wendy was pregnant. He also took extra precautions while x-raying her foot. You will report these codes:
>
> S92.424A Nondisplaced fracture of distal phalanx of right great toe, initial encounter
> Z33.1 Pregnant state, incidental

YOU CODE IT! CASE STUDY

Genesa Thurston, a 31-year-old female, G1 P0, came to see Dr. Mallard for her routine 20-week prenatal checkup. Dr. Mallard noted that Genesa's blood pressure was elevated and told her to come back in 10 days for a recheck.

You Code It!

Go through the steps of coding, and determine the code or codes that should be reported for this encounter between Dr. Mallard and Genesa.

Step #1: Read the case carefully and completely.

Step #2: Abstract the scenario. Which key words or terms describe why the physician cared for the patient during this encounter?

Step #3: Are there any details missing or incomplete for which you would need to query the physician? [If so, ask your instructor.]

Step #4: Check for any relevant guidance, including reading all of the symbols and notations in the Tabular List and the appropriate sections of the Official Guidelines.

Step #5: Determine the correct diagnosis code or codes to explain why this encounter was medically necessary.

Step #6: Double-check your work.

Answer:

Did you determine these to be the correct codes?

Z34.02	Encounter for supervision of normal first pregnancy, second trimester
R03.0	Elevated blood pressure reading, without diagnosis of hypertension

Good job!

Labor and Delivery

The time has come for the baby to make its way into the world (see Figure 17-3). When the event goes picture-perfectly, requiring minimal or very little assistance from the obstetrician, everything is simpler, including the coding. On the mother's chart, every encounter that results in the birth of a baby requires at least two codes:

- The delivery itself.
- The outcome of that delivery—number of babies, alive or not (Z37.-).

Additional codes may be required if there are any complications.

Normal Delivery

When a baby comes by the old-fashioned route—spontaneous, full-term, vaginal, live-born, single infant—and there are *no current* complications or issues related to the pregnancy, your principal diagnostic code will be

O80 Encounter for full-term uncomplicated delivery

GUIDANCE CONNECTION

Read the ICD-10-CM Official Guidelines for Coding and Reporting, section **I. Conventions, General Coding Guidelines and Chapter Specific Guidelines**, subsection **C. Chapter-Specific Coding Guidelines**, chapter **15. Pregnancy, Childbirth, and the Puerperium**, subsections **b.4) When a delivery occurs** and **n. Normal Delivery, Code O80**.

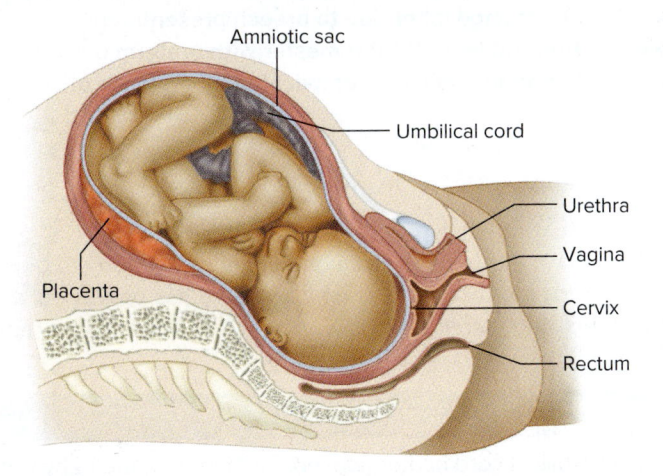

FIGURE 17-3 An illustration identifying the anatomical sites of a pregnant uterus and related parts of the female anatomy Roiger, Deborah, *Anatomy & Physiology: Foundations for the Health Professions*, 1/e. ©2013 McGraw-Hill Education. Figure 16.20, pg. 619. Used with permission.

Vertex presentation Breech presentation

Shoulder presentation

FIGURE 17-4 Illustrations of various birth presentations

Antepartum conditions may have been a concern; however, in order to use code O80, they must have been resolved prior to the big event.

When a pregnant woman is admitted into the hospital and delivers the baby during this admission, the principal diagnosis code should be the reason documented for admitting her, whether or not it is related to the delivery of the baby.

Special Circumstances Related to Delivery

The process of labor and the ultimate delivery of a baby is a natural and joyous occasion. Of course, things don't always happen as they should. There may be an issue that requires ongoing observation, admission into the hospital, or some other factor requiring a change to the original delivery plan (see Figure 17-4). For example:

O64.1xx-	Obstructed labor due to breech presentation
O60.14xx-	Preterm labor third trimester with preterm delivery third trimester
O69.0xx-	Labor and delivery complicated by prolapse of cord

> **GUIDANCE CONNECTION**
>
> Read the ICD-10-CM Official Guidelines for Coding and Reporting, section **I. Conventions, General Coding Guidelines and Chapter Specific Guidelines,** subsection **C. Chapter-Specific Coding Guidelines,** chapter **15. Pregnancy, Childbirth, and the Puerperium,** subsection **a.6) 7th character for Fetus Identification.**

LET'S CODE IT! SCENARIO

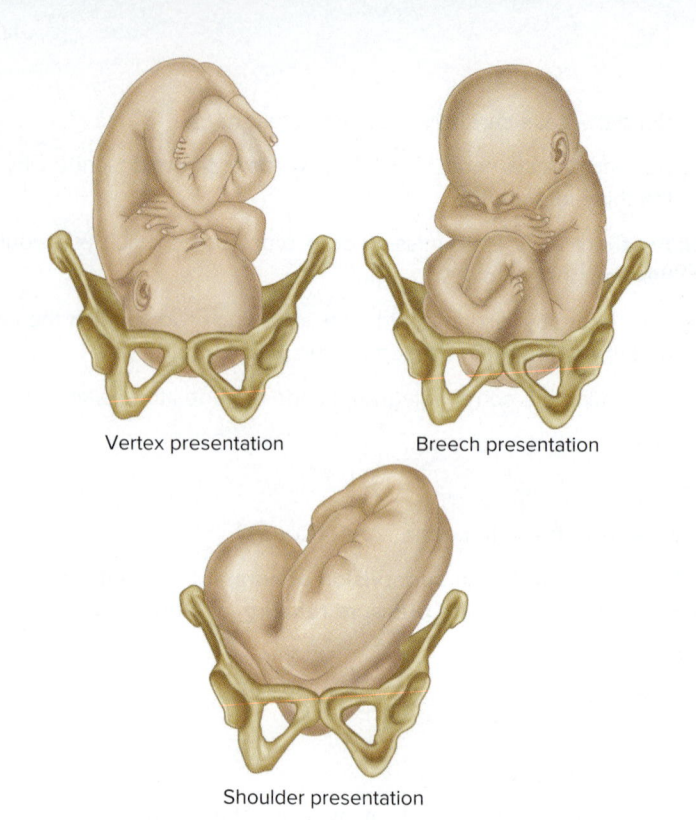

Annette Spearman, a 33-year-old female, G1 P0, is in the birthing room and in full labor, ready to give birth to her baby vaginally. All of a sudden, Dr. Tatum tells her to stop pushing. The umbilical cord has prolapsed, and they cannot seem to move it. Dr. Tatum immediately orders Annette into the OR, where he performs a c-section. Annette's baby girl was born without further incident.

Let's Code It!

Dr. Tatum performed a c-section because the umbilical cord had *prolapsed,* endangering the baby's well-being. This is an example of a complication of childbirth. How should you look it up in the Alphabetic Index? Looking up the word *complication* won't work, so let's take a look at the key diagnostic words, the reason *why* Dr. Tatum performed the c-section (the procedure)—*prolapsed umbilical cord.*

> Prolapse, prolapsed
>   umbilical cord
>   complicating delivery O69.0

Let's check this out in the Tabular List. You find

> ✓4th O69   Labor and delivery complicated by umbilical cord complications

There is a notation about the seventh character required. First, you must determine the first six characters, so continue reading down. The code suggested by the Alphabetic Index is the first one:

> ✓7th O69.0xx-   Labor and delivery complicated by prolapse of cord

Notice that the code requires a seventh character. Go back up to the list shown directly below the O69 category. Which is the most accurate seventh character? A single baby was delivered:

> O69.0xx0   Labor and delivery complicated by prolapse of cord, single gestation

Good job! You will also need to report an outcome-of-delivery code. Keep reading to learn all about this.

Outcome of Delivery

As stated earlier in this chapter, *every* time a patient gives birth during an encounter, you have to code the birth process (the delivery code) *and* you have to report the result of that birth process (the outcome-of-delivery code).

The very last code on the mother's chart that will have anything to do with the baby is a code chosen from the Z37 Outcome of delivery category. The fourth character for the code is determined by two elements:

1. How many babies were born during this delivery.
2. Live-born, stillborn (dead), or, if a multiple birth, a combination.

CODING BITE

Once a baby is born, the baby gets his or her own chart. From that point forward, anything having to do with the baby is coded for the baby and stays off the mother's chart.

Remember that the very last code directly relating to the baby that is placed on the mother's chart is a code from category **Z37 Outcome of delivery**. The *very first code on the baby's chart* will be from code category **Z38 Liveborn infants according to place of birth and type of delivery**. This Z code is used to report that a newborn baby has arrived, and it is always the principal (first-listed) code. A code from this category can be used only once, for the date of birth.

GUIDANCE CONNECTION

Read the ICD-10-CM Official Guidelines for Coding and Reporting, section **I. Conventions, General Coding Guidelines and Chapter Specific Guidelines,** subsection **C. Chapter-Specific Coding Guidelines,** chapter **15. Pregnancy, Childbirth, and the Puerperium,** subsection **b.5) Outcome of delivery.**

LET'S CODE IT! SCENARIO

Shoshanna Betterman, a 29-year-old female, had some third-trimester bleeding, so she went to her doctor. Dr. Patterson performed a pelvic examination and was concerned. A transvaginal ultrasound scan confirmed that she was suffering from total placenta previa. Because she is in her 36th week, Dr. Patterson arranged to do a c-section immediately. Shoshanna's baby girl was born without further incident.

(continued)

> ### Let's Code It!
>
> Dr. Patterson performed a c-section on Shoshanna because she had *total placenta previa with bleeding*. Go to the Alphabetic Index and look up
>
> > **Placenta, placental** — *see* **Pregnancy, complicated by (care of) (management affected by), specified condition**
>
> So let's turn to
>
> > **Pregnancy**
> >   **complicated by (care of) (management affected by)**
> >   **placenta previa O44.0-**
>
> In the Tabular List, you confirm it is an appropriate code. Start reading at
>
> > ☑4 **O44**   **Placenta previa**
>
> There are no notations or directives, so keep reading down the column to determine the most accurate fourth character:
>
> > ☑5 **O44.0-**   **Complete placenta previa NOS or without hemorrhage**
> > ☑5 **O44.1-**   **Complete placenta previa with hemorrhage**
>
> Be certain not to go too fast, or you might miss that the first code, O44.0, states, "without hemorrhage." Shoshanna was hemorrhaging (bleeding). This makes O44.1 more accurate.
>
> Now, you need to determine the required fifth character. As with all codes in this chapter of ICD-10-CM, you will need to determine, from the documentation, which trimester Paula was in at this encounter. Dr. Patterson stated, "some third-trimester bleeding."
>
> Put it all together and your code for this encounter is
>
> > **O44.13**   **Complete placenta previa with hemorrhage, third trimester**
>
> That's good. But coding for the encounter with Shoshanna is not complete.
>
> Shoshanna is in only her 36th week of gestation. Therefore, you need to include this detail. Turn to the Alphabetic Index and look up *weeks*—nothing there. Try *gestation*—not there either. Let's turn to
>
> > **Pregnancy**
> >   **weeks of gestation**
> >   **36 weeks Z3A.36**
>
> Turn to the Tabular List to confirm, as is required by the Official Guidelines:
>
> > ☑4 **Z3A**   **Weeks of gestation**
> >   **Z3A.36**   **36 weeks gestation**
>
> Terrific! You need one more code, to report the outcome of delivery. Shoshanna had one live-born baby.
>
> > ☑4 **Z37**   **Outcome of delivery**
>
> There are no notations or directives, so read down the column to determine the required fourth character that will accurately report Shoshanna's outcome of delivery:
>
> > **Z37.0**   **Outcome of delivery, single live birth**
>
> Excellent!
>
> > **O44.13**   **Placenta previa with hemorrhage, third trimester**
> > **Z3A.36**   **36 weeks gestation**
> > **Z37.0**   **Outcome of delivery, single live birth**

> **CODING BITES**
>
> The last code on the mother's chart regarding the baby is a code from category **Z37 Outcome of delivery.** Once the baby is born, he or she will get his or her own chart. The first code on the baby's chart is a code from category **Z38 Liveborn infants according to place of birth and type of delivery.** More information about coding for the baby's medical record is coming up later in this chapter.

> **CODING BITES**
>
> *Preterm labor* is defined as the spontaneous onset of labor before 37 completed weeks of gestation.

> ### YOU CODE IT! CASE STUDY
>
> Charles Wallace drove his wife, Angela, a 30-year-old female, to the hospital. She had gone into labor, but she was only at 35 weeks gestation. Dr. Callahan assisted in the delivery of her twin girls. However, there was a problem, and one of the twins was stillborn.
>
> #### You Code It!
>
> Review Dr. Callahan's notes on this encounter with Angela and the birth process, and determine the most accurate codes.
>
> Step #1: Read the case carefully and completely.
>
> Step #2: Abstract the scenario. Which key words or terms describe why the physician cared for the patient during this encounter?
>
> Step #3: Are there any details missing or incomplete for which you would need to query the physician? [If so, ask your instructor.]
>
> Step #4: Check for any relevant guidance, including reading all of the symbols and notations in the Tabular List and the appropriate sections of the Official Guidelines.
>
> Step #5: Determine the correct diagnosis code or codes to explain why this encounter was medically necessary.
>
> Step #6: Double-check your work.
>
> **Answer:**
>
> Did you determine these to be the correct codes?
>
> | | |
> |---|---|
> | O60.14x1 | Preterm labor third trimester with preterm delivery third trimester, fetus 1 |
> | O60.14x2 | Preterm labor third trimester with preterm delivery third trimester, fetus 2 |
> | Z3A.35 | 35 weeks gestation |
> | Z37.3 | Outcome of delivery, twins, one liveborn and one stillborn |
>
> Good job!

17.6 Pregnancies with Complications

A complication of pregnancy is considered to be any condition or illness that may

- Threaten the pregnant state, such as an ectopic pregnancy or an abortion.
- Affect or threaten the health of the woman, such as hemorrhage or vomiting.
- Influence the manner in which the woman will be treated, such as preexisting cardiovascular disease or chromosomal abnormality in the fetus.

A complication may be something as common as mild hyperemesis gravidarum (code O21.0), commonly known as *morning sickness,* or something of concern, such as a kidney infection (e.g., O23.03 Infections of kidney in pregnancy, third trimester).

> **YOU CODE IT! CASE STUDY**
>
> Vitalita Meadows, a 31-year-old female, G2 P1, is 17 weeks pregnant. Dr. Kramer is meeting with her to discuss her lab test results, which indicate that Vitalita has anemia. Dr. Kramer is concerned about how the anemia will affect her pregnancy.
>
> ### You Code It!
>
> Go through the steps of coding, and determine the code or codes that should be reported for this encounter between Dr. Kramer and Vitalita.
>
> Step #1: Read the case carefully and completely.
>
> Step #2: Abstract the scenario. Which key words or terms describe why the physician cared for the patient during this encounter?
>
> Step #3: Are there any details missing or incomplete for which you would need to query the physician? [If so, ask your instructor.]
>
> Step #4: Check for any relevant guidance, including reading all of the symbols and notations in the Tabular List and the appropriate sections of the Official Guidelines.
>
> Step #5: Determine the correct diagnosis code or codes to explain why this encounter was medically necessary.
>
> Step #6: Double-check your work.
>
> **Answer:**
>
> Did you determine this to be the correct code?
>
> O99.012   Anemia complicating pregnancy, second trimester
>
> Good work!

GUIDANCE CONNECTION

Read the ICD-10-CM Official Guidelines for Coding and Reporting, section **I. Conventions, General Coding Guidelines and Chapter Specific Guidelines,** subsection **C. Chapter-Specific Coding Guidelines,** chapter **15. Pregnancy, Childbirth, and the Puerperium,** subsections **c. Pre-existing conditions versus conditions due to the pregnancy, d. Pre-existing hypertension in pregnancy,** and **g. Diabetes mellitus in pregnancy.**

Preexisting Conditions Affecting Pregnancy

Some diseases and illnesses are coded differently when the only thing that has changed is that the woman is now pregnant. Such cases most often involve conditions, such as diabetes mellitus or hypertension, that are systemic (involving the whole body) and, therefore, will complicate the pregnancy, childbirth, or puerperium:

O10.01-	Pre-existing essential hypertension complicating pregnancy
O11-	Pre-existing hypertension with pre-eclampsia
O24.01-	Pre-existing diabetes mellitus, type 1, in pregnancy
O24.11-	Pre-existing diabetes mellitus, type 2, in pregnancy
O24.81-	Other pre-existing diabetes mellitus in pregnancy
O98.7-	HIV complicating pregnancy, childbirth, and the puerperium

Gestational Conditions

Other conditions solely related to pregnancy may make caring for a woman and her unborn baby more challenging. Gestational conditions develop as a result of any of the many changes a woman's body goes through and are typically transient, meaning they are expected to go away once the pregnancy is complete.

O13-	Gestational [pregnancy-induced] hypertension without significant proteinuria
O22.43	Hemorrhoids in pregnancy, third trimester
O24.4-	Gestational diabetes mellitus

Multiple Gestations

Code category O30 provides you with the code options available to report a multiple gestation. In addition to determining the number of fetuses from the documentation, you will also need to determine

- The number of placentae (monochorionic, dichorionic, or more).
- The number of amniotic sacs (monoamniotic, diamniotic, or more).
- The specific trimester the gestation is in during this encounter.

> ### EXAMPLES
>
> O30.032   Twin pregnancy, monochorionic/diamniotic, second trimester
> O30.111   Triplet pregnancy with two or more monochorionic fetuses, first trimester

Fetal Abnormalities

When a woman is pregnant, all care for both her and the baby is provided to the woman herself. Therefore, if there is a change to the treatment or care plan of the mother that is prompted by an issue with the fetus, it must be documented and reported. This may be necessary to support medical necessity for admission to the hospital, for example. Code categories O35 Maternal care for known or suspected fetal abnormality and damage and O36 Maternal care for other fetal problems provide you with the options.

> ### EXAMPLES
>
> O36.593-   Maternal care for other known or suspected poor fetal growth, third trimester
> This diagnosis would explain the medical necessity for the mother being referred to a nutritionist for a special diet.
>
> O35.3XX-   Maternal care for (suspected) damage to fetus from viral disease in mother
> This diagnosis would explain the medical necessity for the mother to have special laboratory tests or an amniocentesis.
>
> *Note:* The seventh character reports which fetus is, or may be, damaged or abnormal. The number 0 (zero) is used for a single gestation, the number 1 for the first of a multiple gestation, the number 2 for the second fetus, and so on.

Seventh Character

You may have noticed that many pregnancy complication codes require a seventh character. If the pregnancy is a single gestation, you will report a zero (0). However, when there is more than one fetus, you will need to determine, from the documentation, which specific fetus is having the problem described by the code. For example:

O64.2xx3   Obstructed labor due to face presentation, fetus 3
O69.1xx2   Labor and delivery complicated by cord around neck, with compression, fetus 2

Postpartum and Peripartum Conditions

After the birth, the woman's body continues to go through changes. In some cases, treatment of an antepartum condition extends into the postpartum period. On other occasions, health care concerns develop during or after delivery. The *postpartum* period begins at delivery and extends for 6 weeks. The *peripartum* period runs from the beginning of the last month of pregnancy and ends 5 months after delivery.

GUIDANCE CONNECTION

Read the ICD-10-CM Official Guidelines for Coding and Reporting, section **I. Conventions, General Coding Guidelines and Chapter Specific Guidelines,** subsection **C. Chapter-Specific Coding Guidelines,** chapter **15. Pregnancy, Childbirth, and the Puerperium,** subsection **e. Fetal Conditions Affecting the Management of the Mother.**

> **GUIDANCE CONNECTION**
>
> Read the ICD-10-CM Official Guidelines for Coding and Reporting, section **I. Conventions, General Coding Guidelines and Chapter Specific Guidelines**, subsection **C. Chapter-Specific Coding Guidelines**, chapter **15. Pregnancy, Childbirth, and the Puerperium**, subsection **o. The Peripartum and Postpartum Periods**.

Routine postpartum care, just like routine prenatal care, is reported with a Z code:

Z39.0   Encounter for care and examination of mother immediately after delivery
Z39.1   Encounter for care and examination of lactating mother
Z39.2   Encounter for routine postpartum follow-up

Whenever the health care concern arises—even if the diagnosis falls outside the 6-week period—if the physician's notes document that it is a postpartum complication, or pregnancy-related, you are to code it as a postpartum condition.

Sequelae (Late Effects) of Obstetric Complications

Late effects of obstetric complications, as identified by the attending physician in his or her notes, are coded the same way as all other sequelae. The late effect code—O94 Sequelae of complication of pregnancy, childbirth, and the puerperium—is added when a condition begins during pregnancy but requires continued treatment. The code is placed after the code describing the actual health condition. Notice the notation beneath this code:

> *Code first* condition resulting from (sequela) of complication of pregnancy, childbirth, and the puerperium

YOU CODE IT! CASE STUDY

Marjorie Ableman, a 31-year-old female, gave birth, vaginally, to a beautiful baby girl 3 weeks ago. She comes today to see Dr. Beale because of feelings of fatigue. After exam and blood tests, Dr. Beale diagnoses her with postpartum cervical infection caused by Enterococcus.

You Code It!

Go through the steps of coding, and determine the code or codes that should be reported for this encounter between Dr. Beale and Marjorie.

Step #1: Read the case carefully and completely.

Step #2: Abstract the scenario. Which key words or terms describe why the physician cared for the patient during this encounter?

Step #3: Are there any details missing or incomplete for which you would need to query the physician? [If so, ask your instructor.]

Step #4: Check for any relevant guidance, including reading all of the symbols and notations in the Tabular List and the appropriate sections of the Official Guidelines.

Step #5: Determine the correct diagnosis code or codes to explain why this encounter was medically necessary.

Step #6: Double-check your work.

Answer:

Did you determine these to be the correct codes?

O86.11   Cervicitis following delivery
B95.2   Enterococcus as the cause of diseases classified elsewhere
O94   Sequela of complication of pregnancy, childbirth, and the puerperium

Abortive Outcomes

The term **abortion** should not automatically start a political or religious discussion. Abortions can be spontaneous (caused by a biological or natural trigger) or be induced (initiated by an artificial or therapeutic source). What is commonly known as a *miscarriage* is clinically known as an *abortion*.

Many different situations can result in the loss of the fetus:

- O00.-   Ectopic pregnancy
- O01.-   Hydatidiform mole
- O02.-   Other abnormal products of conception
- O03.-   Spontaneous abortion
- O04.-   Complications following (induced) termination of pregnancy
- O07.-   Failed attempted termination of pregnancy

> **Abortion**
> The end of a pregnancy prior to or subsequent to the death of a fetus.

> **GUIDANCE CONNECTION**
>
> Read the ICD-10-CM Official Guidelines for Coding and Reporting, section **I. Conventions, General Coding Guidelines and Chapter Specific Guidelines,** subsection **C. Chapter-Specific Coding Guidelines,** chapter **15. Pregnancy, Childbirth, and the Puerperium,** subsection **q. Termination of Pregnancy and Spontaneous Abortions.**

> **GUIDANCE CONNECTION**
>
> Read the ICD-10-CM Official Guidelines for Coding and Reporting, section **I. Conventions, General Coding Guidelines and Chapter Specific Guidelines,** subsection **C. Chapter-Specific Coding Guidelines,** chapter **16. Certain Conditions Originating in the Perinatal Period,** subsection **a. General Perinatal Rules.**

EXAMPLE

Nellie, a 22-year-old female who was 10 weeks pregnant, was reading a text message while driving her SUV in slow traffic and didn't notice that the car in front of her had stopped. She hit it. The steering wheel struck and severely bruised her abdomen. This trauma caused her to hemorrhage, resulting in a complete miscarriage. You would report these codes:

- O03.6   Delayed or excessive hemorrhage following complete or unspecified spontaneous abortion
- V47.5xxA   Car driver injured in collision with fixed or stationary object in traffic accident initial encounter

17.7 Neonates and Congenital Anomalies

Neonates

Once a baby is born, the baby gets his or her own chart. From that point forward, anything having to do with the baby is coded for the baby and stays off the mother's chart.

Remember that the very last code directly relating to the baby that is placed on the mother's chart is a code from category Z37 Outcome of delivery. The *very first code on the baby's chart* will be from code category Z38 Liveborn infants according to place of birth and type of delivery. This Z code is used to report that a newborn baby has arrived, and it is always the principal (first-listed) code. A code from this category can be used only once, for the date of birth.

> **LET'S CODE IT! SCENARIO**
>
> Tristan Allen Montegro was born via vaginal delivery in the McGraw Birthing Center at 10:58 a.m. on September 1. He weighed 8 pounds 5 ounces and was 21 inches long, with Apgar scores of 9 and 9. Dr. Grall, a pediatrician, performed a comprehensive examination immediately following Tristan's birth. Baby Tristan was sent home at 6:30 p.m. in the care of his mother, Arashala.
>
> *(continued)*

> ### Let's Code It!
>
> Tristan was just born, and this is his first health care chart. As you learned, his very first code must be from the Z38 range. As with all other cases, begin in the Alphabetic Index. What should you look up? *Birth* would be a logical choice. However, when you turn to this term in the Alphabetic Index, you are going to see a long list of adjectives, none of which applies to Tristan, or any other baby being born without a problem. As you look down the list, you may notice this item:
>
> **Birth**
>
> There is nothing here that fits. Let's go look up the term *newborn*.
>
> **Newborn (infant) (liveborn) (singleton) Z38.2**
>
> Check Dr. Smith's notes. It is documented that Tristan was a *single, liveborn* baby.
> Let's go to the Tabular List and look at our choices. Begin with
>
> ☑4 **Z38**   **Liveborn infants according to place of birth and type of delivery**
>
> As you read down, you can see that code Z38.2 reports *Single liveborn infant, unspecified as to place of birth*. The documentation clearly indicates where Tristan was born—in the McGraw Birthing Center (not a part of a hospital). So this code is not accurate. Keep reading. The answer from the documentation will bring you to the correct code:
>
> **Z38.1**   **Single liveborn infant, born outside the hospital**
>
> Good work!

> **GUIDANCE CONNECTION**
>
> Read the ICD-10-CM Official Guidelines for Coding and Reporting, section **I. Conventions, General Coding Guidelines and Chapter Specific Guidelines,** subsection **C. Chapter-Specific Coding Guidelines,** chapter **16. Certain Conditions Originating in the Perinatal Period,** subsection **b. Observation and Evaluation of Newborns for Suspected Conditions not Found.**

Clinically Significant
Signs, symptoms, and/or conditions present at birth that may impact the child's future health status.

Suspected Conditions Not Found

After a neonate comes into the world, there may be concerns requiring tests to be run or for the baby to stay in the hospital longer. When there is good news, and it turns out the baby is healthy and all the tests are negative, how will you report the medical necessity for the tests and extended stay in the hospital? You will report code Z05 Encounter for Observation and evaluation of newborns for suspected conditions ruled out to explain the circumstances.

For a readmission to the hospital or an outpatient encounter, Z05 may be used as a principal or first-listed diagnosis code.

Clinically Significant Conditions

The guidelines state that you must code all clinically significant conditions noted on the baby's chart during the standard newborn examination. You may be concerned about how you, as a coder, can determine what is **clinically significant** and what is not. Good news! It is not your decision to make. Only the physician can determine and document this. However, you must ensure that the documentation gives you the diagnostic conditions that support any of the following:

- *Therapeutic treatments performed:* For example, perhaps the baby is placed on a respirator.
- *Diagnostic procedures done:* For example, perhaps additional and specific blood tests are performed on the baby.
- *Keeping the baby in the hospital longer than usual:* Perhaps the physician is concerned about an issue so he or she does not discharge the baby yet.
- *Increased monitoring or nursing care:* Perhaps the physician orders 24-hour private-duty nursing care for continuous monitoring.

- *Any implication that the child will need health care services in the future* as a result of a condition, sign, or symptom that can be identified now: Perhaps there is evidence that there may be brain damage as a result of the birth process; however, this cannot be confirmed until the child is about 2 years old.

When a congenital or **perinatal** condition has been resolved and no longer has an impact on the child's health and well-being, you will need to assign a code from the range Z85–Z87, Personal history of . . . .

Maternal Conditions Affecting the Infant

When the physician's notes specify that a mother's illness, injury, or condition had a direct impact on the baby's health, you will include a code on the baby's chart from the subsection code range P00–P04 Newborn affected by maternal factors and by complications of pregnancy, labor, and delivery.

Conditions in the mother, such as nutrition, smoking, high blood pressure, the presence of certain infections, or an abnormal uterus or cervix, can increase the possibilities that the baby might be born **prematurely** and/or with a **low birth weight (LBW)**. A mother's heart, kidney, and/or lung problems might also affect the baby's health.

While the reasons are not completely understood by physicians, a woman may experience spontaneous *premature rupture of the membranes* (PROM), which results in spontaneous preterm labor. There is virtually nothing that can be done to prevent the situation that so often leads to the birth of a premature, LBW baby.

A preterm (premature) neonate is one who has been in gestation for at least 28 completed weeks but less than 37 completed weeks (or between 196 and 258 completed days). While the baby's chart will almost always include a notation of the number of weeks gestation at birth, you are permitted to code "prematurity" only when it is specifically documented by the physician.

A weight of less than 2,500 grams at birth is also an indicator of prematurity. When a fetus has not had the prescribed length of time to grow, the neonate can be susceptible to certain health concerns, realized in the near or distant future.

Premature, LBW babies are more likely to be at risk for developing certain conditions now and later in life. Incomplete growth of the fetus's central nervous system can result in feeding difficulties for the neonate/infant, recurrent apnea, and/or poor vasomotor control. Testing for neonatal hyperbilirubinemia, especially when jaundice is visible, can indicate that the liver did not develop sufficiently to create and excrete bilirubin (a yellowish component of bile that is made by the liver). This is why it is so important that the documentation and the coding accurately report the baby's situation from the beginning. Some of the most common conditions include these:

- Breathing problems, including respiratory distress syndrome (RDS).
- Periventricular and/or intraventricular hemorrhage (bleeding in the brain).
- Patent ductus arteriosus (PDA), a dangerous heart problem.
- Necrotizing enterocolitis (NEC), an intestinal problem that leads to difficulties in feeding.
- Retinopathy of prematurity (ROP).
- Low body temperature (caused by a lack of body fat used by newborns to maintain normal body temperature), which promotes slow growth, breathing problems, and other complications.
- Apnea, an interruption in breathing.
- Jaundice, a result of incomplete liver development.
- Anemia.
- Bronchopulmonary dysplasia, also known as *chronic lung disease*.
- Infections, due to the inability of immature immune systems to fight off bacteria and viruses.

Perinatal
The time period from before birth to the 28th day after birth.

Prematurity
Birth occurring prior to the completion of 37 weeks gestation.

Low Birth Weight (LBW)
A baby born weighing less than 5 pounds 8 ounces, or 2,500 grams.

GUIDANCE CONNECTION

Read the ICD-10-CM Official Guidelines for Coding and Reporting, section **I. Conventions, General Coding Guidelines and Chapter Specific Guidelines**, subsection **C. Chapter-Specific Coding Guidelines**, chapter **16. Certain Conditions Originating in the Perinatal Period**, subsections **a.6) Code all clinically significant conditions** and **c. Coding Additional Perinatal Diagnoses**.

CODING BITES

Usually, the physician will write the baby's birth weight in grams. However, you should learn how to convert from pounds and ounces to grams:

1 ounce = 28.350 gm
1 pound = 16 oz
= 453.6 gm

Mortality
Death.

Morbidity
Unhealthy.

> **CODING BITES**
>
> Codes from category P05 and category P07 may not be reported on the same claim at the same time.

Respiratory distress syndrome (RDS) is the leading cause of **mortality** and **morbidity** of premature neonates. The immature lungs have an insufficient quantity of surfactant—the secretion within the lungs that supports the alveoli and keeps them from collapsing. Maternal diabetes and neonatal asphyxia are known contributing factors. RDS causes hypoxia, which can then lead to pulmonary ischemia, pulmonary capillary damage, and fluid leaking inappropriately into the alveoli. Cyanosis, increased respiratory effort, anoxia, and acidosis are signs and complications. Report a diagnosis of RDS with code P22.0 Respiratory distress syndrome of newborn.

You will find the codes needed to report an infant's prematurity and/or LBW, as well as long gestation and high birth weight, as documented in the physician's notes, within these code categories:

P05	Disorders of newborn related to slow fetal growth and fetal malnutrition
P07	Disorders of newborn related to short gestation and low birth weight, not elsewhere classified
P08	Disorders of newborn related to long gestation and high birth weight

GUIDANCE CONNECTION

Read the ICD-10-CM Official Guidelines for Coding and Reporting, section **I. Conventions, General Coding Guidelines and Chapter Specific Guidelines**, subsection **C. Chapter-Specific Coding Guidelines**, chapter **16. Certain Conditions Originating in the Perinatal Period**, subsections **d. Prematurity and Fetal Growth Retardation** and **e. Low birth weight and immaturity status**.

YOU CODE IT! CASE STUDY

Harper Anne Glosick was born today at 27 weeks 2 days gestation by cesarean section at Hillside Hospital. She weighed 945 grams at birth, and her lungs are immature. Dr. McArthur admits Harper into the neonatal intensive care unit (NICU) with a diagnosis of extreme immaturity.

You Code It!

Read through Dr. McArthur's notes on Harper, and determine the correct diagnosis code or codes.

Step #1: Read the case carefully and completely.

Step #2: Abstract the scenario. Which key words or terms describe why the physician cared for the patient during this encounter?

Step #3: Are there any details missing or incomplete for which you would need to query the physician? [If so, ask your instructor.]

Step #4: Check for any relevant guidance, including reading all of the symbols and notations in the Tabular List and the appropriate sections of the Official Guidelines.

Step #5: Determine the correct diagnosis code or codes to explain why this encounter was medically necessary.

Step #6: Double-check your work.

Answer:

Did you determine these to be the correct codes?

Z38.01	Single liveborn, infant, delivered by Cesarean
P07.03	Extremely low birth weight newborn, 750–999 grams
P07.26	Extreme immaturity of newborn, gestational age 27 completed weeks

Well-Baby Checks

These encounters, just like adult physicals and other checkups, are scheduled by the age of the child: 2 to 4 days, 1 month, 2 months, 4 months, 6 months, 9 months, 1 year, 15 months, 18 months, 2 years, 2.5 years, 3 years, and then annually. The age of the child also influences which codes are reported for the well-baby encounter:

Z00.110	Health examination for newborn under 8 days old
Z00.111	Health examination for newborn 8 to 28 days old
Z00.121	Encounter for routine child health examination with abnormal findings
	Use additional code to identify abnormal findings
Z00.129	Encounter for routine child health examination without abnormal findings

> **CODING BITES**
>
> See the notation beneath code category P07:
>
> *Note: When both birth weight and gestational age of the newborn are available, both should be coded with birth weight sequenced before gestational age.*

LET'S CODE IT! SCENARIO

Roseanna Glassman brought her 39-day-old daughter, Marisol, to Dr. Granger for her routine health check. During the examination, Roseanna related that Marisol's head accidentally was banged into the table and she was worried about neurologic problems. Dr. Granger checked her head and found no bruise or laceration. To calm Roseanna, he took Marisol down the hall to have a special neurologic screening for traumatic brain injury. Fortunately, the scan was negative.

Let's Code It!

What key words in the notes provide you with the information you need to report this encounter? Why did Dr. Granger care for Marisol? Marisol was brought in for her "*routine health check*"—her regular well-baby visit. What will you look up in the Alphabetic Index? *Routine*? Nothing there. *Well-baby*? Nothing there. Try a term that is not technically a diagnosis: *examination*. Take a look and find

Examination (for) (following) (general) (of) (routine) Z00.00

Read down the long list of additional descriptors and find

Child (over 28 days old) Z00.129

That sounds accurate. So let's turn to the Tabular List and check it out:

☑4 **Z00** Encounter for general examination without complaint, suspected or reported diagnosis

There are no notations or directives, so read down the column to determine the most accurate fourth character:

☑6 **Z00.12** Encounter for routine child health examination

Read the notations beneath this code. First, notice that it states "Health check (routine) for child over 28 days old." How old is Marisol? She is 39 days, so this is the correct code. Carefully read the **EXCLUDES1** notation, and ask yourself: Does this apply to Dr. Granger's caring for Marisol during this encounter? No, it doesn't. Read down to review the sixth-character choices. The notes state that he did a neurologic screening because of the bang to her head. You will need to check the documentation for the results of this screening so you can report "abnormal findings" or not. The documentation states that "the scan was negative," so you will report this code:

Z00.129 Encounter for routine child health examination without abnormal findings

You still need to report the neurologic screening. Go back to the Alphabetic Index and look up

Screening (for) Z13.9
  neurological condition Z13.89

That's really the only suggested code, so let's take a look at it in the Tabular List:

☑4 **Z13** Encounter for screening for other diseases and disorders

(continued)

Go back to the notes and see that Dr. Granger wrote "neurologic screening for traumatic brain injury." Therefore, you know that **Z13.850 Encounter for screening for traumatic brain injury** is accurate and matches what Dr. Granger wrote in the notes.

One more code—remember, you need to report a code for the bang on the head because this led Dr. Granger to do the screening. Check the notes and see that Dr. Granger found no bruises or lacerations and that Roseanna did not report any other signs or symptoms, such as vomiting or seizure. The bang on the head will have to be reported with an external cause code because it is an external factor that explains why Dr. Granger screened Marisol for a TBI. Check the External Causes Code Alphabetic Index and look up *strike, striking* because Marisol's head struck the table (furniture). Code W22.03 is suggested. Let's check the Tabular List:

W22	Striking against or struck by other objects
W22.03x-	Walked into furniture

This cannot be accurate because Marisol is only 39 days old and she cannot walk yet. Review all of the other codes in this subsection to determine the code that will report what happened:

W22.8xxA	Striking against or struck by other objects, initial encounter

So for Marisol's visit to Dr. Granger, you have three codes to report:

Z00.129	Encounter for routine child health examination without abnormal findings
Z13.850	Encounter for screening for traumatic brain injury
W22.8xxA	Striking against or struck by other objects, initial encounter

YOU CODE IT! CASE STUDY

Ines Nancy Mulle was born, full term, vaginally at Barton Hospital. Her mother has been an alcoholic for many years and would not stop drinking during the pregnancy. Ines weighed only 1,575 grams, small for a full-term neonate. After testing, she was diagnosed at birth with fetal alcohol syndrome and admitted into the NICU.

You Code It!

Read the notes on Ines, and determine the most accurate diagnosis code(s).

Step #1: Read the case carefully and completely.

Step #2: Abstract the scenario. Which main words or terms describe why the physician cared for the patient during this encounter?

Step #3: Are there any details missing or incomplete for which you would need to query the physician? [If so, ask your instructor.]

Step #4: Check for any relevant guidance, including reading all of the symbols and notations in the Tabular List and the appropriate sections of the Official Guidelines.

Step #5: Determine the correct diagnosis code or codes to explain why this encounter was medically necessary.

Step #6: Double-check your work.

Answer:

Did you determine these to be the correct codes?

Z38.00	Single liveborn infant, delivered vaginally
P05.16	Newborn small for gestational age, 1500–1749 grams
Q86.0	Fetal alcohol syndrome (dysmorphic)

Terrific!

Genetics

Genetics is the study of diseases passed from parent to child, a process known as *hereditary transmission*. There are more than 1,000 diseases that might be inherited. A genetic disorder may be *dominant*—the result of one defective gene in a pair—or it may be *recessive*—the result of both alleles being defective. Some examples of dominant genetic disorders are *familial hypercholesterolemia* (code E87.8) and *familial retinoblastoma* (code C69.2-). Examples of recessive genetic disorders include *cystic fibrosis* (code E84.9) and *Gaucher's disease* (code E75.22). Certain diseases that have been correlated to genetics cause accelerated aging, such as *Hutchinson-Guilford progeria* (code E34.8), an inherited endocrine disorder.

If the patient is diagnosed with a specific genetic condition, you will need to report the code for the confirmed diagnosis. However, there are times when the patient does not exhibit any signs or symptoms of the condition. In these cases, it may be important to document the *family history* of the condition to support more frequent screenings or other preventive or early detection services, such as Family history of alcohol abuse and dependence, reported with code Z81.1.

Genetic Conditions versus Congenital Malformations

The term **congenital anomaly** means an abnormality present at birth and therefore refers to any variation from the norm for a neonate. The abnormality may be genetic in nature or may be a malformation that occurred during gestation. A genetic condition may indicate that a chromosomal alteration has been inherited—passed down from parent to child via chromosomal and cell structures. Or the condition may be a congenital malformation, or damage to a chromosome during formation. A congenital **malformation** means that something went awry during the gestational process. Such alterations can occur spontaneously or can be an adverse reaction to a pathogen, drug, radiation, or chemical.

Congenital
A condition existing at the time of birth.

Anomaly
An abnormal, or unexpected, condition.

Malformation
An irregular structural development.

EXAMPLES

Q91.2 Trisomy 18, translocation
Q93.3 Deletion of short arm of chromosome 4

Inherited Conditions

Your blue eyes and brown hair are the products of genetics—qualities in the chromosomes you received from your father and mother. Sadly, a genetic abnormality will negatively affect the health of a child. An inherited mutation in the DNA causes a permanent alteration that will affect each and every cell as it multiplies during the maturation of the zygote to embryo to fetus to neonate. There is also a strong probability that this person will pass this condition along to his or her children.

Congenital Anomalies

A congenital malformation, also known as a *birth defect*, is a permanent physical defect—the incomplete development of an anatomical structure—that is identified in a neonate. It may be the effect of a genetic mutation, or it may have been caused by a prenatal event. The fetal development of many organs, including the brain, heart, lungs, liver, bones, and/or intestinal tract, may have been altered by alcohol or drugs used by the mother at a particular point during gestation, by exposure to an environmental factor, or by an injury sustained during delivery.

EXAMPLES

Q14.1 Congenital malformation of retina
Q64.4 Malformation of urachus

> **GUIDANCE CONNECTION**
>
> Read the ICD-10-CM Official Guidelines for Coding and Reporting, section **I. Conventions, General Coding Guidelines and Chapter Specific Guidelines,** subsection **C. Chapter-Specific Coding Guidelines,** chapter **17. Congenital malformations, deformations, and chromosomal abnormalities.**

Testing

Health care research has found ways to identify the presence or the likelihood of genetic disorders and congenital anomalies.

Genetic testing can be performed prior to fertilization so the potential parents can gain insights on the possibility of passing along certain diseases to their future children. A family tree analysis, called a *pedigree,* is a diagram of the individual's family that includes diseases and causes of death. A geneticist (a physician specializing in the study of genetics) can use this diagram to identify *inheritance patterns* and probabilities. In addition, a blood test known as a *karyotype* can be used. During this test, multiple staining techniques can illuminate each chromosomal band to enable visualization of a mutation.

Prenatal blood and DNA tests can currently detect more than 600 genetic disorders prior to the baby's birth. This information can allow parents to make informed decisions and to become prepared emotionally, intellectually, and financially for the birth of a child with a genetic disorder. In addition, the physician can make certain appropriate arrangements, such as method of delivery and timing of delivery, that may reduce the severity or impact of the condition.

Amniocentesis is the process of collecting a sample of amniotic fluid via needle aspiration from a pregnant uterus. *Chorionic villus sampling* is the process of obtaining tissues from the placenta for prenatal testing by passing a catheter through the vagina and threading it up to the placenta.

Genetic tests are not limited to potential or impending parents. Adults can use this information as well. For example, many women are tested for the BRCA1 or BRCA2 gene that identifies a potential for the development of breast and/or ovarian cancer.

> **EXAMPLES**
>
> Z14.1   Cystic fibrosis carrier
> Z15.01   Genetic susceptibility to malignant neoplasm of breast

Gene Therapy

Researchers continue to experiment with gene therapy to prevent or treat these types of diseases. The goal is to find a safe and effective way to correct a malfunctioning gene. Methods currently being investigated include

- Placing a normal gene into the genome in a nonspecific place so it can provide the correct function of the nonfunctional gene.
- Using homologous recombination to remove the abnormal gene and replace it with a normal gene.
- Using selected reverse mutation to actually repair the gene so it will function properly.

In such cases, the term *placed* or *inserted* does not mean the same as it typically does in the context of other health care procedures. One method is to put the therapeutic gene into a carrier molecule, known as a *vector,* which is a genetically altered virus. Nonviral methods include the injection of the therapeutic gene directly into its target cell. However, this can be accomplished only with a limited number of tissue types. Studies are being conducted on the effectiveness of using an artificial liposome and/or certain chemicals to achieve the successful delivery of the therapeutic gene.

Genetic Disorders

Chromosomal Abnormalities

Down syndrome (trisomy 21) is a spontaneous **genetic abnormality** and is not inherited. Manifestations include mental retardation, unusual facial features including

---

Genetic Abnormality
An error in a gene (chromosome) that affects development during gestation; also known as a *chromosomal abnormality.*

slanted eyes and protruding tongue, and congenital heart defects, as well as respiratory and related complications. *Mosaicism* is possible in a child with Down syndrome. This is the occurrence of cells with two different genetic makeups within one person. The possibility of having a child with Down syndrome increases with the age of the mother at the time of delivery. Treatment of manifestations can improve the patient's quality of life and extend the life span. Use code category Q90 Down syndrome (trisomy 21), with an additional character to report nonmosaicism, mosaicism, or translocation. An additional code to identify specific physical and intellectual disabilities is required.

Klinefelter's syndrome is a genetic abnormality that results in the inclusion of an extra X chromosome in a male child. Testicular changes occur at puberty, including eventual infertility due to the deterioration of the testicles. In addition, gynecomastia may develop, learning disabilities may become apparent, facial hair may be sparse, and reduced libido causing impotence will become evident. There is a mosaic form of Klinefelter's. Report this syndrome with a code from category Q98 Other sex chromosome abnormalities, male phenotype, not elsewhere classified.

Autosomal Recessive Inherited Diseases

Cystic fibrosis is seen most often in Caucasian children and rarely seen in black or Asian populations. This disease causes chronic pulmonary disease and deficient exocrine pancreatic function, development of thickened mucus that can block bile flow from the liver, and other manifestations. Use code category E84 Cystic fibrosis, with an additional character to identify manifestations.

Tay-Sachs disease (Tay-Sachs amaurotic familial idiocy) is an inherited disease that results in the child's death before the age of 4. Symptoms include increasing deterioration of motor skills and mental acuity, identifiable in the infant at 6 to 10 months of age. Genetic tests can screen potential parents. Report this disease with code E75.02 Tay-Sachs disease.

Phenylketonuria (PKU) is a genetic disorder that causes a gradual deterioration of the patient's mental faculties, often discernable by 1 year of age. Many hospitals perform a simple blood test for PKU as a part of the birth evaluation. This condition can be treated with a semisynthetic diet. Outcomes improve with early detection. Report PKU with code E70.0 Classical phenylketonuria or E70.1 Other hyperphenylalaninemias (maternal).

Sickle cell anemia is an inherited hemolytic anemia that develops as the result of a defective hemoglobin molecule that causes the red blood cells to be misshapen. This half-moon- (sickle-) shaped cell (instead of the rounded, button shape) interferes with circulation and manifests itself as fatigue, dyspnea, and swollen joints. Pharmaceutical treatments can reduce ill health. Sickle cell disorders are grouped into code category D57 Sickle-cell disorders. You will need additional characters to identify the specific type of sickle cell, possibly requiring a pathology report at some point, and to identify whether the patient is having a crisis at this time or not. For example: D57.20 Sickle-cell/Hb-C disease without crisis.

Multifactorial Abnormalities

Cleft lip and cleft palate are malformations of the upper lip and/or palate that occur during the first 2 months of gestation. This **deformity** may be seen unilaterally or bilaterally (medial is rare) and may extend into the nasal cavity and/or the maxilla (upper jaw). Use code categories Q35 Cleft palate (additional character to identify hard palate, soft palate, etc.), Q36 Cleft lip (additional character to specify laterality), and Q37 Cleft palate with cleft lip (additional character to specify laterality).

Deformity
A size or shape (structural design) that deviates from that which is considered normal.

X-Linked Inherited Diseases

Hemophilia is an inherited hemostatic disorder that causes difficulty with the occurrence of coagulation. The abnormal bleeding can be problematic, especially after an injury or surgical procedure. On occasion, spontaneous bleeding may occur, causing damage to the brain, nerves, or muscle function, depending upon the location of the hemorrhage. Treatment can extend life expectancy. Report code D66 Hereditary factor VIII deficiency (hemophilia NOS).

Fragile X syndrome is the most frequently diagnosed underlying cause of inherited mental retardation, and it affects both males and females. An accurate pedigree would be important in predicting the likelihood of this condition because probabilities increase with each generation. Males display profound mental retardation, while females may or may not reveal this dysfunction. Use code Q99.2 Fragile X chromosome to report this condition.

Congenital Malformations

Spina bifida is a condition that results from an incomplete closure of the vertebral column, the spinal cord, or both. Presented often by a hole in the skin covering the area of the spine, it is an abnormality in the development of the central nervous system. In the 1990s, researchers discovered that folic acid (a B vitamin), when taken before and during the first trimester of pregnancy, could actually prevent some cerebral and spinal birth defects. In 1996, the U.S. Food and Drug Administration ordered that folic acid be added into breads, cereals, and other grain products. The number of cases of spina bifida dropped from 2,490 in 1995–1996 to 1,640 in 1999–2000. Spina bifida is sometimes accompanied by hydrocephalus. Code category Q05 Spina bifida (aperta) (cystica) requires an additional character to report the location on the spine (cervical, thoracic, lumbar, sacral), as well as to report the presence or absence of hydrocephalus. *Spina bifida occulta* is reported with Q76.0 Spina bifida occulta. This version of spina bifida is evidenced by a tiny gap between vertebrae with no involvement of the nervous system. It can be seen only on an x-ray of the affected area and generally has no signs or symptoms.

Congenital hernia can occur in several locations in the body, just as with adult hernias. The difference with reporting such conditions is the specification in the documentation that the hernia is congenital. Some of the codes include Q79.0 Congenital diaphragmatic hernia, Q40.1 Congenital hiatus hernia, and Q79.51 Congenital hernia of bladder.

Congenital heart defects have been determined by the CDC to affect close to 400,000 babies born in the United States each year. They are the most common type of congenital anomaly and one of the most common causes of death in infants. Research has proved a strong connection between cigarette smoking, especially during the first trimester of gestation, and neonates with pulmonary valve stenosis and type 2 atrial septal defects, among other congenital heart malformations. Code from categories Q20 Congenital malformations of cardiac chambers and connections, Q21 Congenital malformations of cardiac septa, Q23 Congenital malformations of aortic and mitral valves, and Q24 Other congenital malformations of heart. Additional characters are required to provide specific details, such as Q21.1 Atrial septal defect and Q22.1 Congenital pulmonary valve stenosis.

Chapter Summary

The urinary system is designed to remove the urea from the blood, manufacture urine, and perform waste removal by eliminating the urine. It supports many of the other body systems by ensuring fluid balance and eliminating waste products to avoid toxicity. Understanding the components of this system and their functions will help you correctly interpret the documentation to determine the most accurate code or codes. Some conditions affecting organs in the urinary system are the manifestations of other diseases, such as hypertension or diabetes, whereas others may be the result of an infectious organism. Coders must read carefully (as always) to determine the correct coding process.

The anatomical sites included in the female genital system are the definition of the phrase "private places." These organs have important functions and are susceptible to disease and injury, as with other body systems. Female anatomy includes many organs and anatomical sites that can be subject to health concerns. Well-woman exams and preventive tests should be annual events in every woman's life. Each time, a medical necessity for the visit must be documented. Remember that staying healthy or catching illness or disease early is a medical necessity.

Babies are precious and should always be treated with tender loving care. From the moment they are born, babies receive a special version of health care services created especially for them, due to their size and growth patterns. The guidelines for coding the reasons for these services are very specific. Congenital anomalies, whether inherited or caused by an interaction with a chemical, drug, or other environmental factor during gestation, can have a lifelong effect on the child as well as the family. Congenital deficits can cause a minor inconvenience, present a challenge, require years of health care treatments, or result in premature death.

CODING BITES

The *Apgar* test is named for Virginia Apgar, but it also has come to stand for the following:

Activity (muscle tone)
Pulse rate (heart rate)
Grimace (reflex response)
Appearance (skin color)
Respiratory (breathing effort)

Apgar Scoring for Newborns

Score	Interpretation
0–3	Baby needs immediate lifesaving procedures
4–6	Baby needs some assistance; requires careful monitoring
7–10	Normal

CHAPTER 17 REVIEW
Coding Genitourinary, Gynecology, Obstetrics, Congenital, and Pediatrics Conditions

Enhance your learning by completing these exercises and more at connect.mheducation.com!

Let's Check It! Terminology

Match each key term to the appropriate definition.

Part I

1. LO 17.1 The organ system responsible for removing waste products that are left behind by protein, excessive water, disproportionate amounts of electrolytes, and other nitrogenous compounds from the blood and the body.

2. LO 17.1 Inflammation of any part of the urinary tract: kidney, ureter, bladder, or urethra.

A. Anemic
B. Benign Prostatic Hyperplasia (BPH)

CHAPTER 17 REVIEW

3. LO 17.7 An error in a gene that affects development during gestation.
4. LO 17.2 Enlarged prostate that results in depressing the urethra.
5. LO 17.1 Ongoing malfunction of one or both kidneys.
6. LO 17.7 A size or shape that deviates from that which is considered normal.
7. LO 17.1 Glomerular filtration rate, the measurement of kidney function; used to determine the stage of kidney disease.
8. LO 17.2 Inflammation of the prostate.
9. LO 17.7 An irregular structural development.
10. LO 17.1 Malignancy of the urinary bladder.
11. LO 17.1 A compound that results from the breakdown of proteins and is excreted in urine.
12. LO 17.1 Suffering from a low red blood cell count.

C. Bladder Cancer
D. Chronic Kidney Disease (CKD)
E. Deformity
F. Genetic Abnormality
G. GFR
H. Malformation
I. Prostatitis
J. Urea
K. Urinary System
L. Urinary Tract Infection (UTI)

Part II

1. LO 17.4 A health care specialty focusing on the care of women during pregnancy and the puerperium.
2. LO 17.4 A physician specializing in the care of the female genital tract.
3. LO 17.5 The length of time for the complete development of a baby from conception to birth; on average, 40 weeks.
4. LO 17.4 The time period from the end of labor until the uterus returns to normal size, typically 3 to 6 weeks.
5. LO 17.5 Prior to birth; also referred to as *antenatal*.
6. LO 17.6 The end of a pregnancy prior to or subsequent to the death of a fetus.

A. Abortion
B. Gestation
C. Gynecologist
D. Obstetrics
E. Prenatal
F. Puerperium

Part III

1. LO 17.7 An abnormal, or unexpected, condition.
2. LO 17.7 A condition existing at the time of birth.
3. LO 17.7 A baby born weighing less than 5 pounds 8 ounces, or 2,500 grams.
4. LO 17.7 Unhealthy, diseased.
5. LO 17.7 The time period from before birth to the 28th day after birth.
6. LO 17.7 Birth occurring prior to the completion of 37 weeks gestation.
7. LO 17.7 Signs, symptoms, and/or conditions present at birth that may impact the child's future health status.
8. LO 17.7 Death.

A. Anomaly
B. Clinically Significant
C. Congenital
D. Low Birth Weight (LBW)
E. Morbidity
F. Mortality
G. Perinatal
H. Prematurity

Let's Check It! Concepts

Choose the most appropriate answer for each of the following questions.

1. LO 17.1 GFR below 15 is stage _____ CKD and would be coded _____.
   a. 2, N18.2
   b. 3, N18.3
   c. 4, N18.4
   d. 5, N18.5

2. LO 17.2 _____ is a condition that occurs when fluid collects within the tunica vaginalis of the scrotum, the testis, or the spermatic cord.
   a. Erectile dysfunction
   b. Oligospermia
   c. Hydrocele
   d. Benign prostatic hyperplasia

3. **LO 17.3** The patient is diagnosed with endocarditis. Which ICD-10-CM code should be used?
   a. A51.9   b. A52.06   c. A52.03   d. A51.2

4. **LO 17.4** _____ are tumors located in the female reproductive system.
   a. Uterine leiomyomas   b. Uterine fibromyomas
   c. Uterine fibroids   d. All of these

5. **LO 17.5** A woman noted to be G3 P2 has given birth
   a. once.   b. never.   c. twice.   d. four times.

6. **LO 17.5** You would use code Z33.1 for a pregnant woman who came to see the doctor for
   a. a broken leg.
   b. a regular first-pregnancy checkup.
   c. a regular third-pregnancy checkup.
   d. a regular pregnancy checkup for a woman 37 years old.

7. **LO 17.5** The encounter at which a woman gives birth will always have at least
   a. one code.   b. four codes.   c. two codes.   d. three codes.

8. **LO 17.6** All of the following would be considered a complication of a pregnancy except
   a. hyperemesis gravidarum.   b. kidney infection.
   c. hemorrhage.   d. sprained wrist.

9. **LO 17.7** A congenital malformation is also known as a(n)
   a. inherited condition.   b. birth defect.
   c. breech birth.   d. pediatric factor.

10. **LO 17.7** A newborn has been diagnosed with sepsis due to *Staphylococcus aureus*. Which code should be used to report this?
    a. B95.61   b. A41.01   c. P36.8   d. P36.2

Let's Check It! Guidelines

Part I

Refer to the Official Guidelines and fill in the blanks according to the Chapter 14, Diseases of Genitourinary System, Chapter-Specific Coding Guidelines.

mild	2	severe
query	failure or rejection	stage 1-5
based	N18	CKD
sequencing	severity	N18.3
3	relationship	I.C.19.g
Z94.0	N18.4	N18.6
diabetes mellitus and hypertension	end-stage-renal disease (ESRD)	chronic kidney disease (CKD)

1. The ICD-10-CM classifies CKD based on _____.
2. The severity of CKD is designated by _____.
3. Stage _____, code N18.2, equates to _____ CKD.
4. Stage _____, code _____, equates to moderate CKD.
5. Stage 4, code _____, equates to _____ CKD.
6. Code N18.6, End stage renal disease (ESRD), is assigned when the provider has documented _____.

7. If both a stage of CKD and ESRD are documented, assign code _____ only.
8. Patients who have undergone kidney transplant may still have some form of _____ because the kidney transplant may not fully restore kidney function. Therefore, the presence of CKD alone does not constitute a transplant complication. Assign the appropriate _____ code for the patient's stage of CKD and code _____, Kidney transplant status.
9. If a transplant complication such as _____ or other transplant complication is documented, see section _____ for information on coding complications of a kidney transplant. If the documentation is unclear as to whether the patient has a complication of the transplant, _____ the provider.
10. Patients with _____ may also suffer from other serious conditions, most commonly _____.
11. The _____ of the CKD code in _____ to codes for other contributing conditions is _____ on the conventions in the Tabular List.

Part II

Refer to the Official Guidelines and fill in the blanks according to the Chapter 15, Pregnancy, Childbirth, and the Puerperium, Chapter-Specific Coding Guidelines.

never	fetus	every	complications
7th	O09	"in childbirth"	"unspecified trimester"
prompted	Z37	priority	Z34
antepartum	trimester	insufficient	maternal
		no	

1. Chapter 15 codes have sequencing _____ over codes from other chapters.
2. Chapter 15 codes are to be used only on the _____ record, _____ on the record of the newborn.
3. The majority of codes in Chapter 15 have a final character indicating the _____ of pregnancy.
4. Whenever delivery occurs during the current admission, and there is an "in childbirth" option for the obstetric complication being coded, the _____ code should be assigned.
5. In instances when a patient is admitted to a hospital for _____ of pregnancy during one trimester and remains in the hospital into a subsequent trimester, the trimester character for the _____ complication code should be assigned on the basis of the trimester when the complication developed, not the trimester of the discharge.
6. The _____ code should rarely be used, such as when the documentation in the record is _____ to determine the trimester and it is not possible to obtain clarification.
7. Where applicable, a _____ character is to be assigned for certain categories to identify the _____ for which the complication code applies.
8. For routine outpatient prenatal visits when no complications are present, a code from category _____, Encounter for supervision of normal pregnancy, should be used as the first-listed diagnosis.
9. For routine prenatal outpatient visits for patients with high-risk pregnancies, a code from category _____, Supervision of high-risk pregnancy, should be used as the first-listed diagnosis.
10. In episodes when _____ delivery occurs, the principal diagnosis should correspond to the principal complication of the pregnancy which necessitated the encounter.
11. When an obstetric patient is admitted and delivers during that admission, the condition that _____ the admission should be sequenced as the principal diagnosis.
12. A code from category _____, Outcome of delivery, should be included on _____ maternal record when a delivery has occurred.

Part III

Refer to the Official Guidelines and fill in the blanks according to the Chapter 16, Certain Conditions Origination in the Perinatal Period, Chapter-Specific Coding Guidelines.

perinatal	condition	type	28th
life	originate	definitive	once
place	before	newborn	first
continue	not	default	Z38
never	clinically	should	

1. For coding and reporting purposes the perinatal period is defined as _____ birth through the _____ day following birth.
2. Codes in this chapter are _____ for use on the maternal record.
3. Codes from Chapter 15, the obstetric chapter, are never permitted on the _____ record.
4. Chapter 16 codes may be used throughout the _____ of the patient if the _____ is still present.
5. When coding the birth episode in a newborn record, assign a code from category _____, Liveborn infants according to _____ of birth and _____ of delivery, as the principal diagnosis.
6. A code from category Z38 is assigned only _____, to a newborn at the time of birth.
7. Codes for signs and symptoms may be assigned when a _____ diagnosis has _____ been established.
8. If the reason for the encounter is a _____ condition, the code from Chapter 16 should be sequenced _____.
9. Should a condition _____ in the perinatal period, and _____ throughout the life of the patient, the perinatal code should continue to be used regardless of the patient's age.
10. If a newborn has a condition that may be either due to the birth process or community acquired and the documentation does not indicate which it is, the _____ is due to the birth process and the code from Chapter 16 should be used.
11. All _____ significant conditions noted on routine newborn examination _____ be coded.

Let's Check It! Rules and Regulations

Please answer the following questions from the knowledge you have gained after reading this chapter.

1. **LO 17.1** Turn to the Official Guidelines for Chapter 14. Diseases of Genitourinary System—I.C.14.a.2. Discuss chronic kidney disease and kidney transplant status as outlined in the Chapter 14 guidelines.
2. **LO 17.3** Discuss how sexually transmitted diseases (STDs) are spread. Include an example of an STD and how it would be coded.
3. **LO 17.5** Explain coding the birth, including what code category goes on the mother's chart (and its sequence) and what code category goes on the newborn's chart, including its sequence and how many times this code can be reported.
4. **LO 17.7** Explain the differences between genetic conditions and congenital malformations.
5. **LO 17.4** Explain what procreative management is. Include the subcategory code for a general counseling and advice encounter.

YOU CODE IT! Basics

First, identify the condition in the following diagnoses, then code the diagnosis.

Example: Glaucoma of newborn:
a. main term: _Glaucoma_   b. diagnosis: _Q15.0_

1. Acute nephritic syndrome with dense deposit disease:
   a. main term: _____   b. diagnosis: _____
2. Recurrent hematuria with membranoproliferative glomeruloephritis:
   a. main term: _____   b. diagnosis: _____
3. Chronic interstitial nephritis, reflux associated:
   a. main term: _____   b. diagnosis: _____
4. Stricture of ureter:
   a. main term: _____   b. diagnosis: _____

5. Ovarian ectopic pregnancy:
   a. main term: _____   b. diagnosis: _____
6. Cervical shortening, third trimester:
   a. main term: _____   b. diagnosis: _____
7. Spontaneous abortion:
   a. main term: _____   b. diagnosis: _____
8. Embolism following molar pregnancy:
   a. main term: _____   b. diagnosis: _____
9. Respiratory failure of newborn:
   a. main term: _____   b. diagnosis: _____
10. Neonatal tachycardia:
    a. main term: _____   b. diagnosis: _____
11. Dehydration of newborn:
    a. main term: _____   b. diagnosis: _____
12. Neonatal jaundice from breast milk inhibitor:
    a. main term: _____   b. diagnosis: _____
13. Classic hydatidiform mole:
    a. main term: _____   b. diagnosis: _____
14. Hydrocephalus in newborn:
    a. main term: _____   b. diagnosis: _____
15. Thoracic spina bifida:
    a. main term: _____   b. diagnosis: _____

YOU CODE IT! Practice

Using the techniques described in this chapter, carefully read through the case studies and determine the most accurate ICD-10-CM code(s) and external cause code(s), if appropriate, for each case study.

1. Sean Dollarson, an 8-year-old male, is brought in by his parents to see Dr. Greenburg, his pediatrician. Sean has not been feeling well and has had some pinkish colored urine. Dr. Greenburg completed a physical exam noting elevated blood pressure and periobrbital puffiness. Sean is admitted to the hospital. The laboratory tests reveal azotemia, a BUN:Cr ratio of 18, proteinuria of 2.1 g/day, and that RBCs are dysmorphic. After reviewing the results of the tests, Sean is diagnosed with chronic nephritic syndrome with diffused mesangial proliferative glomerulonephritis.

2. Sally Hyman, a 37-year-old female, presents with the complaint of restlessness, nausea, and vomiting. Sally also admits to intermittent abdominal pain. Dr. Moye completes an examination and orders a noncontrast CT scan followed by an intravenous contrast CT scan. The CT results confirmed the diagnosis of a staghorn calculus of kidney.

3. Murphy Jorganson, a 42-year-old male, presents with the complaint of frequent and painful urination. Dr. Reddy completes a physical examination and notes swelling of the testicles. Murphy admits to some soreness and a whitish discharge. Dr. Reddy inserts a cotton swab approximately 3.5 cm into the urethra and rotates it once. Microscopic examination confirmed the diagnosis of non-gonococcal urethritis due to methicillin-resistant *Staphylococcus aureus*.

4. Eugene Applewhite, a 5-year-old male, is brought in by his parents. Eugene is losing weight and his parents are concerned because Eugene prefers drinking water to eating food. Eugene has also been wetting his bed. Dr. Ryant completes a clinical examination and notes mild dehydration and decides to admit Eugene to the hospital. After reviewing the MRI scan and laboratory results, Eugene is diagnosed with nephrogenic diabetes insipidus.

5. Larry Tucker, a 24-year-old male, presents today to see Dr. Dawkins, a urologist, with the complaint of low level of semen with ejaculation. Dr. Dawkins completes a medical history, a physical examination, and the appropriate tests. Larry is diagnosed with azoospemia due to obstruction of efferent ducts.

6. Pamela Cain, a 34-year-old female, presents today 23 weeks pregnant. Pamela has no complaints and states she is feeling well. Pamela was diagnosed with essential hypertension 1 year ago.

7. Gladys Shull, a 17-year-old female, comes in today to see Dr. Henson. Gladys thinks she may be pregnant. Dr. Henson performs a pregnancy test, results positive.

8. Jennifer Addis, a 23-year-old female, presents today with frequent urination and a burning sensation. Jennifer is 25 weeks pregnant. Dr. Pizzuti completes an examination and orders a culture, which reveals *Escherichia coli*. Jennifer is diagnosed with a urinary bladder infection due to *E. coli*.

9. Kreshella Goodpaster, a 29-year-old female, 17 weeks pregnant, presents with heavy vaginal bleeding. Dr. Freedenberg admits Kreshella to the hospital with the diagnosis of antepartum hemorrhage.

10. Mazie Iablonovski, a 32-year-old female, 13 weeks pregnant, comes to see Dr. Minick, her OB-GYN. Mazie states she is feeling well and has no complaints. Dr. Minick is concerned because Mazie has a history of miscarriages. Mazie is G3 P0.

11. Judy Sovde, a 28-year-old female, gave birth to a beautiful baby girl today at Weston Hospital. Dr. Kibler assisted in the full-term vaginal delivery. Dr. Kibler diagnoses baby Sovde with congenital entropion, right eye. Code baby Sovde's chart.

12. Jason Eldridge was born today at Weston Hospital. Jason was delivered by cesarean section, full term, by Dr. DeYoung. Jason's laboratory results were positive for metabolic acidemia.

13. Paula Devan, a 2-week-old female, is brought by her parents to see her pediatrician, Dr. Langer, for a checkup. Dr. Langer documents a pansystolic murmur. Paula is diagnosed with a congenital ventricular septal defect (VSD).

14. Dr. Jeffers, a neonatologist, was called in to treat Saddie Hawkins, born in this hospital 2 days ago. Saddie is showing signs of hypoxia. Dr. Jeffers transferred Saddie to NICU, where the infant pneumogram confirms a diagnosis of apnea of prematurity.

15. Karen Sprague went into labor, and her husband, Allen, was driving her to the hospital when they got caught in a traffic jam. Karen gave birth in the car, and Allen cut the umbilical cord with the utility knife he keeps in the trunk. Upon arrival at the hospital, Dr. Parkerson performed a complete newborn examination and diagnosed the baby with tetanus neonatorum caused by the use of the nonsterile instrument during delivery. Code baby Sprague's chart.

YOU CODE IT! Application

The following exercises provide practice in abstracting physicians' notes and learning to work with documentation from our health care facility, Prader, Bracker, & Associates. These case studies are modeled on real patient encounters. Using the techniques described in this chapter, carefully read through the case studies and determine the most accurate ICD-10-CM code(s) and external cause code(s), if appropriate, for each case study.

WESTON HOSPITAL

629 Healthcare Way • SOMEWHERE, FL 32811 • 407-555-6541

PATIENT: OTTMAN, BELINDA

ACCOUNT/EHR #: OTTMBE001

DATE: 10/17/18

Attending Physician: Renee O. Bracker, MD

S: This 71-year-old female was diagnosed with end-stage renal disease requiring regular dialysis maintenance 6 months ago. She presents today with shortness of breath, nausea, hiccups, and overall weakness. She admits to noncompliance with her dialysis plan.

O: Ht. 5′4″, Wt. 134 lb., P 81, R 28, BP 170/92. HEENT: unremarkable. Serum creatinine of 1.7 mg/dL, GFR 14 mL/min/1.73 m, hemaglobin 6.4, edema pitting 2+.

A: End-stage renal disease with regular dialysis, noncompliance; anemia due to ESRD

P: Admit to inpatient with immediate hemodialysis session and transfusion

ROB/pw   D: 10/17/18 09:50:16   T: 10/19/18 12:55:01

Determine the most accurate ICD-10-CM code(s).

PRADER, BRACKER, & ASSOCIATES
A Complete Health Care Facility
159 Healthcare Way • SOMEWHERE, FL 32811 • 407-555-6789

PATIENT: BANG, PARC

ACCOUNT/EHR #: BANGPA001

DATE: 10/17/18

Attending Physician: Renee O. Bracker, MD

S: This is a 64-year-old male who comes in today with frequent painful urination and feeling the consistent need to void. He states that he smoked cigarettes for 10+ years but has been smoke-free for 2.5 years.

O: Ht. 6′2″, Wt. 215 lb., P 82, R 18, BP 141/83. HEENT: unremarkable, oxygen saturation 100% in RA. Afebrile. Skin: warm and well perfused with no rash. Back exam: no deformities or defects. Neuro exam: normal tone and strength. Urinalysis is positive for hematuria. Cystoscopy results positive for bladder carcinoma.

A: Bladder cancer, anterior wall, primary.

P: Transurethral resection—discussed TUR option with patient. He will think about it and will return in 1 week.

ROB/pw   D: 10/17/18 09:50:16   T: 10/18/18 12:55:01

Determine the most accurate ICD-10-CM code(s).

PRADER, BRACKER, & ASSOCIATES
A Complete Health Care Facility
159 Healthcare Way • SOMEWHERE, FL 32811 • 407-555-6789

PATIENT: VANZELL, LEONORE

ACCOUNT/EHR #: VANZLE001

DATE: 10/17/18

Attending Physician: Oscar R. Prader, MD

S: This is a 58-year-old female who comes in today with concerns about tiredness and urinating during the night. She states that recently she has had interrupted sleep because of being awakened with an urgent need to void. The past 3–4 nights she has gotten up to void at least four times during the night. Patient also admits that during the day she has to urinate a good bit and yesterday she counted voiding 9 times within a 24-hour period. She states that her fluid intake has not changed and she is not on any medications. She denies any incontinence at this time.

O: Ht. 5'6", Wt. 131 lb., P 72, R 16, BP 135/81. HEENT: unremarkable, oxygen saturation 100% in RA. Afebrile. Patient history is noncontributory. Abdomen: flat, soft, nontender. Back exam: no deformities or cutaneous defect. Neuro exam: normal tone, strength, and activity. Finger stick shows glucose levels within normal range. UA is negative for hematuria and infection. Cystourethroscopy ruled out any tumors and kidney stones. Patient denies any pain associated with micturition.

A: Detrusor muscle hyperactivity

P: Rx: Darifenacin

   Restrict fluid intake

ORP/pw   D: 10/17/18 09:50:16   T: 10/18/18 12:55:01

Determine the most accurate ICD-10-CM code(s).

WESTON HOSPITAL

629 Healthcare Way • SOMEWHERE, FL 32811 • 407-555-6541

PATIENT: TERRY, MARIANNA

ACCOUNT/EHR #: TERRMA001

DATE: 9/17/18

Operative Report

Preoperative DX:	1. First trimester missed abortion; 2. Undesired fertility
Postoperative DX:	Same
Operation:	1. Dilation and curettage with suction; 2. Laparoscopic bilateral tubal ligation using Kleppinger bipolar cautery
Surgeon:	Oscar R. Prader, MD
Assistant:	None
Anesthesia:	General endotracheal anesthesia
Findings:	Pt had products of conception at the time of dilation and curettage. She also had normal-appearing uterus, ovaries, fallopian tubes, and liver edge.
Specimens:	Products of conception to pathology
Disposition:	To PACU in stable condition

Procedure: The patient was taken to the operating room, and she was placed in the dorsal supine position. General endotracheal anesthesia was administered without difficulty. The patient was placed in dorsal lithotomy position. She was prepped and draped in the normal sterile fashion. A red rubber tip catheter was placed gently to drain the patient's bladder. A weighted speculum was placed in the posterior vagina and Deaver retractor anteriorly. A single-tooth tenaculum was placed in the anterior cervix for retraction. The uterus sounded to 9 cm. The cervix was dilated with Hanks dilators to 25 French. This sufficiently passed a #7 suction curet. The suction curet was inserted without incident, and the products of conception were gently suctioned out. Good uterine cry was noted with a serrated curet. No further products were noted on suctioning. At this point, a Hulka tenaculum was placed in the cervix for retraction. The other instruments were removed.

Attention was then turned to the patient's abdomen. A small vertical intraumbilical incision was made with the knife. A Veress needle was placed through that incision. Confirmation of placement into the abdominal cavity was made with instillation of normal saline without return and a positive handing drop test. The abdomen was then insufflated with sufficient carbon dioxide gas to cause abdominal tympany. The Veress needle was removed and a 5-mm trocar was placed in the same incision. Confirmation of placement into the abdominal cavity was made with placement of the laparoscopic camera. Another trocar site was placed two fingerbreadths above the pubic symphysis in the midline under direct visualization. The above-noted intrapelvic and intraabdominal findings were seen. The patient was placed in steep trendelenburg. The fallopian tubes were identified and followed out to the fimbriated ends. They were then cauterized four times on either side. At this point, all instruments were removed from the patient's abdomen. This was done under direct visualization during the insufflation. The skin incisions were reapproximated with 4-0 Vicryl suture. The Hulka tenaculum was removed without incident.

The patient was placed back in the dorsal supine position. Anesthesia was withdrawn without difficulty. The patient was taken to the PACU in stable condition. All sponge, instrument, and needle counts were correct in the operating room.

ORP/pw   D: 9/17/18 09:50:16   T: 9/19/18 12:55:01

Determine the most accurate ICD-10-CM code(s).

PRADER, BRACKER, & ASSOCIATES

A Complete Health Care Facility

159 Healthcare Way • SOMEWHERE, FL 32811 • 407-555-6789

PATIENT: FAIRBANKS, GREGORY

ACCOUNT/EHR #: FAIRGR001

DATE: 09/17/18

Attending Physician: Renee O. Bracker, MD

Consultant: Vivian D. Pixar, MD

Reason for Consultation: Screening for retinopathy of prematurity

S: The patient was born on 08/19/18, with a birth weight of 2,740 grams, gestational age of 36 weeks; given oxygen in NICU for the first 60 minutes of life. Child discharged third day postpartum with oxygen saturation of 98%.

O: Retinal follow-up examination this date shows normal external exam, well-dilated pupils. Indirect exam shows clear media, normal optic nerves both eyes, with normal right retinal vessel extension to the periphery without evidence of retinopathy. Left retinal vessel extension shows a faint demarcation line at the junction between the vascularized and avascular border.

A: Prematurity retinopathy, stage 1, left eye

P: Follow-up 1 week

ROB/mg   D: 09/17/18 09:50:16   T: 09/18/18 12:55:01

Determine the most accurate ICD-10-CM code(s).

Factors Influencing Health Status (Z Codes)

18

Learning Outcomes

After completing this chapter, the student should be able to:

LO 18.1 Abstract details about preventive services to report their medical necessity.

LO 18.2 Determine the medical reasons for early detection testing.

LO 18.3 Demonstrate how to report encounters related to genetic susceptibility.

LO 18.4 Identify the reasons for observation services to determine the correct code or codes.

LO 18.5 Apply the Official Guidelines for reporting aftercare and follow-up care.

LO 18.6 Evaluate the specific services provided for organ donation and report the medical necessity.

LO 18.7 Distinguish indications of antimicrobial drug resistance to report this accurately.

LO 18.8 Employ Z codes accurately.

Key Terms

Abnormal Findings
Allogeneic
Autologous
Carrier
Isogeneic
Preventive Care
Prosthetic
Screening
Xenogeneic

STOP! Remember, you need to follow along in your ICD-10-CM code book for an optimal learning experience.

Preventive Care
Health-related services designed to stop the development of a disease or injury.

18.1 Preventive Care

In several chapters throughout this textbook, you got an overview of Z codes, which are codes used to report a reason for a visit to a physician for something other than an illness or injury. As you have learned, there must always be a valid, medical reason for a patient's encounter with a health care professional. And there are occasions for patients to seek attention even when they are not currently ill. These codes give you the opportunity to explain.

Science and research have provided us with a better understanding of disease and disease progression, as well as etiology (underlying cause of disease). This knowledge has resulted in improved **preventive care** services to stop the onset of illness or injury.

The provision of preventive care services is likely to increase. The enacting of the Affordable Care Act enables more patients to take advantage of more preventive services than ever before. Since September 2010, new health insurance policies must cover preventive services, with no copayment, no coinsurance payments, and no requirement for deductible fulfillment.

Reporting the provision of preventive care will require a Z code to explain the specific reason for the encounter, such as a flu shot or measles vaccination (Z23 Encounter for immunization).

> **GUIDANCE CONNECTION**
>
> Read the ICD-10-CM Official Guidelines for Coding and Reporting, section **I. Conventions, General Coding Guidelines and Chapter Specific Guidelines,** subsection **C. Chapter-Specific Coding Guidelines,** chapter **21. Factors influencing health status and contact with health services,** subsection **c.2) Inoculations and vaccinations.**

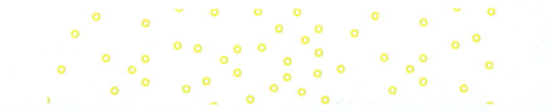

The physician or other health care professional may also be able to provide counseling for the patient and/or family members. This type of counseling is not the same as that provided by a psychiatrist or psychologist; instead, the physician would take the time to discuss options for preventing the development of disease or injury. Perhaps this may include dietary counseling and surveillance (Z71.3) to prevent the onset of hypertension, heart disease, obesity, or other nutrition-related conditions, or a discussion about the patient's tobacco use (Z72.0) could focus on various methodologies available to quit smoking to prevent the patient from developing lung disease. Couples may come in for genetic counseling (Z31.5) to prevent passing chromosomal abnormalities to their future children; for those who do not want to have children yet, general counseling and advice on contraception (Z30.09) may be provided.

LET'S CODE IT! SCENARIO

Bonnie Poggio, a 15-year-old female, came into the clinic with her mother. While searching for seashells at the beach, she went up on the boardwalk barefooted to get ice cream and stepped on a nail, puncturing the sole of her left foot. After checking the puncture wound, cleaning it, and dressing it, Dr. Baldwin gave Bonnie a tetanus shot as a precaution.

Let's Code It!

You are reviewing how to determine Z codes in this chapter, so here's the first code for this encounter: **S91.332A Puncture wound without foreign body, left foot, initial encounter**. Dr. Baldwin's notes state that Bonnie received a preventive tetanus shot. You have learned that, in medical terminology, this is known as an *immunization*. When you turn to the Alphabetic Index, you see

    Immunization — *see also* **Vaccination**
        Encounter for Z23

When you turn to the Tabular List, you confirm:

    Z23   **Encounter for immunization**

This is great. However, the reason Bonnie went to see Dr. Baldwin was care for the wound. The tetanus shot was secondary. So, you will not report Z23. But you do need an external cause code to explain why Bonnie needed this immunization. Turn to the *Alphabetic Index to External Causes*. Did you find this?

    Puncture, puncturing — *see also* **Contact, with, by type of object or machine**

Let's turn to

    Contact (accidental)
        with
            nail W45.0

Now let's find code category W45 in the Tabular List:

    ✓4 **W45**   **Foreign body or object entering through skin**

That sounds right. First, read carefully the **EXCLUDES2** *notation* listing several diagnoses. Take a minute to review them, and determine whether any apply to Bonnie's condition. No, none of them do, so you are in the correct location. Notice the seventh-character options here. You will need them for later. First, you need to determine the first six characters, so continue down and review all of the fourth-, fifth-, and sixth-character choices. Which matches Dr. Baldwin's notes?

    W45.0   **Nail entering through skin**

Perfect! And the seventh character? The choices are listed at the top of this code category:

> W45.0XXA   Nail entering through skin, initial encounter
>
> Next, you need the place of occurrence (the beach) and the status code. (Refer to the chapter **Coding Injury, Poisoning, and External Causes** to remind yourself about reporting external cause codes whenever you are reporting an injury or poisoning.)
> Take a look. Did you find these codes:
>
> Y92.832   Beach as the place of occurrence of the external cause
> Y99.8   Other external cause status
>
> Fantastic! You have determined all of the codes required for this encounter:
>
> S91.332A   Puncture wound without foreign body, left foot, initial encounter
> W45.0XXA   Nail entering through skin, initial encounter
> Y92.832   Beach as the place of occurrence of the external cause
> Y99.8   Other external cause status
>
> You have got this!

18.2 Early Detection

The reason for routine and administrative exams is to ensure continued good health by looking for signs of disease as early as detection may be possible, using a physician's knowledge and technological advancement. Commonly, these health care encounters are known as *annual physicals, well-baby checks,* or *well-woman exams.* These routine encounters, most often prompted by the calendar rather than the way the patient feels, are reported with Z codes, such as code Z00.00 Encounter for general adult medical examination without abnormal findings or Z00.129 Encounter for routine child health examination without abnormal findings.

Many schools and organizations require that a physician examine a child before the child joins a sports team (Z02.5), companies may require preemployment exams (Z02.1), and virtually all surgeons will order pre-procedural exams (Z01.81-) for the patient prior to surgery. These are all considered administrative health encounters because they are determined by a specific circumstance, rather than the calendar or the way the patient feels.

Certain conditions, even after being resolved, may continue to identify the patient as being at risk of a recurrence. The patient had a previous condition; however, prudent health care standards require that the physician keep a watchful eye to catch and treat a recurrent episode. Codes such as Z86.11 Personal history of tuberculosis and Z87.11 Personal history of peptic ulcer may provide medical necessity for an extra screening test or encounter.

> ### YOU CODE IT! CASE STUDY
>
> *Kathryn Rogers, a 49-year-old female, came in to see Dr. Apter to get a colonoscopy. Dr. Apter explained last week that this was an important screening for malignant neoplasms of the colon and was recommended for all adults aged 50 and over. After the screening, Dr. Apter told Kathryn she was fine and there were no abnormalities.*
>
> #### You Code It!
> Go through the steps of coding, and determine the code or codes that should be reported for this encounter between Dr. Apter and Kathryn.
>
> *(continued)*

> Step #1: Read the case carefully and completely.
>
> Step #2: Abstract the scenario. Which main words or terms describe why the physician cared for the patient during this encounter?
>
> Step #3: Are there any details missing or incomplete for which you would need to query the physician? [If so, ask your instructor.]
>
> Step #4: Check for any relevant guidance, including reading all of the symbols and notations in the Tabular List and the appropriate sections of the Official Guidelines.
>
> Step #5: Determine the correct diagnosis code or codes to explain why this encounter was medically necessary.
>
> Step #6: Double-check your work.
>
> **Answer:**
>
> Did you determine this to be the correct code?
>
> > Z12.11   Encounter for screening for malignant neoplasm of colon

Screening
An examination or test of a patient who has no signs or symptoms that is conducted with the intention of finding any evidence of disease as soon as possible, thus enabling better patient outcomes.

A **screening** is a test or examination, such as routine lab work or imaging services, administered when there are no current signs, symptoms, or related diagnosis. Report a visit for a screening with a Z code such as code Z13.22 Encounter for screening for metabolic disorder or Z13.820 Encounter for screening for osteoporosis.

The standards of care have established important examinations and tests to detect illnesses at the earliest possible time. However, these tests are typically recommended for specific population subgroups determined to be at the greatest risk, such as mammograms for women over 40 or prostate examinations for men over 50. These encounters would be reported with a Z code such as code Z12.5 Encounter for screening for malignant neoplasm of prostate or Z13.6 Encounter for screening for cardiovascular disorders.

Society, especially in the United States, is designed for interaction between individuals. Shopping malls, concert halls and festival venues, public transport sites, classrooms, playgrounds, and other locations draw friends, families, and strangers together in close proximity to one another. Close physical proximity can put someone in contact with a potential health hazard and facilitate (suspected) exposure to a communicable disease. Think of this: Two children, Jane and Mary, were playing together, and the next day Jane is diagnosed with rubella. This means that Mary was exposed. When Mary's mom takes her to the doctor, this visit will include code Z20.4 Contact with and (suspected) exposure to rubella. Another example: Kenny works for County Animal Control. As he was placing a wild raccoon into his vehicle, the raccoon bit him. Kenny went to the emergency clinic immediately, and code Z20.3 Contact with and (suspected) exposure to rabies was included on the claim.

Abnormal Findings
Test results that indicate a disease or condition may be present.

With all these tests being done to confirm the patient's good health, there are times when the documentation includes **abnormal findings**, meaning the results indicate something is wrong. This is not the same thing as a confirmed diagnosis, necessarily. It may be a signal that a condition is potential or that more extensive and specific examinations must be done.

> **EXAMPLES**
>
> Z00.01   Encounter for general adult medical examination with abnormal findings
>
> Z01.411   Encounter for gynecological examination (general) (routine) with abnormal findings

> **GUIDANCE CONNECTION**
>
> Read the ICD-10-CM Official Guidelines for Coding and Reporting, section **I. Conventions, General Coding Guidelines and Chapter Specific Guidelines**, subsection **C. Chapter-Specific Coding Guidelines**, chapter **21. Factors influencing health status and contact with health services**, subsections **c.1) Contact/exposure, c.4) History (of), c.5) Screening,** and **c.13) Routine and administrative examinations**, plus section **IV. Diagnostic Coding and Reporting Guidelines for Outpatient Services,** subsection **P. Encounters for general medical examinations with abnormal findings.**

> **YOU CODE IT! CASE STUDY**
>
> Dallas Rossi, a 66-year-old male, came in to see his regular physician, Dr. DeGusipe, for his annual physical. Dallas said he has been feeling great and working out about twice a week. During the digital rectal exam, Dr. DeGuisipe noted a palpable nodule on the posterior of Dallas's prostate. Dr. DeGuispe told Dallas that he appears in good health except for the nodule. They discussed this and scheduled an appointment for a biopsy.
>
> ### You Code It!
>
> Go through the steps of coding, and determine the code or codes that should be reported for this encounter between Dr. DeGusipe and Dallas.
>
> Step #1: Read the case carefully and completely.
>
> Step #2: Abstract the scenario. Which main words or terms describe why the physician cared for the patient during this encounter?
>
> Step #3: Are there any details missing or incomplete for which you would need to query the physician? [If so, ask your instructor.]
>
> Step #4: Check for any relevant guidance, including reading all of the symbols and notations in the Tabular List and the appropriate sections of the Official Guidelines.
>
> Step #5: Determine the correct diagnosis code or codes to explain why this encounter was medically necessary.
>
> Step #6: Double-check your work.
>
> **Answer:**
>
> Did you determine these to be the correct codes?
>
> | | |
> |---|---|
> | Z00.01 | Encounter for general adult medical examination with abnormal findings |
> | N40.2 | Nodular prostate without lower urinary tract symptoms |
>
> You did great!

18.3 Genetic Susceptibility

A patient might be a **carrier** or suspected carrier of a disease. He or she needs to know this so the condition is not unintentionally passed on. Or the patient may have an abnormal gene that may increase a patient's chances of developing a disease. This is of particular concern when there is a known family history for conditions that are, or may be, inherited.

In most cases, the documentation will note that the patient has a family history of a condition, such as code Z80.6 Family history of leukemia or Z83.3 Family history of diabetes

Carrier
An individual infected with a disease who is not ill but can still pass it to another person; an individual with an abnormal gene that can be passed to a child, making the child susceptible to disease.

> **GUIDANCE CONNECTION**
>
> Read the ICD-10-CM Official Guidelines for Coding and Reporting, section I. **Conventions, General Coding Guidelines and Chapter Specific Guidelines,** subsection **C. Chapter-Specific Coding Guidelines,** chapter **21. Factors influencing health status and contact with health services,** subsections **c.3), Status** and **c.14) Miscellaneous Z codes—Prophylactic Organ Removal.**

> **CODING BITES**
>
> Notice that these codes are used when the physician determines observation is required "to be sure" and the result is nothing is wrong [ruled out]. If the determination is that there *is* a problem, you would then report the code for the problem, not the observation.

> **GUIDANCE CONNECTION**
>
> Read the ICD-10-CM Official Guidelines for Coding and Reporting, section I. **Conventions, General Coding Guidelines and Chapter Specific Guidelines,** subsection **C. Chapter-Specific Coding Guidelines,** chapter **21. Factors influencing health status and contact with health services,** subsection **c.6) Observation.**

mellitus. In these cases, no additional genetic testing may be done. However, the knowledge of family members with a particular condition could support more frequent screenings, such as a patient getting a mammogram every 6 months instead of the standard annual test.

A patient may have reason to believe he or she is the carrier of a disease, such as diphtheria (Z22.2) or viral hepatitis B (Z55.51). A carrier is an individual who has been infected with a pathogen yet has no signs or symptoms of the disease. Carriers, while not ill themselves, are still able to pass the condition to another person.

> **EXAMPLE**
>
> Cystic fibrosis, the result of mutations in the CFTR gene, is a common genetic disease. Due to its nature, both parents must each carry a copy of the mutated gene in order for the child to inherit and develop the disease. However, the parents may not show any signs or symptoms.
>
> Risk is measured by family history and ethnic background. If the patient has a family history of CF, then the probability of being a carrier is increased above the risk based on ethnicity alone. The probability increases if the patient is a close relative of an individual with CF, such as a parent, sibling, or child.
>
> To report medical necessity to perform the genetic testing:
>
> Z84.81   Family history of carrier of genetic disease
> Z13.71   Encounter for nonprocreative screening for genetic disease carrier status
>
> or
>
> Z31.430 Encounter of female for testing for genetic diseases carrier status for procreative management
>
> or
>
> Z31.440 Encounter of male for testing for genetic diseases carrier status for procreative management
>
> If the woman is currently pregnant and needs to be screened, use this code:
>
> Z36.-   Encounter for antenatal screening of mother
>
> If the test is positive, report
>
> Z14.1   Cystic fibrosis carrier

You may have heard about genetic susceptibility to malignant neoplasm of the breast (Z15.01) and genetic susceptibility to malignant neoplasm of the ovary (Z15.02), identified by the BRCA1 and BRCA2 tests. These tests may be used to confirm, or deny, the presence of an abnormality in a gene that may have been inherited, which can serve as a prediction of the potential for developing a disease—in these cases, cancer. Some patients have opted for prophylactic (preventive) surgery after a positive finding of an abnormal gene. If a patient had this procedure, you would report it with code Z40.01 Encounter for prophylactic removal of breast.

18.4 Observation

There might be a reason that a physician suspects a patient may be ill despite the absence of signs and symptoms. Code categories Z03 and Z04 enable you to report the reason these types of encounters are medically necessary.

- ☑4 Z03   Encounter for medical observation for suspected diseases and conditions ruled out
- ☑4 Z04   Encounter for examination and observation for other reasons

Imagine that a mother brings her 2-year-old son into the emergency department because she found him in her bathroom with her allergy pill bottle tipped over and pills strewn about the floor. She does not know whether he ingested any of the pills and, if he did, how many. After an examination showing no signs or symptoms of overdose or poisoning, the doctor decides to keep the boy in the hospital for observation, just in case. The next day, the boy appears to be fine, and his blood tests show no signs of the allergy medication at all. He is discharged with a clean bill of health. You would report this with code Z03.6 Encounter for observation for suspected toxic effect from ingested substance, ruled out.

> ### YOU CODE IT! CASE STUDY
>
> Tracey Morales, a 33-year-old male, was brought into the ED after an accident on his construction job site. He tripped and hit his head against a pile of bricks. There was a 3 cm laceration on his temporal lobe scalp, but he did not lose consciousness. CT scan of his head was inconclusive. After the laceration was stitched up with a simple repair, Dr. Tribow placed Tracey into observation status so they could watch for signs of a concussion. After 20 hours with normal vital signs and a normal neurologic exam, he was determined to not have suffered a concussion and released.
>
> #### You Code It!
>
> Review Dr. Tribow's documentation about Tracey's stay in observation. Then, determine the correct ICD-10-CM code or codes to report the reasons why Tracey needed care.
>
> Step #1: Read the case carefully and completely.
>
> Step #2: Abstract the scenario. Which main words or terms describe why the physician cared for the patient during this encounter?
>
> Step #3: Are there any details missing or incomplete for which you would need to query the physician? [If so, ask your instructor.]
>
> Step #4: Check for any relevant guidance, including reading all of the symbols and notations in the Tabular List and the appropriate sections of the Official Guidelines.
>
> Step #5: Determine the correct diagnosis code or codes to explain why this encounter was medically necessary.
>
> Step #6: Double-check your work.
>
> **Answer:**
>
> Did you determine these to be the codes?
>
> | Code | Description |
> |---|---|
> | Z04.2 | Encounter for examination and observation following work accident |
> | S01.01xA | Laceration without foreign body of scalp, initial encounter |
> | W01.198A | Fall on same level from slipping, tripping and stumbling with subsequent striking against other object, initial encounter |
> | Y92.61 | Building [any] under construction as the place of occurrence of the external cause |
> | Y99.0 | Civilian activity done for income or pay |

18.5 Continuing Care and Aftercare

Chronic illness may require long-term use of medication, known as *drug therapy*. When a patient is taking any type of pharmaceutical on an ongoing basis, regular monitoring can identify potential concerns, such as side effects or loss of potency. Some individuals' body chemistry can get used to certain drugs, making them less

> **GUIDANCE CONNECTION**
>
> Read the ICD-10-CM Official Guidelines for Coding and Reporting, section **I. Conventions, General Coding Guidelines and Chapter Specific Guidelines**, subsection **C. Chapter-Specific Coding Guidelines**, chapter **21. Factors influencing health status and contact with health services**, subsection **c.7) Aftercare**.

effective. When coding an encounter for such monitoring, you may begin with Z51.81 Encounter for therapeutic drug level monitoring, along with a code to identify the type of therapeutic drug, such as Z79.01 Long term (current) use of anticoagulants or Z79.811 Long term (current) use of aromatase inhibitors.

Of course, the physician-patient relationship in treating a specific illness or injury does not end at the end of a surgical procedure or other type of therapeutic service. A healing illness or injury may require aftercare, reported with a code such as Z47.1 Aftercare following joint replacement surgery, Z48.00 Encounter for change or removal of nonsurgical wound dressing, or Z45.24 Encounter for aftercare following lung transplant.

Patients with implanted medical devices may need more frequent encounters to check the device to ensure it is working properly, as is the case with a patient with a cardiac pacemaker (Z45.01) or a patient with a cochlear implant (Z45.321).

Follow-up examinations may be necessary for a condition that has already been treated or no longer exists. Examples of such follow-ups include an encounter for the removal of sutures (stitches), reported with code Z48.02, or an encounter after the patient has completed treatment for a malignant neoplasm (Z08), once the patient has finished the chemotherapy or radiation treatment plan.

> **GUIDANCE CONNECTION**
>
> Read the ICD-10-CM Official Guidelines for Coding and Reporting, section **I. Conventions, General Coding Guidelines and Chapter Specific Guidelines**, subsection **C. Chapter-Specific Coding Guidelines**, chapter **21. Factors influencing health status and contact with health services**, subsection **c.8) Follow-up**.

LET'S CODE IT! SCENARIO

Adelina Plenner, a 43-year-old female, came in to see Dr. Buldar, her gastroenterologist. She had a colostomy 6 weeks ago, and this is a standard post-procedural follow-up. He noted that there was some irritation and he applied some ointment and gave Adelina a prescription for more ointment. Dr. Buldar examined the area and told Adelina to return prn.

Let's Code It!

This encounter is a standard follow-up post-surgically to ensure all is well with the patient. Dr. Buldar was checking Adelina's condition post-colostomy.

In the ICD-10-CM Alphabetic Index, find

Aftercare (*see also* Care) Z51.89

Read all of the indented items. Hmm, there doesn't seem to be anything that matches this encounter. Let's try this:

Care (of) (for) (following)

Wow, nothing here seems to fit, either. What about . . .

Encounter (with health service) (for) Z76.89

Not here, either! One more idea. . . . Dr. Buldar paid attention to Adelina's stoma. Take a look at this:

Attention (to)
    artificial

526   PART II | REPORTING DIAGNOSES

> opening (of) Z43.9
>> digestive tract NEC Z43.4
>> colon Z43.3
>
> Finally!!! Success!! This proves that you cannot give up. You must keep thinking and looking because it will always be there . . . somewhere.
> Turn in the ICD-10-CM Tabular List and find
>
> ☑4 **Z43** **Encounter for attention to artificial openings**
>
> Read carefully the diagnoses listed next to the INCLUDES, EXCLUDES1, and EXCLUDES2 notations. Did you check the *artificial opening status only, without need for care (Z93.-)*? Was there a need for care? The ointment could support this. Did you check to see if this qualifies as a *complication of external stoma* . . . particularly K94.-? When on the job, you could query the physician for confirmation. This documentation does not really describe a complication, so let's continue on to confirm this code:
>
> **Z43.3** **Encounter for attention to colostomy**
>
> Good job!

18.6 Organ Donation

The number of organs and tissues that can be successfully transplanted has dramatically increased over the years, and many can be provided by a living donor. Code category Z52 Donors of organs and tissues includes various types of blood donors (Z52.0-), skin donors (Z52.1-), and bone donors (Z52.2-). You will notice that all three of these code subcategories require you, as the professional coder, to determine from the documentation whether the donor is **autologous** or is providing another type of graft or donation (see Table 18-1). It is not unusual for a patient to donate his or her own blood prior to having a surgical procedure so that in the event he or she needs a transfusion, his or her own blood will be used. When an injury to the skin is so severe that a graft is needed, there are times when the surgeon will take the graft from another part of the patient's own body and transfer it to the injured site.

A kidney (Z52.4) and cornea (Z52.5) as well as a part of the liver (Z52.6) may come from a living donor. Fertility issues occur and some women donate their oocytes (eggs) for in vitro fertilization for themselves or someone else (Z52.81-). The donation of any of these organs would almost always be used as an **allogeneic** donation to another individual.

A donation from the recipient's monozygotic twin is called **isogeneic**, while a **xenogeneic** donation involves a donor and recipient who are of different species. Synthetic organ and tissue replacements are referred to as **prosthetics**.

Autologous
The donor tissue is taken from a different site on the same individual's body (also known as an *autograft*).

Allogeneic
The donor and recipient are of the same species, e.g., human → human, dog → dog (also known as an *allograft*).

Isogeneic
The donor and recipient individuals are genetically identical (i.e., monozygotic twins).

Xenogeneic
The donor and recipient are of different species, e.g., bovine cartilage → human (also known as a *xenograft* or *heterograft*).

Prosthetic
Lost tissue that is replaced with synthetic material such as metal, plastic, or ceramic, to take over the function of the lost tissue.

TABLE 18-1 Types of Grafts

Autologous	The donor tissue is taken from a different site on the same individual's body (also known as an *autograft*).
Isogeneic	The donor and recipient individuals are genetically identical (i.e., monozygotic twins).
Allogeneic	The donor and recipient are of the same species, e.g., human → human, dog → dog (also known as an *allograft*).
Xenogeneic	The donor and recipient are of different species, e.g., bovine cartilage → human (also known as a *xenograft* or *heterograft*).
Prosthetic	Lost tissue is replaced with synthetic material such as metal, plastic, or ceramic.

> ### YOU CODE IT! CASE STUDY
>
> Ilani Marhefka, a 31-year-old female, came in to donate her eggs. Her sister, Serita, had lesions on her ovaries and had to have them removed many years ago. Dr. Stark is going to harvest eggs from Ilani to implant in Serita so she and her husband, Jude, can have children. Ilani wanted to help her sister and brother-in-law by donating her eggs.
>
> #### You Code It!
>
> Go through the steps of coding, and determine the code or codes that should be reported for this encounter between Dr. Stark and Ilani.
>
> Step #1: Read the case carefully and completely.
>
> Step #2: Abstract the scenario. Which main words or terms describe why the physician cared for the patient during this encounter?
>
> Step #3: Are there any details missing or incomplete for which you would need to query the physician? [If so, ask your instructor.]
>
> Step #4: Check for any relevant guidance, including reading all of the symbols and notations in the Tabular List and the appropriate sections of the Official Guidelines.
>
> Step #5: Determine the correct diagnosis code or codes to explain why this encounter was medically necessary.
>
> Step #6: Double-check your work.
>
> **Answer:**
>
> Did you determine this to be the correct code?
>
> **Z52.811**   Egg (oocyte) donor under age 35, designated recipient
>
> Very good!

Of course, prior to the actual procedure to harvest the organ or tissue, an examination will need to be done, reported with code Z00.5 Encounter for examination for potential donor of organ or tissue.

18.7 Resistance to Antimicrobial Drugs

You learned about antimicrobial resistance (AMR) in the chapter about coding infectious diseases. Let's review these codes again, just to reinforce how to report these situations using Z codes.

Take a look at code category Z16 Resistance to antimicrobial drugs. You can see that ICD-10-CM provides a note with some direction about the proper use of these Z codes:

> **NOTE:** The codes in this category are provided for use as additional codes to identify the resistance and non-responsiveness of a condition to antimicrobial drugs.

And you can see the *Code first* **the infection** notation that provides sequencing direction.

Z16.10	Resistance to unspecified beta lactam antibiotics
Z16.11	Resistance to penicillins (amoxicillin) (ampicillin)
Z16.12	Extended spectrum beta lactamase (ESBL) resistance
Z16.19	Resistance to other specified beta lactam antibiotics (cephalosporins)

Z16.20	Resistance to unspecified antibiotic (antibiotics NOS)
Z16.21	Resistance to vancomycin
Z16.22	Resistance to vancomycin related antibiotics
Z16.23	Resistance to quinolones and fluoroquinolones
Z16.24	Resistance to multiple antibiotics
Z16.29	Resistance to other single specified antibiotic (aminoglycosides) (macrolides) (sulfonamides) (tetracylines)
Z16.342	Resistance to multiple antimycobacterial drugs
Z16.35	Resistance to multiple antimicrobial drugs

EXCLUDES1 resistance to multiple antibiotics only (Z16.24)

Reporting these conditions is not exclusive to the Z code chapter. When a patient is confirmed to have an infection that is resistant, you might report one of these codes instead:

A41.02	Sepsis due to methicillin resistant Staphylococcus aureus
A49.02	Methicillin resistant Staphylococcus aureus infection, unspecified site
B95.62	Methicillin resistant Staphylococcus aureus infection as the cause of diseases classified elsewhere
J15.212	Pneumonia due to methicillin resistant Staphylococcus aureus

And remember, back in the chapter about infectious diseases, you learned about using the additional codes to identify the bacterial or viral pathogen in a specific other infection, such as a urinary tract infection or infected laceration, by using an additional code from B95–B97, including these:

B95.61	Methicillin susceptible Staphylococcus aureus infection as the cause of diseases classified elsewhere
B95.62	Methicillin resistant Staphylococcus aureus infection as the cause of diseases classified elsewhere

These code descriptions change the language a bit, so you will need to know the difference between "resistant" and "susceptible." In this context:

- *Resistant* means that those certain antibiotics will not be effective in combating this pathogen.
- *Susceptible* (also referred to as *sensitive*) means that the named antibiotic is expected to be successful in killing off the infection.

YOU CODE IT! CASE STUDY

PATIENT: Paulina Stohl

DATE OF CONSULTATION: 011/09/2018

PHYSICIAN REQUESTING THE CONSULT: Ada Carole, MD

REASON FOR CONSULTATION: Resistant infection.

CHIEF COMPLAINT: Fatigue.

HISTORY OF PRESENT ILLNESS: The patient is a 57-year-old female with a history of type 2 diabetes mellitus, pancreatitis, and chronic hepatitis C who presented with complaints of fever and generalized malaise. She was seen and evaluated by Dr. Koehler in the ED and subsequently admitted. Vital signs identified a low grade fever [99.8 F] and blood cultures taken in ED were positive for gram-positive cocci. In addition, urinalysis was positive for MRSA. Patient was given Zosyn, 3.375g q 6 hr. Infectious disease was requested in for a consultation.

(continued)

At bedside, the patient stated a cystoscopy was performed by her urologist for chronic obstructive uropathy. The following biopsy was negative for malignancy. A few days later, the patient began to experience generalized malaise and then experienced fever and chills. The urine culture taken in ED was noted to be positive for MRSA and one of two blood cultures was positive. Since admission 1 day ago, blood cultures were repeated, with positive results in both tests for gram-positive cocci in clusters.

FAMILY HISTORY: No immune dysfunction other than diabetes.

ALLERGIES: No known drug allergies.

REVIEW OF SYSTEMS: A 14-system review is as per history of present illness, otherwise negative.

CURRENT MEDICATIONS: List is reviewed.

PHYSICAL EXAMINATION:

VITAL SIGNS: Upon my initial evaluation, patient has T 100.2 degrees Fahrenheit, pulse 104, respirations 20, and blood pressure 120/70.

GENERAL: Patient is alert and oriented x3, in no apparent distress at rest.

HEENT: Head is normocephalic and atraumatic. Extraocular muscle movements are intact. No scleral icterus. Oropharynx is clear.

NECK: Free of palpable adenopathy.

HEART: Regular at 100. No auscultated rub.

LUNGS: Clear to auscultation and percussion bilaterally. No rhonchi and no wheezing.

ABDOMEN: Positive bowel sounds, soft, nontender, and nondistended. No rebound, rigidity, or guarding.

EXTREMITIES: Lower extremities are without clubbing or cyanosis.

NEUROMUSCULAR: Neurologically, patient is nonfocal with normal cranial nerves. Muscle strength is normal in the upper extremities.

LABORATORY STUDIES: A complete blood count, basic metabolic profile, full microbiologic database, all of which have been reviewed.

IMPRESSION:

1. Methicillin-resistant *Staphylococcus aureus* urinary tract infection in a patient who has recently undergone a genitourinary procedure for outlet obstruction.

2. Type 2 diabetes mellitus with poor control.

3. Fever.

RECOMMENDATIONS:

1. Place the patient in contact isolation.

2. Repeat blood cultures x2.

4. Start vancomycin.

5. Discontinue Zosyn [the extended-spectrum penicillin that has proved ineffective to patient's MRSA].

Thank you for this interesting consult and allowing us to participate in this patient's care.

Allen B. Dechante, MD

You Code It!

Read Dr. Dechante's notes regarding his evaluation of Paulina Stohl and determine the accurate ICD-10-CM diagnosis codes for this encounter.

Step #1: Read the case carefully and completely.

Step #2: Abstract the scenario. Which main words or terms describe why the physician cared for the patient during this encounter?

Step #3: Are there any details missing or incomplete for which you would need to query the physician? [If so, ask your instructor.]

Step #4: Check for any relevant guidance, including reading all of the symbols and notations in the Tabular List and the appropriate sections of the Official Guidelines.

Step #5: Determine the correct diagnosis code or codes to explain why this encounter was medically necessary.

Step #6: Double-check your work.

Answer:

Did you determine these to be the codes?

N39.0	Urinary tract infection, site not specified
B95.62	Methicillin resistant Staphylococcus aureus infection as the cause of diseases classified elsewhere
E11.9	Type 2 diabetes mellitus without complication

18.8 Z Codes as First-Listed/Principal Diagnosis

During most encounters, a Z code may be the only code you report, or it may be reported along with others, determined by the specific circumstances. Except for 20 of the Z codes, sequencing is determined by the facts of the encounter and the Official Guidelines, as explained in Sections II and III. The other 20 Z codes are permitted to be *only* first-listed or principal diagnosis codes:

Z00	Encounter for general examination without complaint, suspected or reported diagnosis
Z01	Encounter for other special examination without complaint, suspected or reported diagnosis
Z02	Encounter for administrative examination
Z03	Encounter for medical observation for suspected diseases and conditions ruled out
Z04	Encounter for examination and observation for other reasons
Z33.2	Encounter for elective termination of pregnancy
Z31.81	Encounter for male factor infertility in female patient
Z31.82	Encounter for Rh incompatibility status
Z31.83	Encounter for assisted reproductive fertility procedure cycle
Z31.84	Encounter for fertility preservation procedure
Z34	Encounter for supervision of normal pregnancy
Z38	Liveborn infants according to place of birth and type of delivery
Z39	Encounter for maternal postpartum care and examination
Z42	Encounter for plastic and reconstructive surgery following medical procedure or healed injury
Z51.0	Encounter for antineoplastic radiation therapy
Z51.1-	Encounter for antineoplastic chemotherapy and immunotherapy
Z52	Donors of organs and tissues *Except:* Z52.9, Donor of unspecified organ or tissue
Z76.1	Encounter for health supervision and care of foundling
Z76.2	Encounter for health supervision and care of other healthy infant and child
Z99.12	Encounter for respirator [ventilator] dependence during power failure

> **GUIDANCE CONNECTION**
>
> Read the ICD-10-CM Official Guidelines for Coding and Reporting, section **I. Conventions, General Coding Guidelines and Chapter Specific Guidelines**, subsection **C. Chapter-Specific Coding Guidelines**, chapter **21: Factors influencing health status and contact with health services**, subsection **c.16) Z Codes That May Only be Principal/First-Listed Diagnosis.**

LET'S CODE IT! SCENARIO

Alfredo "Al" Martinelli, a 43-year-old male, was admitted to the hospital today because he is donating one of his kidneys to his son, Anthony. The surgery is scheduled for this afternoon.

Let's Code It!

Even though he is perfectly healthy, Alfredo Martinelli is admitted into the hospital. Why? Because he is an organ donor. You don't have too much information here, so how will you look this up? Turn in the ICD-10-CM Alphabetic Index to

> **Donor (organ or tissue) Z52.9**

Read down the indented list beneath and find:

> **kidney Z52.4**

This appears to be very straightforward, so go to the code category in the Tabular List:

> ✓4 **Z52   Donors of organs and tissues**

Directly below this you will see INCLUDES and EXCLUDES1 notations. Good that you saw these. Read them carefully. Alfredo is definitely a living donor. Is this "autologous"? In transplantation, the term "autologous" means that the donor and the recipient are the same person. This is not the case here because Alfredo is donating to his son. Does this mean you cannot use a code from this code category? Remember that the term "and" also means "and/or," so because Alfredo is a living donor, this situation is included here. What about the EXCLUDES1 notation? Is Alfredo here to be examined as a "potential" donor? No, it is evident that this has been done previously because Alfredo is here to donate, and the surgery is scheduled. Good! So, you can now read all of the fourth-character options and determine which is accurate for this encounter. . . .

Now you can report, with confidence, this code to specify the medical necessity for Alfredo's admission into the hospital.

> **Z52.4   Kidney donor**

Good job!

Chapter Summary

As a professional coder, you are responsible to ensure that every physician-patient encounter is supported as medically necessary. You probably know from your own personal experience that there are legitimate reasons for a healthy person to seek the attention of a physician or other health care professional. In ICD-10-CM, virtually all of the codes used to explain these valid reasons are found in the Z code chapter. Here, you will find codes to report the medical necessity for providing preventive care services, performing a screening, observing a patient, and checking for the viability of a potential organ donor.

CODING BITES

Free Preventive Services under Affordable Care Act

All marketplace plans and many other plans must cover the following list of preventive services without charging you a copayment or coinsurance. This is true even if you haven't met your yearly deductible. This applies only when these services are delivered by a network provider.

1. *Abdominal aortic aneurysm one-time screening* for men of specified ages who have ever smoked.
2. *Alcohol misuse screening and counseling.*
3. *Aspirin use* to prevent cardiovascular disease for men and women of certain ages.
4. *Blood pressure screening* for all adults.
5. *Cholesterol screening* for adults of certain ages or at higher risk.
6. *Colorectal cancer screening* for adults over 50.
7. *Depression screening* for adults.
8. *Diabetes (type 2) screening* for adults with high blood pressure.
9. *Diet counseling* for adults at higher risk for chronic disease.
10. *HIV screening* for everyone ages 15 to 65, and other ages at increased risk.
11. *Immunization vaccines* for adults—doses, recommended ages, and recommended populations vary:
    - Hepatitis A
    - Hepatitis B
    - Herpes zoster
    - Human papillomavirus
    - Influenza (flu shot)
    - Measles
    - Mumps
    - Rubella
    - Meningococcal
    - Pneumococcal
    - Tetanus
    - Diphtheria
    - Pertussis
    - Varicella
12. *Obesity screening and counseling* for all adults.
13. *Sexually transmitted infection (STI) prevention counseling* for adults at higher risk.
14. *Syphilis screening* for all adults at higher risk.
15. *Tobacco use screening* for all adults and cessation interventions for tobacco users.

Source: Preventive care benefits. https://www.healthcare.gov/what-are-my-preventive-care-benefits/

CHAPTER 18 REVIEW
Factors Influencing Health Status (Z Codes)

Let's Check It! Terminology

Match each key term to the appropriate definition.

1. **LO 18.6** The donor and recipient individuals are genetically identical.
2. **LO 18.3** An individual infected with a disease who is not ill but can still pass it to another person; an individual with an abnormal gene that can be passed to a child, making the child susceptible to disease.

A. Abnormal Findings
B. Allogeneic

CHAPTER 18 REVIEW

3. LO 18.2 Test results that indicate a disease or condition may be present.
4. LO 18.6 The donor and recipient are of different species.
5. LO 18.2 An examination or test of a patient who has no signs or symptoms that is conducted with the intention of finding any evidence of disease as soon as possible, thus enabling better patient outcomes.
6. LO 18.6 Lost tissue that is replaced with synthetic materials such as metal, plastic, or ceramic.
7. LO 18.6 The donor tissue is taken from a different site on the same individual's body.
8. LO 18.1 Health-related services designed to stop the development of a disease or injury.
9. LO 18.6 The donor and recipient are of the same species.

C. Autologous
D. Carrier
E. Isogeneic
F. Preventive Care
G. Prosthetic
H. Screening
I. Xenogeneic

Let's Check It! Concepts

Choose the most appropriate answer for each of the following questions.

1. LO 18.2 The patient, a 38-year-old adult, presents for an annual physical examination, without abnormal findings. You would use code _____.
   a. Z00.00   b. Z01.00   c. Z00.2   d. Z00.70

2. LO 18.1 When the patient has a preventive care encounter, you will use a _____ code.
   a. W   b. Z   c. X   d. Y

3. LO 18.6 If the donor and recipient are of different species, the graft is
   a. isogeneic.   b. allogeneic.
   c. xenogeneic.   d. autologous.

4. LO 18.2 Abnormal findings are
   a. test results that indicate a disease or condition may be present.
   b. test results that are negative.
   c. test results showing that the donor and recipient are of the same species.
   d. test results that are inconclusive.

5. LO 18.8 All of the following "Z" codes can be reported as the principal diagnosis except _____.
   a. Z00   b. Z33.2   c. Z76.2   d. Z46.0

6. LO 18.6 James Davis presents today to donate his bone marrow. How would you code this?
   a. Z52.3   b. Z52.21   c. Z52.29   d. Z52.20

7. LO 18.3 An individual has been found to be a typhoid carrier. How would you code this?
   a. Z22.1   b. A01.00   c. A01.03   d. Z22.0

8. LO 18.5 The patient presents today to have his surgical wound dressing changed. What code would you use?
   a. Z48.00   b. Z48.01   c. Z48.02   d. Z48.03

9. LO 18.4 If a patient is without signs or symptoms and is being watched for a suspected illness, then the patient is under
   a. preventive care.   b. observation.
   c. continuous care.   d. aftercare.

10. LO 18.7 Ben Harris, an 8-year-old male, has an ear infection. Dr. Whitman prescribed a round of penicillin, but Ben's condition has not improved. Ben's infection is resistant to penicillin. You would first code the infection and then code _____.
    a. Z16.10   b. Z16.11   c. Z16.21   d. Z16.22

Let's Check It! Guidelines

Part I

Refer to the Official Guidelines and fill in the blanks according to the Chapter 21, Factors influencing health status and contact with health services, Chapter-Specific Coding Guidelines.

first-listed	secondary	any
screening	present	past
potential	Z	carrier
procedure	specifically	higher
depending	Family	no
sequelae	not	

1. _____ codes are for use in _____ health care setting.
2. Z codes may be used as either a _____ (principal diagnosis code in the inpatient setting) or secondary code, _____ on the circumstances of the encounter.
3. Z codes are _____ procedure codes.
4. A corresponding _____ code must accompany a Z code to describe any procedure performed.
5. Contact/exposure codes may be used as a first-listed code to explain an encounter for testing, or, more commonly, as a _____ code to identify a potential risk.
6. Status codes indicate that a patient is either a _____ of a disease or has the _____ or residual of a past disease or condition.
7. Personal history codes explain a patient's _____ medical condition that _____ longer exists and is not receiving any treatment, but that has the _____ for recurrence, and therefore may require continued monitoring.
8. _____ history codes are for use when a patient has a family member(s) who has had a particular disease that causes the patient to be at _____ risk of also contracting the disease.
9. A _____ code may be a first-listed code if the reason for the visit is _____ the screening exam.
10. The observation codes are not for use if an injury or illness or any signs or symptoms related to the suspected condition are _____.

Part II

Z40	routine	support
surveillance	continued	living
multiple	prophylactic	inital
aftermath	Z52	risk

1. Aftercare visit codes cover situations when the _____ treatment of a disease has been performed and the patient requires _____ care during the healing or recovery phase, or for the long-term consequences of the disease.
2. The follow-up codes are used to explain continuing _____ following completed treatment of a disease, condition, or injury.
3. A follow-up code may be used to explain _____ visits.
4. Codes in category _____, Donors of organs and tissues, are used for _____ individuals who are donating blood or other body tissue.
5. Counseling Z codes are used when a patient or family member receives assistance in the _____ of an illness or injury, or when _____ is required in coping with family or social problems.
6. The Z codes allow for the description of encounters for _____ examinations, such as, a general checkup, or, examinations for administrative purposes, such as, a pre-employment physical.
7. For encounters specifically for _____ removal of an organ (such as prophylactic removal of breasts due to a genetic susceptibility to cancer or a family history of cancer), the principal or first-listed code should be a code

from category _____, Encounter for prophylactic surgery, followed by the appropriate codes to identify the associated _____ factor (such as genetic susceptibility or family history).

Let's Check It! Rules and Regulations

Please answer the following questions from the knowledge you have gained after reading this chapter.

1. LO 18.2 Why is early detection important? Include examples of early detection encounters.
2. LO 18.3 Why is it important for a patient to know if he or she has a genetic susceptibility?
3. LO 18.5 Why would a patient need continuing care or aftercare?
4. LO 18.6 Explain the difference between *autologous, allogeneic,* and *xenogeneic.*
5. LO 18.8 List 10 of the Z codes, including descriptions, that are permitted to be only first-listed or principal codes.

YOU CODE IT! Basics

First, identify the condition in the following diagnoses; then code the diagnosis.

Example: Awaiting organ transplant status:

a. main term: *Status*   b. diagnosis: *Z76.82*

1. Encounter for disability limiting activities:
   a. main term: _____   b. diagnosis: _____
2. Encounter for screening for human papillomavirus:
   a. main term: _____   b. diagnosis: _____
3. Personal history of leukemia:
   a. main term: _____   b. diagnosis: _____
4. Genetic susceptibility to malignant neoplasm:
   a. main term: _____   b. diagnosis: _____
5. Contact with and suspected exposure to rubella:
   a. main term: _____   b. diagnosis: _____
6. Carrier of diphtheria:
   a. main term: _____   b. diagnosis: _____
7. Encounter for surveillance of injectable contraceptive:
   a. main term: _____   b. diagnosis: _____
8. Encounter for procreative management:
   a. main term: _____   b. diagnosis: _____
9. Encounter for fitting and adjustment of external right breast prosthesis:
   a. main term: _____   b. diagnosis: _____
10. Aftercare following explantation of knee joint:
    a. main term: _____   b. diagnosis: _____
11. Cornea donor:
    a. main term: _____   b. diagnosis: _____
12. High-risk bisexual behavior:
    a. main term: _____   b. diagnosis: _____
13. Acquired absence of left upper limb below elbow:
    a. main term: _____   b. diagnosis: _____
14. Encounter for examination of blood pressure without abnormal findings:
    a. main term: _____   b. diagnosis: _____
15. Presence of heart assist device:
    a. main term: _____   b. diagnosis: _____

YOU CODE IT! Practice

Using the techniques described in this chapter, carefully read through the case studies and determine the most accurate ICD-10-CM code(s) and external cause code(s), if appropriate, for each case study.

1. Donald DuFour, an 8-month-old male, is brought in by his mother and Kent Fuller to determine if Kent is the biological father. Don's mother is applying for child support and social welfare benefits and needs proof

of the biological father before she can proceed. Dr. Sanderson completes a paternity test, results 99.99% that Kent is the biological father.

2. Jane Ellerbe, a 36-year-old female, presents today to see Dr. Molly, her dentist. Dr. Molly's dental hygienist cleans Jane's teeth and Dr. Molly completes a dental examination. Dr. Molly notes no abnormalities.

3. Charles Copeland, a 48-year-old male, presents today to see Dr. McElmurray. Charles is scheduled to have a cardiac pacemaker implanted. Dr. McElmurray completes the pre-procedural cardiovascular examination and clears Charles for the implant.

4. Betty Junketer, a 32-year-old female, was plugging in a light fixture at work when it shocked her badly. She was taken to the ER by the office manager. After the appropriate tests were completed, Dr. Peterson, the ER physician, put Betty under observation.

5. Tammy Coco, a 33-year-old female, went on a tour of 19th century buildings last week. The company that conducted the tour just announced asbestos was found in some of these buildings. Tammy comes to see Dr. Kiefer today because she is concerned she might have been exposed to asbestos. Dr. Kiefer completes the appropriate tests, which return a negative result for asbestos exposure.

6. Kelly Richardson, a 46-year-old female, comes in today with the complaints of painful and burning urination. Dr. Keyton completes the appropriate tests and diagnoses Kelly with a UTI due to *Staphylococcus aureus;* the culture shows the UTI is resistant to vancomycin.

7. Connie Burton, a 63-year-old female, presents today for a screening for malignant neoplasm of the ovaries. Connie's mother died at age 58 of ovarian cancer. Dr. Bales performs the screening; results were negative.

8. Bennie Cantrell, a 45-day-old male, is brought in by his parents for a well-baby check. Dr. Davis notes that Bennie's heel prick is slow to coagulate and stop bleeding. After the appropriate tests, Dr. Davis diagnoses Bennie with hemophilia A, symptomatic carrier.

9. Ross Risinger, a 47-year-old male, presents today for screening of a malignant neoplasm of the prostate. Ross's grandfather died of prostate cancer. Dr. Richardson completes the appropriate test; results were negative.

10. Nellie Preacher, a 27-year-old female, is in her second trimester of pregnancy, G2 P1. Nellie presents today for her regular checkup. Dr. Williams notes no abnormalities and tells Nellie she is doing fine.

11. Alexandra Smith, a 31-year-old female, presents today to donate blood platelets for her child, who has been diagnosed with thrombocytopenia.

12. Martha Henry, a 38-year-old female, was diagnosed with breast cancer. Martha had a mastectomy 1 month ago and Dr. Martin chose to delay the breast reconstruction. Martha presents today for the breast reconstruction procedure.

13. Van Poteat, a 59-year-old male, was diagnosed with colon cancer and now has an end colostomy. Van comes to see Dr. Holland, who inspects and cleans the colostomy opening. Dr. Holland tells Van he is doing well.

14. Edwina Henning, a 61-year-old female, was diagnosed with atrial fibrillation and her cardiologist, Dr. Balestrero, prescribed heparin, an anticoagulant. Edwina is taking the heparin as prescribed and presents today for therapeutic drug monitoring.

15. Andrew Medders, a 12-year-old male, is brought in by his parents to see Dr. Hearn, his pediatrician. Andrew has been cross and having some temper tantrums. Dr. Hearn notes Andrew has yawned three times since he has been in the examination room. Dr. Hearn also notes minor periorbital dark circles and slight periorbital puffiness. Andrew admits he has not been sleeping well. Andrew is diagnosed with sleep deprivation.

YOU CODE IT! Application

The following exercises provide practice in abstracting physicians' notes and learning to work with documentation from our health care facility, Prader, Bracker, & Associates. These case studies are modeled on real patient encounters. Using the techniques described in this chapter, carefully read through the case studies and determine the most accurate ICD-10-CM code(s) and external cause code(s), if appropriate, for each case study.

CHAPTER 18 REVIEW

PRADER, BRACKER, & ASSOCIATES

A Complete Health Care Facility

159 Healthcare Way • SOMEWHERE, FL 32811 • 407-555-6789

PATIENT: ELLIOTT, ELLYN

ACCOUNT/EHR #: ELLIEL001

DATE: 10/16/18

Attending Physician: Oscar R. Prader, MD

S: Patient is a 27-year-old female who came in for a physical. I last saw this patient approximately 1 month ago when she received her annual flu shot. She is starting a new job on the first of next month and is required by her employment contract to get a complete physical including blood pressure check, cholesterol screening, blood glucose levels, tetanus-diphtheria and acellular pertussis (TdAP), and flu vaccine.

O: Vital signs charted by the nurse, including BMI. Finger stick glucose test was normal, showing there were no indications of patient being prediabetic. Cholesterol screening is within normal limits. The TdAP immunization was administered on 5/24/2012. The flu vaccine was administered on 09/14/2018.

A: Preemployment examination.

P: Form completed, and attached the documentation showing the TdAP and flu administration dates, and signed it.

ORP/pw   D: 10/16/18 09:50:16   T: 10/18/18 12:55:01

Determine the most accurate ICD-10-CM code(s).

WESTON HOSPITAL

629 Healthcare Way • SOMEWHERE, FL 32811 • 407-555-6541

PATIENT: GALLOP, MICHAEL

ACCOUNT/EHR #: GALLMI001

DATE: 10/16/18

Attending Physician: Renee O. Bracker, MD

S: Neonate was born 8 hours ago via spontaneous vaginal delivery, full-term, this hospital.

O: Newborn screening exam performed in the well-baby nursery included pulse oximetry showing normal percentage of hemoglobin in his blood that is saturated with oxygen. However, the test for hypothyroidism was positive. Prior to discharge, I met with the parents and explained this condition and discussed thyroxine, the medication required so the baby can avoid problems such as slowed growth and brain damage.

A: Congenital hypothyroidism without goiter

P: Rx: Thyroxine

Follow-up in office in 2 days

ROB/pw   D: 10/16/18 09:50:16   T: 10/18/18 12:55:01

Determine the most accurate ICD-10-CM code(s).

PRADER, BRACKER, & ASSOCIATES

A Complete Health Care Facility

159 Healthcare Way • SOMEWHERE, FL 32811 • 407-555-6789

PATIENT: BELLOW, SANDRA

ACCOUNT/EHR #: BELLSA001

DATE: 10/17/18

Attending Physician: Oscar R. Prader, MD

Patient and her husband, Wayne, are thinking about starting a family, so they came in to learn about genetic screenings. They wanted to get all the information possible before Sandra gets pregnant so preparations can be employed to have a healthy child. I counseled them and discussed many options. Both Sandra and Wayne decided to complete a preconception genetic test, and family histories were reviewed.

ORP/pw   D: 10/17/18 09:50:16   T: 10/18/18 12:55:01

Determine the most accurate ICD-10-CM code(s).

PRADER, BRACKER, & ASSOCIATES

A Complete Health Care Facility

159 Healthcare Way • SOMEWHERE, FL 32811 • 407-555-6789

PATIENT: LESZEK, OGLEV

ACCOUNT/EHR #: LESZOG001

DATE: 10/17/18

Attending Physician: Renee O. Bracker, MD

S: This 13-year-old male was last seen in this office for his back-to-school annual exam 3 months ago. This exam revealed a healthy young man without any significant medical history.

Today Oglev presents complaining of a cough and a sore throat, of approximately 1 week duration. He is accompanied by his mother. He and his mother deny fever, nasal congestion, or runny nose. He says he feels more tired than usual, and his mom states that she can't get him out of bed to go to school. Oglev has been truant from school over the last 6 weeks. Patient states that his "mom won't get off my back." He admits that his grades have been dropping and he quit the baseball team. Mom leaves the room, and patient admits to smoking pot every day, sometimes several times a day, for the last month or so. He denies any other drug use and states smoking pot is "no big deal."

O: Physical examination is remarkable only for a mildly erythematous throat without petechiae. Lungs are clear, and the rest of his exam is normal. Vital signs are also unremarkable.

COUNSELING: Patent is assured that doctor-patient confidentiality is secure. We discussed side effects and risks of abusing pot. He states he has tried to quit but can't make it through an entire day without smoking. It is pointed out to him that his pot use is already having a negative impact on his life. He understands that his parents need to know about this but that he must tell them himself. We discussed options and methodologies for his quitting with reduced effects. He agrees to regular surveillance.

A: Marijuana abuse counseling

P: Refer to drug counselor

ROB/pw   D: 10/17/18 09:50:16   T: 10/18/18 12:55:01

Determine the most accurate ICD-10-CM code(s).

PRADER, BRACKER, & ASSOCIATES

A Complete Health Care Facility

159 Healthcare Way • SOMEWHERE, FL 32811 • 407-555-6789

PATIENT: MONETS, ARNOLD

ACCOUNT/EHR #: MONEAR001

DATE: 10/17/18

Attending Physician: Oscar R. Prader, MD

S: Patient is a 37-year-old male who came to our office for his annual physical exam. Blood was taken and processed in our in-house lab while the rest of the exam was completed. The results of his blood work revealed a random elevated transferrin saturation of 82%.

O: Past Medical History: Noncontributory

Family History: Noncontributory

Social History: Active; states he works out in the gym three times a week; apparently healthy; married for 4 years to Valerie, no children. He states that his wife gives him a multivitamin daily, but he is not certain which one or its exact contents. His diet includes raw oysters on the half shell and sushi about once a week; denies eating red meat or organ meat; drinks coffee, about three cups a day, but denies drinking teas or caffeinated beverages.

Physical Exam: Unremarkable; Height: 6'1"; Weight: 215 lb.; Vital signs: within normal limits.

A: Hemochromatosis

P: Quantitative phlebotomy of 500 mL of whole blood per week for an estimated 5 months.

Regular monitoring via blood tests every month: serum ferritin, hemoglobin, and hematocrit over the course of the phlebotomy treatments.

Dietary modifications, including elimination of all iron supplements and multivitamins containing iron, as well as no more consumption of raw shellfish.

ORP/pw   D: 10/17/18 09:50:16   T: 10/19/18 12:55:01

Determine the most accurate ICD-10-CM code(s).

Inpatient (Hospital) Diagnosis Coding

19

Learning Outcomes

After completing this chapter, the student should be able to:

LO 19.1 Evaluate concurrent and discharge coding methodologies.
LO 19.2 Utilize the Official Guidelines specific for inpatient reporting.
LO 19.3 Apply the Present-On-Admission (POA) indicators properly.
LO 19.4 Determine the impact of diagnosis-related groups (DRGs) on the coding process.
LO 19.5 Recognize the importance of the Uniform Hospital Discharge Data Set (UHDDS).

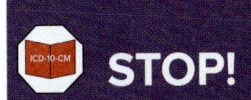

Key Terms

Co-morbidity
Complication
Concurrent Coding
Diagnosis-Related Group (DRG)
Hospital-Acquired Condition (HAC)
Major Complication and Co-morbidity (MCC)
Present-On-Admission (POA)
Uniform Hospital Discharge Data Set (UHDDS)

STOP! Remember, you need to follow along in your ICD-10-CM code book for an optimal learning experience.

19.1 Concurrent and Discharge Coding

Some acute care facilities have patients who may spend weeks or months in the hospital. In these cases, professional coding specialists may do what is called **concurrent coding**. This means that coders actually go up to the nurse's station on the floor of the hospital and code from the patient's chart while the patient is still in the hospital. Concurrent coding enables the hospital to gain reimbursement to date without having to wait until the patient is discharged, improving cash flow for the facility. Figure 19-1 shows you an example of progress notes that might be found in a patient's chart. A coder performing concurrent coding would read these, as well as other documentation, to determine what diagnoses to report.

Once a patient is discharged, you will go through the complete patient record. The most important documentations to look for include:

- *Discharge summary or discharge progress notes*, signed by the attending physician.
- *Hospital course*, which is a summary of the patient's hospital stay.
- *Discharge instructions*, a copy of which is given to the patient.
- *Discharge disposition*, which contains orders for the patient to be transferred home with special services, transferred to another facility, etc.
- *The death/discharge summary*, which is used if the patient expired prior to discharge.

All of these documents should be reviewed to provide you with a complete picture of what procedures, services, and treatments were provided to the patient, along with signs, symptoms, and diagnoses to support medical necessity.

Concurrent Coding
System in which coding processes are performed while a patient is still in the hospital receiving care.

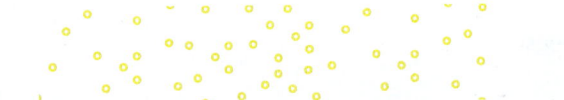

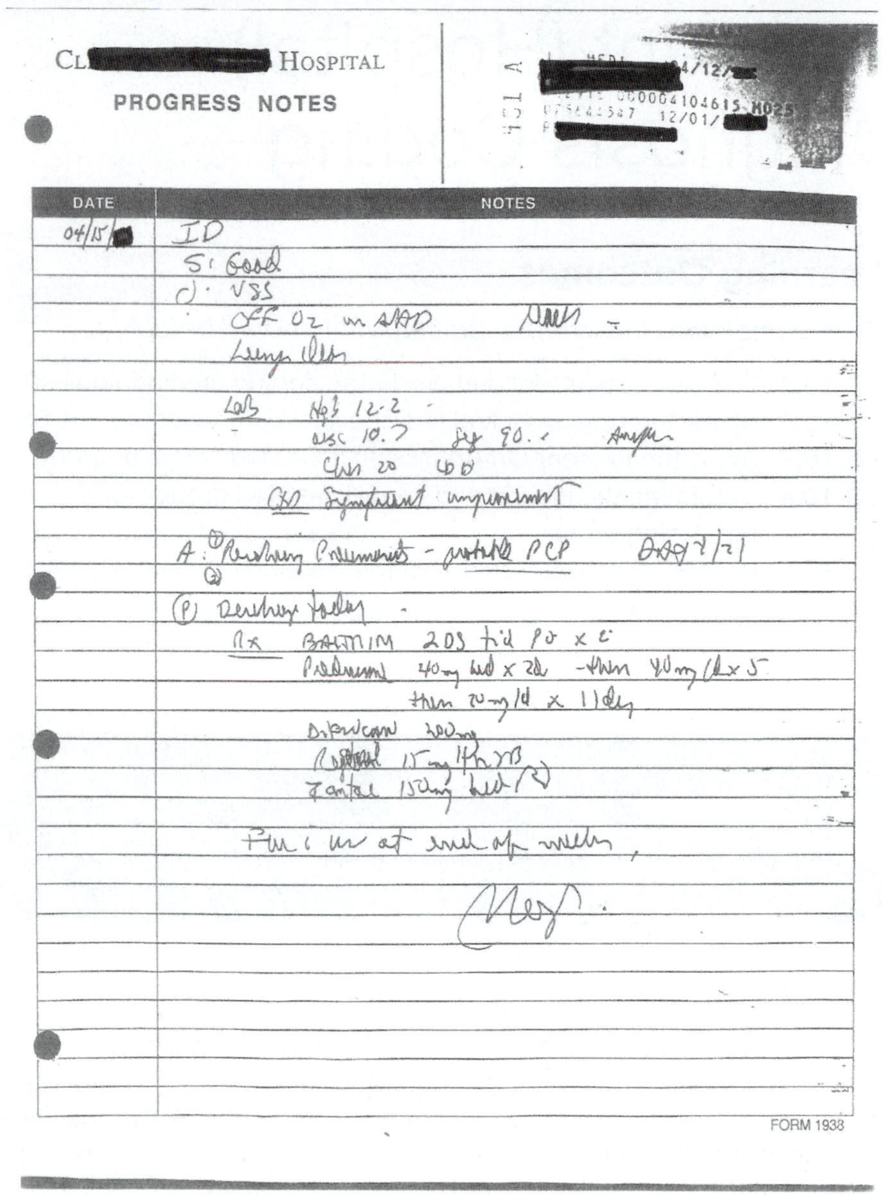

FIGURE 19-1 An example of a handwritten physician's progress note

> ### LET'S CODE IT! SCENARIO
>
> The attending physician, Raymond Morrison, MD, included this in the discharge summary:
>
> Admission Diagnosis: Abdominal pain, status post appendectomy
> Final Diagnosis: Abdominal pain, unknown etiology, status post appendectomy
>
> Brief History: Patient underwent an appendectomy for perforated appendicitis 6 weeks ago. . . . Three days prior to admission, she had a recurrent bout of diffuse, dull abdominal pain in the right upper quadrant with associated nausea and anorexia. She was admitted to the hospital at the time for workup of this pain.
> At this time, the patient has just had a regular meal without difficulty and feels like returning home. She will be discharged home at this time and can follow up with her primary MD. We will see her on an as-needed basis.

> ### Let's Code It!
>
> This discharge documentation provides you the information you need to code the diagnosis supporting this patient's stay in the hospital. (To code the procedures, you would have to review the complete record.)
>
> You have the admitting diagnosis and the final diagnosis. Remember, the Official Guidelines state that the principal diagnosis is "that condition established after study." This tells you that the final diagnosis would be used. You have two conditions to report: *abdominal pain, unknown etiology,* and *status post appendectomy.*
>
> As always, begin in the Alphabetic Index, and find
>
> **Pain(s)** – *see also* **Painful R52**
>   **abdominal R10.9**
>
> Turn to the Tabular List to review the complete code description:
>
> **R10** **Abdomen and pelvis pain**
>
> The **EXCLUDES1** and **EXCLUDES2** notations do not appear to include any diagnosis documented in these notes, so continue reading down the column to determine the most accurate fourth character:
>
> ☑4 **R10.1** **Pain localized to upper abdomen**
>
> Virtually all of the choices you have for the fifth character are specific to the location of the pain in the abdomen. Dr. Morrison did state that when the patient was admitted, she had "abdominal pain in the right upper quadrant," leading you to the fifth character 1. So, here is how this diagnosis code will be reported:
>
> **R10.11** **Right upper quadrant pain**
>
> Are you done? Do you need to report that the patient was status post appendectomy? Yes, you do. It is not known if the pain is related to the surgical procedure or the condition for which it was performed. So let's turn back to the Alphabetic Index and look up
>
> **Status (post)** – *see also* **Presence (of)**
>
> *Appendectomy* is not listed. What can you look up? Think about the patient status post: What exactly is an appendectomy? Surgery. No, *surgery* is not listed in this index either. Hmmmm. Try looking at *postsurgical.* Aha!
>
> **Status (post)** – *see also* **Presence (of)**
>   **postsurgical (postprocedural) NEC Z98.890**
>
> (*Postoperative NEC* is also shown, leading to the same code.)
>
> Let's turn to the Z code section and check this code out:
>
> ☑4 **Z98** **Other postprocedural states**
>
> The **EXCLUDES2** notes don't relate to this discharge summary, so continue reading down the column to find the correct fourth character. No other fourth character is accurate to report postappendectomy, so let's take a look at what the Alphabetic Index suggested:
>
> ☑5 **Z98.8** **Other specified postprocedural status**
>   ☑6 **Z98.89** **Other specified postprocedural states**
>   **Z98.890** **Other specified postprocedural states**
>
> When you review the other procedures included in this classification, none seem to relate to an appendectomy. This code description is the most accurate of those available. Therefore, these are the diagnosis codes you will report for this case:
>
> **R10.11** **Right upper quadrant pain**
> **Z98.890** **Other specified postprocedural states**
>
> Good job!

> **CODING BITES**
>
> What about the part of the diagnosis where Dr. Morrison wrote "Abdominal pain, *unknown etiology*"? How is that reported? Notice that the code R10.11 for the abdominal pain is located in **Symptoms, signs, and abnormal clinical and laboratory conditions, not elsewhere classified** (ICD-10-CM's chapter 18). This is the part that reports the physician could not determine the cause (etiology) of the pain. Had the cause of the pain been identified, you would be reporting that with a different code.

19.2 Official Coding Guidelines

In the front of your ICD-10-CM code book are the Official Coding Guidelines. Included are some specific directions that focus on inpatient coding, rather than on outpatient coding or both. They are always at your fingertips, right there in your code book, but please become familiar with them, so you can gain confidence to use them correctly.

Uncertain Diagnosis

Remember, you learned for *out*patient coding (as shown in Section IV, Subsection H. Uncertain diagnosis) that you are *not permitted* to ever code something identified by the physician in his or her documentation as "rule out," "probable," "possible," "suspected," or other similar terms of an unconfirmed nature.

For *in*patient coding, this guidance (as shown in Section II, Subsection H. Uncertain diagnosis) is different.

> **GUIDANCE CONNECTION**
>
> Read the ICD-10-CM Official Guidelines for Coding and Reporting, section II. **Selection of Principal Diagnosis**, subsection **H. Uncertain diagnosis.**

The guidance for inpatient coders is that you *are permitted* to "code the condition as if it existed or was established." This is done so that medical necessity can be reported for tests, observation, or other services and resources used to care for the patient whether or not these efforts resulted in a confirmed diagnosis.

Patient Receiving Diagnostic Services Only

In the outpatient world, the guidelines instruct you to wait until the test results have been determined and interpreted by the physician as documented in the final report before coding. At that time, confirmed diagnoses, or the signs and symptoms that were documented as the reason for ordering the test, are reported.

> **GUIDANCE CONNECTION**
>
> Read the ICD-10-CM Official Guidelines for Coding and Reporting, section III. **Reporting Additional Diagnoses**, subsection **B. Abnormal findings.**

When you are coding for inpatient services, abnormal test results are not reported unless the physician has documented the clinical significance of those results. Interestingly, in this section of the guidelines, it is reiterated that if the coding professional notices abnormal test results and documentation is unclear from the physician, it is "appropriate to ask the provider whether the abnormal finding should be added."

> ### YOU CODE IT! CASE STUDY
>
> The attending physician, Thomas Talbott, MD, included this in the discharge summary:
>
> Admission Diagnosis: Acute cervical pain, admitted through ED after MVA
>
> Final Diagnosis: Acute cervical pain and radiculitis secondary to degenerative disc disease with posttraumatic activation of pain
>
> Brief History: Patient is a 41-year-old male who was involved in a motor vehicle accident, admitted after being brought to the ED by the ambulance that responded to the accident scene. Patient showed signs of neck and arm pain associated with cervical radiculopathy, radiating into the shoulders along with constant headaches. He has numbness and tingling into the hands and fingers.
>
> Radiology: X-rays AP and lateral cervical spinal x-rays demonstrate evidence of significant degenerative disc disease at C5–6 and C6–7 levels. MRI of cervical spine demonstrates evidence of significant degenerative disc disease at the C5–6 and C6–7 levels with osteophyte formation and canal compromise with the spinal canal diameter reduced to approximately 9 mm. Lumbar spine MRI demonstrates mild degenerative disc disease; otherwise normal.
>
> Recommendation to patient is to undergo an anterior cervical diskectomy and fusion utilizing an autologous iliac bone grafting and placement of anterior titanium plate. After reviewing with patient regarding risks and benefits of surgery, the patient refused and requested to be discharged immediately.
>
> #### You Code It!
>
> In this case, the patient received only diagnostic services. Determine the most accurate diagnosis codes for this inpatient encounter.
>
> **Answer:**
>
> Did you determine the accurate codes?
>
> | | |
> |---|---|
> | M50.122 | Cervical disc disorder at C5-C6 level with radiculopathy |
> | M50.123 | Cervical disc disorder at C6-C7 level with radiculopathy |
> | G89.11 | Acute pain due to trauma |
> | V43.92xA | Unspecified car occupant injured in collision with other type car in traffic accident, initial encounter |
>
> Good job!

19.3 Present-On-Admission Indicators

Present-On-Admission (POA) indicators are required for each diagnosis code reported on UB-04 and 837 institutional claim forms. They are used to report additional detail about the patient's condition.

Centers for Medicare and Medicaid Services (CMS), in CR5499, requires a POA indicator for every diagnosis appearing on a claim from an acute care facility. Claims are returned stamped "unpaid" to the facility if POA indicators are not included. Hospitals are permitted to enter the POA indicators and refile the claim; however, think about all the time and work wasted by having to do this.

Present-On-Admission (POA)
A one-character indicator reporting the status of the diagnosis at the time the patient was admitted to the acute care facility.

> ### GUIDANCE CONNECTION
>
> Read the ICD-10-CM Official Guidelines for Coding and Reporting, **Appendix I. Present on Admission Reporting Guidelines.**

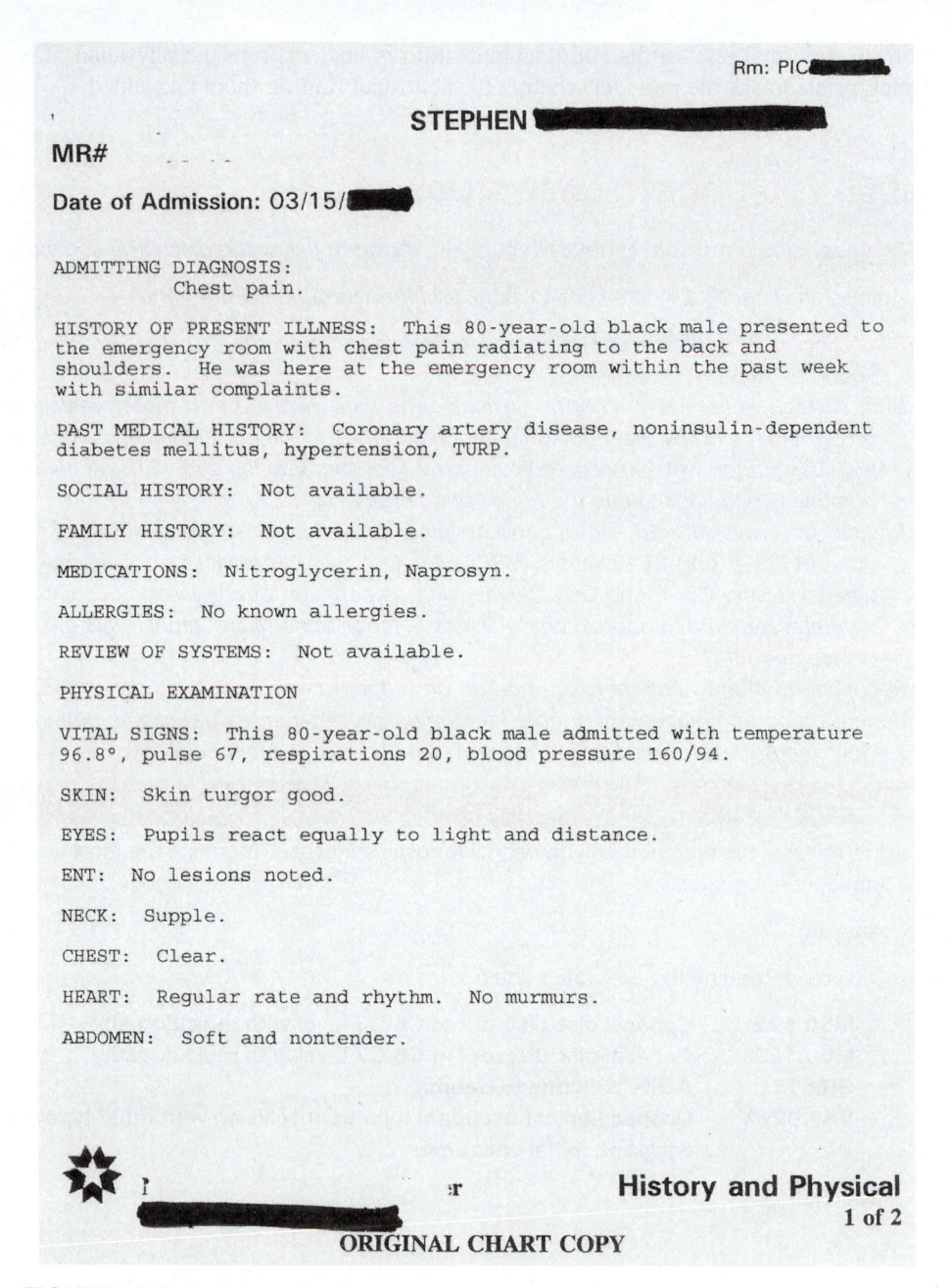

```
                                                          Rm: PIC
                    STEPHEN
    MR#

    Date of Admission: 03/15/

    ADMITTING DIAGNOSIS:
          Chest pain.
    HISTORY OF PRESENT ILLNESS:  This 80-year-old black male presented to
    the emergency room with chest pain radiating to the back and
    shoulders.  He was here at the emergency room within the past week
    with similar complaints.
    PAST MEDICAL HISTORY:  Coronary artery disease, noninsulin-dependent
    diabetes mellitus, hypertension, TURP.
    SOCIAL HISTORY:  Not available.
    FAMILY HISTORY:  Not available.
    MEDICATIONS:  Nitroglycerin, Naprosyn.
    ALLERGIES:  No known allergies.
    REVIEW OF SYSTEMS:  Not available.
    PHYSICAL EXAMINATION
    VITAL SIGNS:  This 80-year-old black male admitted with temperature
    96.8°, pulse 67, respirations 20, blood pressure 160/94.
    SKIN:  Skin turgor good.
    EYES:  Pupils react equally to light and distance.
    ENT:  No lesions noted.
    NECK:  Supple.
    CHEST:  Clear.
    HEART:  Regular rate and rhythm.  No murmurs.
    ABDOMEN:  Soft and nontender.


                                                    History and Physical
                                                            1 of 2
                    ORIGINAL CHART COPY
```

FIGURE 19-2 An example of an admitting history and physical (H&P) (Page 1 of 2)

CODING BITES

A POA indicator is required to be assigned to the principal diagnosis codes as well as all secondary diagnoses, including external cause of injury codes.

Hospital-Acquired Condition (HAC)
A condition, illness, or injury contracted by the patient during his or her stay in an acute care facility; also known as *nosocomial condition*.

General Reporting Guidelines

According to CMS Publication 100-04, "*Present on admission is defined as present at the time the order for inpatient admission occurs—conditions that develop during an outpatient encounter, including emergency department, observation, or outpatient surgery, are considered as present on admission.*"

What does this mean? This means professional coders must carefully review the admitting physician's history and physical (H&P)—the documentation that supports the order to admit the patient into the hospital (see Figure 19-2 for an example)—to determine whether or not the condition was identified at that time. Then you will assign the POA indicator to report this fact: Yes—this diagnosis was present when the patient was admitted; No—it was not present; and so on.

One reason for the importance of gathering POA data is to identify **hospital-acquired conditions (HACs)**. A hospital-acquired condition is exactly what it sounds

```
                                                    Rm: PIC
                    STEPHEN
MR#


GENITALIA:  Not done.

RECTAL:  Not done.

EXTREMITIES:  No edema.

NEUROLOGIC:  Intact.

ADMISSION IMPRESSION:
    1.  Chest pain.
    2.  Noninsulin-dependent diabetes mellitus.
    3.  Hypertension.

TREATMENT PLAN:  The patient went to the telemetry floor.  He was seen
in consultation by Dr. Dennis, cardiologist.  CPK, LDH, troponin,
q.8h. x 3, EKG daily x 3.  He was given an inch of nitro paste q.6h.
Further recommendations to follow.

PROGNOSIS:  Guarded.


                                            STEPHEN

SMS:rd  3847
d: 03/15/         5:29 P
t: 03/16/         7:09 A
cc:  STEPHEN
```

                                    History and Physical
                                    2 of 2
                    ORIGINAL CHART COPY

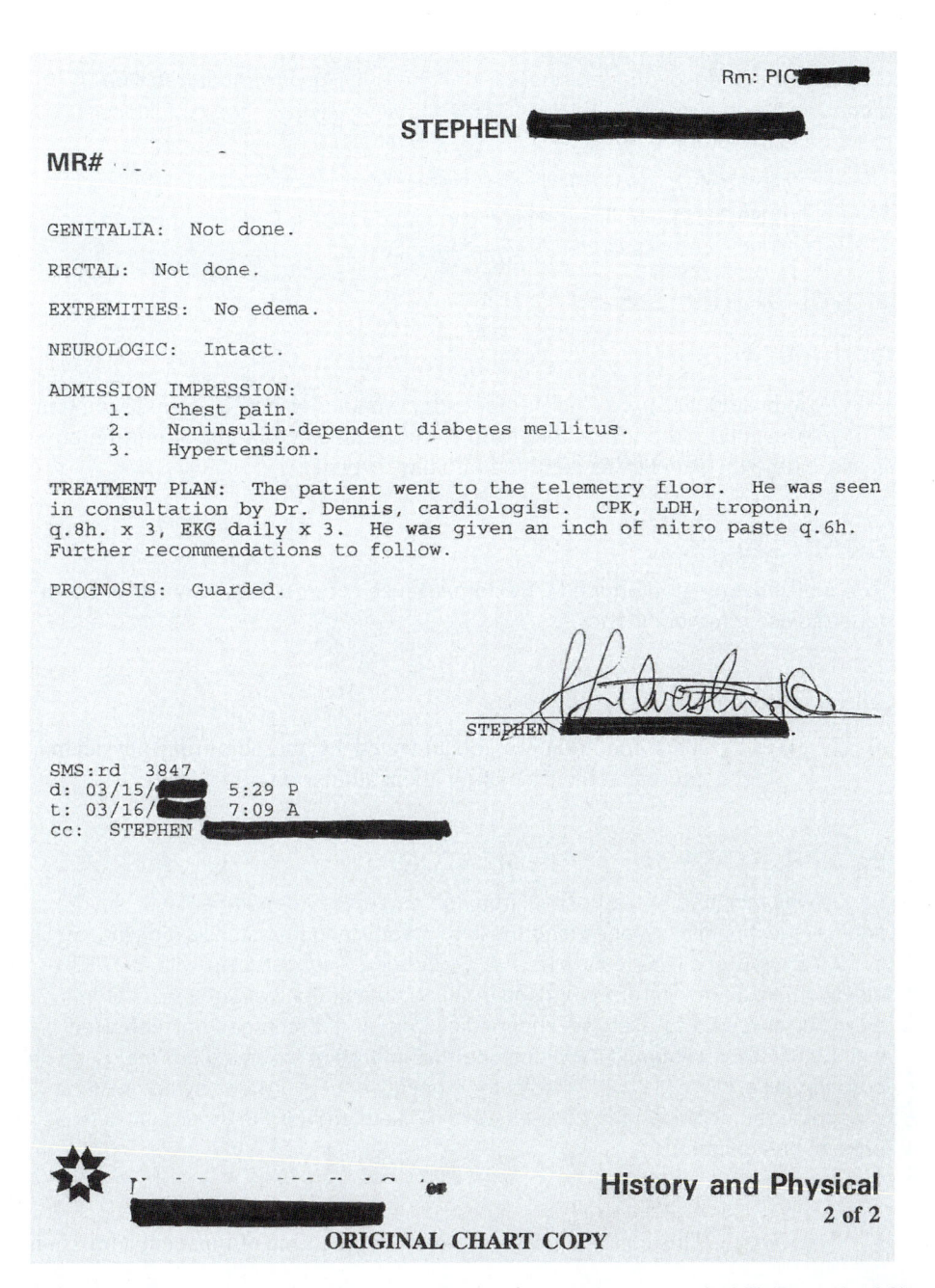

FIGURE 19-2 An example of an admitting history and physical (H&P) (Page 2 of 2)

like: an illness or injury that the patient contracted solely due to the fact that he or she was in the hospital at the time. HAC data are used for many different purposes, including evaluating patient safety directives and limiting payment to a facility for errors it may have made that caused the problem.

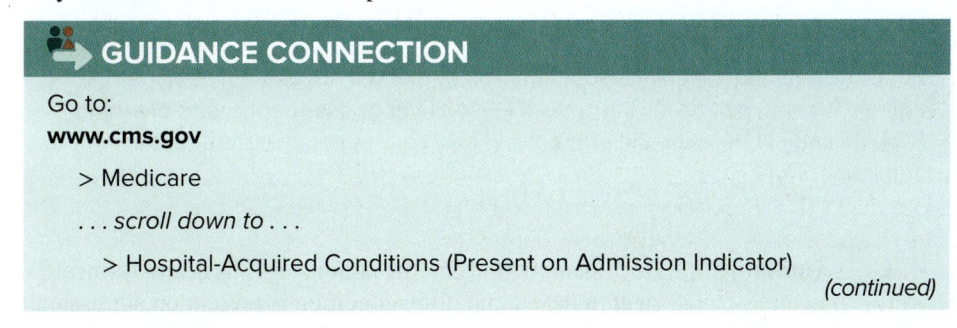

GUIDANCE CONNECTION

Go to:
www.cms.gov

> Medicare

...scroll down to...

> Hospital-Acquired Conditions (Present on Admission Indicator)

(continued)

> On the next screen, on the left side, click on the link: **Hospital-Acquired Conditions** and then click on **ICD-10 HAC LIST** for a current list of the conditions included in this program.
>
> https://www.cms.gov/Medicare/Medicare-Fee-for-Service-Payment/HospitalAcqCond/icd10_hacs.html
>
> The ICD-10 HAC LIST actually shows you the diagnosis and then the procedures, with ICD-10-PCS codes included. Very interesting!

POA Indicators

The POA indicators are used to clearly identify whether or not the signs, symptoms, and diagnoses reported on the claim form were documented by the admitting physician at the time the patient was admitted into the hospital.

> **CODING BITES**
>
> POA indicators are not required for external cause codes unless the code is being reported as an "other diagnosis."

The indicators are Y, N, U, W, and 1:

- **Y   Yes**   This condition was documented by the admitting physician as present at the time of inpatient admission.

> **EXAMPLE OF POA—"Y" INDICATOR**
>
> Felicia was admitted to the hospital from the emergency department with severe angina (chest pains), dyspnea (shortness of breath), and paresthesia (tingling) in her left arm. After all the tests were run, Dr. Gordon diagnosed her with an ST elevation, acute myocardial infarction (AMI) of the anterior wall, left main coronary artery; discussed diet, exercise, and medications; and discharged her. Reported with **I21.01 ST elevation (STEMI) myocardial infarction involving left main coronary artery** would be POA indicator Y because the signs and symptoms that caused her admission to the hospital were those of an AMI. Her heart attack was present on admission.

- **N   No**   This condition was *not* present at the time of inpatient admission.

> **CODING BITES**
>
> If any part of the diagnosis code description was NOT present at the time of admission, report this with an N.

> **EXAMPLE OF POA—"N" INDICATOR**
>
> Porter was admitted with an esophageal ulcer that did not begin bleeding until after admission. Reported with code **K22.11 Ulcer of esophagus with bleeding** is POA indicator N because the entire description of this code was not present at admission.

- **U   Unknown**   Documentation from the admitting physician is insufficient to determine if the condition is present on admission.

EXAMPLE OF POA—"U" INDICATOR

David was admitted to the hospital to have his tonsils removed due to his chronic tonsillitis. The second day, the physician noted a diagnosis of urinary tract infection (UTI) and ordered antibiotics. Upon discharge, code **J35.01 Chronic tonsillitis** will get POA indicator Y; however, code **N39.0 Urinary tract infection, site not specified,** would receive a U because the documentation is not clear whether the UTI was not present and developed while he was in the hospital or was present and not diagnosed when David was admitted.

CODING BITES

It is the responsibility of the physician or health care provider admitting the patient into the hospital to clearly document which conditions are POA. However, it is the professional coder's responsibility to query the physician if the documentation is incomplete with regard to this issue.

- **W**   **Clinically Undetermined**   Provider is unable to clinically determine whether the condition was present on admission or not.

EXAMPLE OF POA—"W" INDICATOR

Torrie was admitted with diabetic gangrene. After a blood workup early on her third day in the hospital, the physician documented an additional diagnosis of septicemia. Upon discharge, the code for the diabetic gangrene (E11.52) would be reported with a POA of Y; however, the septicemia (A41.9) would receive POA indicator W because the physician documented that there is no way to be certain clinically whether the septicemia was not present and developed while she was in the hospital or present and not diagnosed when Torrie was admitted.

👥 GUIDANCE CONNECTION

Read the ICD-10-CM Official Guidelines for Coding and Reporting, **Appendix I, Present on Admission Reporting Guidelines,** subsection **Condition is on the "Exempt from Reporting" list.**

- **1**   **Exempt**

You can find a list of the conditions, and their diagnosis codes, that are exempt from POA reporting in the Official Coding Guidelines in your ICD-10-CM book or on the CMS website. (*Note:* Some third-party payers prefer this box remain blank instead of using the numeral 1.)

EXAMPLE OF POA—"EXEMPT" DIAGNOSES

Belinda was admitted to the hospital in full labor and delivered a beautiful baby boy the next morning. Upon discharge, both codes **O80 Normal delivery** and **Z37.0 Outcome of delivery, single liveborn,** are reported with POA indicator 1. You will notice that both of these codes are on the *Categories and Codes Exempt from Diagnosis Present on Admission Requirement* list shown in the Official Coding Guidelines in ICD-10-CM, Appendix I.

> **CODING BITES**
>
> The CDC website has the detailed list of ICD-10-CM codes that are exempt from (do not require) the use of a POA indicator:
>
> ftp://ftp.cdc.gov/pub/Health_Statistics/NCHS/Publications/ICD10CM/2017/
>
> *The conditions on this exempt list represent categories and/or codes for circumstances regarding the health care encounter or factors influencing health status that do not represent a current disease or injury or are always present on admission.*

LET'S CODE IT! SCENARIO

Kimberly Byner was admitted into the hospital because she was suffering acute exacerbation of her obstructive chronic bronchitis. After 2 days of treatment, while still in the hospital, she tried to get out of bed without help, fell, and broke her left wrist.

Let's Code It!

The reason Kimberly was admitted into the hospital was because she was having exacerbation of her bronchitis. Therefore, the documentation (the physician's H&P) identifies this as being present when she was admitted:

J44.1   Chronic obstructive pulmonary disease with (acute) exacerbation
             POA: Y

When she was discharged, Kimberly also had her wrist in a cast, due to the break suffered from her fall. This is very clearly a condition she did not have when she was admitted:

S62.102A   Fracture of unspecified carpal bone, left wrist, initial encounter
             POA: N

19.4 Diagnosis-Related Groups

Diagnosis-Related Group (DRG)
An episodic care payment system basing reimbursement to hospitals for inpatient services upon standards of care for specific diagnoses grouped by their similar usage of resources for procedures, services, and treatments.

In addition to dealing with diagnosis and procedure codes, hospitals must work with **diagnosis-related groups (DRGs)** for Medicare reimbursement, under Medicare Part A—Hospital Insurance. To determine how much an acute care facility will be paid, the Inpatient Prospective Payment System (IPPS) was developed. Within IPPS, each and every patient case is sorted into a DRG.

Each DRG has a payment weight assigned to it determined by the typical resources used to care for the patient in that case. This calculation includes the labor costs, such as nurses and technicians, as well as nonlabor costs, such as maintenance for equipment and supplies.

> **GUIDANCE CONNECTION**
>
> Go to:
>
> **www.cms.gov**
>
> > Medicare
>
> . . . scroll down to. . .
>
> > Acute Inpatient PPS
>
> Here, along with the links on the left side, you will find up-to-date information on the Inpatient Prospective Payment System.

Typically, professional coding specialists do not have to worry about assigning the DRG for a patient's case. This is determined, most often, by a special software program known as a "DRG grouper."

Medicare-Severity Diagnosis-Related Groups (MS-DRGs) are a subset of 745 subclassifications used in the IPPS (Inpatient Prospective Payment System) that Medicare uses to determine reimbursement for services provided to Medicare beneficiaries by acute care health care facilities (hospitals). MS-DRGs are subdivided into three payment tiers based on the presence (or lack) of major complications and co-morbidities (MCC) and/or complications and co-morbidities (CC).

> **EXAMPLE**
>
> There are several other versions of DRG systems that focus on different details:
>
> APR-DRG = All-Patient Refined Diagnosis-Related Group
> APS-DRG = All-Patient Severity-Adjusted DRG
> MS-LTC-DRG = Medicare-Severity—Long-Term Care DRG
> R-DRG = Refined DRG
> AP-DRG = All Patient DRG
> S-DRG = Severity DRG
> IR-DRG = International-Refined DRG

Principal Diagnosis

So why do you need to know all this? The *principal* diagnosis assigned is one of the factors used to determine which DRG is most accurate. Particularly when it comes to coding for reporting inpatient services to a Medicare beneficiary, the sequence in which you place the diagnosis codes can make a big difference in how accurately the hospital will be reimbursed.

Remember that the principal, or first-listed, diagnosis as defined by the guidelines is "that condition established after study to be chiefly responsible for occasioning the admission of the patient to the hospital for care." This is the diagnosis that explains the most serious reason for the patient to be in the hospital. This might be the reason for admission, it might be the most serious condition, or it might be the condition that required the greatest number of services, treatments, or procedures during the patient's stay in the hospital.

> **GUIDANCE CONNECTION**
>
> Read the ICD-10-CM Official Guidelines for Coding and Reporting, section **II. Selection of Principal Diagnosis.**

Complications and Co-morbidities

As each diagnosis is evaluated for its standard of care, CMS understands that a patient in a hospital may have multiple conditions or concerns (signs, symptoms, diagnoses) that are interrelated and create a more complex need for care. These may be *complications and/or co-morbidities (CCs)*.

In some cases, regardless of the precautions that may be taken, **complications** of a procedure or treatment may arise during the patient's stay. Such a condition must be coded and reported to support the medical necessity for the treatment provided to resolve the concern.

Complication
An unexpected illness or other condition that develops as a result of a procedure, service, or treatment provided during the patient's hospital stay.

> **EXAMPLE**
>
> Lori had surgery this morning and is now having a bronchospasm, a reaction to the general anesthesia. This bronchospasm is a complication of the administration of general anesthesia and must be coded and reported to identify the medical necessity for the treatments to help alleviate this condition.

You have learned that a patient may have, or end up with, several different conditions treated during a stay in the hospital. The individual may also have preexisting conditions that have nothing to do with the reason for admission but still need attention by hospital personnel.

> **EXAMPLE**
>
> Henry was admitted into the hospital with appendicitis. During his stay, the physician had to order and the nurses had to continue to give Henry his Lipitor, prescribed for his preexisting hypercholesterolemia (high cholesterol). Even though this condition has nothing to do with the appendicitis or the appendectomy (surgery to remove the infected appendix), this **co-morbidity** must be coded and reported to support the medical necessity for the hospital supplying the medication.

Co-morbidity
A separate condition or illness present in the same patient at the same time as another, unrelated condition or illness.

Major Complications and Co-morbidities

Conditions, illnesses, and injuries come in all shapes and sizes, as well as severities, and so do complications and co-morbidities. Typically, a **major complication and co-morbidity (MCC)** is a condition that is systemic, making treatment for the principal diagnosis more complex and/or making the health concern life-threatening.

Major Complication and Co-morbidity (MCC)
A complication or co-morbidity that has an impact on the treatment of the patient and makes care for that patient more complex.

> **EXAMPLES**
>
> | | | |
> |---|---|---|
> | MS-DRG 799 | Splenectomy with MCC | Weight: 4.7488 |
> | MS-DRG 800 | Splenectomy with CC | Weight: 2.7250 |
> | MS-DRG 801 | Splenectomy without CC or MCC | Weight: 1.7473 |
>
> You can see how the presence, or absence, of MCC and/or CC alters the weight applied to the reimbursement for this procedure.

> **GUIDANCE CONNECTION**
>
> Read the ICD-10-CM Official Guidelines for Coding and Reporting, section **III. Reporting Additional Diagnoses.**

19.5 Uniform Hospital Discharge Data Set

The **Uniform Hospital Discharge Data Set (UHDDS)** is a collection of specific data gathered about hospital patients at discharge. No, this is not an invasion of privacy, nor is it a collection of personal data. The information pulled from hospital claim forms is related to demographic and clinical details.

Demographic data include

Uniform Hospital Discharge Data Set (UHDDS)
A compilation of data collected by acute care facilities and other designated health care facilities.

- *Gender.*
- *Age.*
- *Race and ethnicity.*
- *Geographic location.*
- *Provider information,* such as the hospital facility National Provider Identifier (NPI) as well as attending and operating physician(s).
- *Expected sources of payment,* including primary and other sources of payment for this care.

- *Length of stay (LOS),* determined by date of admission and date of discharge.
- *Total charges billed by the hospital* for this admission (this will not include physician and other professional services billed).

Clinical data collected evaluate

- *Type of admission,* described as *scheduled* (planned in advance with preregistration at least 24 hours prior) or *unscheduled.*
- *Diagnoses,* including principal and additional diagnoses.
- *Procedures, services, and treatments provided* during this admission period.
- *External causes of injury,* determined by the reporting of external cause codes.

Definitions of these, and other, categories as determined by the UHDDS are used by ICD-10-CM in the Official Coding Guidelines. Over the years that the UHDDS has been in place, these definitions have been used to assist the reporting of patient data not only in acute care facilities (hospitals) but also for inpatient short-term care, long-term care, and psychiatric hospitals. Outpatient providers including home health agencies, nursing homes, and rehabilitation facilities also use these definitions for their data.

Chapter Summary

The coding process remains the same for inpatient and outpatient services for which coders are determining and reporting accurate diagnosis codes. The same code set, ICD-10-CM, is used; the same guidelines are used (with the exception of the two specific guidelines). Therefore, with the additional knowledge provided in this chapter, a professional coder can be successful in any type of facility.

CODING BITES

POA Reporting Options

Y = Yes
N = No
U = Unknown
W = Clinically undetermined
Unreported/Not used = Exempt from POA reporting

POA Reporting Definitions

Y = Present at the time of inpatient admission
N = Not present at the time of inpatient admission
U = Documentation is insufficient to determine if condition is present on admission
W = Provider is unable to clinically determine whether condition was present on admission or not

---

CHAPTER 19 REVIEW
Inpatient (Hospital) Diagnosis Coding

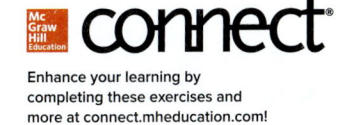

Let's Check It! Terminology

Match each key term to the appropriate definition.

CHAPTER 19 REVIEW

1. LO 19.4 A complication or co-morbidity that has an impact on the treatment of the patient and makes care for that patient more complex.
2. LO 19.4 A separate condition or illness present in the same patient at the same time as another, unrelated condition or illness.
3. LO 19.5 A compilation of data collected by acute care facilities and other designated health care facilities.
4. LO 19.1 System in which coding processes are performed while a patient is still in the hospital receiving care.
5. LO 19.3 A condition, illness, or injury contracted by the patient during his or her stay in an acute care facility; also known as a *nosocomial condition*.
6. LO 19.4 An unexpected illness or other condition that develops as a result of a procedure, service, or treatment provided during the patient's hospital stay.
7. LO 19.4 An episodic-care payment system basing reimbursement to hospitals for inpatient services upon standards of care for specific diagnoses grouped by their similar usage of resources for procedures, services, and treatments.
8. LO 19.3 A one-character indicator reporting the status of the diagnosis at the time the patient was admitted to the acute care facility.

A. Co-morbidity
B. Complication
C. Concurrent Coding
D. Diagnosis-Related Group (DRG)
E. Hospital-Acquired Condition (HAC)
F. Major Complication and Co-morbidity (MCC)
G. Present-On-Admission (POA)
H. Uniform Hospital Discharge Data Set (UHDDS)

Let's Check It! Concepts

Choose the most appropriate answer for each of the following questions.

1. LO 19.1 Which of the following is signed by the attending physician?
   a. Hospital course
   b. Discharge instructions
   c. Discharge summary
   d. Discharge disposition

2. LO 19.2 Martha Jameson was found to have a breast lump during a mammogram last month. She is admitted today for a breast biopsy of her left breast. The pathology report returns with lower-inner quadrant breast carcinoma of the left breast. Martha's mother had breast cancer in her fifties. What is the correct code assignment?
   a. D05.12
   b. D05.12, Z80.3
   c. C50.312
   d. C50.912, Z80.3

3. LO 19.3 All of the following are POA indicators except
   a. X.
   b. Y.
   c. W.
   d. 1.

4. LO 19.5 The UHDDS is a new code set that will replace ICD-10-CM in 2020.
   a. True
   b. False

5. **LO 19.3** Bobby was admitted into the hospital with a compound fracture of the left femur head. Three days later, during his stay, he developed pneumonia. The POA indicator for the pneumonia is
   a. Y.
   b. 1.
   c. W.
   d. N.
6. **LO 19.4** An example of a complication is a
   a. known allergy to penicillin.
   b. family history of breast cancer.
   c. high-risk pregnancy.
   d. postoperative wound infection.
7. **LO 19.2** Inpatient coders are not permitted to ever code something identified in the physician's notes as "suspected" or "probable."
   a. True
   b. False
8. **LO 19.5** The UHDDS collects all of these data elements except
   a. gender.
   b. credit card number.
   c. geographic location.
   d. age.
9. **LO 19.1** Once a patient is discharged, the coder will go through the complete patient record. The most important documentation to look for includes all of the following except
   a. the discharge summary.
   b. the hospital course.
   c. the discharge disposition.
   d. all of these documentations are important.
10. **LO 19.4** DRGs are used for reimbursement from Medicare to
    a. physician offices.
    b. acute care facilities.
    c. ambulatory surgical centers.
    d. walk-in clinics.

Let's Check It! Guidelines

Part I

Refer to the Official ICD-10-CM Guidelines and fill in the blanks according to Sections II and III.

inpatient	diagnostic	Abnormal
outside	one	principal
admitted	complete	discharge
not	unusual	worsens
ask	existed	established
equally	overemphasized	led

CHAPTER 19 REVIEW

1. The circumstances of _____ admission always govern the selection of principal diagnosis.

2. The principal diagnosis is defined in the Uniform Hospital Discharge Data Set (UHDDS) as "that condition _____ after study to be chiefly responsible for occasioning the admission of the patient to the hospital for care."

3. The importance of consistent, _____ documentation in the medical record cannot be _____.

4. Codes for symptoms, signs, and ill-defined conditions from Chapter 18 are _____ to be used as _____ diagnosis when a related definitive diagnosis has been established.

5. In the _____ instance when two or more diagnoses _____ meet the criteria for principal diagnosis as determined by the circumstances of admission, diagnostic workup and/or therapy provided, and the Alphabetic Index, Tabular List, or another coding guidelines does not provide sequencing direction, any _____ of the diagnoses may be sequenced first.

6. If the diagnosis documented at the time of _____ is qualified as "probable," "suspected," "likely," "questionable," "possible," or "still to be ruled out," or other similar terms indicating uncertainty, code the condition as if it _____ or was established.

7. When a patient is _____ to an observation unit for a medical condition, which either _____ or does not improve, and is subsequently admitted as an inpatient of the same hospital for this same medical condition, the principal diagnosis would be the medical condition which _____ to the hospital admission.

8. If the provider has included a diagnosis in the final _____ statement, such as the discharge summary or the face sheet, it should ordinarily be coded.

9. _____ findings (laboratory, x-ray, pathologic, and other diagnostic results) are not coded and reported unless the provider indicates their clinical significance.

10. If the findings are _____ the normal range and the attending provider has ordered other tests to evaluate the condition or prescribed treatment, it is appropriate to _____ the provider whether the abnormal finding should be added.

Part II

Go to www.cms.gov and click on the Medicare tab in the upper yellow navigation bar. In the right column, look for Medicare Fee-for-Service Payment. Under this subtitle you will see Acute Inpatient PPS. Now click on it and fill in the blanks accordingly.

(IPPS)	add-on	approved	prospectively
census	diagnosis-related group	unusually	outlier
multiplied	added	divided	low-income
inpatient	qualify	wage	ratio
disproportionate	prospective	cost of living	average

1. Section 1886(d) of the Social Security Act (the Act) sets forth a system of payment for the operating costs of acute care hospital _____ stays under Medicare Part A (Hospital Insurance) based on _____ set rates.

2. This payment system is referred to as the inpatient _____ payment system _____.

3. Under the IPPS, each case is categorized into a _____ (DRG). Each DRG has a payment weight assigned to it, based on the _____ resources used to treat Medicare patients in that DRG.

4. The base payment rate is _____ into a labor-related and nonlabor share.

5. The labor-related share is adjusted by the _____ index applicable to the area where the hospital is located, and if the hospital is located in Alaska or Hawaii, the nonlabor share is adjusted by a _____ adjustment factor.

6. This base payment rate is _____ by the DRG relative weight.

7. If the hospital treats a high-percentage of _____ patients, it receives a percentage _____ payment applied to the DRG-adjusted base payment rate.

8. This add-on, known as the _____ share hospital (DSH) adjustment, provides for a percentage _____ in Medicare payment for hospitals that _____ under either of two statutory formulas designed to identify hospitals that serve a disproportionate share of low-income patients.

9. Also if the hospital is an _____ teaching hospital it receives a percentage add-on payment for each case paid through IPPS.

10. This add-on known as the indirect medical education (IME) adjustment, varies depending on the _____ of residents-to-beds under the IPPS for operating costs, and according to the ratio of residents-to-average daily _____ under the IPPS for capital costs.

11. Finally, for particular cases that are _____ costly, known as _____ cases, the IPPS payment is increased.

12. Any outlier payment due is _____ to the DRG-adjusted base payment rate, plus any DSH or IME adjustments.

Let's Check It! Rules and Regulations

Please answer the following questions from the knowledge you have gained after reading this chapter.

1. **LO 19.3** Define "Present-On-Admission" according to CMS Publication 100-04.
2. **LO 19.2** What are the two instances in which the ICD-10-CM guidelines direct inpatient coders differently than outpatient?
3. **LO 19.4** Explain what DRG stands for and what it is.
4. **LO 19.4** Differentiate between a co-morbidity and a complication.
5. **LO 19.5** What does UHDDS stand for and what is its function? Include the type of data UHDDS collects.

YOU CODE IT! Application

The following exercises provide practice in abstracting physicians' notes and learning to work with documentation from our health care facility, Westward Hospital. These case studies are modeled on real patient encounters. Using the techniques described in this chapter, carefully read through the case studies and determine the most accurate ICD-10-CM code(s) and external cause code(s), if appropriate, for each case study.

WESTWARD HOSPITAL

591 Chester Road

Masters, FL 33955

DISCHARGE SUMMARY

PATIENT: FALSONE, LEWIS

DATE OF ADMISSION: 05/30/18

DATE OF SURGERY: 05/31/18

DATE OF DISCHARGE 06/01/18

CHAPTER 19 REVIEW

ADMITTING DIAGNOSIS: Right breast mass

DISCHARGE DIAGNOSIS: Malignant neoplasm of areola, right breast, estrogen receptor status negative; postsurgical respiratory congestion

This 52-year-old African American male was admitted to the hospital with a palpable 2.25-cm nodule in the right breast in the superficial aspect of the right breast in the 4 o'clock axis near the periphery.

Excision of the right breast mass with an intermediate wound closure of 3 cm was accomplished. Patient tolerated the procedure well; however, some respiratory complications were realized as a result of the general anesthesia so the patient was kept in the facility for an extra day.

Patient is discharged home with his wife. Discharge orders instruct him to make a follow-up appointment with Dr. Facci, the oncologist, to discuss treatment.

Benjamin Johnston, MD

556839/mt98328: 06/01/18 09:50:16   T: 06/01/18 12:55:01

Determine the most accurate ICD-10-CM code(s).

WESTWARD HOSPITAL

591 Chester Road

Masters, FL 33955

DISCHARGE SUMMARY

PATIENT: FRIZZELLI, ALLISON

DATE OF ADMISSION: 07/15/18

DATE OF DISCHARGE: 08/01/18

ADMITTING DIAGNOSIS: Schizoaffective disorder

DISCHARGE DIAGNOSIS: Schizoaffective disorder; hypothyroidism; hypercholesterolemia; borderline hypertension

The patient is a 34-year-old white female with a long history of schizoaffective disorder with numerous hospitalizations, brought in by ambulance for increasing paranoia; increasing arguments with other people; and, in general, an exacerbation of her psychotic symptoms, which had been worsening over the previous 2 weeks.

She is now discharged to return to her home at the YMCA and also to return to her weekly psychiatric appointments with Dr. Mulford. The patient also is advised to follow up with her medical doctor for her hypertension.

The patient was advised during this admission to start on hydrochlorothiazide 12.5 mg daily, but she refused.

She has been compliant with her medication until the recently refused hydrochlorothiazide. She is irritable at times, but overall she is redirectable and is considered to be at or close to her best baseline. She is considered in no imminent danger to herself or to others at this time.

Roxan Kernan, MD

556848/mt98328: 08/01/18 09:50:16   T: 08/01/18 12:55:01

Determine the most accurate ICD-10-CM code(s).

WESTWARD HOSPITAL

591 Chester Road

Masters, FL 33955

DISCHARGE SUMMARY

PATIENT: TAPPEN, KENNETH

DATE OF ADMISSION: 03/05/18

DATE OF DISCHARGE: 03/17/18

ADMITTING DIAGNOSIS: Major depressive disorder

DISCHARGE DIAGNOSIS: Alcohol dependence; cocaine dependence; major depressive disorder, recurrent; HIV positive; hepatitis C; and history of asthma

This 39-year-old single male was referred for this admission, his second lifetime rehabilitation. The patient has a history of alcohol and cocaine dependence since age 17.

During the course of admission, the patient was placed on hydrochlorothiazide 25 milligrams for hypertension, to which he responded well. He participated in this rehabilitation program and worked rigorously throughout.

On discharge, the patient is alert and oriented ×3. Mood is euthymic. Affect is full range. The patient denies SI, HI, denies AH, VH. Thought process is organized. Thought content—no delusions elicited. There is no evidence of psychosis. There is no imminent risk of suicide or homicide.

Benjamin Johnston, MD

556845/mt98328: 03/17/18 09:50:16   T: 03/17/18 12:55:01

Determine the most accurate ICD-10-CM code(s).

WESTWARD HOSPITAL

591 Chester Road

Masters, FL 33955

DISCHARGE SUMMARY

PATIENT: ENGELS, WARREN

DATE OF ADMISSION: 01/15/18

DATE OF DISCHARGE: 01/17/18

ADMITTING DIAGNOSIS: Mass in bladder

DISCHARGE DIAGNOSIS: High-grade transitional cell carcinoma of the left bladder wall; low-grade transitional cell carcinoma in situ, bladder; underlying mild chronic inflammation, bladder

This 59-year-old male was admitted with a suspicious mass identified in the lateral bladder wall. Biopsy was performed, and upon pathology report of malignancy, a transurethral resection of the bladder tumors was performed. Patient was kept overnight. Foley catheter removed second day, and discharged with orders to make appointment to be seen in the office in about 2 weeks to start weekly BCG bladder installation treatments for recurrent bladder tumors.

Kenzi Bloomington, MD

556839/mt98328: 01/17/18 09:50:16   T: 01/17/18 12:55:01

Determine the most accurate ICD-10-CM code(s).

WESTWARD HOSPITAL

591 Chester Road

Masters, FL 33955

DISCHARGE SUMMARY

PATIENT: BROCKTON, BRIAN

DATE OF ADMISSION: 10/07/18

DATE OF DISCHARGE: 10/09/18

ADMITTING DIAGNOSIS: Hematuria

DISCHARGE DIAGNOSIS: Benign prostatic hypertrophy; hematuria

This 51-year-old male had a transurethral resection of prostate 10 years ago, complicated by a postoperative bleed as well as evaluation with an attempted ureteroscopy. This hematuria is secondary to prostatic varices.

Flexible cystoscopy demonstrated a normal urethra and obstructed bladder outlet secondary to a very large nodular regrowth of the prostate at the medium lobe.

A transurethral resection of prostate was performed with success.

Phillip Carlsson, MD

556845/mt98328: 10/09/18 09:50:16   T: 10/09/18 12:55:01

Determine the most accurate ICD-10-CM code(s).

WESTWARD HOSPITAL

591 Chester Road

Masters, FL 33955

DISCHARGE CLINICAL RESUME

PATIENT: LOGAN, PETER

DATE OF ADMISSION: 05/09/18

DATE OF DISCHARGE: 05/14/18

ADMITTING DIAGNOSES:

1. Dyspnea
2. Congestive heart failure (CHR) exacerbation
3. Hypertension
4. Heart murmur
5. Inferior vena cava filter placed July 2010 secondary to lower extremity deep venous thrombosis (DVT)
6. Hypothyroidism with TSH 9.1
7. Peripheral vascular disease—peripheral arterial disease

DISCHARGE DIAGNOSES:

1. Dyspnea, resolved
2. Diastolic CHR, ejection fraction 70%
3. Hypertension, controlled
4. Aortic stenosis with insufficiency
5. Catheter placed secondary to deep venous thrombosis, on Coumadin, INR in 2 on discharge
6. Hypothyroidism
7. Peripheral vascular disease
8. Renal ultrasound with medical disease

HISTORY: A 76-year-old male was admitted with dyspnea. He was found with diastolic CHF exacerbation. The patient was seen by Dr. Shah, vascular surgeon, who believed that he had some mild arterial insufficiency and continued anticoagulation. He wants to see him in his office as an outpatient. During admission, on and off he was having numbness in bilateral feet and hands and cyanosis that resolved by themselves with no problems. Probably Raynaud phenomenon. During the admission he also was seen by cardiologist, who diuresed the patient with no complications. He believes that the patient needs to be started on 1 mg po Bumex. Weigh every day. If the weight gain is more than 3 pounds, Bumex is to be increased by 1 mg po. The patient also was seen by Dr. Almeada, who believed that the patient can go home and continue follow-up as an outpatient. Pulmonology saw the patient as well and believed the same thing. The patient has been stable. Vital signs stable, afebrile, 98% O_2 stat on room air. He was complaining of some biting itching. The daughter had taken him to the dermatologist and wants to continue follow-up with the dermatologist as an outpatient.

RECOMMENDATIONS: Discharge patient home. Follow up with Dr. Yablakoff in the nursing home.

DISCHARGE MEDICATIONS

1. The patient is going with alendronate 70 mg every week, bumetanide 1 mg twice a day if the weight gain is more than 3 pounds

2. Diovan 80 mg once a day

3. Levothyroxine was increased to 200 mcg every day, and check TSH in 4 weeks with Dr. Yablakoff

4. Metolazone 2.5 mg once a day

5. Potassium 20 mEq prn every day

6. Warfarin 5 mg every day. Check INR every day and let Dr. Yablakoff know if the INR is more than 2.5

7. Medrol Dosepak as directed

The outpatient care plan was discussed with the patient and his daughter. They understood, had no questions, and agreed with the plan.

Keith Kappinski, MD

556842/mt98328 05/14/18 12:13:56 05/14/18 17:51:58

cc. Carole Yablakoff, MD

Determine the most accurate ICD-10-CM code(s).

WESTWARD HOSPITAL

591 Chester Road

Masters, FL 33955

DISCHARGE CLINICAL RESUME

PATIENT: DRYLER, ARTHUR

DATE OF ADMISSION: 06/03/18

DATE OF DISCHARGE: 06/06/18

ADMITTING DIAGNOSIS: Ischemia, transient ischemic attack, rule out myocardial infarction, arrythmia

DISCHARGE DIAGNOSES: Transient ischemic attack (TIA)
Hyperlipidemia
Coronary artery disease, status post coronary artery bypass graft and cardioversion
Urinary tract infection

CONSULTATIONS: Dr. Jenson for neurology and Dr. Balmer for cardiology

PROCEDURES: Echocardiogram, TEE, Thallium stress test

COMPLICATIONS: None

INFECTIOUS: None

HISTORY: Eighty-one-year-old white male with significant history of coronary artery disease, status post coronary artery bypass graft 3 years ago and cardioversion in February 2016, who presented with difficulty speaking. He stated that he had difficulty obtaining the right words when he spoke. This lasted about 15 minutes; however, when the patient came to the emergency room he was completely okay. He did not have any deficits. The patient was admitted and consultants were called in to provide evaluation of possible TIA with rule out cardiac source. Carotid Doppler was done. Echocardiogram was done. This showed dilated left ventricle, severe global left ventricular dysfunction, estimated ejection fraction 20% and left atrial enlargement, mitral annular calcification with severe mitral regurgitation, aortic sclerosis with moderate aortic insufficiency, and severe tricuspid regurgitation with estimated pulmonary study pressure of 70 mm. Thallium stress test was uneventful. Persantine infusion protocol and no clinical EKG changes of ischemia and radionuclide showed fixed defect anteroseptal, anteroapical, and adjacent inferior wall with hypokinesis; no ischemia seen. The ejection fraction was calculated 40%. CT of the brain showed white matter ischemic changes and atrophy, no acute intracranial abnormalities. MRI showed extensive periventricular white matter ischemia changes. MRA was normal. EKG was within normal limits, showing sinus bradycardia with average of 50 to 56.

The patient went to TEE to rule out cardiac source. The TEE was not conclusive and there was no hypokinesis, as described in the previous echocardiogram, and it was considered the patient needs to have lifetime Coumadin because of previous events.

The hospital course was uneventful. He never presented with any other new deficit or any new symptoms.

Today, the patient is asymptomatic; vital signs are stable. Monitor shows sinus rhythm, and he is discharged in stable condition to be followed by Dr. Curran in 1 week, by Dr. Jenson in 2 weeks, and by Dr. Balmer in 2 weeks. He will have home health nurse to inject him Lovenox until PT and INR reach therapeutic levels of 2/3. He will be on Coumadin 5 mg po qd, and home health nurse will draw PT and INR daily until Dr. Roman thoroughly assesses the patient. He will receive the last dose of Bactrim today for urine; however, urine culture has been negative.

Rudolph Langer, MD

556842/mt98328 06/06/18 1:23:36 06/06/18 10:11:59

cc. Karyn Curran, MD

Determine the most accurate ICD-10-CM code(s).

WESTWARD HOSPITAL

591 Chester Road

Masters, FL 33955

DISCHARGE DOCUMENT SUMMARY

PATIENT: WESTCOTT, ROSEANNE

DATE OF ADMISSION: 02/09/18

DATE OF DISCHARGE: 02/10/18

ADMISSION DIAGNOSIS: Abdominal pain, status postappendectomy

DISCHARGE DIAGNOSIS: Abdominal pain, unknown etiology, status postappendectomy

BRIEF HISTORY: The patient is a 21-year-old female who, 6 weeks ago, underwent an appendectomy for perforated appendicitis. About 3 weeks following that, she had episodes of nausea and vomiting and diffuse abdominal pain. This was worked up at Kinsey Urgent Care Center, including CT scan, Meckel scan, and laboratory, which were unremarkable. It resolved spontaneously over a 3-day period. Three days prior to admission, she had a recurrent bout of diffuse, dull, abdominal pain with associated nausea and anorexia. She was admitted to our hospital at the time for workup of this pain.

CLINICAL COURSE: On examination, the patient was found to have a diffuse, mild tenderness without any rebound or peritoneal signs. Plain radiographs of the abdomen were obtained, which were within normal limits. A CT scan of the abdomen and pelvis was also obtained, which was unremarkable. She was without leukocytosis. Dr. Pointer of GI saw the patient in consultation, and an upper GI with small bowel follow-through was obtained. This was performed today and was found to be normal.

At this time, the patient has just had a regular meal without difficulty and feels like returning home. She will be discharged home at this time and can follow up with her primary MD. We will see her on an as-needed basis.

Robyn Charne, MD

6582411/mt98328 02/10/18 12:13:56 02/10/18 17:51:58

Determine the most accurate ICD-10-CM code(s).

WESTWARD HOSPITAL

591 Chester Road

Masters, FL 33955

DISCHARGE DOCUMENT SUMMARY

PATIENT: ROMANSKI, CESAR

DATE OF ADMISSION: 08/01/18

DATE OF DISCHARGE: 08/22/18

FINAL DIAGNOSES:

1. Alcohol dependence, methamphetamine dependence

2. Major depressive disorder, recurrent, current episode severe

3. HIV

4. Tuberculosis of the lung, primary

5. Hepatitis C, chronic

DISCHARGE MEDICATIONS:

1. Zoloft 100 mg po qam

2. Seroquel 50 mg po qhs

3. Truvade 1 tab qam

4. Regataz 300 mg po qam

5. Norvir 100 mg po qam with breakfast

6. Dapsone 100 mg po qam

7. Hydrochlorothiazide 25 mg po qam

DISPOSITION: The patient will return to his residence at the Daylight Hotel. He will attend the hospital continuing day treatment program.

PROGNOSIS: Guarded

HISTORY: He is noted to have significant immunosuppression related to his HIV. Currently there is no stigmata of opportunistic infection.

During the course of admission, the patient was placed on hydrochlorothiazide 25 mg for hypertension, which he responded well to.

CONDITION ON DISCHARGE: The patient is a 43-year-old single black male referred for his first BRU admission, his second lifetime rehabilitation. The patient has a history of alcohol and methamphetamine dependence since age 21. Prior to this admission, he had attained no significant period of sobriety other than time spent incarcerated.

The patient participated in a 21-day MICA rehabilitation program. He worked rigorously throughout the entire program. He had perfect attendance and participated well as a peer support provider. The patient attended eight groups daily. He worked well in individual therapy with his nurse practitioner and social worker.

On discharge, the patient is alert and oriented ×3. Mood is euthymic. Affect is full range. The patient denies SI, HI, denies AH, VH. Thought process is organized. Thought content—no delusions elicited. There is no evidence of psychosis. There is no imminent risk of suicide or homicide.

Kelsey Berge, MD

517895221/mt98328 08/22/18 12:13:56 08/22/18 17:51:58

Determine the most accurate ICD-10-CM code(s).

WESTWARD HOSPITAL

591 Chester Road

Masters, FL 33955

DISCHARGE CLINICAL RESUME

PATIENT: MORETTA, TERACIA

DATE OF ADMISSION: 11/05/18

DATE OF DISCHARGE: 11/18/18

This is a 36–37-week-old female neonate delivered to a 25-year-old, gravida 2, para 1, who was a known breech presentation. Mother presented with complaint of vaginal bleeding, rupture of membranes, and abdominal pain and cramping. On exam found to be complete with large fecal impaction. Fetal heart rate 120 by monitor. To c-section room for disimpaction and cesarean section for breech. Delivered precipitously immediately after impaction was removed, breech presentation. OB moved baby to warmer. She was pale with no respiratory effort or heart rate. Ambu bagged with mask for 30 seconds. Intubation attempted. Code called. UAC was placed. ENT in place and bagged. No heart rate, no breath sounds, pale, cyanotic. Reintubated with chest rise, heart rate about 60. Chest compression stopped when heart rate above 120, color improved. Apgar 0 at 1 minute, 1 at 5 minutes, and 4 at 10 minutes. No spontaneous respiratory effort. Received sodium bicarbonate, epinephrine, and calcium. No grimace, no spontaneous movements. Pupils midpoint, nonreactive to light. NG placed for distended abdomen. Cord pH 7.33. Mother noted to have 50% abruptio placenta. Transferred to Neo. UAC was removed and replaced. UVC also placed.

Physical exam: weight 2,620 grams, pink, fontanelle soft, significant clonus of extremities, tone decreased. Pupils 2 cm and round, nonreactive to light. No movement, no grimace, no suck, good chest rise. Equal breath sounds, no murmur. Pulses 2+. Perfusion good. Abdomen soft and full. No masses. Normal female genitalia externally. Anus patent. Extremities no edema. Skin—Mongolian spot sacrum and both arms, single café-au-lait spot left flank 1.5 cm × 0.5 cm. Palate intact.

IMPRESSION:

1. 36–37 week AGA female

2. Status postcardiopulmonary arrest

3. Rule out sepsis

4. At risk for hypoxic ischemic encephalopathy

PHYSICAL EXAM: 23 days of age, weight 2,520 grams, head circumference 35, pink. Anterior fontanelle soft. Heart—II/VI murmur radiating to the axilla. Chest clear. Abdomen soft, positive bowel sounds, gastrostomy tube intact, wound is okay. Neuro—irritable. The infant has an anal fissure at 12 o'clock that has caused some blood streaks in the stool.

FINAL DIAGNOSES:

1. 36–37 week appropriate for gestational age female

2. History post cardiac arrest

3. Respiratory arrest

4. Rule out sepsis

5. Hypoxic ischemic encephalopathy, mild

6. Seizures

7. Gastroesophageal reflux and feeding problems

8. Postoperative cesarean wound disruption

Nancy Odom, MD

2564821/mt98328 11/18/18 12:13:56 11/18/18 17:51:58

Determine the most accurate ICD-10-CM code(s).

20 Diagnostic Coding Capstone

> **Learning Outcomes**
>
> *After completing this chapter, the student should be able to:*
>
> **LO 20.1** Apply the techniques learned, carefully read through the case studies, and determine the accurate ICD-10-CM code(s) and the external cause code(s), as required.

As you worked your way through the last 19 chapters, you have learned how to abstract documentation and interpret the reasons *WHY* a physician needed to care for a patient—known as the diagnosis—into ICD-10-CM codes. You also learned to distinguish signs and symptoms, and other conditions, and when to code those—or not. Now, this chapter provides you with case studies so you can get some hands-on practice.

For each of the following case studies, read through the documentation and:

- Determine what code or codes report these reasons, to their most specific level.
- Determine how many ICD-10-CM codes you will need to tell the whole story as to WHY the patient required care.
- Identify external cause codes in cases of injury or poisoning.
- If more than one code is required, determine the sequence in which to report the codes.

Remember, the notations, symbols, and Official Guidelines are there to help you get it correct.

YOU CODE IT! DIAGNOSIS CAPSTONE

CASE STUDY 1: JELYSA HANSON

JeLysa Hanson, a 41-year-old female, presents to the ED complaining of shortness of breath and tightness in her chest. Following examination, she is discharged with a diagnosis of musculoskeletal pain due to overexertion while practicing her new hobby, kickboxing in her backyard.

CASE STUDY 2: HARRIS TEAL

Harris Teal, a 19-year-old male, reports to the hospital-based urgent care clinic for headache and wheezing. Following examination, he is discharged with an acute frontal sinus infection, recurrent, and exacerbated asthma due to environmental dust allergies.

CASE STUDY 3: ROGER GILL

Roger Gill, a 39-year-old retired professional athlete, comes in with complaints of intermittent joint pain, particularly in his left shoulder. He was a pitcher on a AA league baseball team. He also states he feels tenderness at the outer aspect of the left shoulder, most often when he raises his arm. He states that simply putting on his shirt is very painful. Dr. Jeaneau asks Roger if he suffered any shoulder injuries while playing baseball. Roger admitted that his left proximal humerus was fractured when hit by a thrown ball during a game. Roger quickly added that it healed OK. Dr. Jeaneau confirms a diagnosis of abscess of the bursa of his shoulder.

CASE STUDY 4: ANGEL DUNBAR

Angel Dunbar, a 27-year-old male, presents to see his physician, Dr. Davison, with the complaints of difficulty breathing, muscle weakness, and fatigue. Following a complete examination, Dr. Davison notes ataxia and sudden muscle spasms in Angel's legs. The lab results are positive for lactic acidosis. CSF results show elevated protein and the muscle biopsy is positive for ragged red fiber. Angel is diagnosed with MERRF syndrome.

CASE STUDY 5: RENAY GRIFFITH

Renay Griffith, a 25-year-old female, recently returned from working for the Red Cross overseas. She presents to the clinic for an evaluation of a rash. Dr. Leisom evaluates the patient and diagnoses her with cutaneous leishmaniasis related to her recent deployment to Iraq.

CASE STUDY 6: MARYBELLE OSTENKOWSKY

Patient: Marybelle Ostenkowsky

Physician: Fiona McNally, MD

December 17, 2018

History

This 87-year-old female has been a patient of the McGraw Health Center and Clinic since 2005. Chronic conditions: pernicious anemia, osteoarthritis, and urinary incontinency. She is fully functional and fully independent. She provides care for her homebound husband, who has severe COPD. They live in a home chosen because it was "close to the hospital" to ensure access to house calls for her husband.

In September 2005, the husband died as a result of respiratory arrest. Her only relative is a niece who talks with her about once a month. In October 2007, her home was broken into and our patient was raped and robbed. She was taken to a local hospital specializing in rape. Here, she was distressed, delusional, and reported to be very emotionally distraught.

Examination

I saw the patient about 3 weeks after the rape in a community nursing home, where she was moved after a 4-day stay at the hospital. She was very distressed, delusional, and confused. She slowly improved over 2 months and was discharged to a senior living center.

In March of 2018, the patient was seen in the office. She is still very emotionally unstable. She is crying, depressed (not suicidal), and stressed about her new home. She wants to move to a different Senior Housing unit because it would be on the bus route, making it easier to get around. She has also hired a middle-aged woman as a caregiver.

In November 2018, 9 months after moving to the new facility, she becomes acutely ill with psychotic symptoms and severe paranoia. She hallucinates that men and women are in her bed and calls others all hours of the day. I admitted her into a hospitalized psychiatric unit and she shows improvement over about 14 days without antipsychotic medication.

Today, 1 week following discharge from the hospital, symptoms rapidly recurred when she returned to the senior apartment. She was disruptive and threatened with eviction unless something was done rapidly. An emergency petition was prepared because she refused medical care. With the help of her companion, we were finally able to persuade her to take a neuroleptic drug (Haloperidol 0.025 – 1.0 mg/day) for her recurrent incapacitating hallucinations. Initial injection was administered IM 5 mg. Our office nurse and staff called her later in the day to guide her through the process of taking her medicines. She slowly but steadily improved and became stabilized.

Diagnosis: Chronic Post Traumatic Stress Disorder

Rx: Haloperidol 0.025 – 1.0 mg/day

CASE STUDY 7: RAYONNETTA CALHOUN

Patient: Rayonnetta Calhoun

Physician: Robert Morgan, MD

ADMISSION to McGraw Hill Hospital

History
A fully functional, independent female who is nearly 89 years old; lives with her two sons. A history finds that she has

- high blood pressure
- CAD
- congestive heart failure
- cataracts
- hearing impairments
- knee osteoarthritis

Current Medications: lisinopril, furosemide, ASA, and metoprolol.

Examination
Patient develops abdominal pain increasing over 4 days; obstipation for 1 day. She is acutely ill and appears uncomfortable and volume depleted. On exam, she has abdominal distention, she has hypoactive bowel sounds, and no mass is found. Her heart is enlarged and no S3.

Laboratory findings:
- WBC . . . 13290
- HCT . . . 42

- Na ... 128
- K ... 2.6
- Bun/creatinine ... normal

An abdominal CT scan shows the cecum is very dilated to 13 cm and the left image shows a possible mass in the descending colon.

Recognizing the seriousness of her illness, she was quickly stabilized with volume repletion due to her hypertonic dehydration. She was in the emergency department 2 hours, then admitted to a non-intensive care surgical unit and cared for by a general surgeon, Herman Canton, MD, and a geriatrician, Kyla Mondolano, MD.

Upon Admission
Protocol calls for endoscopy, but to do so would require a delay before surgery that is clearly needed. There was an urgency to get her to surgery as delays would likely lead to complications. Accordingly, no colonoscopy was performed. Prior to surgery, careful anesthesia planning and intra-operative management were designed. A shortened bowel prep was initiated.

A left hemicolectomy was performed on day 2 with pathology confirmation of malignant neoplasm of the sigmoid colon. Pain was controlled with low doses of morphine and fluid management was tightly managed. She was provided a single, quiet room and a family member stayed with her continuously. The patient was discharged to subacute rehabilitation on day 5, and then to home on day 10.

CASE STUDY 8: WINSTON WALLER

Patient: Winston Waller

Physician: Morris Johnston, MD

August 1, 2018

History:

This patient is a 73-year-old male nonsmoker with type 2 diabetes mellitus and hypertension. He presented to this ED with shortness of breath and was found to have an acute infarction of the anterior wall of his heart showing an ST elevation. He developed several complications, including renal failure from a combination of cardiogenic shock and toxicity from the dye used for emergency catheterization of his heart.

Hemodialysis was started during this hospitalization because of his renal failure. After spending almost a month in the hospital and developing severe deconditioning, he was discharged to a subacute rehabilitation facility.

Examination

While he was there he was noted to have symptoms consistent with mild depression, as well as a prior history of a major depressive episode in 2016. Mirtazapine (Remeron) 25 mg/day was started.

He was transferred to a skilled nursing unit for another month of rehabilitation management of his medical conditions and then discharged home to the care of his wife.

CASE STUDY 9: GERALD YOUNG

Patient: Gerald Young

Physician: Hannah Cohen, MD

This 37-year-old man presents to the psychiatry emergency room for inappropriate behavior and confusion. He works as a janitor and has had reasonably good work attendance. His coworkers say that he has appeared "fidgety" for several years. They specifically mention jerky movements that seem to affect his entire body more recently. His mother is alive and well, although his father died at age 28 in an auto accident.

On examination, he is alert but easily distracted. His speech is fluent without paraphasias but is noted to be tangential. He has trouble with spelling the word "world" backwards and serial seven's, but recalls three objects at 3 minutes. His constructions are good. When he walks, there is a lot of distal hand movement, and his balance is precarious, although he can stand with both feet together. His reflexes are increased bilaterally, and there is bilateral ankle clonus. A urine drug screen is negative.

Most likely diagnosis: Huntington disease.

Next diagnostic step: Genetic counseling and genetic testing for Huntington disease. Review the history very carefully with patient and his relatives and assess medications—either illicit or licit that could be responsible.

Molecular or genetic basis: Repeat CAG triplets present in a gene called huntingtin located on chromosome 4p16.3. Repeat lengths greater than 40 are nearly always associated with clinical Huntington's disease. Confirmed Huntington's disease.

CASE STUDY 10: LORRAINE PARNETE

Patient: Lorraine Parnete

Physician: Jason Nuouri, MD

July 16, 2018

History

A well-established, 67-year-old female patient (since 1991) has controlled hypertension with no complications. She is a smoker [cigarettes, about one pack a day] and takes clonidine and HCTZ for her hypertension, and estrogen to address menopausal symptoms. Overall, she is well and fully active.

Examination

Patient presents with fatigue, about 1 month duration, associated with the withdrawal from estrogen because of published data suggesting an increased risk of breast cancer and other complications. Exam includes complete review of systems. CXR [chest x-ray] and PPD (tuberculin skin test) are negative except for the following:

- cough with minimal sputum
- a low grade fever to about 100°F
- 5 pound weight loss

Plan

Order for CBC, glucose tolerance test, TSH.
Patient to return to discuss lab results.

CASE STUDY 11: BLAIZE MASTERS

PATIENT: Blaize Masters

IMPRESSION: This is a 49-year-old male who has significant multivessel coronary artery disease. He has atypical anginal symptoms, suspected to be secondary to his type 1 diabetes mellitus. Still it is believed that he is at risk for ischemia. To reduce this risk, surgical myocardial revascularization is recommended.

The patient is given complete details about the procedure, the risks, and the benefits. We also discuss alternative treatments that may be viable. The patient signs the informed consent and the surgery is scheduled.

PLAN: Proceed with coronary artery bypass graft operation utilizing the left internal mammary artery as conduit to the left anterior descending. The remaining conduit will come from the greater saphenous veins.

CASE STUDY 12: CAROLINA SPENCER

PATIENT: Carolina Spencer

REASON FOR ENCOUNTER: Assistance with tracheostomy management.

HISTORY OF PRESENT ILLNESS: The patient is a 73-year-old female admitted to McGraw Hospital on July 17th with acute ischemic CVA and DKA. The patient has a very complicated medical history, including respiratory failure, on prolonged mechanical ventilation. She underwent tracheostomy placement on July 19th and was weaned from mechanical ventilation within 12 hours. She was also diagnosed with hospital-acquired pneumonia, multi-organism, and pulmonary embolism by CTPA. She is currently on heparin drip, while started on Warfarin. She also has end-stage renal disease and is on hemodialysis.

PAST MEDICAL HISTORY: In addition to the above, the patient was found to have some type of intracardiac shunt per echocardiogram, not otherwise defined; atherosclerosis of the internal carotid arteries; positive lupus anticoagulants; and long-standing history of diabetes mellitus, type II.

SOCIAL HISTORY: Tobacco and alcohol use are unknown.

MEDICATIONS: Sliding scale insulin, Reglan, Lantus insulin, diltiazem, Timentin, heparin drip, Warfarin, Bactrim, Pepcid, and iron sulfate.

ALLERGIES: No known allergies.

REVIEW OF SYSTEMS: Not available.

FAMILY HISTORY: Not available.

PHYSICAL EXAMINATION:

GENERAL: She is an unresponsive female, in no acute distress.

VITAL SIGNS: Temperature is 98.6 degrees; respiratory rate is 21 to 25, somewhat irregular; pulse is 102; blood pressure is 122/80; and pulse oximetry is 97% on 50% cuffless tracheostomy.

HEENT: Unable to visualize posterior pharynx secondary to the patient's resistance to mouth opening. The patient does have some natural dentition anteriorly. No coating of the tongue is appreciated. The patient has an eschar on the left upper lip, presumably secondary to ET tube. Conjunctivae are clear. Gaze is conjugate. The patient has a size 8 Portex cuffless tracheostomy tube in the midline.

CHEST: The patient has a few crackles at the right base, few anterior coarse rhonchi. No wheeze or stridor with the tracheostomy tube, patent. With finger occlusion of the cuffless #8 Portex, the patient does have stridor and increased respiratory rate. Unable to adequately percuss the chest.

CARDIOVASCULAR: The patient has regular rate and rhythm. No murmur or gallop is appreciated. No heaves or thrills.

ABDOMEN: Soft and obese. The patient has G-tube in position and normoactive bowel sounds. No guarding.

EXTREMITIES: She has decreased pulse in lower extremities bilaterally. No discrepancy in calf size is appreciated. No clubbing, cyanosis, or edema.

NEUROLOGIC: The patient does withdraw, on the left side; grimaces to pain. She is not cooperative with exam at this time.

LABORATORY DATA: BUN 16 and creatinine 3.3 on July 18th with venous CO_2 of 24, calcium 9.1, white count 9200, hemoglobin 9.2, and platelets 515,000. Chest x-ray is not available for review.

IMPRESSION: The patient is a 73-year-old female, status post respiratory failure, prolonged mechanical ventilation, necessitating tracheostomy tube placement. She has had multiple complications including pulmonary embolism, for which she is now anticoagulated with heparin and reportedly intracardiac shunt, which would help explain her Aa gradient. She also reported she had a right-sided cavitary lesion and had negative AFB on bronchoalveolar lavage.

RECOMMENDATIONS:

1. Change to #8 Portex cuffless tracheostomy tube. Would not plan on downsizing, capping tracheostomy at this time secondary to poor patient cough, decreased mental status, and inability to protect airway. She does have some evidence with occlusion of the tracheostomy of possible upper airway obstruction, and so, if her ability to protect her airway improves, she may need evaluation of the upper airway before considering progressing toward decannulation as well.

2. Repeat chest x-ray to evaluate right cavitary lesion and obtain films from the primary care physician for comparison.

CASE STUDY 13: LINDA BROTHERS

This is a 33-year-old female, primigravida, who came in experiencing early labor. The patient had been scheduled for a cesarean section due to breech presentation.

This patient has had no significant problems during first, second, or third trimester. The patient's past medical history is noncontributory. The patient's LMP was 06/22/2017, placing her EDC at 04/05/2018. Ultrasounds were performed throughout the pregnancy and revealed adequate growth during the pregnancy and EDC remained technically the same.

The patient's initial blood work showed blood type to be A positive, VDRL was nonreactive, rubella titer indicated immunity, hepatitis B surface antigen (HbsAg) was negative, HIV screen was negative, GC and *Chlamydia* cultures were negative. Pap smear was normal. Her 1-hour glucose tolerance test was within normal parameters. The patient's blood count also remained well within normal parameters. Her quad screen for maternal serum alpha-fetoprotein (MSAFP) was normal. Strep culture was likewise negative at 34–35 weeks.

The patient, upon admission, was having contractions approximately every 4–5 minutes, moderate in intensity. The patient had no dilation; presenting part was still in a breech presentation, per bedside ultrasound; and the patient was therefore made ready for primary cesarean section.

The patient was taken to surgery, where primary classical cesarean section was performed with delivery of a breech infant from left sacral anterior positioning, male weighing 6 pounds 10 ounces with Apgars 8 and 8 at 1 and 5 minutes. Placenta delivered intact. Membranes were removed. The patient tolerated the procedure quite well. Estimated blood loss was less than 600 mL.

The patient has had an uneventful postoperative period. She is ambulating well and moving well at this time. The patient is passing gas, moving her bowels, and urinating well; moderate lochia is present; uterus is firm. The patient is discharged from the hospital, being given careful instructions to avoid douching, intercourse, strenuous activity, going up and down stairs, and traveling by car. She is to keep her incision clean with peroxide. She was discharged with Darvocet-N 100 as needed for pain. She will be followed up in 1 week for staple removal. The patient was given information and instructions. Should she experience unusual bleeding; difficulty urinating, voiding, or having a bowel movement; or temperature elevation, she is to contact this physician. The patient's baby is showing some jaundice and may be kept for another 24–48 hours to evaluate bilirubin levels.

CASE STUDY 14: STEWART ALLEN

DATE OF ADMISSION: 11/15/2018
DATE OF DISCHARGE: 11/25/2018

DISCHARGE DIAGNOSES:

AXIS I:

1. Bipolar disorder, depressed, with psychotic features, symptoms in remission.
2. Attention deficit hyperactivity disorder, symptoms in remission.

AXIS II: Deferred.
AXIS III: None.
AXIS IV: Moderate.
AXIS V: Global assessment of functioning 65 on discharge.

REASON FOR ADMISSION: The patient was admitted with a chief complaint of suicidal ideation. The patient was brought to the hospital after his guidance counselor found a note the patient wrote, which detailed to whom he was giving away his possessions when he dies. The patient told the counselor that he hears voices telling him to hurt himself and others. The patient reports over the last month these symptoms have exacerbated. The patient had a fight in school recently, which the patient blames on the voices. Three weeks ago, he got pushed into a corner at school and threatened to shoot himself and others with a gun. The patient was suspended for that remark.

PROCEDURES AND TREATMENT:

1. Individual and group psychotherapy.
2. Psychopharmacologic management.
3. Family therapy with the patient and the patient's family for the purpose of education and discharge planning.

HOSPITAL COURSE: The patient responded well to individual and group psychotherapy, milieu therapy, and medication management. As stated, family therapy was conducted.

DISCHARGE ASSESSMENT: At the time of discharge, the patient is alert and fully oriented. Mood euthymic. Affect broad range. He denies any suicidal or homicidal ideation. IQ is at baseline. Memory intact. Insight and judgment good.

PLAN: The patient may be discharged as he no longer poses a risk of harm towards himself or others.

The patient will continue on the following medications: Ritalin LA 60 mg q.a.m., Depakote 500 mg q.a.m. and 750 mg q.h.s., Abilify 20 mg q.h.s. Depakote level on date of discharge was 110. Liver enzymes drawn were within normal limits.

The patient will follow up with Dr. Wallace for medication management and Dr. Deiter for psychotherapy. All other discharge orders per the psychiatrist, as arranged by social work.

CASE STUDY 15: NOAH LOGAN

PATIENT: Noah Logan
PREOPERATIVE DIAGNOSIS: Midface deficiency.
POSTOPERATIVE DIAGNOSIS: Cleft hard palate with cleft soft palate
OPERATIVE PROCEDURE: LeFort I osteotomy with advancement.
ANESTHESIA: General via nasal intubation.
BLOOD LOSS: 200.
FLUIDS: 600.
URINE OUTPUT: 125.
DRAINS: No drains.
COMPLICATIONS: No complications.

BRIEF HISTORY: The patient is an 8-month-old male who has been under the care of Dr. Grayson for his pre-surgical orthodontics in order to address a midface deficiency. He was also found to have a maxillary midline deficit of approximately 3 mm to his left side. It was determined that he would benefit from a maxillary advancement of approximately 6 mm with rotation in order to set the midline straight.

OPERATIVE PROCEDURE: He was seen in the preop area, brought to the operating room, placed in supine position. General anesthesia was induced. Head and neck were prepped and draped in normal fashion. Time-out was performed. An NG was placed. The external reference marks were made using the right and left medial canthal tendon areas. The nasal width was also measured.

Next, a vestibular incision was made between the right and left first molars in the maxilla. Subperiosteal dissection was performed, as well as dissection around the piriform rim into the nasal fossa. Next, using a reciprocating saw, a standard LeFort 1 osteotomy was made. The osteotomy was taken posteriorly into the pterygomaxillary junction. Next, using a series of guarded chisels, the osteotomies were completed. The nasal septum was disarticulated as were the lateral nasal walls and finally pterygomaxillary disjunction was completed with chisels. The maxilla was brought down quite easily without any bleeding. All bony interferences were removed. The maxilla was then mobilized appropriately.

Next, the maxilla was placed into intermaxillary fixation, and four 1.5 mm KLS plates were placed across the right and left piriform rims as well as the zygomaticomaxillary buttresses in order to plate the LeFort 1 osteotomy. Once this was done, the intermaxillary fixation was released and the occlusion was found to be stable and repeatable. This was approximately a 6-mm advancement move with about a 2-mm rotation to the left. At this point, a V-Y closure of the upper lip was performed. An alar cinch suture was also used to reestablish the alar width. The vestibular incision was then irrigated and closed. The throat pack was removed. NG was maintained. The patient was extubated and taken to the recovery room.

PART VI

REIMBURSEMENT, LEGAL, AND ETHICAL ISSUES

INTRODUCTION

A professional coding specialist's responsibilities may not stop when the last code is determined. Remember, the codes you determine are used on requests for payment, known as reimbursement *claims*. Whenever money is involved, there are always legal and ethical issues attached, and you must familiarize yourself with all of the aspects for doing a complete and professional job for your facility, whether it is a small physician's office or a huge hospital. Understanding these components ensures that you will have a career draped in honesty, integrity, and success.

39 Reimbursement

Key Terms

Automobile Insurance
Capitation Plans
Centers for Medicare & Medicaid Services (CMS)
Dependents
Diagnosis-Related Group (DRG)
Disability Compensation
Discounted FFS
Electronic Media Claim (EMC)
Electronic Remittance Advice (ERA)
Eligibility Verification
Episodic Care
Explanation of Benefits (EOB)
Fee-for-Service (FFS) Plans
Gatekeeper
Health Care
Health Maintenance Organization (HMO)
Insurance Premium
Liability Insurance
Managed Care
Point-of-Service (POS)
Preferred Provider Organization (PPO)
Remittance Advice (RA)
Third-Party Payer
Tracer
TriCare
Usual, Customary, and Reasonable (UCR)
Workers' Compensation

Learning Outcomes

After completing this chapter, the student should be able to:

LO 39.1 Define the role of health insurance and managed care plans in the delivery of health care services.
LO 39.2 Identify and define the types of health insurance plans.
LO 39.3 Explain the types of compensation used in health care reimbursement.
LO 39.4 Describe the information available for proper coding from NCCI edits and NCD and LCD.
LO 39.5 Utilize Place-of-Service and Type-of-Service codes as required.
LO 39.6 Create a system for organizing claims, understanding denials, and filing appeals.

39.1 The Role of Insurance in Health Care

A health insurance policy is a contractual agreement between an insurance carrier (company) and an individual related to health care issues. And the basis of this contract is risk. Insurance is just like gambling in Las Vegas. Basically, the insurance company is betting that a certain event will *not* happen to you, such as you getting sick. If that happens, it would have to pay your medical bills. On the other side of the table, you are betting (by paying an **insurance premium**) that you *will* have a major illness or health catastrophe. Think about it—if you knew for a fact that you would never get ill or have any injury, and would only have to go to the doctor for your annual checkups, would you pay all that money every month for insurance premiums? Of course not. You are betting that you will, at some point, get all that money back, when you need it to pay for some type of treatment.

When **managed care** was developed, the health insurance industry realized that it could lower its risk (and save money) if it could keep people healthy by encouraging them to go to the doctor for regular checkups, tests, and so forth. This thinking created a major change in the health insurance industry and in the medical care industry, increasing the focus of health care delivery to include preventive care, rather than only therapeutic (medical) care.

Medical care is the identification and treatment of illnesses and injuries—in other words, whatever a health care provider does to help you with a health problem or concern that you have (Figure 39-1).

Preventive care is provision of services designed to prevent the problem from manifesting (developing) or to discover it in early stages when it is more easily corrected. Preventive care includes well-baby visits (Figure 39-2), screenings, diagnostics, and routine checkups.

The term **health care** refers to a combination of these two types of services.

Insurance Premium
The amount of money, often paid monthly, by a policyholder or insured, to an insurance company to obtain coverage.

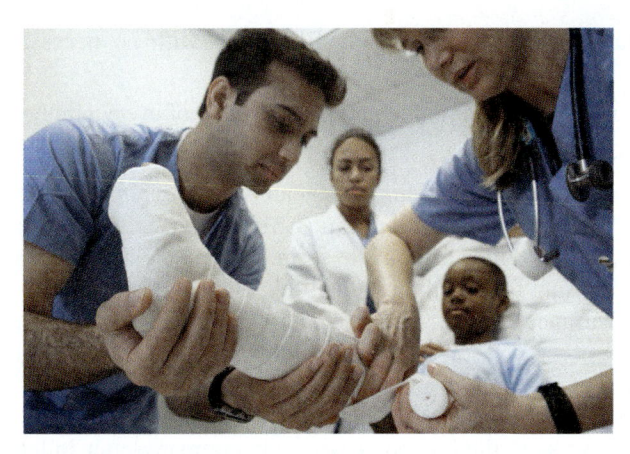

FIGURE 39-1 Treatment of a broken leg is an example of medical care
©ERproductions Ltd/Blend Images LLC RF

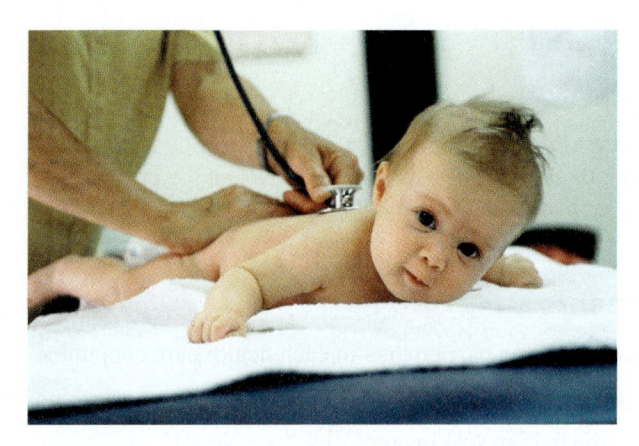

FIGURE 39-2 Well-baby visits are an example of preventive care
©Picture Partners/AGE Fotostock RF

Managed Care
A type of health insurance coverage that controls the care of each subscriber (or insured person) by using a primary care provider as a central health care supervisor.

Health Care
The total management of an individual's well-being by a health care professional.

CODING BITES
Medical Care + Preventive Care = Health Care

EXAMPLES
Dr. Michaelson examines Paul and gives him a shot of antibiotics to help Paul get rid of an infection. The doctor has identified Paul's illness and is treating that illness. This is medical care.

Dr. Calavari knows Katrina works at a day care center and gives her a flu shot to help her avoid getting the flu. The doctor is preventing Katrina from becoming ill. This is preventive care.

We all know that every organization needs to have money coming in so that it can stay in business. The physician provides a service to his or her patients and expects to be paid for those services. That money is what keeps a practice open and allows it to pay your salary. If enough people don't pay their bills, then an office must lay off people (and that could mean you!). Or you might not be able to get that next raise, even if you deserve it.

By now, you understand how important all of this information is and how you have a personal stake in completing claim forms correctly. As you transfer information from patient registration forms and other documents, be certain to

- Double-check your work to make sure it is accurate.

CODING BITES
The process of getting information and submitting claims to the third-party payer is key to the survival of your health care facility and all the people it employs.

- Confirm that the form is completely filled out, with no necessary information missing.
- Verify the spelling of every name and the accuracy of every number.

It all must be absolutely correct.

Most third-party payers, including Medicare, prefer claim forms to be submitted electronically. An **electronic media claim** (**EMC**), also called an electronic claim, is evaluated more quickly than a print claim form. Accepted claims are paid faster. Years ago, it was not unusual for health care facilities to wait 4 to 6 months to receive payment from an insurance company. With electronic claims, this time has been reduced to 2 to 3 weeks.

Increased use of technology in this process also means that there is an excellent chance a computer will be reviewing your claim form. During the initial processing of a claim you have sent, the computer will only compare letter to letter and number to number, looking for an exact match to the letters and numbers in their files. Then, claims with errors, such as invalid policy numbers or missing information, will be rejected and returned to you.

> **Electronic Media Claim (EMC)**
> A health care claim form that is transmitted electronically.

EXAMPLE
The computer cannot scan your claim form and say, "Oh, I can see this is a typo. They really meant to put a *W* instead of a *U*." No, all the computer knows is that the letter is supposed to be a *U* and it is not. And the claim will be rejected.

The Participants
Essentially, there are three participants in each health care encounter, or visit:

1. The physician or health care provider.
2. The patient—the person seeking services.
3. The insurance carrier covering the costs of health care activities for the patient.

Some people get their health insurance policies through a program at their place of employment, some through the government, and others directly with the insurance carriers as individual policyholders. It doesn't matter very much to the health care facility. In any case, a **third-party payer** will pay, in part, the patient's bills for services that your facility will provide. Health insurance carriers are often referred to as third-party payers. This means that someone not directly involved in the health care relationship is paying for the service. The health care provider is party #1, the patient is party #2, and the insurance carrier is party #3—the third party. Therefore, the insurance company is the third-party payer.

> **CODING BITES**
> Party #1: The health care provider
> Party #2: The patient
> Party #3: The insurance carrier

> **Third-Party Payer**
> An individual or organization that is not directly involved in an encounter but has a connection because of its obligation to pay, in full or part, for that encounter.

39.2 Types of Insurance Plans

There are many types of health plans that people may purchase, or contract for, with companies that specialize in insurance.

Health Maintenance Organization (HMO)

In a **health maintenance organization** (**HMO**), members, also called enrollees, prepay for health care services. The members are encouraged to get preventive treatment to promote wellness (and keep medical costs down). In addition, each member has a primary care physician (PCP), also known as a **gatekeeper**. The PCP is responsible for monitoring the individual's well-being and making all decisions regarding care. It is the PCP who determines if a specialist is required for a certain evaluation or procedure. When this occurs, it is the PCP who is responsible for completing the patient

> **Health Maintenance Organization (HMO)**
> A type of health insurance that uses a primary care physician, also known as a gatekeeper, to manage all health care services for an individual.

1158   PART VI | REIMBURSEMENT, LEGAL, AND ETHICAL ISSUES

referral form and getting approval from the HMO for the patient to visit the specialist. Generally, HMOs do not require a patient to satisfy a deductible before benefits begin. (See the section *Individual Insurance Contributions* later in this chapter.)

> **CODING BITES**
>
> HMOs use a "home base" concept, with a primary care physician (PCP), also known as the gatekeeper, serving as the central base to supervise each individual's health care.

Preferred Provider Organization (PPO)

In a **preferred provider organization (PPO)**, physicians, hospitals, and other health care providers join together and agree to offer services to members of a group (often called subscribers) at a lower cost or discount. These plans usually permit the individual subscriber (the patient) to choose the physician or specialist to see, with a discount for staying in the network by using a physician who is a member of the plan. If the individual chooses a physician who does not belong to the network, or is not participating with that PPO, the individual will pay a penalty or receive less of a discount in the cost of those services. This can give the individual more control over his or her health care. It can save time and money, as well.

Some PPO plans require the patient to satisfy a deductible first before benefits begin. (See the section *Individual Insurance Contributions* later in this chapter.) Typically, a higher deductible will translate into a lower monthly premium for this type of insurance coverage.

> **EXAMPLE**
>
> If a person covered under a PPO plan is having problems sneezing and knows the problem is his or her allergies, the individual can choose an allergist—a provider who specializes in the treatment of allergies—from the PPO network without having to go to his or her primary care physician for a referral. If the plan were an HMO, the person would have to make an appointment with the PCP first, in order to get the referral to the allergist. Then, the person could make an appointment to see the allergist.

Point-of-Service (POS) Plan

Giving individuals a little more flexibility, a **point-of-service (POS)** plan is almost a combination of an HMO and a PPO. Each insured person has a primary care physician (PCP) and a list of providers that participate in the HMO. When health care providers within the HMO network are used, the insured pays only a regular co-payment amount or a small charge. There is no deductible or co-insurance payment involved. However, this plan may also include a self-referral option, in which the individual insured can choose to go to an out-of-network provider. In that case, the individual may be responsible for paying both a deductible and a co-insurance payment.

> **CODING BITES**
>
> POS plans combine features of an HMO and a PPO.

Federal Government Plans

Centers for Medicare & Medicaid Services (CMS)

In 1977, the Health Care Financing Administration (HCFA, pronounced hic-fah) was created to coordinate federal health services programs. On July 1, 2001, HCFA

Gatekeeper
A physician, typically a family practitioner or an internist, who serves as the primary care physician for an individual. This physician is responsible for evaluating and determining the course of treatment or services, as well as for deciding whether or not a specialist should be involved in care.

Preferred Provider Organization (PPO)
A type of health insurance coverage in which physicians provide health care services to members of the plan at a discount.

> **CODING BITES**
>
> PPOs typically **P**ermit the **P**atient to **O**pt (or choose) his or her physician or specialist.

Point-of-Service (POS)
A type of insurance plan that will allow an HMO enrollee to choose his or her own nonmember physician at a lower benefit rate, costing the patient more money out-of-pocket.

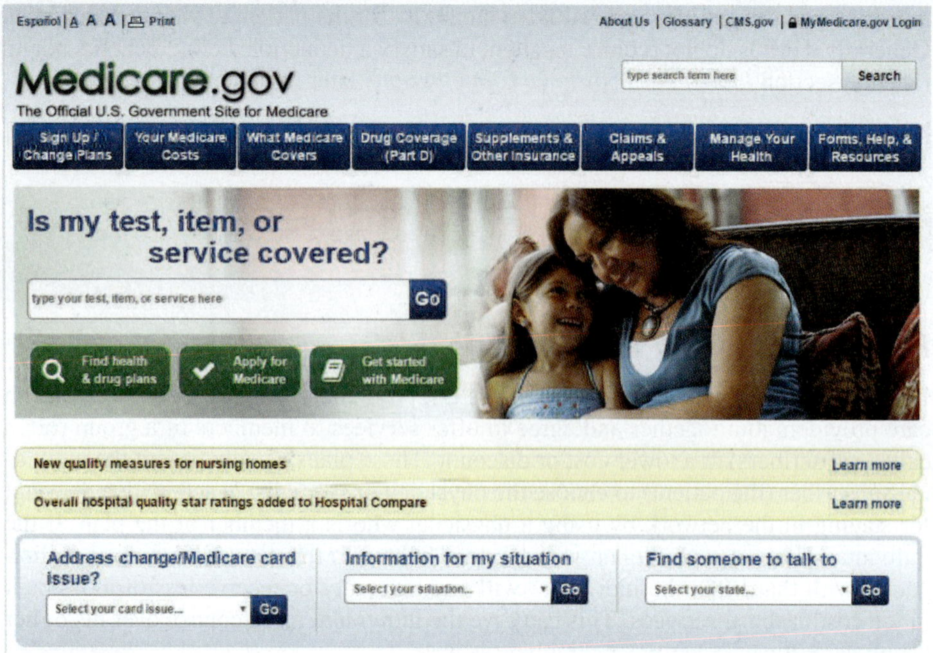

FIGURE 39-3 Medicare.gov, the official U.S. government site for Medicare
Source: Medicare.gov

Centers for Medicare & Medicaid Services (CMS)
The agency under the Department of Health and Human Services (DHHS) in charge of regulation and control over services for those covered by Medicare and Medicaid.

CODING BITES

Medica**RE** = **RE**tired people (who are over the age of 65)

Medica**ID** = **I**n**D**igent, or low-income, individuals

TriCare
A government health plan that covers medical expenses for the dependents of active-duty service members, CHAMPUS-eligible retirees and their families, and the dependents of deceased active-duty members.

Dependents
Individuals who are supported, either financially or with regard to insurance coverage, by others.

became the **Centers for Medicare & Medicaid Services (CMS)**. Many health care professionals still refer to this agency as "HicFah" and to the CMS-1500 claim form as the "HicFah 1500." Old habits take a while to change. At least you now understand that these two acronyms refer to the same federal organization.

Medicare is a national health insurance program that pays, or reimburses, for health care services provided to those over the age of 65 (see Figure 39-3). In addition, this plan may cover individuals who are under the age of 65 and are permanently disabled (such as the blind), as well as those with end-stage renal disease (ESRD) who are suffering from permanent kidney failure and require either dialysis or a kidney transplant.

Medicaid is a plan that pays for, or reimburses, medical assistance and health care services for people who are indigent (low-income) (see Figure 39-4). The program is jointly funded by the federal and state governments. Each state government then administers its own plan. This means that each state determines who is eligible and what services are covered. It is important to know that each state has its own requirements, in case you have a patient that has just moved to your state. Each state may even have a unique name or term for its program. For example, in California the program is called Medi-Cal.

TriCare

TriCare offers the most common health care plans you will encounter when caring for individuals in the military and their families (see Figure 39-5). This program was formerly known as CHAMPUS.

TriCare was created to help the following individuals receive better access to improved health care services:

- Active-duty service members (ADSM), also known as sponsors.
- The **dependents** (spouses and children) of ADSMs.
- Surviving spouses and surviving children of deceased ADSMs.
- Retired service members, their spouses, and their children.
- Surviving spouses and children of deceased retired members.

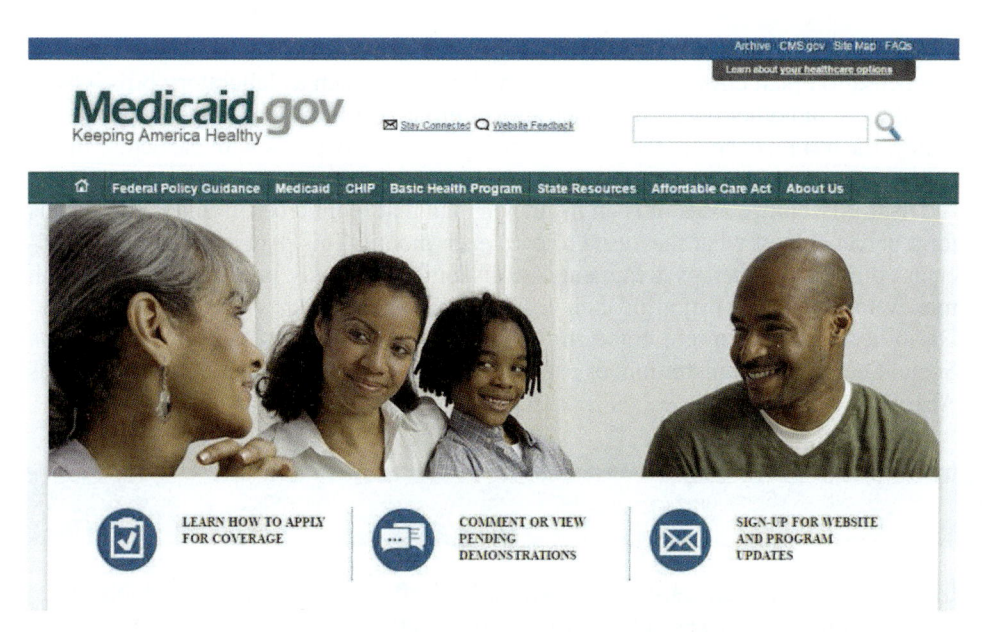

FIGURE 39-4 Medicaid.gov, the official U.S. government website of Medicaid
Source: Medicaid.gov

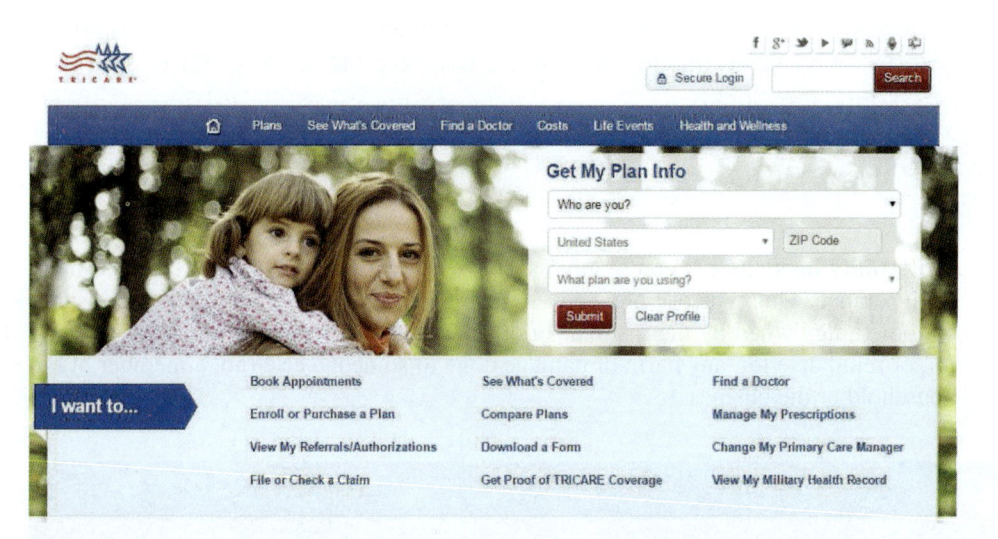

FIGURE 39-5 TriCare.mil, the official U.S. government website of TRICARE
Source: Tricare.mil

TriCare was created to provide health care benefits for the dependents of those serving in the uniformed services and retirees. ADSMs are those from any of the seven uniformed services, including the U.S. military (the Army, Navy, Air Force, Marine Corps, and Coast Guard), as well as those serving in the Public Health Service, National Guard and Reserve, and the National Oceanic and Atmospheric Administration (NOAA). Eligibility for TriCare is determined by the services and information is maintained in the Defense Enrollment Eligibility Reporting System (DEERS).

Other Insurance Plans

Workers' compensation is an insurance program designed to pay the medical costs for treating those injured, or made ill, at their place of work or by their job. This includes injuries resulting from a fall off a ladder while performing a job-related task, getting hurt in an accident while driving a company car on a business trip, or

Workers' Compensation
An insurance program that covers medical care for those injured or for those who become ill as a consequence of their employment.

developing a lung disorder caused by toxic fumes in the office. Generally, a workers' compensation plan covers only specific medical bills, such as laboratory bills, physicians' fees, and other medical services. Most often, lost income is not covered by this policy. Each state oversees the workers' compensation contracts with particular insurance carriers.

Disability Compensation
A plan that reimburses a covered individual a portion of his or her income that is lost as a result of being unable to work due to illness or injury.

Disability compensation is an insurance plan that reimburses disabled individuals for a percentage of what they used to earn each month. This plan does not pay physicians' bills or for therapy treatments. A disability plan only provides insureds with money to replace a portion of their lost paycheck because they are unable to work. Disability payments might come through a federal government agency such as the Social Security Administration, or patients may have a private insurance plan (such as AFLAC).

YOU INTERPRET IT!

Joe Hines works as an electrician for a small company. One day, he falls off a ladder at work and injures his back severely. He is taken to the emergency room by ambulance, and the attending physician orders x-rays and a CT scan. The tests confirm that Joe's spine is broken in two places and a cast is applied around Joe's entire torso. After a week in the hospital, Joe is discharged. The physician's discharge orders state that Joe is to stay in bed for 7 months, in traction, while the fracture heals. A home health agency is contracted to provide a trained health care professional to go to Joe's house to care for him and attend to his needs around the clock.

1. In this scenario, what type of insurance will be responsible for the payment of each of Joe's expenses due to this accident?

Liability Insurance
A policy that covers loss or injury to a third party caused by the insured or something belonging to the insured.

Liability insurance is commonly part of a person's homeowners or business owners insurance. This type of policy covers losses to a third party caused by the insured or something owned by the insured. In other words, the insurance company will pay for, or reimburse for, any harm or damage done to someone else (not a member of the household or the business).

YOU INTERPRET IT!

Sarah goes over to Margaret's house for dinner. After a delicious meal, Sarah walks toward the door to leave and go home. As she turns to say goodnight to Margaret, Sarah trips and falls. Margaret calls the paramedics, and, at the hospital, the x-rays ordered by the attending physician confirm that Sarah has indeed broken her wrist. A cast is applied, and Sarah is sent home with a prescription for pain medication. The attending physician advises Sarah to see her primary care physician in 1 week for a follow-up.

2. What type of insurance will cover Sarah's medical expenses?

YOU INTERPRET IT!

Kyle, a fifth-grade student, slipped down the stairs at school. Typically, the school's liability policy would cover the damage, or medical expenses. The school is the insured, and the student is the third party.

3. If a faculty member and a student are walking through the cafeteria of the school and both slip and fall, what types of policies will cover any injuries that might be caused by the fall?

Automobile insurance might become an issue for your office if you treat someone for an injury that was caused by the individual's involvement in an automobile accident. Full-coverage automobile policies usually include liability insurance that covers these expenses.

Details Are Required

As you can see from all this information, different types of insurance policies might be responsible for an individual's medical treatment. Therefore, in your job as medical insurance coder/biller, you must make certain that if an individual comes to the provider for treatment for an *injury* (rather than an *illness*), you must find out the *details* of how and where the injury occurred. This will help determine which carrier will cover the charges.

> **Automobile Insurance**
> Auto accident liability coverage will pay for medical bills, lost wages, and compensation for pain and suffering for any person injured by the insured in an auto accident.

> **CODING BITES**
> And you need these details for determining the external cause codes, too!

39.3 Methods of Compensation

There are several payment plans that insurance carriers (third-party payers) use to pay physicians and other health care providers for their services.

Fee-for-Service (FFS) Plans

In **fee-for-service (FFS) plans**, the insurance company pays the health care provider for each individual service supplied to the patient, as reported by the procedure codes listed on the claim, according to an agreed-upon price list (also known as a fee schedule). When the physician's office agrees to participate in the plan, it is also agreeing to provide services and accept the amount of money indicated on that schedule for each of those services. This is like going to a restaurant with an à la carte menu. The menu lists a price for each item: the salad, the roast beef, the apple pie. The restaurant accepts the amount of money the guest pays for each item received. Different plans may pay different amounts of money for one particular service, just as different restaurants may charge different amounts for a similar dish.

Sometimes, when one insurance carrier pays a provider at a lower rate than other carriers, it is referred to as a **discounted FFS**. In a typical discounted FFS, the payments are reduced from the physician's regular rate. This is similar to the discount you might get at a store when showing your student ID card—you get a discount because you are a member of the school.

> **Fee-for-Service (FFS) Plans**
> Payment agreements that outline, in a written fee schedule, exactly how much money the insurance carrier will pay the physician for each treatment and/or service provided.

> **Discounted FFS**
> An extra reduction in the rate charged to an insurer for services provided by the physician to the plan's members.

> **EXAMPLE**
> Three people, each with a different insurance carrier, go to the same physician for a flu shot (injection). Insurance carrier #1 has agreed to pay the physician $20 for giving the injection. Insurance carrier #2 has agreed to pay the physician $22.50, and insurance carrier #3 has agreed to pay the physician $18 for the same injection. Your office should charge all patients the same amount. This is known as the *charged amount*. However, insurance carriers working with your office on a fee-for-service contract will pay only the amount stated on their fee schedule. That's all they will pay and no more. This is called the *allowed amount*.

Capitation Plans

With **capitation plans**, the insurance company pays the physician a fixed amount of money for every individual covered by that plan (often called members or subscribers) being seen by that physician. Physicians get this amount of money every month, as long as they are listed as the physician of record (primary care physician (PCP)) for that individual. Whether the insured person goes to see that physician once, three

> **Capitation Plans**
> Agreements between a physician and a managed care organization that pay the physician a predetermined amount of money each month for each member of the plan who identifies that provider as his or her primary care physician.

<aside>
CODING BITES

CAPitation plans pay by the *cap*. One cap goes on one head, and the insurance carrier is going to pay the physician for each cap, or head—that is, per person.
</aside>

times, or not at all during a particular month, the physician's office will be paid the same amount. This plan is like the dinner special at your local restaurant. You pay one price, which includes soup, salad, all-you-can-eat entrée, and dessert. If you don't eat your soup, you do not pay any less; if you get seconds on the entrée, you do not pay any more.

Episodic Care

An **episodic care** agreement between insurer and physician means the provider is paid one flat fee for the expected course of treatment for a particular injury or illness. This is like the meal deal of health care. One package price includes all of the services and treatments necessary for the proper care of the patient's condition in accordance with the accepted standards of care.

<aside>
Episodic Care
An insurance company pays a provider one flat fee to cover the entire course of treatment for an individual's condition.
</aside>

> **EXAMPLE**
>
> Audrey Callahan fell off her bicycle and broke her arm. The x-ray shows that it is a simple, clean fracture and the physician applies a cast. The doctor schedules a follow-up appointment for her and expects that she will not need much other attention until the cast comes off in 6 weeks. At that time, an x-ray will confirm that the fracture has healed properly and the cast will be removed. This entire sequence of events, and treatment, is very predictable for a routine simple fracture. Therefore, the insurance company has agreed to pay the physician one flat fee for this event, rather than having the physician's office file a claim for each procedure and service individually: the first encounter; the first x-ray; the application of the cast; the follow-up encounter; the last encounter; the last x-ray; and removal of the cast.
>
> Audrey Callahan's physician is being reimbursed under an episodic care agreement with the insurance carrier.

<aside>
Diagnosis-Related Group (DRG)
An episodic care payment system basing reimbursement to hospitals for inpatient services upon standards of care for specific diagnoses grouped by their similar usage of resources for procedures, services, and treatments.
</aside>

Diagnosis-related groups (DRGs) are a type of episodic care payment plan used by Medicare to pay for treatments and services provided to beneficiaries who have been admitted into an acute care hospital (inpatients). DRGs are categorized by the principal (first-listed) diagnosis code and take into consideration elements such as the patient's age and gender and the presence of any complications or manifestations (additional diagnoses or conditions). You read more about DRGs in the chapter titled *Inpatient (Hospital) Diagnosis Coding*.

Patient/Beneficiary Out-of-Pocket Contributions

Patients with insurance policies often contribute to reimbursing providers for their health care services, in addition to paying monthly premiums. The following are the most common methods used for the individual's payments:

1. *Co-payment (also known as the co-pay).* The co-payment is usually a fixed amount of money that the individual will pay each time he or she goes to a health care provider. It may be $10, $15, $20, or more. Each policy is different. As a matter of fact, the co-pay on the same policy for the same patient may be different, depending on whether this is a visit to a family physician, a specialist, or the hospital.

<aside>
Usual, Customary, and Reasonable (UCR)
The process of determining a fee for a service by evaluating the *usual* fee charged by the provider, the *customary* fee charged by most physicians in the same community or geographical area, and what is considered *reasonable* by most health care professionals under the specific circumstances of the situation.
</aside>

2. *Co-insurance.* Co-insurance is different from the co-payment because it is based on a percentage of the total charge rather than a fixed amount. The percentage that the patient pays is most often calculated on the **usual, customary, and reasonable (UCR)** charge that has been determined for this type of visit or procedure. Frequently, the individual is required to pay 20% of the total allowed amount by the physician or facility, but that might differ for various types of policies and carriers.

3. *Deductible.* This is the amount of money that patients must pay, out of their own pockets, before the insurance benefits begin. The deductible might be as little as $250 or as much as $1,000 or more. Patients have to pay the total amount until they have paid the whole deductible for that calendar year. After that, they will usually pay just the co-payment and/or the co-insurance amount.

> **CODING BITES**
>
> The various amounts for the co-pay, the co-insurance, and the deductible are good examples of why it is so essential that you contact the insurance carrier for every patient to verify the patient's coverage and eligibility for certain procedures and treatments and to see if the deductible has been met for the year.

MACRA

Medicare Access and CHIP Reauthorization Act (MACRA) has been designed to reward health care providers for quality patient care and to ultimately reduce costs. As a part of this, the Quality Payment Program was also implemented. This program incorporates important advances to ensure that electronic health information will be available when and where clinicians need it so optimal care can be provided.

The Quality Payment Program includes two paths:

- Advanced Alternative Payment Models (APMs)
- Merit-Based Incentive Payment System (MIPS)

Both of these paths require use of certified EHR technology to exchange information across providers and with patients to support improved care delivery, including patient engagement and care coordination. In addition, this program requires EHR manufacturers to publish application programming interfaces (API), which increase interoperability (making it easier for software programs such as smartphone apps to access information from other programs) for certified health IT.

Physicians have options and began participating in this program as early as January 2017.

39.4 NCCI Edits and NCD/LCD

National Correct Coding Initiative (NCCI)

The CMS developed the National Correct Coding Initiative (NCCI) to reinforce accurate and proper coding in addition to preventing reimbursement of inaccurate amounts as the result of noncompliance coding methods in Part B claims (physician and outpatient services). This system was founded with coding policies based on

- The official coding guidelines, as published in American Medical Association's CPT code book.
- National (NCD) and local (LCD) policies and edits.
- Coding guidelines developed by national societies.
- Analysis of standard medical and surgical practices.
- Review of current coding practices.

There are two types of edits within the NCCI focus: PTP and MUE.

Procedure-to-Procedure (PTP) Edits

Within the long lists of procedures, services, and treatments performed by health care providers, there are those that cannot, or should not, be provided to the same patient on the same date of service. CMS computers evaluate submitted claims to look for pairs of codes being reported that are known to be mutually exclusive procedures, also known as procedure-to-procedure (PTP) edits.

> ### EXAMPLE
>
> 23680   Open treatment of shoulder dislocation, with surgical or anatomical neck fracture, with manipulation
>
> 20690   Application of a uniplane (pins or wires in 1 plane), unilateral, external fixation system
>
> These codes report two procedures that would not be performed at the same time for the same patient, according to the standards of care. This is an example of a PTP edit.

Medically Unlikely Edits (MUE)

The purpose of the NCCI medically unlikely edits (MUE) is to prevent improper payments when services are reported with incorrect units of service. An MUE for a HCPCS/CPT code is the maximum units of service that a provider would report under most circumstances for a single beneficiary on a single date of service.

> ### EXAMPLE
>
> 72270   Myelography, 2 or more regions, radiological supervision and interpretation
>
> The MUE edit for this code is a maximum of one for a patient per date of service because the code description states "two or more." Therefore, reporting this code more than once for the same patient on the same date would not be accurate.

National Coverage Determinations (NCD) and Local Coverage Determinations (LCD)

In some circumstances, a National Coverage Determination (NCD) is created to clearly establish the criteria for coverage of an item or service applicable to all Medicare beneficiaries nationwide. When there is no NCD, there may be a Local Coverage Determination (LCD) in effect. An LCD is a decision by a fiscal intermediary (FI) or carrier as to when and for what reasons a particular service or item is covered in that area (a state or region). The Medicare Coverage Database (MCD), available at www.cms.gov (see Figure 39-6), contains all NCDs and LCDs in a searchable database.

Virtually all third-party payers issue coverage determinations valid nationally or in a particular state or locale. Therefore, you should have the ability to verify coverage for an item or service *prior* to providing it, and certainly before creating and submitting the claim.

Once you find a coverage determination on the service or item the physician wants to provide to the patient, you can obtain the details about the criteria for coverage. In this Medicare NCD on Adult Liver Transplantation (Figure 39-7), the procedure would be categorized (**BENEFIT CATEGORY**) as an Inpatient Hospital Service.

Next, the section **ITEM/SERVICE DESCRIPTION** is provided to ensure that everyone understands precisely what procedure, service, or item is being discussed. Read further down the page to the section **INDICATIONS** AND **LIMITATIONS OF COVERAGE**: **B. NATIONALLY COVERED INDICATIONS** and you can see the diagnoses considered as medically necessary for this procedure. Earlier in this text, you learned about medical necessity in the chapter *Introduction to the Languages of Coding*. The next section clarifies what types of **FOLLOW-UP CARE** will be covered, as well.

> **CODING BITES**
>
> Submitting a claim for a service or item not covered by the patient's policy is considered fraud . . . even if it gets paid. It is your responsibility to know! Not the patient. Not the doctor. You, the professional coding specialist.

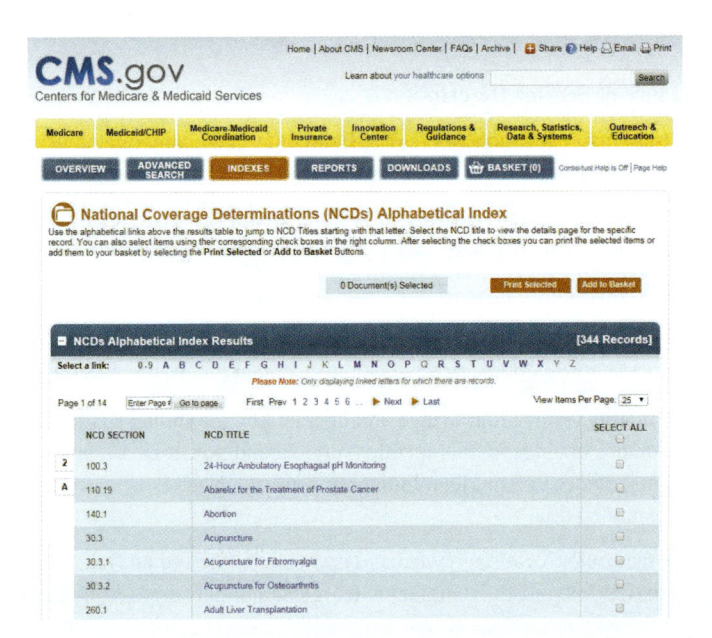

FIGURE 39-6 National Coverage Determinations (NCDs) Alphabetic Index Source: CMS.gov

> **GUIDANCE CONNECTION**
>
> Go to the **Medicare Coverage Database:**
>
> https://www.cms.gov/medicare-coverage-database/overview-and-quick-search.aspx
>
> On the right side is the Quick Search bar to sort through all National Coverage Determinations (NCDs) and Local Coverage Determinations (LCDs).

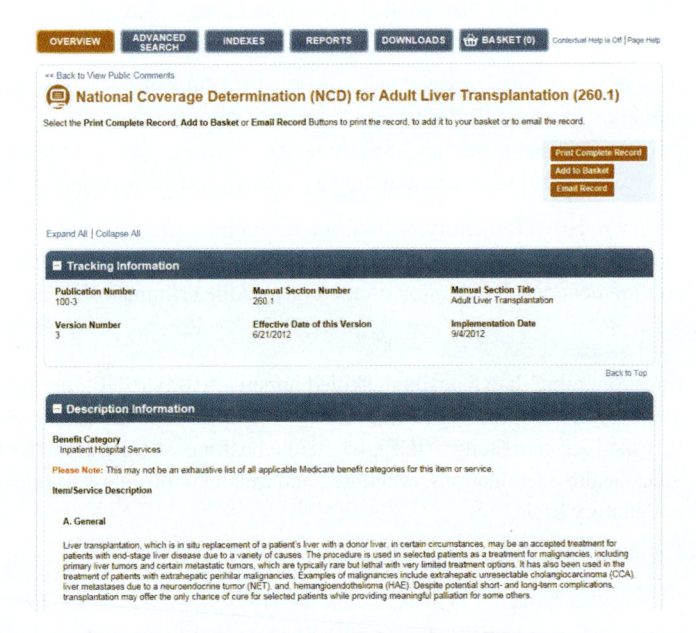

FIGURE 39-7 NCD for Adult Liver Transplantation (in part) Source: CMS.gov

39.5 Place-of-Service and Type-of-Service Codes

Place-of-Service Codes

Place-of-Service (POS) codes are used on professional claims to identify the specific location where procedures, services, and treatments were provided to the patient.

CHAPTER 39 | REIMBURSEMENT **1167**

Place of Service Code(s)	Place of Service Name	Place of Service Description
01	Pharmacy	A facility or location where drugs and other medically related items and services are sold, dispensed, or otherwise provided directly to patients.
02	Telehealth	The location where health services and health-related services are provided or received, through a telecommunication system.
03	School	A facility whose primary purpose is education.
04	Homeless Shelter	A facility or location whose primary purpose is to provide temporary housing to homeless individuals (e.g., emergency shelters, individual or family shelters).
05	Indian Health Service Free-Standing Facility	A facility or location, owned and operated by the Indian Health Service, that provides diagnostic, therapeutic (surgical and nonsurgical), and rehabilitation services to American Indians and Alaska Natives who do not require hospitalization.
06	Indian Health Service Provider-Based Facility	A facility or location, owned and operated by the Indian Health Service, that provides diagnostic, therapeutic (surgical and nonsurgical), and rehabilitation services rendered by, or under the supervision of, physicians to American Indians and Alaska Natives admitted as inpatients or outpatients.
07	Tribal 638 Free-Standing Facility	A facility or location, owned and operated by a federally recognized American Indian or Alaska Native tribe or tribal organization under a 638 agreement, that provides diagnostic, therapeutic (surgical and nonsurgical), and rehabilitation services to tribal members who do not require hospitalization.
08	Tribal 638 Provider-Based Facility	A facility or location, owned and operated by a federally recognized American Indian or Alaska Native tribe or tribal organization under a 638 agreement, that provides diagnostic, therapeutic (surgical and nonsurgical), and rehabilitation services to tribal members admitted as inpatients or outpatients.
09	Prison/Correctional Facility	A prison, jail, reformatory, work farm, detention center, or any other similar facility maintained by either federal, state, or local authorities for the purpose of confinement or rehabilitation of adult or juvenile criminal offenders.
10	Unassigned	
11	Office	Location, other than a hospital, skilled nursing facility (SNF), military treatment facility, community health center, state or local public health clinic, or intermediate care facility (ICF), where the health professional routinely provides health examinations, diagnosis, and treatment of illness or injury on an ambulatory basis.
12	Home	Location, other than a hospital or other facility, where the patient receives care in a private residence.
13	Assisted Living Facility	Congregate residential facility with self-contained living units providing assessment of each resident's needs and on-site support 24 hours a day, 7 days a week, with the capacity to deliver or arrange for services including some health care and other services.
14	Group Home	A residence, with shared living areas, where clients receive supervision and other services such as social and/or behavioral services, custodial service, and minimal services (e.g., medication administration).
15	Mobile Unit	A facility/unit that moves from place-to-place equipped to provide preventive, screening, diagnostic, and/or treatment services.
16	Temporary Lodging	A short-term accommodation such as a hotel, camp ground, hostel, cruise ship, or resort where the patient receives care, and that is not identified by any other POS code.

Place of Service Code(s)	Place of Service Name	Place of Service Description
17	Walk-in Retail Health Clinic	A walk-in health clinic, other than an office, urgent care facility, pharmacy, or independent clinic and not described by any other Place-of-Service code, that is located within a retail operation and provides, on an ambulatory basis, preventive and primary care services.
18	Place of Employment-Worksite	A location, not described by any other POS code, owned or operated by a public or private entity where the patient is employed, and where a health professional provides ongoing or episodic occupational medical, therapeutic, or rehabilitative services to the individual.
19	Off-Campus Outpatient Hospital	A portion of an off-campus hospital provider-based department that provides diagnostic, therapeutic (both surgical and nonsurgical), and rehabilitation services to sick or injured persons who do not require hospitalization or institutionalization.
20	Urgent Care Facility	Location, distinct from a hospital emergency room, an office, or a clinic, whose purpose is to diagnose and treat illness or injury for unscheduled, ambulatory patients seeking immediate medical attention.
21	Inpatient Hospital	A facility, other than psychiatric, that primarily provides diagnostic, therapeutic (both surgical and nonsurgical), and rehabilitation services by, or under, the supervision of physicians to patients admitted for a variety of medical conditions.
22	On-Campus Outpatient Hospital	A portion of a hospital's main campus that provides diagnostic, therapeutic (both surgical and nonsurgical), and rehabilitation services to sick or injured persons who do not require hospitalization or institutionalization.
23	Emergency Room—Hospital	A portion of a hospital where emergency diagnosis and treatment of illness or injury is provided.
24	Ambulatory Surgical Center	A freestanding facility, other than a physician's office, where surgical and diagnostic services are provided on an ambulatory basis.
25	Birthing Center	A facility, other than a hospital's maternity facilities or a physician's office, that provides a setting for labor, delivery, and immediate post-partum care as well as immediate care of newborn infants.
26	Military Treatment Facility	A medical facility operated by one or more of the Uniformed Services. Military Treatment Facility (MTF) also refers to certain former U.S. Public Health Service (USPHS) facilities now designated as Uniformed Service Treatment Facilities (USTF).
27–30	Unassigned	N/A
31	Skilled Nursing Facility	A facility that primarily provides inpatient skilled nursing care and related services to patients who require medical, nursing, or rehabilitative services but does not provide the level of care or treatment available in a hospital.
32	Nursing Facility	A facility that primarily provides to residents skilled nursing care and related services for the rehabilitation of injured, disabled, or sick persons, or, on a regular basis, health-related care services above the level of custodial care to other than individuals with intellectual disabilities.
33	Custodial Care Facility	A facility that provides room, board, and other personal assistance services, generally on a long-term basis, and that does not include a medical component.
34	Hospice	A facility, other than a patient's home, in which palliative and supportive care for terminally ill patients and their families are provided.
35–40	Unassigned	N/A

(continued)

Place of Service Code(s)	Place of Service Name	Place of Service Description
41	Ambulance—Land	A land vehicle specifically designed, equipped, and staffed for lifesaving and transporting the sick or injured.
42	Ambulance—Air or Water	An air or water vehicle specifically designed, equipped, and staffed for lifesaving and transporting the sick or injured.
43–48	Unassigned	N/A
49	Independent Clinic	A location, not part of a hospital and not described by any other Place-of-Service code, that is organized and operated to provide preventive, diagnostic, therapeutic, rehabilitative, or palliative services to outpatients only.
50	Federally Qualified Health Center	A facility located in a medically underserved area that provides Medicare beneficiaries preventive primary medical care under the general direction of a physician.
51	Inpatient Psychiatric Facility	A facility that provides inpatient psychiatric services for the diagnosis and treatment of mental illness on a 24-hour basis, by or under the supervision of a physician.
52	Psychiatric Facility—Partial Hospitalization	A facility for the diagnosis and treatment of mental illness that provides a planned therapeutic program for patients who do not require full-time hospitalization, but who need broader programs than are possible from outpatient visits to a hospital-based or hospital-affiliated facility.
53	Community Mental Health Center	A facility that provides the following services: outpatient services, including specialized outpatient services for children, the elderly, individuals who are chronically ill, and residents of the CMHC's mental health services area who have been discharged from inpatient treatment at a mental health facility; 24-hour-a-day emergency care services; day treatment, other partial hospitalization services, or psychosocial rehabilitation services; screening for patients being considered for admission to state mental health facilities to determine the appropriateness of such admission; and consultation and education services.
54	Intermediate Care Facility/ Individuals with Intellectual Disabilities	A facility that primarily provides health-related care and services above the level of custodial care to individuals but does not provide the level of care or treatment available in a hospital or SNF.
55	Residential Substance Abuse Treatment Facility	A facility that provides treatment for substance (alcohol and drug) abuse to live-in residents who do not require acute medical care. Services include individual and group therapy and counseling, family counseling, laboratory tests, drugs and supplies, psychological testing, and room and board.
56	Psychiatric Residential Treatment Center	A facility or distinct part of a facility for psychiatric care that provides a total 24-hour therapeutically planned and professionally staffed group living and learning environment.
57	Nonresidential Substance Abuse Treatment Facility	A location that provides treatment for substance (alcohol and drug) abuse on an ambulatory basis. Services include individual and group therapy and counseling, family counseling, laboratory tests, drugs and supplies, and psychological testing.
58–59	Unassigned	N/A
60	Mass Immunization Center	A location where providers administer pneumococcal pneumonia and influenza virus vaccinations and submit these services as electronic media claims, paper claims, or using the roster billing method. This generally takes place in a mass immunization setting, such as a public health center, pharmacy, or mall but may include a physician office setting.

Place of Service Code(s)	Place of Service Name	Place of Service Description
61	Comprehensive Inpatient Rehabilitation Facility	A facility that provides comprehensive rehabilitation services under the supervision of a physician to inpatients with physical disabilities. Services include physical therapy, occupational therapy, speech pathology, social or psychological services, and orthotics and prosthetics services.
62	Comprehensive Outpatient Rehabilitation Facility	A facility that provides comprehensive rehabilitation services under the supervision of a physician to outpatients with physical disabilities. Services include physical therapy, occupational therapy, and speech pathology services.
63–64	Unassigned	N/A
65	End-Stage Renal Disease Treatment Facility	A facility, other than a hospital, that provides dialysis treatment, maintenance, and/or training to patients or caregivers on an ambulatory or home-care basis.
66–70	Unassigned	N/A
71	Public Health Clinic	A facility maintained by either state or local health departments that provides ambulatory primary medical care under the general direction of a physician.
72	Rural Health Clinic	A certified facility that is located in a rural medically underserved area that provides ambulatory primary medical care under the general direction of a physician.
73–80	Unassigned	N/A
81	Independent Laboratory	A laboratory certified to perform diagnostic and/or clinical tests independent of an institution or a physician's office.
82–98	Unassigned	N/A
99	Other Place of Service	Other place of service not identified above.

Type-of-Service Codes

In addition to providing pre-categorization of procedures, Type-of-Service (TOS) codes are also used to ensure that procedures, services, and treatments, along with the Place-of-Service codes, are used to determine appropriateness of location and service.

Type of Service Indicators

0   Whole Blood
1   Medical Care
2   Surgery
3   Consultation
4   Diagnostic Radiology
5   Diagnostic Laboratory
6   Therapeutic Radiology
7   Anesthesia
8   Assistant at Surgery
9   Other Medical Items or Services
A   Used DME
B   High Risk Screening Mammography
C   Low Risk Screening Mammography
D   Ambulance
E   Enteral/Parenteral Nutrients/Supplies

Type of Service Indicators

F	Ambulatory Surgical Center (Facility Usage for Surgical Services)
G	Immunosuppressive Drugs
H	Hospice
J	Diabetic Shoes
K	Hearing Items and Services
L	ESRD Supplies
M	Monthly Capitation Payment for Dialysis
N	Kidney Donor
P	Lump Sum Purchase of DME, Prosthetics, Orthotics
Q	Vision Items or Services
R	Rental of DME
S	Surgical Dressings or Other Medical Supplies
T	Outpatient Mental Health Treatment Limitation
U	Occupational Therapy
V	Pneumococcal/Flu Vaccine
W	Physical Therapy

39.6 Organizing Claims: Resubmission, Denials, and Appeals

One thing that is very important for a professional insurance biller to do is to keep track of all the claims sent out on behalf of his or her medical facility, whether it is a physician's office or a hospital. Even with the help of computers and clearinghouses, a claim can get lost. It happens on occasion with letters sent through the post office, and it can happen electronically as well. One little power surge or a computer with a virus can make your claim disappear. The only way you may know about this happening is the absence of a response, such as a payment, a statement of rejection, or a denial. Therefore, you have to keep track of every claim form you submit.

The following are two simple steps for staying organized.

1. Keep a log of every claim as you send it. If you are using a clearinghouse, you will receive a report, listing all the claims sent (complete with date and time sent) and to which payer they were forwarded. Place these notices in a file folder on your computer's desktop or print out these reports and place them in a three-ring binder or another type of file. If you are sending claims directly from your office, you should create a separate master index for logging in this information. If you prefer, you can keep a master index in a notebook on your desk and handwrite a notation for each claim you send, indicating the following:

    - Carrier name (the third-party payer to whom you sent the claim)
    - Patient name
    - Date of service
    - Date and time you sent the claim

2. Build into your schedule a specific day and time each week for following up claims. When you set an appointment with yourself, such as every Friday at 9 a.m., or Mondays after the morning staff meeting, you will reduce the number of times that your workday will prevent you from doing this. It is so easy to say, "Once a week I am going to follow up on the claims" and just never have the time for this very important task. Each week, or as often as required by the number of claims you send out, go over the list and separate the claims into three "piles":

> **CODING BITES**
>
> You are responsible for following up on every claim you send.

- Pile 1: Claims that have been paid by the insurers
- Pile 2: Claims for which you have received rejection or denial notices
- Pile 3: Claims for which you have received no notices or payment

Pile 1: Claims That Have Been Paid by the Insurers

The HIPAA Health Care Payment and Remittance Advice is the electronic transmission of this payment, using HIPAA-approved secure data sets. The transmission has two parts: the transaction and the document.

- The document is a **remittance advice (RA)** or an **electronic remittance advice (ERA)**. Some health care professionals also refer to this document as an **explanation of benefits or EOB**. However, an EOB is sent to the patient or beneficiary, not the provider.
- The transaction is an electronic funds transfer (EFT) that sends the payment directly into your facility's bank account, like a direct deposit.

The RA will provide all the details of this payment, including

- The exact amount of monies your office is receiving
- For which patient
- For which procedures performed
- On which service dates

Remittance Advice (RA)
Notification identifying details about a payment from the third-party payer.

Electronic Remittance Advice (ERA)
Remittance advice that is sent to the provider electronically.

Explanation of Benefits (EOB)
Another type of paper remittance advice, more typically sent to the policyholder. However, some in the industry use the term *EOB* interchangeably with *RA*.

Once you are certain that a claim has been approved and your office has received payment from the third-party payer, the first thing you should do is mark this claim as paid in your master index. Be very careful when doing this.

When you enter the deposits into the computer (and into the bank, if the funds were not electronically transferred), you must be very diligent. You might have two claims for the same patient for different dates or two patients with the same name or similar names. You do not want to mark the wrong claim paid and leave the wrong claim marked unpaid. This will cause a lot of confusion and aggravation in dealing with the insurance carrier.

Pile 2: Claims for Which You Have Received Denial Notices

You have learned how to avoid many denied claims by checking, double-checking, and triple-checking your work. Make certain that

1. Insurance coverage is confirmed (eligibility verification).
2. All the information (such as policyholder and policy number) is entered correctly.
3. The best, most appropriate codes are used.
4. Medical necessity has been established by those codes.
5. All the information has been correctly placed on the correct claim form.

Despite doing everything correctly, some claims are denied and come back unpaid. However, this does not mean that you either have to go after the guarantor for the money or have your office go without the money it deserves. There are many reasons an insurance carrier, or payer, may deny a claim. Let's review some of the most common reasons for a claim to be denied and what you can do about it.

Denied Due to Office Personnel Error

If you discover that the claim has been denied by the insurance carrier due to an error made by you or someone in your office, this can be fixed. Simply find out what the error was and correct it.

Compare the policy number on the claim to the copy of the insurance card that you made when the patient was seen in your office for this encounter. It is important that

> **CODING BITES**
>
> Get into the habit of dating the copy you make of the insurance card each time the patient comes in to see the physician.

> **CODING BITES**
>
> Make certain that you mark a resubmission with the words "Corrected Claim" so there is no mistake that you are not double billing (which is against the law).

Eligibility Verification
The process of confirming with the insurance carrier that an individual is qualified for benefits that would pay for services provided by your health care professional on a particular day.

you specifically check it against the copy taken at the encounter for which this claim form is billing the insurance company. The patient may have been in your office more recently with a new policy because his or her insurance changed between the most recent visit and the visit for which this claim was submitted.

You might find that, when you keyed the number into the computer, you inadvertently switched two numbers. It can happen when you are in a busy, hectic, noisy office with many people talking to you at the same time.

If you find that the policy number matches the ID card, you will have to continue looking for the typo, going over the claim form one box at a time to check every piece of information that was entered. Once you find the error, all you have to do is correct it and resubmit a corrected claim form.

You should have caught the error when you double-checked your work, but . . . OK. It happens. You have wasted time (and if you are using a clearinghouse, you have wasted money as well), and you have delayed payment to your office, but follow the third-party payer's procedure for resubmitting corrected claims and the money will arrive.

> **EXAMPLES**
>
> The policy number or a CPT code is invalid (nonexistent) because it was entered improperly.
>
> Anyone could look at the number 546998823 and accidentally key in 546999823.

Denied Due to Lack of Coverage

You look at the denial notice and it doesn't make sense. You have documentation in the file that, when you called for **eligibility verification**, the insurance carrier representative confirmed that the patient's coverage was valid and the policy carried no exclusions. The co-payment, co-insurance, and deductible were also confirmed. However, the claim was returned as denied, with the reason that the patient was not covered.

What may have happened is that, between your verification of the patient's coverage and the arrival of the claim at the insurance carrier's office, the policy was canceled or changed. When your claim arrived, the computer, or the person, simply looked at the file, saw that the policy was no longer in effect, and therefore denied the claim. If this is the case:

1. You will need to send a letter, not make a phone call, to the insurance carrier. In the letter, carefully state the date and time of the eligibility verification and the name of the insurance representative who told you the patient was covered for services by your office. (Make certain your office's procedure for eligibility verification includes the documentation of all of these details for just this reason.) Emphasize the date of the phone call or print out the electronic verification, as well as the date(s) of treatment or service, and attach a fresh printout of the claim form.

2. Before you mail this letter, call the company and confirm the name, title, and address of the employee responsible for receiving your appeal request. If you send this information to the wrong person, it may get lost within the company or, at the very least, it will delay your satisfaction of this issue.

3. Make certain you keep copies of everything, and follow up in a week or two if you have not heard from the insurer.

In other cases, claims have been denied because the individual's policy was canceled prior to your treatment and the insurance representative did not have (or did not tell you) up-to-date information. Therefore, your office provided treatment based on misinformation. As a matter of policy, typically the insurance carrier will claim that its staff member's confirmation of coverage does not represent a guarantee that your office will be paid. Again, you do not want to take no for an answer.

Both federal and state courts have ordered insurance carriers to pay claims based on their statements of eligibility at the time treatment and services were provided. These courts have established that the insurance representative's, or the electronic, confirmation of benefits serves as encouragement to the physician, or other provider, to offer that treatment or service.

When you think about it, if the insurance carrier had stated that the patient did not have coverage at the time you called for verification, your office may have chosen to not see the patient, to not take an x-ray, or to ask the patient to pay cash at that time. The fact that the insurance carrier told you, or a member of your office, that they would pay the claim encouraged your physician to treat the individual and reasonably expect to be paid for his or her work. Again, you must do the following:

1. Write a letter of appeal to the appropriate person at the insurance company, stating all the details of the verification conversation.
2. If your office does eligibility verification electronically, you should copy the printout of the electronic confirmation and attach it to the letter.
3. Always keep hard copy (paper) documentation or notes indicating to whom you spoke, what was said, and the date and time of the conversation.

If your appeal is denied again, your office may need to enlist the services of an attorney. The bottom line is that your office is entitled to this payment, but there are times you may need to fight for it.

Denied Due to Lack of Medical Necessity

Should your office receive a denial based on lack of medical necessity, there are some things you must do:

1. Go back and confirm the diagnosis (ICD-10-CM) and procedure (CPT or ICD-10-PCS) codes that appear on the claim form are the best, most accurate codes.
   a. There is a possibility that there was a simple error in keying in the code (such as transposing two of the numbers or leaving off a digit). More than once, a health care office and a patient have gone through months of arguing with the insurance carrier for the coverage of a procedure, only to find that the entire problem was a simple typographical error.
   b. Perhaps there was an error in coding. Go back and look at the physician's notes. Start from the beginning and recode the encounter. If there is another coder in your office, you might ask him or her to look at the notes and code the diagnosis and procedure(s). Then compare the other coder's determination of the best, most appropriate codes with yours. If you come up with different and/or additional codes this time, you might go ahead and resubmit the claim with the new codes. Or this review might confirm that the codes were correct on the original claim.
   c. Review the linking of the procedure codes to diagnosis codes (CMS-1500 Box 24E). Confirm the links are correct.
2. Contact the insurance carrier and get a written copy of its definition of medical necessity, or check its website and print it out. Often the list of criteria for medical necessity consists of any treatment or service that
   a. Is commonly performed by health care practitioners (considered accepted standard of care) for the treatment of the condition, illness, or injury as indicated by the diagnosis code(s) provided.
   b. Is provided at the most efficient level of care that ensures the patient's safety.
   c. Is not experimental.
   d. Is not elective.

   Using the criteria for medical necessity from the insurance carrier that denied the claim (different carriers may have different criteria), review the patient's health record to confirm that this individual and this particular encounter meet all of the requirements. Again,

- Double-check the diagnosis and procedure codes to make certain they all accurately represent what occurred during that visit.
- Call and speak with the claims examiner to identify exactly what he or she thought the problem was with the claim. This conversation may give you some insight into what you should be looking for as you review the patient's chart.
- Get support materials from your health care professionals, particularly the attending physician on this case. Copies of articles or pages from credible sources, such as *The Merck Manual,* the *New England Journal of Medicine,* or other qualified sources of research, will help support your claim.
- If this patient encounter was the result of another provider referring the individual to your physician for additional treatment, the referring physician might agree to write a letter supporting your office.

3. Write a letter to the third-party payer's appeals board, or to whomever the claims representative instructs you to send the documentation, outlining all of the information you have gathered to corroborate specifically why the denial should be overturned.

   a. Include copies of supporting documentation, such as pages from the National Library of Medicine's website or a letter from the referring provider.

   b. In addition, request that a qualified health care professional licensed in the area of treatment or service under discussion be the one to review your appeal. This may provide a more agreeable opinion as to the medical necessity of your claim and get it approved.

> **EXAMPLE**
>
> Christopher Novack, a 67-year-old male, is seen by his family physician after stating that he was driving to his office earlier and felt so dizzy he had to pull over. While waiting for the dizziness to pass, he felt his heart beating rapidly, and he began to sweat. He was worried that he was having a heart attack and came right over to see Dr. Bennetti.
>
> Dr. Bennetti, knowing that Chris had been diagnosed with type 2 diabetes mellitus, checked his glucose levels and found them to be grossly abnormal, causing the dizziness and sweating. He administered an injection of insulin. Then, Dr. Bennetti checked Chris's heart with a 12-lead EKG. The results were negative.
>
> When you perform your medical necessity review, you can see that the code for type 2 diabetes mellitus will justify the glucose test and the injection of the insulin.
>
> However, if you do not have a second diagnosis code for his rapid heartbeat, the claim would be rejected. Without the code for rapid heartbeat, there is no medical justification provided on the claim form for performing an EKG.

Denied Due to Preexisting Condition

A denial on the grounds that the patient was treated for a preexisting excluded condition or illness reinforces the need for accurate confirmation of eligibility before the patient is seen and treated by the physician. If, in fact, your physician is about to treat a patient for a specific diagnosis, you must determine if the insurance carrier has excluded that condition, illness, or injury from coverage. This should be done during the eligibility verification. However, if you get to the point at which a submitted claim has been denied due to a preexisting condition that has been excluded, you still have several options to try to get your claim paid:

1. Start by reviewing the diagnosis code. There may be a difference in the diagnosis codes, now and for past treatment, making your claim valid.

2. Request a copy of the insurance carrier's definition of a preexisting condition. Once you clearly understand the requirements, you will be able to better analyze the details of this claim and its validity.
3. A review of the patient's past medical records may also assist you in appealing this denial. Examining specific diagnosis codes and physician's notes' diagnostic statements may find an opportunity to justify the insurance carrier's coverage of this claim.

When you have the information to support your claim, write an appeal letter outlining why the denial should be reversed.

Denied Due to Benefit Limitation on Treatment by an Assistant

Some medical offices have physician's assistants and nurse practitioners treat patients for routine examinations, vaccinations, and other medical services. However, some insurance carriers limit the types of treatments and services for which they will pay when provided by a health care worker who is not a licensed physician. There are a couple of approaches to appeal this type of denial.

1. Begin by authenticating the qualifications of the person who provided the service or treatment. You will also want to reinforce, in your appeal, that having this health care professional perform this procedure, under the supervision of the licensed physician, was the most cost-efficient way to provide the service to the patient.
2. Obtain a copy of the carrier's written policy regarding treatment to patients by assistants and search for language that specifically denies payment for services provided by a professional with the credentials of your staff member. If you do not find any such language, your appeal letter should include that the insurance carrier's policy does not specifically exclude services provided by this level of professional.

Subsequent Denials

There are additional steps that can be taken to appeal a second or third denial. Sometimes an insurance carrier will deny a claim, hoping that you will give up and it will not have to pay. However, most of the time, subsequent denials are just a matter of poor communication between the insurance carrier and the health care facility. Remember, although it is an insurance carrier's responsibility and obligation to pay claims, it is also its responsibility and obligation to protect its assets from fraud. Primarily, it is this intention that creates the circumstance of a falsely denied claim. However, after you have exhausted all efforts within the insurance carrier's organization to get the carrier to see your side and pay the claim, you have additional options:

1. Many states have state boards and/or review panels for this type of situation. Experienced health care providers, with varying areas of specialization, sit on these review boards. Their duty is to go over all the details of the case; examine the patient's health record, the claim form, and all other documentation; and evaluate the insurance carrier's basis for denying the claim. They have the right, empowered by the state government, to override the insurance carrier's decision and force the carrier to pay the claim. Bringing an appeal to this type of review board is an option to both health care professionals and individuals alike.
2. If the patient is covered under an employer's self-insured health plan, the state board is usually not an option for appeal. However, the federal government oversees and regulates self-insured plans and can provide you with an appeals process. At the very least, these insurers are required to have an in-house appeal board that will hear your case.

Surprisingly, you have an excellent chance of winning an appeal when you handle it properly. Researchers have found very high success rates for providers who file appeals. Therefore, if a claim is denied, it is worth the time to look into the reasons for denial and possibly exercise the right to appeal.

Writing Letters of Appeal

When a claim has been denied and you have gathered all the documentation to support your position that the denial is incorrect, you need to write a formal letter of appeal. This letter should contain the following:

Recipient: Call the third-party payer and get the name, title, and address of the person to whom you should address this letter. Make certain you double-check the spelling of the person's name—don't assume. Even a name as straightforward as John can also be spelled Jon or Jahn. Just ask!

RE: In the space between the recipient's name and address, and the salutation, you need to include identification regarding the person to whom this letter refers. This should be indented to your one-inch tab position. The details that should be shown in this area of the letter are

> Patient Name:
> Policyholder Name:
> Policy Number:
> Date(s) of Service:
> Claim Number:
> Total Amount of Claim: $

Salutation: Always begin the letter with a proper business salutation to the recipient by name. For example, Dear Mr. Smith: or Dear Ms. Jones (followed by a colon). Avoid generic salutations such as To Whom It May Concern unless the insurance carrier will not release the name of the person designated to receive appeal letters and has instructed you to address this letter to a department or title.

Paragraph 1: State briefly and directly why you are writing this letter. This is a summary or condensed version of the rest of the letter. Be factual, not emotional. Be specific about when and/or how you were informed that the claim was denied and the reasons stated by the insurance carrier for the denial. This paragraph is to make certain that you and the reader of this letter are on the same page (pardon the pun!). It is difficult to capture and retain someone's attention to what you are saying if he or she doesn't know to what or whom you are referring.

> **EXAMPLES**
> 1. Our claims service representative, Raul Vega, told us that the above claim was denied due to a lack of medical necessity. This letter is an official notice that we wish to appeal this decision.
> 2. On November 3, 2018, our office received a notice stating that the above-mentioned claim was denied because of lack of coverage. This letter is to appeal this decision.

Paragraph 2: Itemize all the facts/evidence you have to support your position that you should be paid. Explain what documentation you have to encourage them to change their minds and approve/pay your claim. This list may contain highlights from the physician's notes outlining why the procedure was medically necessary. You might include statistics proving that this procedure is no longer considered experimental but is now widely accepted as the new standard of care. Attach copies (never originals) of documents that contain the information and refer to those attachments in this portion of the letter. In reality, this section of the letter may need to be longer than one paragraph. Write what you need to establish your rationale, but remember that this is not creative writing. Do not use flowery language or get long in your explanation. Be direct and to the point and include just the facts.

> **EXAMPLES**
> 1. As you can see in the attached documentation, the x-rays confirmed that the patient had a compound fracture requiring immediate surgery.
> 2. On Thursday, September 4, 2018, at 1:35 p.m. Eastern, I spoke with Emma Longwood in your Eligibility Verification department, who confirmed that Mr. Smith was fully covered by your HMO plan for the following procedures. . . .

<u>Paragraph 3</u>: Use paragraph 3 (the last paragraph) to clearly define where this discussion should go next. Of course, you want them to just reconsider and pay the claim; however, you will need to keep this a bit more open-ended. Offer to provide any additional documentation the insurance carrier may feel necessary. Supply your contact information (office phone number, e-mail address, fax number) even if it is right there on the letterhead. Set an appointment generally (i.e., "I will call you next week") to follow up with this person. The purpose of this statement is to keep this appeal moving in a direction toward acceptance and payment. You do not want this letter to get buried on a busy desk. In addition, mark your calendar and call when you said you would. It is your responsibility to keep this issue on the top of the insurance carrier's priority list. You know that old saying, "The squeaky wheel gets the grease." This means that those that speak up get the attention.

> **EXAMPLES**
> 1. If you need any more information, to bring this to a quick resolution, please contact me at . . . .
> 2. I will call you at the end of the week to discuss this matter further. In the meantime, if you need to contact me, please do so at . . . .

<u>Closing and Signature</u>: All business letters should contain a closing, as well as the signature and title of the person sending the correspondence. *Sincerely* or *Sincerely yours* (followed by a comma) are the most common closings. After leaving four lines blank to make room for your signature, key in your full name. Directly underneath your name, key in your title (e.g., Insurance Specialist). If you are going to attach copies of important documentation to this letter, you need to note this under your signature. Leave one empty line under your title, and key in Enclosure or Enclosures or Enc. This notation points the recipient to the additional pages included in the envelope.

Pile 3: Claims for Which You Have Received No Notices or Payment

If a reasonable time has passed after sending a claim and you have received no notices or payment, you will need to follow up with the insurance carrier. (The term *reasonable time* is specifically defined by each third-party payer.)

1. Go to the third-party payer's website and check the status of the claim, or call and speak with someone in customer service to determine which examiner or representative will be handling your claim. Try to confirm that he or she has received your claim by getting a date and time of receipt and ask which staff member received it. If you cannot get this information, or you get a vague statement, such as "Oh, I'm sure we have it somewhere. We are very busy. We'll get to it soon," you will need to take the next step.
2. Go back over all the paperwork that accompanied claims paid by this carrier in the same time frame, such as an electronic remittance advice (ERA), or a remittance

Tracer
An official request for a third-party payer to search its system to find a missing health claim form. It is also a term used for a replacement health claim form resubmitted to replace one that was lost.

advice (RA). There may have been a mistake and the wrong claim was marked paid in your file (meaning that this claim has really already been paid) and it is another claim that is still outstanding.

3. Once you are certain the insurance company has not responded to this claim in any way, you may need to send a **tracer**, also known as a duplicate billing or second submission.

Most insurance carriers require you to wait a specific number of days or weeks after the original date of submission before you are permitted to send a tracer claim. Check with the carrier, as each may have a different waiting period. This second version of the same claim must be marked "Tracer." This is to make sure that the insurance carrier knows you are not attempting to bill a second time for the same services. Double billing is against the law; however, sending a bill a second time because you believe that the first claim has been lost is good business.

Make a note in your master index of the date and time that you refiled the claim. That way, you can follow up again if you need to.

Chapter Summary

A fundamental part of an insurance coding and medical billing specialist's job is to work with the insurance companies that will reimburse your health care facility for the services and procedures you provide to your patients. You need to understand how your facility will be paid (such as fee-for-service, capitation, or episodic care); be able to distinguish among the types of policies (such as HMOs, PPOs, and managed care policies, as well as Medicare, Medicaid, and TriCare plans); and quickly identify which is responsible for sending payment to you. This will help your billing efforts be more efficient and get paid more quickly.

The procedures you develop and abide by for tracking the health insurance claim forms you submit is almost as important as the coding process itself. Some health care offices do not have a routine for handling situations, such as lost claims or denied claims. However, you must realize how important this is to the overall financial well-being of your facility.

When you are organized, and keep a tracking log of all the claims you submit, your work is easier and your success rate is higher. Appealing denied claims is a part of your career, and it is an important part of the entire medical billing and insurance claims process.

> **CODING BITES**
>
> The basic reimbursement methods are applicable across all types of health care, and include capitation, fee for service, episodic (global) payment, and cost reimbursement.
>
> It is the provider's responsibility to confirm the method of reimbursement prior to providing services.
>
> For more information on the newest program, MACRA, go to
> https://www.cms.gov/Medicare/Quality-Initiatives-Patient-Assessment-Instruments/Value-Based-Programs/MACRA-MIPS-and-APMs/MACRA-MIPS-and-APMs.html

You Interpret It! Answers

1. Workers' compensation and disability compensation, **2.** Margaret's liability insurance, **3.** Facility member = workers' compensation; student = school's liability insurance

CHAPTER 39 REVIEW
Reimbursement

Let's Check it! Terminology

Match each term to the appropriate definition.

Part I

1. LO 39.2 — **I** — A physician, typically a family practitioner or an internist, who serves as the primary care physician for an individual. This physician is responsible for evaluating and determining the course of treatment or services, as well as for deciding whether or not a specialist should be involved in care.
2. LO 39.1 — **N** — A type of health insurance coverage that controls the care of each subscriber (or insured person) by using a primary care provider as a central health care supervisor.
3. LO 39.2 — **K** — A type of health insurance that uses a primary care physician, also known as a gatekeeper, to manage all health care services for an individual.
4. LO 39.2 — **M** — A policy that covers loss or injury to a third party caused by the insured or something belonging to the insured.
5. LO 39.1 — **J** — The total management of an individual's well-being by a health care professional.
6. LO 39.3 — **G** — An insurance company pays a provider one flat fee to cover the entire course of treatment for an individual's condition.
7. LO 39.2 — **C** — The agency under the Department of Health and Human Services (DHHS) in charge of regulation and control over services for those covered by Medicare and Medicaid.
8. LO 39.3 — **H** — Payment agreements that outline, in a written fee schedule, exactly how much money the insurance carrier will pay the physician for each treatment and/or service provided.
9. LO 39.3 — **F** — An extra reduction in the rate charged to an insurer for services provided by the physician to the plan's members.
10. LO 39.1 — **L** — The amount of money, often paid monthly, by a policyholder or insured, to an insurance company to obtain coverage.
11. LO 39.2 — **A** — Auto accident liability coverage will pay for medical bills, lost wages, and compensation for pain and suffering for any person injured by the insured in an auto accident.
12. LO 39.3 — **B** — Agreements between a physician and a managed care organization that pay the physician a predetermined amount of money each month for each member of the plan who identifies that provider as his or her primary care physician.
13. LO 39.2 — **E** — A plan that reimburses a covered individual a portion of his or her income that is lost as a result of being unable to work due to illness or injury.
14. LO 39.2 — **D** — Individuals who are supported, either financially or with regard to insurance coverage, by others.

A. Automobile Insurance
B. Capitation Plans
C. Centers for Medicare & Medicaid Services (CMS)
D. Dependents
E. Disability Compensation
F. Discounted FFS
G. Episodic Care
H. Fee-for-Service (FFS) Plans
I. Gatekeeper
J. Health Care
K. Health Maintenance Organization (HMO)
L. Insurance Premium
M. Liability Insurance
N. Managed Care

Part II

1. LO 39.6 — **I** — An official request for a third-party payer to search its system to find a missing health claim form. It is also a term used for a replacement health claim form resubmitted to replace one that was lost.
2. LO 39.3 — **K** — The process of determining a fee for a service by evaluating the *usual* fee charged by the provider, the *customary* fee charged by most physicians in the same community or geographical area, and what is considered *reasonable* by most health care professionals under the specific circumstances of the situation.
3. LO 39.6 — **B** — Remittance advice that is sent to the provider electronically.
4. LO 39.2 — **E** — A type of insurance plan that will allow an HMO enrollee to choose his or her own nonmember physician at a lower benefit rate, costing the patient more money out-of-pocket.
5. LO 39.1 — **H** — An individual or organization that is not directly involved in an encounter but has a connection because of its obligation to pay, in full or part, for that encounter.
6. LO 39.6 — **D** — Another type of paper remittance advice, more typically sent to the policyholder. However, some in the industry use the term *EOB* interchangeably with *RA*.
7. LO 39.2 — **F** — A type of health insurance coverage in which physicians provide health care services to members of the plan at a discount.
8. LO 39.2 — **J** — A government health plan that covers medical expenses for the dependents of active-duty service members, CHAMPUS-eligible retirees and their families, and the dependents of deceased active-duty members.
9. LO 39.2 — **L** — An insurance program that covers medical care for those injured or for those who become ill as a consequence of their employment.
10. LO 39.1 — **A** — A health care claim form that is transmitted electronically.
11. LO 39.6 — **C** — The process of confirming with the insurance carrier that an individual is qualified for benefits that would pay for services provided by your health care professional on a particular day.
12. LO 39.6 — **G** — Notification identifying details about a payment from the third-party payer.

A. Electronic Media Claim (EMC)
B. Electronic Remittance Advice (ERA)
C. Eligibility Verification
D. Explanation of Benefits (EOB)
E. Point-of-Service (POS)
F. Preferred Provider Organization (PPO)
G. Remittance Advice (RA)
H. Third-Party Payer
I. Tracer
J. TriCare
K. Usual, Customary, and Reasonable (UCR)
L. Workers' Compensation

Part III

1. LO 39.2 — **F** — May cover medical expenses caused by a car accident.
2. LO 39.2 — **D** — Preferred provider organization.
3. LO 39.3 — **A** — A fixed amount paid each visit by the individual.
4. LO 39.3 — **C** — Payment, per service provided, from the insurance company.
5. LO 39.2 — **E** — A government program for indigent and needy people.
6. LO 39.3 — **B** — An episodic-care payment system basing reimbursement to hospitals for inpatient services upon standards of care for specific diagnoses grouped by their similar usage of resources for procedures, services, and treatments.

A. Co-payment
B. DRG
C. Fee-for-Service
D. PPO
E. Medicaid
F. Auto Insurance Policy

Let's Check It! Concepts

Choose the most appropriate answer for each of the following questions.

1. LO 39.1 Medical care is defined as
   a. identification and treatment of illness and/or injury.
   b. services to prevent illness such as a routine checkup or wellness visit.
   c. laboratory services.
   d. only those services performed by a medical doctor.

2. LO 39.2 An organization that depends on the services of a gatekeeper is
   a. a preferred provider organization.
   b. Medicare.
   c. a health maintenance organization.
   d. a not-for-profit hospital.

3. LO 39.3 A capitation plan pays the provider
   a. per specific service.
   b. per member every month.
   c. for treatments in a hospital only.
   d. one flat fee per illness or condition.

4. LO 39.2 Medicare is a government plan that covers primarily
   a. military personnel.
   b. poor and needy.
   c. those over the age of 65.
   d. government employees.

5. LO 39.4 When CMS computers evaluate submitted claims to look for pairs of codes being reported that are known to be mutually exclusive procedures, this is also known as _____ edits.
   a. LCD
   b. NCD
   c. PTP
   d. MUE

6. LO 39.2 TriCare provides health care benefits for the dependents of
   a. state workers.
   b. those serving in the uniformed services.
   c. athletes.
   d. health care workers.

7. LO 39.5 What specific location does POS code 23 identify?
   a. Urgent Care Facility
   b. Assisted Living Facility
   c. Telehealth
   d. Emergency Room—Hospital

8. LO 39.6 The HIPAA Health Care Payment and Remittance Advice is the electronic transmission of payment, using HIPAA-approved secure data sets. The transmission has two parts: the _____ and the _____.
   a. claim, transaction
   b. transaction, document
   c. document, claim
   d. date, carrier name

9. LO 39.3 When an individual pays a percentage of the total charge, it is called the
   a. deductible.
   b. co-payment.
   c. co-insurance.
   d. premium.

10. LO 39.2 CMS stands for
    a. Centers for Medical Services.
    b. Corporation of Medical Systems.
    c. Centers for Medicare & Medicaid Services.
    d. Cycle of Medical Selections.

CHAPTER 39 REVIEW

Let's Check It! Which Type of Insurance?

Match the situation with the type of insurance that would cover the expenses. Answers may be used more than once.

A. Health Insurance
B. Workers' Compensation
C. Medicaid
D. Disability Compensation
E. Liability Insurance
F. TriCare
G. Automobile Insurance
H. Medicare

B 1. LO 39.2 Mrs. Matthews, a teacher at Medical Coder Academy, slipped in her office, fell, and hurt her back.

D 2. LO 39.2 Ralph broke his leg and must be in traction for 9 months. What plan will help him pay his rent and electric bill?

E 3. LO 39.2 Mary Lou was at the mall, shopping for a birthday present, when she slipped on a wet floor and broke her hip.

A 4. LO 39.1 Keith was walking down the stairs in his house, fell over his son's toy, and twisted his ankle.

G 5. LO 39.2 Marlene was driving to work when another car hit her from behind. The EMTs took her to the hospital with a sprained ankle and sore neck.

A 6. LO 39.2 Harvey caught a cold when he went fishing last weekend.

E 7. LO 39.2 Jared enrolled in the insurance coding program at the local college. While leaving after his first class, another student bumped into him, he banged his head on a shelf, and he got a scalp laceration.

H 8. LO 39.2 At home after his 85th birthday party, Jack tripped on the rug, fell, and broke his hip.

F 9. LO 39.2 Suzette's husband is in the Marines. She is pregnant with their first child.

C 10. LO 39.2 James is out of work and has no prospects. He is broke and has a really bad sore throat.

Let's Check It! Rules and Regulations

Please answer the following questions from the knowledge you have gained after reading this chapter.

1. LO 39.4 What does NCCI stand for and what is its purpose? pg. 1165
2. LO 39.4 What is a procedure-to-procedure edit, who performs it, and when is it performed? pg 1165
3. LO 39.4 What is the purpose of medically unlikely edits? pg 1166
4. LO 39.6 What does it mean when a claim is denied due to an office personnel error and can it be corrected? pg. 1174
5. LO 39.6 What should you do if your office receives a claim denial due to lack of medical necessity? pg 1175

Introduction to Health Care Law and Ethics

40

Learning Outcomes

After completing this chapter, the student should be able to:

- **LO 40.1** Identify the sources for directives governing behavior.
- **LO 40.2** Understand the rules for ethical and legal coding.
- **LO 40.3** Apply the requirements of the False Claims Act.
- **LO 40.4** Translate the components of the Health Insurance Portability and Accountability Act's Privacy Rule.
- **LO 40.5** Elaborate the responsibilities of the Health Care Fraud and Abuse Control Program.
- **LO 40.6** Adhere to the codes of ethics of our industry.
- **LO 40.7** Analyze the reasons for creating a compliance plan.

Key Terms

Administrative Laws
Civil Law
Coding for Coverage
Common Law
Covered Entities
Criminal Law
Disclosure
Double Billing
Executive Orders
HIPAA's Privacy Rule
Mutually Exclusive Codes
Protected Health Information (PHI)
Release of Information (ROI)
Statutory Laws
Supporting Documentation
Unbundling
Upcoding
Use

40.1 Sources for Legal Guidance

The health care industry is responsible for providing services to maintain and repair the human body. For all of those providing health care services, the federal and state governments have crafted and enacted laws and regulations designed to ensure honest, safe, and appropriate behaviors from all involved. In addition, these laws and regulations provide a remedy—compensation or restitution—when individuals step outside of these approved boundaries. As a health care professional, you must be familiar with the government's directives so you can conduct yourself and your facility accordingly. This text is written to provide you with the necessary foundation of legal and ethical knowledge and understanding to support a successful career in health care. This chapter will introduce you to the basic concepts.

The Federal Register

The *Federal Register* is the daily journal of the U.S. federal government. The Office of the Federal Register (OFR), in conjunction with the U.S. Government Printing Office (GPO), created and maintains the website version of this publication.

Created in 1935, the *Federal Register*'s purpose is to inform *"citizens of their rights and obligations, documents the actions of Federal agencies, and provides a forum for public participation in the democratic process."* Included in its contents are executive orders, presidential proclamations, policy statements, proposed rules, notices of scheduled hearings, and other government actions.

Take a look at a small section of the *Federal Register* in Figure 40-1 and access the full *Federal Register* at https://www.federalregister.gov/.

Sources of Directives

Many different types of laws and regulations exist to direct certain behaviors of those individuals working in health care, on both the clinical side and the administrative side. Federal and state governments and their agencies initiate these directives.

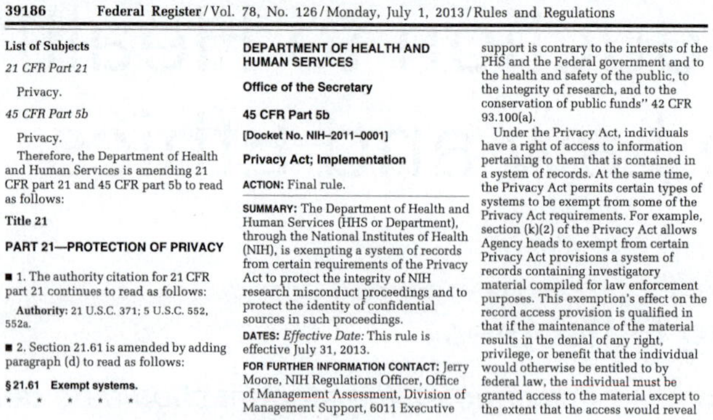

39186 **Federal Register** / Vol. 78, No. 126 / Monday, July 1, 2013 / Rules and Regulations

List of Subjects

21 CFR Part 21

Privacy.

45 CFR Part 5b

Privacy.

Therefore, the Department of Health and Human Services is amending 21 CFR part 21 and 45 CFR part 5b to read as follows:

Title 21

PART 21—PROTECTION OF PRIVACY

■ 1. The authority citation for 21 CFR part 21 continues to read as follows:

Authority: 21 U.S.C. 371; 5 U.S.C. 552, 552a.

■ 2. Section 21.61 is amended by adding paragraph (d) to read as follows:

§ 21.61 Exempt systems.

* * * * *

DEPARTMENT OF HEALTH AND HUMAN SERVICES

Office of the Secretary

45 CFR Part 5b

[Docket No. NIH–2011–0001]

Privacy Act; Implementation

ACTION: Final rule.

SUMMARY: The Department of Health and Human Services (HHS or Department), through the National Institutes of Health (NIH), is exempting a system of records from certain requirements of the Privacy Act to protect the integrity of NIH research misconduct proceedings and to protect the identity of confidential sources in such proceedings.

DATES: *Effective Date:* This rule is effective July 31, 2013.

FOR FURTHER INFORMATION CONTACT: Jerry Moore, NIH Regulations Officer, Office of Management Assessment, Division of Management Support, 6011 Executive

support is contrary to the interests of the PHS and the Federal government and to the health and safety of the public, to the integrity of research, and to the conservation of public funds" 42 CFR 93.100(a).

Under the Privacy Act, individuals have a right of access to information pertaining to them that is contained in a system of records. At the same time, the Privacy Act permits certain types of systems to be exempt from some of the Privacy Act requirements. For example, section (k)(2) of the Privacy Act allows Agency heads to exempt from certain Privacy Act provisions a system of records containing investigatory material compiled for law enforcement purposes. This exemption's effect on the record access provision is qualified in that if the maintenance of the material results in the denial of any right, privilege, or benefit that the individual would otherwise be entitled to by federal law, the individual must be granted access to the material except to the extent that the access would reveal

FIGURE 40-1 U.S. Congress's *Federal Register* showing official details relating to the Privacy Act (in part) Source: gpo.gov

There is a hierarchy established that sets the level of authority, which begins at the top with the U.S. Constitution as the first and foremost directive. In 1787, at the Constitutional Convention in Philadelphia, Pennsylvania, the Constitution of the United States was determined to be the highest and foremost of enacted law. Article VI of the Constitution states:

> *"This Constitution, and the Laws of the United States which shall be made in Pursuance thereof; and all Treaties made, or which shall be made, under the Authority of the United States, shall be the supreme Law of the Land; and the Judges in every State shall be bound thereby, any Thing in the Constitution or Laws of any State to the Contrary notwithstanding."*

Following the U.S. Constitution is federal law—those laws established by the U.S. Congress. State constitutions, state statutory laws, and then local laws complete the bottom tiers.

Statutory Laws
Laws that are enacted by federal and state legislature.

Statutory laws, most often referred to as *statutes,* are created and enacted by the federal and state legislatures (Congress). Members of Congress are responsible for writing the law. Then, once passed by votes in the House and the Senate, it is said to be "enacted." Because federal statutes take precedence over state statutory laws, state and local legislatures are not permitted to enact a law that contradicts any current federal law. This way, no one has to worry about which law takes dominance because this order of priority is already established.

There are circumstances, however, where the federal law provides some flexibility in behavior and the state law is more exact about the required behavior. In these cases, the state law would take precedence. For example, the federal law commonly called HIPAA's Privacy Rule (Health Insurance Portability and Accountability Act) empowers a health care provider to use his or her judgment whether or not to reveal protected health information to authorities when a patient is diagnosed with a contagious disease. However, virtually every state has a law that makes the reporting to authorities of a patient diagnosed with a contagious disease mandatory. The state law does not conflict with the federal law; it is actually more specific in its directive about behavior, so it overrules the federal law. This example is one that illustrates how important it is for all health care professionals to be familiar with both federal and state laws that govern their job responsibilities.

EXAMPLES

The Emergency Medical Treatment and Active Labor Act (EMTALA)

The Affordable Care Act (ACA)

Equal Employment Opportunity Act (EEO)

Executive orders are official documents issued by the president of the United States to set policy. They do not require approval from the legislature (Congress); however, they are issued, typically, under statutory authority and, therefore, have the full effect and force of a federal statute. The federal courts have upheld this.

Common law, also referred to as case law, is created by a judicial decision made during a court trial. These decisions, documented in law books for local, state, and federal court cases, create precedence—they establish a position. If you have ever watched a television show or movie with a court scene, you might remember the attorneys stating something like, "In *Brown v. the Board of Education*. . . ." This statement refers to a specific court case (*Brown v. the Board of Education*) and the decision made by that presiding judge. Those decisions are already accepted by the court, and therefore provide the current presiding judge with an established opinion.

You can see an example of the use of case law in the small portion of the Supreme Court opinion shown in Figure 40-2, the last three lines. A previous case—*PLIVA, Inc. v. Mensing,* 564 U.S. __ —is cited and this document goes on to explain the decision determined in that case and how it is related to this current case.

Executive Orders
Official policies issued by the president of the United States.

Common Law
Also known as case law, this is created by judicial decisions made during court trials.

> **EXAMPLES**
> *United States v. Windsor*
> *Mutual Pharmaceutical Co. v. Bartlett*
> *Adoptive Couple v. Baby Girl*

Administrative laws are those created and monitored by administrative agencies that have been given the responsibility to oversee specific areas, such as health care. The creation and implementation of specific rules and regulations have been delegated to those agencies created by Congress, under the Administrative Procedures Act, so each agency can ensure its assigned tasks can be accomplished. For example, Congress created the Centers for Disease Control and Prevention (CDC) as an administrative agency of the federal government to oversee issues related to contagious diseases. The CDC, therefore, has the authority to establish rules and regulations and to enforce those regulations (as long as they are consistent with the statute under which the agency was created). One of these rules is the mandated reporting of infectious diseases. Several surveillance information systems are used to enable the required reporting of these diagnoses; some are direct to the CDC while others are channeled through state departments of health first. However, if a particular diagnosis of an infectious disease is not reported, as required, the CDC has the authority to take action for noncompliance.

In Figure 40-3, you can see a screen shot of the website Regulations.gov. This website provides you with a searchable database of all federal agency regulations.

Administrative Laws
Also known as rules and regulations, these are created and adjudicated by administrative agencies given authority by Congress.

> **EXAMPLE**
> Centers for Medicare & Medicaid Services (CMS) has established its "rules of participation" for health care participating providers.

Criminal law seeks to control the behavior of people and companies when their actions are related to the health, welfare, and safety of an individual or property with the intention of protecting public order. Criminal activity is divided into two types, determined by the severity of the infraction: misdemeanors and felonies.

- A *misdemeanor* is a lesser offense, such as driving under the influence, public nuisances, and certain traffic violations. These infractions are adjudicated in local courts and are punishable with fines, penalties, and possible sentences of incarceration to county jail for up to 364 days.

Criminal Law
Laws governing the behavior of the actions of the population related to health and well-being.

> (Slip Opinion) OCTOBER TERM, 2012 1
>
> **Syllabus**
>
> NOTE: Where it is feasible, a syllabus (headnote) will be released, as is being done in connection with this case, at the time the opinion is issued. The syllabus constitutes no part of the opinion of the Court but has been prepared by the Reporter of Decisions for the convenience of the reader. See *United States v. Detroit Timber & Lumber Co.*, 200 U.S. 321, 337.
>
> **SUPREME COURT OF THE UNITED STATES**
> Syllabus
>
> MUTUAL PHARMACEUTICAL CO., INC. *v.* BARTLETT
>
> CERTIORARI TO THE UNITED STATES COURT OF APPEALS FOR THE FIRST CIRCUIT
>
> No. 12-142. Argued March 19, 2013—Decided June 24, 2013
>
> Federal Food, Drug, and Cosmetic Act (FDCA) requires manufacturers to gain Food and Drug Administration (FDA) approval before marketing any brand-name or generic drug in interstate commerce. 21 U.S.C. §355(a). Once a drug is approved, a manufacturer is prohibited from making any major changes to the "qualitative or quantitative formulation of the drug product, including active ingredients, or in the specifications provided in the approved application." 21 CFR §314.70(b)(2)(i). Generic manufacturers are also prohibited from making any unilateral changes to a drug's label. See §§314.94(a)(8)(iii), 314.150(b)(10).
>
> In 2004, respondent was prescribed Clinoril, the brand-name version of the nonsteroidal anti-inflammatory drug (NSAID) sulindac, for shoulder pain. Her pharmacist dispensed a generic form of sulindac manufactured by petitioner Mutual Pharmaceutical. Respondent soon developed an acute case of toxic epidermal necrolysis. She is now severely disfigured, has physical disabilities, and is nearly blind. At the time of the prescription, sulindac's label did not specifically refer to toxic epidermal necrolysis. By 2005, however, the FDA had recommended changing all NSAID labeling to contain a more explicit toxic epidermal necrolysis warning. Respondent sued Mutual in New Hampshire state court, and Mutual removed the case to federal court. A jury found Mutual liable on respondent's design-defect claim and awarded her over $21 million. The First Circuit affirmed. As relevant, it found that neither the FDCA nor the FDA's regulations pre-empted respondent's design-defect claim. It distinguished *PLIVA, Inc. v. Mensing*, 564 U.S. ___—in which the Court held that failure-to-warn claims against generic manufacturers are pre-empted by the FDCA's prohibition on changes to generic drug labels—by . . .

FIGURE 40-2 The use of case law is cited in this Supreme Court opinion regarding a drug approval case Source: Supreme Court of the United States Syllabus

- A *felony* is much more serious. This is a crime in violation of state or federal law and often carries a sentence of anywhere from 1 year to life in prison. Health care claims that are fraudulent and abusive of the reimbursement system constitute criminal activity and are an example of a felony. The Department of Justice, in conjunction with states' attorneys general, investigates accusations of these improper actions.

In Figure 40-4, you can see a release from the FBI reporting a guilty plea from a man in Ohio who was investigated and found guilty of criminal activity—involving billing Medicare and Medicaid for home health care services.

Civil law governs the conduct of those involved in a relationship: between private companies, individuals, and sometimes the government. Most often, a civil complaint

Civil Law
Laws that govern the relationships between people, and between businesses.

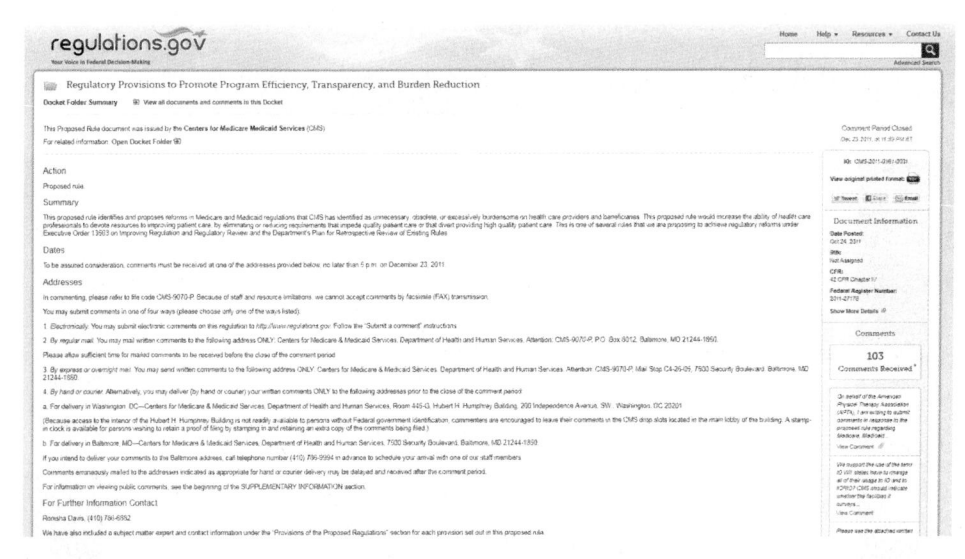

FIGURE 40-3 A snapshot of the website Regulations.gov, which offers a searchable database of federal agency rules and regulations Source: Regulations.gov

---

Orange Man Pleads Guilty to Health Care Fraud Charges Related to Overbilling Medicaid and Medicare by $2.5 Million

U.S. Attorney's Office   **Northern District of Ohio**
April 15, 2013   (216) 622-3600

A man who lives in Orange, Ohio, admitted to overbilling Medicaid and Medicare by more than $2.5 million, said Steven M. Dettelback, United States Attorney for the Northern District of Ohio.

Divyesh "Davis" C. Patel, age 39, pleaded guilty to one count of conspiracy to commit health care fraud and four counts of health care fraud. Patel is expected to be sentenced later this year.

"This defendant enriched himself and his company by flouting rules designed to protect the public," Dettelbach said.

"Mr. Patel defrauded the taxpayers by scamming Medicaid and Medicare," said Stephen D. Anthony, Special Agent in Charge of the FBI's Cleveland Field Office. "Waste, fraud, and abuse take critical resources out of our health care system and contribute to the rising cost of health care for all Americans."

Patel was the owner and president of Alpine Nursing Care, Inc.

FIGURE 40-4 A brief summary of a case where a man pleads guilty to health care fraud Source: "Orange Man Pleads Guilty to Health Care Fraud Charges Related to Overbilling Medicaid and Medicare by $2.5 Million," FBI, U.S. Attorney's Office, April 15, 2013.

---

or lawsuit will result from one party accusing the other of failure to comply with the terms of a contract. There are many instances of contractual relationships throughout the health care industry. Physicians and health care facilities may contract with a managed care organization; some facilities use contract workers to fill in for staff members on vacation; a family may contract with a home health care agency for services to a homebound patient; and the federal government may contract for health care services from a professional that does not include direct patient care. Figure 40-5 shows specific language that may be included in one of these contracts. The violation of a patient's confidentiality falls into this category because, in the United States, privacy

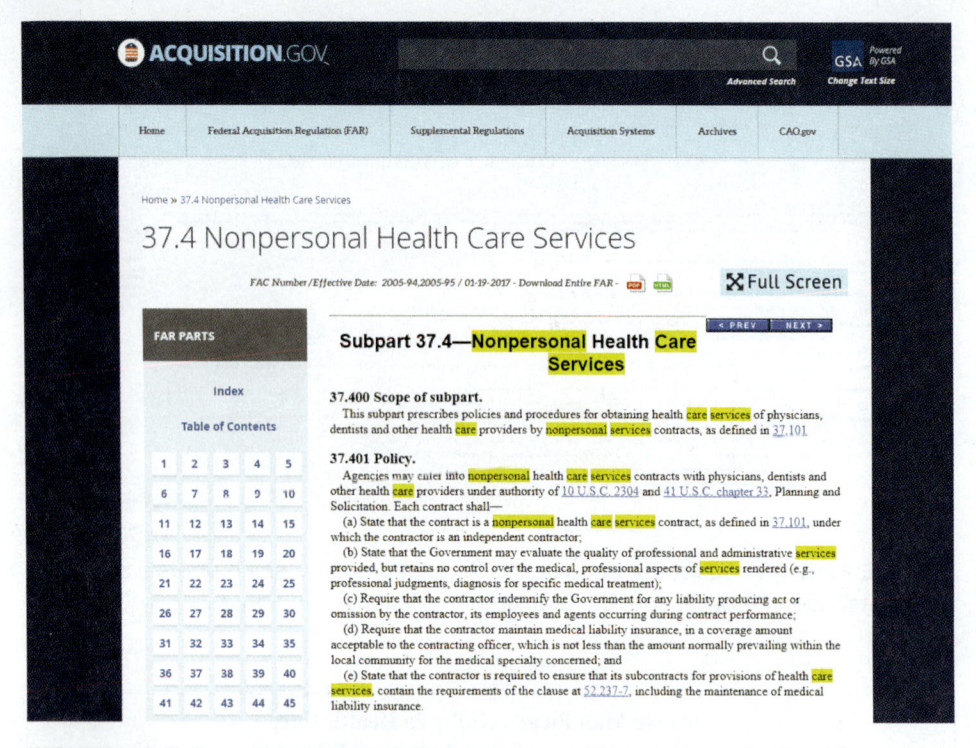

FIGURE 40-5 A partial example of language used in a contract for health care services that does not always include direct patient contact Source: Acquisition.gov

is considered a civil right. This is why an alleged violation of privacy laws is handled through the Office of Civil Rights (OCR) within the Department of Health and Human Services (DHHS) of the federal government.

40.2 Rules for Ethical and Legal Coding

As a coder, you have a very important responsibility—to yourself, your patients, and your facility. The work you do results in the creation of health claim forms and other reports that are legal documents. What you do can contribute to your facility staying healthy (businesswise) or being fined and possibly shut down by the Office of the Inspector General and your state's attorney general. You might make an error that could cause a patient to be unfairly denied health insurance coverage. It is important that you clearly understand the ethical and legal aspects of your position. Following are some issues, with regard to the ethics and legalities of coding, with which you should become very familiar.

1. It is very important that the codes indicated on the health claim form represent the services actually performed and the reasons why they are provided as supported by the documentation in the patient's health record. Don't use a code on a claim form without ensuring the **supporting documentation** is there in the file.

Supporting Documentation
The paperwork in the patient's file that corroborates the codes presented on the claim form for a particular encounter.

> **EXAMPLE**
> Coral Robinson's file indicates that Dr. Longmire ordered a blood test to determine whether or not she is pregnant. There is no report showing the results of the test. You see Dr. Longmire, and he tells you that Coral is pregnant and you should go ahead and code that diagnosis so the claim can be sent in. He promises to place the lab report and update the notes in her file later. Until the physician documents in the patient's chart that the patient is pregnant, you are not permitted to code the pregnancy.

2. Some health care providers may improperly encourage **coding for coverage**. This term refers to the process of determining diagnostic and procedural codes not by the accuracy of the code but with regard to what the insurance company will pay for or "cover." That is dishonest and is considered fraud. If you find yourself in an office or facility that insists you "code for coverage" rather than code to accurately reflect the documentation and the services actually performed, you should immediately discuss your situation with someone you trust. Some providers will rationalize the process by saying they are doing it so the patients can get the treatment they really need paid for by the insurance company. Altruism aside, it is still illegal and, once discovered, financial penalties and possible jail time can be assessed.

Coding for Coverage
Choosing a code on the basis of what the insurance company will cover (pay for) rather than accurately reflecting the truth.

> **EXAMPLE**
> Corbin Bloom wants a nose job (rhinoplasty); however, he cannot afford it. The insurance carrier will not pay for cosmetic surgery, so the coder changes the code to indicate that Corbin has a deviated septum requiring surgical correction so that the insurance carrier will pay for the procedure. That is *coding for coverage* and is fraud.

3. If you find yourself in an office or facility that insists that you include codes for procedures that you know, or believe, were never performed at a level of intensity or complexity as described by the code, this might be fraudulent behavior known as **upcoding**—the process of using a code that claims a higher level of service, or a more severe illness, than is true. Upcoding is considered falsifying records. Even if all you do is fill out the claim form, you are participating in something unethical and illegal.

Upcoding
Using a code on a claim form that indicates a higher level of service or a more severe aspect of disease or injury than that which was actual and true.

> **EXAMPLE**
> Erica Forney, a 69-year-old female, in the hospital for a broken hip, had her glucose level checked by the nurse, and it was at an abnormal level. Dr. Magnus ordered additional tests to rule out diabetes mellitus. Coding that Erica has diabetes is *upcoding* her condition and will fraudulently increase reimbursement from Medicare by changing the diagnosis-related group (DRG). In addition, placing a chronic disease on her health chart when she doesn't have it will cause her problems later on.

4. It is not permissible to code and bill for individual (also known as *component*) elements when a comprehensive or combination (bundle) code is available. This is referred to as **unbundling** and is illegal.

   For Medicare billing, refer to the Medicare National Correct Coding Initiative (CCI), which lists standardized bundled codes. The CCI is used to find coding conflicts, such as unbundling, the use of **mutually exclusive codes**, and other unacceptable reporting of CPT codes. When these errors are discovered, those claims are pulled for review and may be subject to possible suspension or rejection.

Unbundling
Coding the individual parts of a specific diagnosis or procedure rather than one combination or bundle that includes all of those components.

Mutually Exclusive Codes
Codes that are identified as those that are not permitted to be used on the same claim form with other codes.

Double Billing
Sending a claim for the second time to the same insurance company for the same procedure or service, provided to the same patient on the same date of service.

> **EXAMPLE**
> Dr. Hayden's notes indicate that Rico was experiencing nausea and vomiting. Instead of coding **R11.2 Nausea with vomiting**, the coder unbundles, coding **R11.0 Nausea** alone and **R11.11 Vomiting** alone.

5. If you resubmit a claim that has been lost, identify it as a "tracer" or "second submission." If you don't, you might be found guilty of **double billing**, billing the insurance company twice for a service provided only once. This also constitutes fraud.

CODING BITES

Always read the complete description in the provider's notes in addition to referencing the encounter form or superbill, and then carefully find the best available code that supports medical necessity according to the documentation.

6. You must code all conditions or complications that are relevant to the current encounter. Separating the codes relating to one specific encounter and placing them on several different claim forms over the course of several different days is neither legal nor ethical. It not only indicates a lack of organization of the office but also can cause suspicion of duplicating service claims, known as double billing. Even if you are reporting procedures that were actually done for diagnoses that actually exist, remember that the claim form is a legal document. All data on that claim form, including dates of service, must be accurate. Do not submit the claim form until you are certain it is complete, with all diagnoses and procedures listed. If it happens that, after you submit a claim, an additional service provided comes to light (such as a lab report with an extra charge that didn't come across your desk until after you filed the claim), then you must file an amended claim. While not illegal because you are identifying that the claim contains an adjustment, most third-party payers really dislike amended claims. You can expect an amended claim to be scrutinized.

All the activities mentioned here are considered fraud and are against the law.

It is not worth breaking the law and being charged with any of these penalties just to hang onto a job.

Office of the Inspector General (OIG) Workplan

The Office of the Inspector General (OIG), in the Department of Health and Human Services, is the agency that investigates and prosecutes failure to comply with the legal requirements for coding. The OIG plans in advance, for the upcoming year, what specific violations will be reviewed and investigated. This is valuable information to support the development of internal policies and procedures as well as foci for internal audits. When you can uncover and correct coding and billing errors *BEFORE* the federal or state auditors show up, this lessens fines and penalties considerably.

The workplan is released each year by October 1 for the upcoming calendar year. It is subsectioned by the type of facility affected, so you don't have to read through everything to find that which applies to your organization. Sometimes the issue is directly related to billing and coding; others may be more administrative.

CODING BITES

Office of the Inspector General (OIG)
https://oig.hhs.gov/reports-and-publications/workplan/index.asp

EXAMPLES

Hospitals

Intensity-Modulated Radiation Therapy
We will review Medicare outpatient payments for intensity-modulated radiation therapy (IMRT) to determine whether the payments were made in accordance with Federal requirements. IMRT is an advanced mode of high-precision radiotherapy that uses computer-controlled linear accelerators to deliver precise radiation doses to a malignant tumor or specific areas within the tumor. Prior OIG reviews have identified hospitals that have incorrectly billed for IMRT services. In addition, IMRT is provided in two treatment phases: planning and delivery. Certain services should not be billed when they are performed as part of developing an IMRT plan.

Selected Inpatient and Outpatient Billing Requirements
We will review Medicare payments to acute care hospitals to determine hospitals' compliance with selected billing requirements and recommend recovery of overpayments. Prior OIG reviews and investigations have identified areas at risk for noncompliance with Medicare billing requirements. Our review will focus on those hospitals with claims that may be at risk for overpayments.

> **EXAMPLE**
>
> *Home Health Services*
>
> Medicare Home Health Fraud Indicators
> We will describe the extent that potential indicators associated with home health fraud are present in home health billing for 2014 and 2015. We will analyze Medicare claims data to identify the prevalence of potential indicators of home health fraud. The Medicare home health benefit has long been recognized as a program area vulnerable to fraud, waste, and abuse. OIG has a wide portfolio of work involving home health fraud, waste, and abuse.

40.3 False Claims Act

The federal False Claims Act (FCA) was enacted by Congress to make the submission of a claim to a federal agency containing false information an illegal act. After this law was put into place, virtually every individual state passed its own version. This means that an individual may be charged with violation of both the federal law *AND* the state law, magnifying the fines, penalties, and consequences of this fraudulent behavior.

Who Is Liable?

Which staff members are responsible for ensuring that a facility or provider complies with FCA? All individuals and facilities that are involved in the creation and submission of claims—requests for reimbursement—based on coverage provided by governmental programs, such as Medicare or Medicaid, are responsible for complying with this law. Legally, these entities are referred to as federal contractors. Some people read the word *contractor* and immediately think of construction projects. However, in these cases, this phrase refers to one signing a contract to do business with a government program, that is, a participating provider. The Department of Justice takes enforcement of the FCA seriously. (See Figure 40-6 for just one example.)

Department of Justice Office of Public Affairs FOR IMMEDIATE RELEASE Monday, February 6, 2017

Healthcare Service Provider to Pay $60 Million to Settle Medicare and Medicaid False Claims Act Allegations

A major U.S. hospital service provider, TeamHealth Holdings, as successor in interest to IPC Healthcare Inc., f/k/a IPC The Hospitalists Inc. (IPC), has agreed to resolve allegations that IPC violated the False Claims Act by billing Medicare, Medicaid, the Defense Health Agency and the Federal Employees Health Benefits Program for higher and more expensive levels of medical service than were actually performed (a practice known as "up-coding"), the Department of Justice announced today. Under the settlement agreement, TeamHealth has agreed to pay $60 million, plus interest.

"This settlement reflects our ongoing commitment to ensure that health care providers appropriately bill government programs vital to patient health care," said Acting Assistant Attorney General Chad A. Readler of the Justice Department's Civil Division. The government contended that IPC knowingly and systematically encouraged false billings by its hospitalists, who are medical professionals whose primary focus is the medical care of hospitalized patients. Specifically, the government alleged that IPC encouraged its hospitalists to bill for a higher level of service than actually provided. IPC's scheme to improperly maximize billings allegedly included corporate pressure on hospitalists with lower billing levels to "catch up" to their peers.

FIGURE 40-6 An extract from a press release from the Department of Justice concerning a case enforcing the False Claims Act Source: "Justice Department Recovers Nearly $6 Billion from False Claims Act Cases in Fiscal Year 2014," Department of Justice, Office of Public Affairs, November 20, 2014.

What Is a Claim?

Needless to say, this law requires the proper behavior of individuals filing claims for reimbursement. So, let's begin with the FCA's specific definition of what a claim is: *"a demand for money or property made directly to the Federal Government or to a contractor, grantee, or other recipient."**

Under the requirements of the individual state governments, this would be a demand for reimbursement from the state government or other entity within.

The Knowledge Requirement

In addition, this law includes a "knowledge requirement." This portion of the law states that the simple action of submitting a claim with false information is not a violation. The individual must *know* that the information on the claim is false. What does "*know*" mean?

- *Actual knowledge* . . . knowing for a fact that the information is false.
- *Willful ignorance,* also known as deliberate ignorance . . . those who should know due to their job position, training, or responsibilities within the organization with regard to filing the claim but purposely don't ask about the validity of the information, or ignore the falsity of the information.
- *Disregard* of the truth or falsity . . . behavior that exhibits an indifference to confirming that the information is true.

> ### EXAMPLES
> Actual knowledge:
>> "I know that the procedures documented in the patient's record were not actually performed."
>
> Willful ignorance:
>> "I don't know for a fact, and I don't want to know."
>
> Disregard of the truth:
>> "It's not my concern. I just do what I am told."

Essentially, this means that an individual is required to comply with this law if, as part of his or her job, the individual *knows* the accuracy of the information on the claim, or *should know* the accuracy of the information. If your job involves anything to do with the creation and submission of a claim to any third party, it is your responsibility to know for a fact that the information is true. And no court will accept your excuse that you "didn't know."

The Qui Tam Provision

The *qui tam provision* within the FCA, commonly known as the *Whistleblower Statute,* empowers private citizens (typically those who work within organizations that do not comply) to file a lawsuit on behalf of the federal or state government against the facility for noncompliance. Sadly, there are health care professionals who will not listen to a staff member explaining that a particular behavior or sequence of actions is not legal. The intent of this statute is to recruit those honest individuals who witness an organization that is committing, or encouraging, fraudulent activities to step up and help to stop the illegal actions by reporting the fraud or filing a qui tam suit.

The government knows how scary and difficult it can be to come forward. Therefore, they reward the person or persons reporting the fraud with a percentage of the total amount recovered by the federal or state government as a result of the qui tam lawsuit. This reward can be anywhere from 15% to 30%.

*Source: Federal False Claims Act, Department of Justice.

> **EXAMPLE**
>
> "Of the $3.8 billion the department recovered in fiscal year 2013, $2.9 billion related to lawsuits filed under the qui tam provisions of the False Claims Act. During the same period, the department paid out more than $345 million to the courageous individuals who exposed fraud and false claims by filing a qui tam complaint."
>
> http://www.justice.gov/opa/pr/justice-department-recovers-38-billion-false-claims-act-cases-fiscal-year-2013

40.4 Health Insurance Portability and Accountability Act (HIPAA)

The Health Insurance Portability and Accountability Act of 1996, known as HIPAA (pronounced *hip-aah*), was enacted by the federal government and directly applies to you as a coding professional. Like most federal laws, HIPAA covers many different issues and concerns. The Privacy Rule is one part of this law that you are obligated to know and understand.

HIPAA's Privacy Rule

HIPAA's Privacy Rule was written to protect an individual's privacy with regard to personal health information, without getting in the way of the flow of data that is necessary to provide appropriate care for that patient. Essentially, the lawmakers tried to make certain that *a patient's information is easily accessible to those who should have access to it* [such as the physician, insurance coder and biller, and therapist] *and, at the same time, keep it secured against unauthorized people* [such as potential employers, coworkers, or neighborhood gossips] so that they do not see things they have no business seeing.

Who Is Responsible for Obeying This Law

HIPAA's Privacy Rule went into effect on April 14, 2003, and concerns every physician's office, clinic, hospital, and health insurance carrier—every type of business that is directly involved in the delivery of and/or payment for health care services, no matter how big or small. The largest of corporations owning hundreds of hospitals around the country and an office with one physician working alone are all included. HIPAA calls these businesses **covered entities**, and they all must comply with the terms of the law.

Covered entities are divided into three categories:

- Health care providers
- Health plans
- Health care clearinghouses

You probably already know the definition of a *health care provider:* any person or organization that gives health care services as the primary business purpose.

> **EXAMPLE**
>
> Health care providers as defined by HIPAA: physicians, dentists, hospitals, clinics, pharmacies, laboratories, and so on.

Health plans are described as organizations that provide and/or pay for health care services as their main reason for being in business. They include health insurance carriers, HMOs, employee welfare benefit plans, government health plans (such as

---

CODING BITES

Want more details about qui tam lawsuits? Here is an interesting article: "**Top 10 Tips for Qui Tam Whistleblowers,**" from the *National Law Review:*

http://www.natlawreview.com/article/top-10-tips-qui-tam-whistleblowers

CODING BITES

Be very careful when writing or typing this acronym. It is HIPAA . . . one P and two As.

HIPAA's Privacy Rule
A portion of HIPAA that ensures the availability of patient information for those who should see it while protecting that information from those who should not.

Covered Entities
Health care providers, health plans, and health care clearinghouses—businesses that have access to the personal health information of patients.

> **CODING BITES**
>
> Respecting a patient's privacy is also a sign of respect for the person. When you are the patient, you want to be treated with respect. So following HIPAA's Privacy Rule is not just the law of the United States; it is the law of treating people fairly.

TriCare, Medicare, and Medicaid), and group health plans provided through employers and associations. It doesn't matter whether the plan is offered to an individual or a group—all companies offering this coverage are included.

> ### EXAMPLE
> Health care plans as defined by HIPAA: Medicare, Medicaid, TriCare, BlueCross BlueShield, Prudential, and so on.

In addition, technology has created another type of organization involved in this process, called a *health care clearinghouse.* These companies help process electronic health insurance claims. Medical billing services, medical review services, and health information management system companies are included in this definition.

> ### EXAMPLE
> Health care clearinghouses as defined by HIPAA: National Clearinghouse, NDC Electronic Claims, WebMD Network Services, and others.

The workforces of covered entities are also included under HIPAA. A covered entity's workforce consists of every person who is involved with the company—full time, part time, volunteer, intern, extern, physician, nurse, assistant—and this has nothing to do with whether they are paid. Everyone must comply with the terms of this law.

> **CODING BITES**
>
> HIPAA's Privacy Rule is mostly about protecting your patient's privacy.

> ### EXAMPLE
> A covered entity's workforce as defined by HIPAA: full-time staff members, part-time staff members, volunteers, interns, externs, janitorial staff members, and so on.

What This Law Covers

You are certainly familiar with the topic of doctor–patient confidentiality. It means that anything a patient tells his or her doctor must be kept private. The doctor is not allowed, under most circumstances, to reveal to anyone what was said. This includes family members, parents (in many cases), and friends. This is important so that an individual will feel comfortable being open and honest and tell the physician things that are very, very personal, possibly even embarrassing or private facts that this person has never told anyone else. However, in order for the physician to properly treat this individual, the physician must know everything.

In order for you to do your job properly, you have access to all this confidential information. You need to know very personal and private facts about every one of your patients in order to accurately report the data.

You know what is wrong with them (their diagnoses) now and in the past; you know why they came to see this health care provider and why they saw others before they came to your facility; and you know what the health care provider thinks (observations and impressions) about these patients, as well as what has been done, is being done, and will be done to treat them. You know all these things because you have access to patients' health care records, including all the physician's notes. HIPAA calls this personal health care information (past, present, and future conditions) individually identifiable health information. In other words, it is information that anyone could look at and know exactly which individual is being discussed—one specific person. Specific pieces of data, called **protected health information (PHI)**, are pieces of information related to an individual that must be kept confidential, the grouping of facts that might have someone say, "Oh, I know him! Oh, and he has that!"

Protected Health Information (PHI)
Any patient-identifiable health information regardless of the form in which it is stored (paper, computer file, etc.).

> **EXAMPLE**
>
> Nicholas is a patient of Dr. Molinaro, and the information inside his chart (paper or electronic) consists of his records, charts, lab reports, and physician's notes documenting everything Nicholas has ever discussed with his physician. Karyn needs all this information to do her job as the office's coding specialist. At this moment, Karyn has stepped away from her desk. Nicholas's file is sitting on Karyn's desk, lying open.
>
> From the color of the folder, even from a distance, it is obvious that this is a patient of Dr. Molinaro's. The top piece of paper indicates that his patient has been diagnosed with a sexually transmitted disease. *At this point, any unauthorized person couldn't really know whose chart this is because Dr. Molinaro has hundreds of patients.*
>
> Right above the diagnosis anyone can see that this patient is a male. Although this will eliminate some of Dr. Molinaro's patients, there are still too many to know for certain.
>
> Upon closer examination of the paperwork in the folder, anyone could see that this male patient with the sexually transmitted disease lives on Main Street in Our Town, Florida. *The list of Dr. Molinaro's patients that is being referred to is getting very short now.*
>
> In the upper right corner, anyone can see Dr. Molinaro's male patient, who lives on Main Street, Our Town, Florida, who has a sexually transmitted disease, was born on June 13, 1985. *Oh my, did you know Nicholas lives on Main Street in Our Town, and his birthday is June 13th? It must be Nicholas who has that terrible disease!*
>
> Did Karyn fulfill her responsibility to protect Nicholas's privacy? What could she have done differently to ensure that this patient's PHI was protected?

Nicholas's private health record is no longer private. His diagnosis of a sexually transmitted disease is health information. After discovering his gender, address, and birth date, someone can connect this diagnosis directly to one particular person. All these details, and any other pieces of information like these, are protected to be private under the law. This means that all this information is confidential, and it is against the law for you to reveal any of it, with only a few exceptions:

1. You can tell other health care professionals who are directly involved in the course of doing your job.
2. You can tell someone when given written permission from the patient to do so.
3. You can tell in situations, as outlined in the law, based on "best professional judgment."

The Use and Disclosure of PHI

HIPAA's Privacy Rule is very specific as to how you can handle the PHI that you work with every day. The guidelines offer two terms to describe how you might deal with these data.

The term **use** (with regard to HIPAA) means that the information is being shared between people who work together in the same office and need to exchange PHI in order to better serve the patient.

> **EXAMPLE**
>
> You are getting ready to code the diagnosis for Herman Farber's recent visit and need additional information. You speak with the attending physician, Dr. Yaw, to discuss Herman's PHI so that you can make certain you find the best, most appropriate diagnosis code. You are using that patient's PHI because the information is being shared between you and the physician in the same office for the benefit of the patient.

The second term is **disclosure**. HIPAA defines the term *disclosure* to mean that PHI is being revealed to someone outside the health care office or facility. For example, you

Use
The sharing of information between people working in the same health care facility for purposes of caring for the patient.

Disclosure
The sharing of information between health care professionals working in separate entities, or facilities, in the course of caring for the patient.

prepare a health insurance claim form to send to the patient's insurance company so it will pay your office for the procedures provided. On that claim form, you must put the patient's full name and address, birth date, diagnosis codes, and procedure codes. As you learned earlier in this chapter, each piece of data is not necessarily confidential. When you put all this information together in one place, it becomes PHI because this health information (diagnosis and procedure codes) is now connected to a specific person (identified by the name, address, birth date, etc.) on one piece of paper. However, you must disclose this information to the insurance carrier in order to get paid. You are disclosing the information because the insurance company personnel who will read this claim form do not work for your health care facility—they are an outside company.

> **EXAMPLE**
>
> Dr. Royan indicates that his patient, Caleb Carter, needs some lab work. Dr. Royan will use Mr. Carter's PHI in his orders for which tests should be performed. Then you need to call the laboratory and disclose Mr. Carter's PHI (his name and diagnosis) along with what specific tests should be performed by the lab.

Remember that everyone in your office and everyone at the insurance carrier and the lab is a member of a covered entity's workforce. You are all bound by the same terms of the HIPAA law and cannot reveal any patient's PHI, except under particular circumstances (such as use and disclosure), unless you have the patient's written permission (Figure 40-7).

Getting Written Approval

In most situations, other than those already mentioned, the health care provider must get a patient's written permission to disclose the PHI. Although there are many preprinted **Release of Information (ROI)** forms that your office or facility may purchase, the Privacy Rule of HIPAA insists that all these documents have the following characteristics:

1. Are written in plain language (not legalese) so that the average person can understand what he or she is signing.
2. Are very specific as to exactly what information will be disclosed or used.
3. Specifically identify the person or organization that will be disclosing the information.
4. Specifically identify the person(s) who will be receiving the information.
5. Have a definite expiration date.
6. Clearly explain that the person signing this release may retract this authorization in writing at any time.

Figure 40-8 is an example of a form that your facility might use for this purpose.

Release of Information (ROI)
The form (either on paper or electronic) that a patient must sign to give legal permission to a covered entity to disclose that patient's PHI.

HHS.gov	Health Information Privacy	U.S. Department of Health & Human Services
$750,000 HIPAA SETTLEMENT UNDERSCORES THE NEED FOR ORGANIZATION WIDE RISK ANALYSIS		
The University of Washington Medicine (UWM) has agreed to settle charges that it potentially violated the Health Insurance Portability and Accountability Act of 1996 (HIPAA) Security Rule by failing to implement policies and procedures to prevent, detect, contain, and correct security violations. The settlement includes a monetary payment of $750,000, a corrective action plan, and annual reports on the organization's compliance efforts.		

FIGURE 40-7 A partial summary of a case where HIPAA violations cost a health care facility big money Source: "$750,000 HIPAA Settlement Underscores the Need for Organization Wide Risk Analysis," HHS Press Office, December 14, 2015.

IHS-810 (4/09) DEPARTMENT OF HEALTH AND HUMAN SERVICES FORM APPROVED: OMB NO. 0917-0030
FRONT Indian Health Service Expiration Date: 4/30/2016
  See OMB Statement on Reverse.

AUTHORIZATION FOR USE OR DISCLOSURE OF PROTECTED HEALTH INFORMATION

COMPLETE ALL SECTIONS, DATE, AND SIGN

I. I, _____, hereby voluntarily authorize the disclosure of information from my health record. *(Name of Patient)*

II. The information is to be disclosed by: | And is to be provided to:

NAME OF FACILITY	NAME OF PERSON/ORGANIZATION/FACILITY
ADDRESS	ADDRESS
CITY/STATE	CITY/STATE

III. The purpose or need for this disclosure is:
- ☐ Further Medical Care ☐ Attorney ☐ School ☐ Research
- ☐ Personal Use ☐ Insurance ☐ Disability ☐ Other *(Specify)* _____

IV. The information to be disclosed from my health record: *(check appropriate box(es))*
- ☐ Only information related to *(specify)* _____
- ☐ Only the period of events from _____ to _____
- ☐ Other *(specify) (CHS, Billing, etc.)* _____
- ☐ Entire Record

If you would like any of the following sensitive information disclosed, check the applicable box(es) below:
- ☐ Alcohol/Drug Abuse Treatment/Referral ☐ HIV/AIDS-related Treatment
- ☐ Sexually Transmitted Diseases ☐ Mental Health *(Other than Psychotherapy Notes)*
- ☐ Psychotherapy Notes ONLY (by checking this box, I am waiving any psychotherapist-patient privilege)

V. I understand that I may revoke this authorization in writing submitted at any time to the Health Information Management Department, except to the extent that action has been taken in reliance on this authorization. If this authorization was obtained as a condition of obtaining insurance coverage or a policy of insurance, other law may provide the insurer with the right to contest a claim under the policy. If this authorization has not been revoked, it will terminate one year from the date of my signature unless a different expiration date or *expiration event* is stated.

_____
(Specify new date)

I understand that IHS will not condition treatment or eligibility for care on my providing this authorization except if such care is: (1) research related or (2) provided solely for the purpose of creating Protected Health Information for disclosure to a third party.

I understand that information disclosed by this authorization, except for Alcohol and Drug Abuse as defined in 42 CFR Part 2, may be subject to redisclosure by the recipient and may no longer be protected by the Health Insurance Portability and Accountability Act Privacy Rule [45 CFR Part 164], and the Privacy Act of 1974 [5 USC 552a].

SIGNATURE OF PATIENT OR PERSONAL REPRESENTATIVE *(State relationship to patient)* | DATE

SIGNATURE OF WITNESS *(If signature of patient is a thumbprint or mark)* | DATE

This information is to be released for the purpose stated above and may not be used by the recipient for any other purpose. Any person who knowingly and willfully requests or obtains any record concerning an individual from a Federal agency under false pretenses shall be guilty of a misdemeanor (5 USC 552a(i)(3)).

PATIENT IDENTIFICATION

NAME *(Last, First, MI)*	RECORD NUMBER
ADDRESS	
CITY/STATE	DATE OF BIRTH

FIGURE 40-8 Example of authorization form to release health information Source: Department of Health and Human Services, Form IHS-810 (4/09)

CHAPTER 40 | INTRODUCTION TO HEALTH CARE LAW AND ETHICS **1199**

Permitted Uses and Disclosures

The Privacy Rule outlines six circumstances in which health care professionals are permitted, with or without written patient permission, to use their best professional judgment as to whether or not they should use and/or disclose a patient's PHI.

1. *To the individual.* Health care professionals can *use their best professional judgment to decide whether or not a patient should be told* certain things contained in his or her health care record. Questions come up especially when mental health issues and terminal conditions (when a patient is almost certain to die in the near future) are concerned and there is doubt if the patient can deal with the medical facts. In almost all cases, providing patients with their own PHI is allowed.

2. *Treatment, payment, and/or operations (TPO).* This means that health care professionals are free to use and/or disclose PHI when it comes to making decisions, coordinating, and managing the *treatment* of a patient's condition.

    In addition, PHI can be disclosed for *payment* activities, such as billing and claims processing, as mentioned earlier in this chapter. In this description, the term *operations* refers to the health care facility's own management of case coordination and quality evaluations.

> ### EXAMPLE
> A physician needs to be able to discuss PHI details with a therapist so that, together, they can establish a proper course of treatment for the patient.

3. *Opportunity to agree or object.* This relates to a more informal situation where the patient is present and alert and has the ability to give verbal permission or not with regard to a specific disclosure.

    One important point to remember: Although it is much easier to simply ask someone for his or her oral approval than to go get a form and make the patient sign first, it is in your best interest to get written approval whenever possible. People's memories may fail, or they may change their mind later about what they really did tell you. If there is nothing on paper, you cannot prove what was said. For your own protection, get it in writing whenever possible!

> ### EXAMPLE
> Asher Grimm is about to hear Dr. Brant explain his test results. Asher's wife is in the waiting room. Dr. Brant may ask Asher if it is okay to invite his wife in and permit her to hear this information, too. Asher can then say, "Yes, that is fine" or "No, I don't want her to know about this." Dr. Brant then must abide by what the patient requests.

4. *Incidental use and disclosure.* As long as reasonable safeguards are in place, this portion of the rule addresses the fact that information might accidentally be used or disclosed during the regular course of business.

> **CODING BITES**
>
> *Incidental* is close to the word *accidental*—if someone accidentally overhears what you say.

> ### EXAMPLE
> Dr. Holloway comes out of an examining room and approaches Nurse Miller standing at the desk. This is a back area, and patients are not generally in this hallway, so Dr. Holloway speaks to the nurse in a normal tone of voice to instruct her on preparing Mrs. Hunter for a procedure. All of a sudden, another patient comes around the corner, lost on her way back to the waiting room, and overhears the conversation.

This is called incidental use and is understandable in a working environment; therefore, it is not considered a violation of the law.

However, it is important for conversations like this to include only the minimum necessary PHI to accomplish the goal. *Minimum necessary* refers to the caution that should be used to release only the smallest amount of information required to accomplish the task and no more. Not only is it unnecessary to release more, it is unprofessional.

> **EXAMPLE**
>
> In the hallway outside the exam room, the physician would only need to say, "Serita, please prepare Mrs. Hunter for her examination." She would not need to include other details about Mrs. Hunter, such as, "Serita, please prepare Mrs. Hunter for her examination. You know she has a terrible rash on her thighs. I suspect that it's poison ivy. However, it could be a sexually transmitted disease. We'll have to find out how many sexual partners she has had in the last 6 months." All that extra information is unnecessary to the proper care of Mrs. Hunter at this moment.

5. *Public interest.* There are times when the public's best interest may prompt disclosing what you know about a patient. Very often, this is mandated by state laws, which would then take priority over the federal HIPAA law. In other words, if the federal law says you are allowed to tell, and your state's law says you must tell—then, you must! These situations include the reporting of suspected abuse (child abuse, elder abuse, neglect, domestic violence) and the reporting of sexually transmitted and other contagious diseases. You are included in the health care team and must think about the community, which must be warned if someone is walking around with a contagious (communicable) disease. Most states require notification to the police in cases where the patient has been shot or stabbed. It is your responsibility to find out what the laws are in your state and how to correctly file a report.

   If the physician does not report suspected child abuse of one of your patients, it is your obligation to pick up the phone and call.

6. *Limited data set.* For research, public health statistics, or other health care operations, PHI can be revealed, but only after it has been depersonalized. In other words, if the data that connect this information to a specific individual are removed or blacked out, the information is no longer individually identifiable health information, so it does not need to be protected any longer.

> **CODING BITES**
>
> Remember that, when there is a state or federal mandate to report (that means you have no choice; you must report to the proper authorities), this does not apply *only* to the physician of your practice but also applies to you.

> **EXAMPLE**
>
> You can release a health record that has no name, address, telephone number, e-mail address, Social Security number, or photographs attached to it. Even certain physician's notes can be released after they have been stripped of personal data. Following is a sample portion of a record that can be shown without fear of violating anyone's privacy:
>
> "_____ is 33 years old. Back in April, _____ was in a motor vehicle accident while he was on the job. _____ is complaining about some neck pain. _____ has tingling into the left hand."
>
> The example above is a direct quote from the medical record of an actual patient after the specified direct identifiers have been removed. You cannot connect this health information to any one particular person. Therefore, the information is no longer protected and can be used for research and in other ways that may help the community.

> **CODING BITES**
>
> This law simply assures every person coming to your health care facility that his or her personal and private information will be protected and treated with respect.

Privacy Notices

HIPAA instructs all its covered entities to create policies and procedures with regard to the use and disclosure of PHI. In addition, the law actually states that, once policies and procedures are developed, the facilities must follow these policies. Copies of the written policy must be given to every patient and posted in a general area where it can be seen by all patients.

Notices of Privacy written in compliance with HIPAA's Privacy Rule must contain the following points:

1. A full description of how the covered entity may use and/or disclose a patient's PHI.
2. A statement about the covered entity's responsibility to protect a patient's privacy.
3. Complete information about the patient's rights, including contact information for the Department of Health and Human Services (DHHS), should the patient wish to lodge a complaint that his or her privacy was violated.
4. The name of a specific employee of the covered entity, who must be named as *privacy officer*. This person's name, as well as contact information, must be included in the written notice to handle patients' questions and complaints.

The covered entity must receive written acknowledgment from each patient stating that he or she received the written privacy practices notice. This is usually one of the papers that a patient has to sign when going to a health care facility for the first time.

One of the most important aspects of this portion of the Privacy Rule is that the law specifically says that the covered entity not only has to create these policies and procedures but also has to abide by them. If it doesn't, it is considered to be in violation of federal law and punishable by fines and/or imprisonment.

Although some health care staff members feel that HIPAA and its Privacy Rule are a pain in the neck, think about what this law actually means: respecting your patients' privacy and dignity. Isn't that what you expect from your health care professionals when you go for help? It is not enough that only the doctor be bound to protect the patient's information as confidential because the doctor is no longer the only person who has access. Your health care facility is no place for gossip. You might find this person's hemorrhoids funny or that person's rash gross. As a professional, you should not be concerned with entertaining your friends with your patients' private circumstances. How would you feel if it were *your* personal problem that your health care team members were giggling about with their friends? Or you might consider telling your brother that his girlfriend came in with a sexually transmitted disease. You cannot! Everyone is entitled to privacy. As difficult as it may be, you must remain a professional.

CODING BITES

Just because you *can* take a look at any patient's chart doesn't mean you should. In your facility, you will probably be granted permission to access patients' charts so you can do your work. Under certain circumstances you may be tempted to look, not for your job but because the patient is your friend or neighbor or a celebrity. You may think no harm is being done, just caring or curiosity. But there is harm, and you are prohibited, by law, to do this.

Back in October 2007, 27 employees of a New Jersey hospital were fired or put on suspension for looking at George Clooney's file after he was brought into the emergency department (ED) following a motorcycle accident.

You could be the president of the hospital and have your best friend come into the ED of your hospital. Without specific permission from that patient, you would be forbidden from looking at the record. Every individual has the right to make his or her own decision about who should know what about his or her own health information.

Violating HIPAA's Privacy Rule

Any individual who discovers that his or her privacy has been misused or disclosed without permission can file a complaint with the Department of Health and Human Services (DHHS) that the health care provider, health plan, or clearinghouse has not followed HIPAA's regulations. When writing this law, Congress included specifications for both civil and criminal penalties to be applied against any covered entity that fails to protect its patients' PHI. These penalties include fines—up to $250,000—and up to 10 years in prison (Figure 40-9).

A covered entity is responsible for any violation of HIPAA requirements by any of its employees, business associates, or other members of its workforce, such as interns and volunteers. Generally, the senior officials of the covered entity may be punished for the lack of compliance; however, middle managers and staff members are not exempt.

HHS requires California medical center to protect patients' right to privacy

FOR IMMEDIATE RELEASE
Thursday, June 13, 2013

HHS Press Office
(202) 690-6343

News Release

Shasta Regional Medical Center (SRMC) has agreed to a comprehensive corrective action plan to settle a U.S. Department of Health and Human Services (HHS) investigation concerning potential violations of the Health Insurance Portability and Accountability Act (HIPAA) Privacy Rule.

The HHS Office for Civil Rights (OCR) opened a compliance review of SRMC following a Los Angeles Times article which indicated two SRMC senior leaders had met with media to discuss medical services provided to a patient. OCR's investigation indicated that SRMC failed to safeguard the patient's protected health information (PHI) from impermissible disclosure by intentionally disclosing PHI to multiple media outlets on at least three separate occasions, without a valid written authorization. OCR's review indicated that senior management at SRMC impermissibly shared details about the patient's medical condition, diagnosis and treatment in an email to the entire workforce. In addition, SRMC failed to sanction its workforce members for impermissibly disclosing the patient's records pursuant to its internal sanctions policy.

"When senior level executives intentionally and repeatedly violate HIPAA by disclosing identifiable patient information, OCR will respond quickly and decisively to stop such behavior," said OCR Director Leon Rodriguez. "Senior leadership helps define the culture of an organization and is responsible for knowing and complying with the HIPAA privacy and security requirements to ensure patients' rights are fully protected."

In addition to a $275,000 monetary settlement, a corrective action plan (CAP) requires SRMC to update its policies and procedures on safeguarding PHI from impermissible uses and disclosures and to train its workforce members. The CAP also requires fifteen other hospitals or medical centers under the same ownership or operational control as SRMC to attest to their understanding of permissible uses and disclosures of PHI, including disclosures to the media.

The Resolution Agreement can be found on the OCR website at:
http://www.hhs.gov/ocr/privacy/hipaa/enforcement/examples/shasta-agreement.pdf

FIGURE 40-9 A press release from the Department of Health and Human Services with details about violators of HIPAA facing consequences Source: "HHS requires California medical center to protect patients' right to privacy," *U.S. Department of Health and Human Services*, June 13, 2013.

Civil Penalties

1. $100 with no prison for each single violation of a HIPAA regulation with a maximum of $25,000 for multiple violations of the same portion of the regulation during the same calendar year.

> **EXAMPLE**
>
> You tell your best friend that Oliver Tesca, whom you both went to school with, came into your physician's office and tested positive for a sexually transmitted disease. You, of course, swear her to secrecy. Later that day, she bumps into Oliver's fiancée and feels obligated to tell her about Oliver's condition. Oliver puts two and two together, after his fiancée breaks up with him, and he files a complaint that you disclosed his PHI without permission. You and/or your physician is fined $100.

Criminal Penalties

2. Up to $50,000 *and* up to 1 year in jail for the unauthorized or inappropriate disclosure of individually identifiable health information.

> **EXAMPLE**
>
> After you are fined the $100 civil penalty for the inappropriate disclosure of Oliver Tesca's PHI, you and/or your physician is charged with criminal penalties for the same disclosure, including a fine of $50,000 and a year in jail.

3. Up to $100,000 *and* up to 5 years in prison for the unauthorized or inappropriate disclosure of individually identifiable health information through deception.

> **EXAMPLE**
>
> Your best friend since high school, Sally-Anne Hoskins, just got a great job as a pharmaceutical representative. To help her, you give her a list of 250 patients from your facility who have been diagnosed with diabetes so she can advertise her company's new drug to them. You and she both know this is illegal, so you tell Sally-Anne that you got permission from each of the patients to release the information (and that is a lie). After a patient complains to DHHS, the investigation discovers your relationship with Sally-Anne. You and your physician are fined $100,000 per occurrence (that's for each person on the list), as well as sentenced to 5 years in prison. FYI: 250 × $100,000 = $25 million!

4. Up to $250,000 *and* up to 10 years in prison for the unauthorized or inappropriate disclosure of individually identifiable health information through deception with intent to sell or use for business-related benefit, personal gain, or hateful detriment.

> **EXAMPLE**
>
> A famous television star is a patient of the physician's office down the hall from yours. You get a call from a tabloid newspaper offering you $50,000 for any information on the celebrity's health. So you call the manager of the pathology lab and tell him you are filling in at the other physician's office and need test results for Mr. TV. Then you call the tabloid reporter and tell him what you found out. You used deception (you lied about working in the other physician's office) to gain PHI, which you then sold for personal financial gain. You (and possibly your physician) are fined a quarter of a million dollars and sentenced to 10 years in prison—definitely not worth it!

Refusing to Release Patient Information

Sometimes, it seems that everyone agrees with the importance of protecting a patient's privacy until he or she asks for someone's details and is refused. It happens with parents and spouses all too often, and you must be prepared for how to say "no" and deal with the impact that may ensue.

When asked *why* you will not release details about a man's wife or mother's teenage daughter, educate the individual with the facts. Frequently, simply replying, "That is our policy" accomplishes little more than infuriating them, so instead, explain why you cannot share the information. Explain that health care staff are all required, by federal law, to protect our patients' privacy with no exceptions. Say that, as soon as possible, he or she should speak with the patient and enable the patient to tell the story about his or her health care encounter. Ask nicely for the individual's understanding.

40.5 Health Care Fraud and Abuse Control Program

The Health Insurance Portability and Accountability Act (HIPAA) created the Health Care Fraud and Abuse Control Program (HCFACP). This program, under the direction of the attorney general and the secretary of the DHHS, acts in accordance with the Office of the Inspector General (OIG) and coordinates with federal, state, and local law enforcement agencies to discover those who attempt to defraud or abuse the health care system, including Medicare and Medicaid patients and programs.

By catching those who submitted fraudulent claims, approximately $2.3 billion was won or negotiated by the federal government during fiscal year 2014. The federal government deposited approximately $1.9 billion to the Medicare Trust Fund in fiscal year 2014, plus more than $523 million of federal Medicaid funds were brought into the U.S. Treasury. Since it was created in 1997, the HCFACP has collected more than $27.8 billion for the Medicare Trust Fund—money improperly received by health care professionals filing fraudulent claims. The statistics show that for every $1 spent to pay for these investigations and prosecutions, the government actually brings in about $4 in money returned.

Also, in 2014, 496 criminal indictments were filed in health care fraud cases, and 805 defendants were convicted for health care fraud–related crimes, resulting in 734 defendants convicted of health care fraud–related crimes. In addition, 782 new civil cases were filed and 957 more civil matters were pending during this same year. These investigations also prohibited 4,017 individuals and organizations from working with any federally sponsored programs (such as Medicare and Medicaid). Most of these were as a result of convictions for Medicare- or Medicaid-related crimes, including patient abuse and patient neglect, or as a result of providers' licenses having been revoked.

When you look at these 2014 numbers, you can see that people are being caught trying to get money for health care services to which they are not entitled. This is an important reminder that if individuals try to get you to participate in illegal or unethical behaviors, the question is not "Will you be caught?" but "*When* will you be caught?"

> **CODING BITES**
>
> From *Fact Sheet: The Health Care Fraud and Abuse Control Program Protects Consumers and Taxpayers by Combating Health Care Fraud,* dated February 26, 2016.
>
> "In Fiscal Year (FY) 2015, the government recovered $2.4 billion as a result of health care fraud judgements, settlements and additional administrative impositions in health care fraud cases and proceedings. Since its inception in 1997, the Health Care Fraud and Abuse Control (HCFAC) Program has returned more than $29.4 billion to the Medicare Trust Funds. In this past fiscal year, the HCFAC program has returned $6.10 for each dollar invested."
>
> Source: justice.gov

40.6 Codes of Ethics

There are two premier trade organizations for professional coding specialists. Each has published a code of ethics to guide members of our industry on the best professional way to conduct themselves.

American Health Information Management Association Code of Ethics

The American Health Information Management Association (AHIMA) is the preeminent professional organization for health information workers, including insurance coding specialists. The AHIMA House of Delegates designated the elements as being critical to the highest level of honorable behavior for its members.

In this era of reimbursements based on diagnostic and procedural coding, the professional ethics of health information coding professionals continue to be challenged. Standards of ethical coding practices for coding professionals were developed by AHIMA's Coding Policy and Strategy Committee and approved by AHIMA's board of directors.

> **GUIDANCE CONNECTION**
>
> **AHIMA Code of Ethics**
>
> This Code of Ethics sets forth ethical principles for the health information management profession. Members of this profession are responsible for maintaining and promoting ethical practices. This Code of Ethics, adopted by the American Health Information Management Association, shall be binding on health information management professionals who are members of the Association and all individuals who hold an AHIMA certification.
>
> The following ethical principles are based on the core values of the American Health Information Management Association and apply to all health information management professionals. Health information management professionals must:
>
> 1. Advocate, uphold, and defend the individual's right to privacy and the doctrine of confidentiality in the use and disclosure of information.
> 2. Put service and the health and welfare of persons before self-interest and conduct themselves in the practice of the profession so as to bring honor to themselves, their peers, and the health information management profession.
> 3. Preserve, protect, and secure personal health information in any form or medium and hold in the highest regard the contents of the records and other information of a confidential nature, taking into account the applicable statutes and regulations.
> 4. Refuse to participate in or conceal unethical practices or procedures.
> 5. Advance health information management knowledge and practice through continuing education, research, publications, and presentations.
> 6. Recruit and mentor students, peers, and colleagues to develop and strengthen a professional workforce.
> 7. Represent the profession accurately to the public.
> 8. Perform honorably health information management association responsibilities, either appointed or elected, and preserve the confidentiality of any privileged information made known in any official capacity.
> 9. State truthfully and accurately their credentials, professional education, and experiences.
> 10. Facilitate interdisciplinary collaboration in situations supporting health information practice.
> 11. Respect the inherent dignity and worth of every person.
>
> Reprinted with permission from the American Health Information Management Association. Copyright ©2015 by the American Health Information Management Association. All rights reserved. No part of this may be reproduced, reprinted, stored in a retrieval system, or transmitted, in any form or by any means, electronic photocopying, recording, or otherwise, without the prior written permission of the association.

AHIMA Standards of Ethical Coding

Coding is one of the foundational functions of the health information management department. As complex as is the process of coding accurately, there are multipart, intricate regulations that impact that process. In addition, professional coding specialists must make ethical decisions that would benefit from an appropriate and knowledgeable source. The AHIMA Standards of Ethical Coding are presented to all members of the industry to support their ethical and legal decisions and behaviors, as well as to reinforce and evidence the commitment of coding professionals to integrity. These Standards are offered for use to all AHIMA members or nonmembers, in all types of health care facilities and organizations.

> ### GUIDANCE CONNECTION
>
> **AHIMA Standards of Ethical Coding**
>
> Coding professionals should:
>
> 1. Apply accurate, complete, and consistent coding practices that yield quality data.
> 2. Gather and report all data required for internal and external reporting, in accordance with applicable requirements and data set definitions.
> 3. Assign and report, in any format, only the codes and data that are clearly and consistently supported by health record documentation in accordance with applicable code set and abstraction conventions, and requirements.
> 4. Query and/or consult as needed with the provider for clarification and additional documentation prior to final code assignment in accordance with acceptable healthcare industry practices.
> 5. Refuse to participate in, support, or change reported data and/or narrative titles, billing data, clinical documentation practices, or any coding related activities intended to skew or misrepresent data and their meaning that do not comply with requirements.
> 6. Facilitate, advocate, and collaborate with healthcare professionals in the pursuit of accurate, complete and reliable coded data and in situations that support ethical coding practices.
> 7. Advance coding knowledge and practice through continuing education, including but not limited to meeting continuing education requirements.
> 8. Maintain the confidentiality of protected health information in accordance with the Code of Ethics.
> 9. Refuse to participate in the development of coding and coding related technology that is not designed in accordance with requirements.
> 10. Demonstrate behavior that reflects integrity, shows a commitment to ethical and legal coding practices, and fosters trust in professional activities.
> 11. Refuse to participate in and/or conceal unethical coding, data abstraction, query practices, or any inappropriate activities related to coding and address any perceived unethical coding related practices.
>
> Reprinted with permission from the American Health Information Management Association. Copyright ©2015 by the American Health Information Management Association. All rights reserved. No part of this may be reproduced, reprinted, stored in a retrieval system, or transmitted, in any form or by any means, electronic photocopying, recording, or otherwise, without the prior written permission of the association.

AAPC Code of Ethical Standards

American Academy of Professional Coders (AAPC) is an influential organization in the health information management industry. Its members, and their certifications, are well respected throughout the United States and the world. Its Code of Ethical Standards also illuminates the importance of an insurance coding and billing specialist's exhibiting the most ethical and moral conduct.

> **GUIDANCE CONNECTION**
>
> **AAPC Code of Ethical Standards**
>
> Members of the American Academy of Professional Coders shall be dedicated to providing the highest standard of professional coding and billing services to employers, clients and patients. Professional and personal behavior of AAPC members must be exemplary.
>
> AAPC members shall maintain the highest standard of personal and professional conduct. Members shall respect the rights of patients, clients, employers and all other colleagues.
>
> Members shall use only legal and ethical means in all professional dealings and shall refuse to cooperate with, or condone by silence, the actions of those who engage in fraudulent, deceptive or illegal acts.
>
> Members shall respect and adhere to the laws and regulations of the land and uphold the mission statement of the AAPC.
>
> Members shall pursue excellence through continuing education in all areas applicable to their profession.
>
> Members shall strive to maintain and enhance the dignity, status, competence and standards of coding for professional services.
>
> Members shall not exploit professional relationships with patients, employees, clients or employers for personal gain.
>
> Above all else we will commit to recognizing the intrinsic worth of each member.
>
> This code of ethical standards for members of the AAPC strives to promote and maintain the highest standard of professional service and conduct among its members. Adherence to these standards assures public confidence in the integrity and service of professional coders who are members of the AAPC.
>
> Failure to adhere to these standards, as determined by AAPC, will result in the loss of credentials and membership with the American Academy of Professional Coders.
>
> Copyright © 2014, American Academy of Professional Coders. All rights reserved. Reprinted with permission.

40.7 Compliance Programs

A formal compliance program has been strongly recommended by the OIG (Office of Inspector General) of the DHHS (Department of Health and Human Services) to help all health care facilities establish their organizations' respect for the laws and their agreement to follow the direction from those laws. However, there are certain health care providers for whom this is not only suggested but mandated by law.

The Deficit Reduction Act of 2005, which went into effect January 1, 2007, mandates a compliance program for all health care organizations that receive $5 million or more a year from Medicaid. This law is very specific that the facility's compliance program include written guidance and policies about employees' responsibilities under the False Claims Act.

On March 23, 2010, President Obama signed the Patient Protection and Affordable Care Act into law. Among the many other elements of health care covered by this law, there is a provision in Section 6401 that providers participating in Medicare and Medicaid create compliance programs. This includes physicians' offices and suppliers.

A compliance program will officially create policies and procedures, establish the structure to adhere to those policies, set up a monitoring system to ensure that it works, and correct conduct that does not comply. The foundation of the compliance program is the creation of an organizational culture of honesty and compliance with the laws; the discouragement of fraud, waste, and abuse; the discovery of any fraudulent activities as soon as possible using internal policies and audits; and immediate corrective action when fraud and abuse do occur.

The federal sentencing guidelines manual provides a seven-step list of the components of an effective compliance program.

> **GUIDANCE CONNECTION**
>
> **Federal Sentencing Guidelines Manual: The Seven Steps to Due Diligence**
>
> 1. Establish compliance standards and procedures
> 2. Assign overall responsibility to specific high-level individual(s)
> 3. Use due care to avoid delegation of authority to individuals with an inclination to get involved in illegal actions
> 4. Effectively communicate standards and procedures to all staff
> 5. Utilize monitoring and auditing system to detect non-compliant conduct
> 6. Enforce adequate disciplinary sanctions when appropriate
> 7. Respond to episodes of non-compliance by modifying program, if necessary
>
> Source: United States Sentencing Commission. (2014, November 1). 2014 USSC Guidelines Manual, ussc.gov

Chapter Summary

Knowing your legal and ethical responsibilities as a health care professional will give you a strong foundation for a healthy career. HIPAA's Privacy Rule, along with the codes of ethics from both AHIMA and AAPC, should help guide you through any challenges.

For all of those providing health care services, the federal and state governments have crafted and enacted laws and regulations designed to ensure honest, safe, and appropriate behaviors from all involved. The *Federal Register* is the daily journal of the U.S. federal government, used to inform citizens of the actions of the federal government. The hierarchy established for the levels of authority begin with the U.S. Constitution, followed by federal statutory law, state constitutions, state statutory laws, and local laws. Executive orders, issued by the president of the United States, have the same authority as federal statutes. Common law, also known as case law, is created by a judicial decision made during a court trial and it establishes precedence. Administrative laws are the rules and regulations established by administrative agencies in their efforts to encourage compliance so they can complete their assigned tasks. The violation of criminal law may be a misdemeanor (lessor offense) or a felony (more serious offense). Civil laws govern the conduct of two individuals or entities in a contractual agreement or a civil wrongdoing, known as a tort.

Confidentiality, honesty, and accuracy are the watchwords that all health information management professionals should live by.

> **CODING BITES**
>
> Medical records, also known as patient charts, whether in paper or electronic form, are legal documents. As business records, they can be used as evidence in a court of law, and can be required by issuance of a *subpoena duces tecum*.
>
> As per the HIPAA Privacy Rule, a "designated record set" must be specified by each health care organization. Essentially, this is a collection of files (paper or electronic) that include:
>
> - the medical records and billing records about individuals maintained by, or for, a covered health care provider;
> - the enrollment, payment, claims adjudication, case study, or medical management record systems maintained by or for a health plan; or
> - documentation used for the provider or plan to make decisions about individuals.

CHAPTER 40 REVIEW
Introduction to Health Care Law and Ethics

Let's Check It! Terminology

Match each term to the appropriate definition.

B 1. LO 40.2 Choosing a code on the basis of what the insurance company will cover (pay for) rather than accurately reflecting the truth.

E 2. LO 40.1 Laws governing the behavior of the actions of the population related to health and well-being.

M 3. LO 40.2 Coding the individual parts of a specific diagnosis or procedure rather than one combination or bundle that includes all of those components.

H 4. LO 40.1 Official policies issued by the president of the United States.

A 5. LO 40.1 Also known as rules and regulations, these are created and adjudicated by administrative agencies, given authority by Congress.

D 6. LO 40.4 Health care providers, health plans, and health care clearinghouses—businesses that have access to the personal health information of patients.

J 7. LO 40.4 Any patient-identifiable health information regardless of the form in which it is stored (paper, computer file, etc.).

K 8. LO 40.1 Laws that are enacted by federal and state legislature.

N 9. LO 40.2 Using a code on a claim form that indicates a higher level of service or a more severe aspect of disease or injury than that which was actual and true.

I 10. LO 40.4 A portion of HIPAA that ensures the availability of patient information for those who should see it while protecting that information from those who should not.

O 11. LO 40.4 The sharing of information between people working in the same health care facility for purposes of caring for the patient.

F 12. LO 40.4 The sharing of information between health care professionals working in separate entities, or facilities, in the course of caring for the patient.

C 13. LO 40.1 Also known as case law, this is created by judicial decisions made during court trials.

L 14. LO 40.2 The paperwork in the patient's file that corroborates the codes presented on the claim form for a particular encounter.

G 15. LO 40.2 Sending a claim for the second time to the same insurance company for the same procedure or service, provided to the same patient on the same date of service.

A. Administrative Law
B. Coding for Coverage
C. Common Law
D. Covered Entities
E. Criminal Law
F. Disclosure
G. Double Billing
H. Executive Orders
I. HIPAA's Privacy Rule
J. Protected Health Information (PHI)
K. Statutory Laws
L. Supporting Documentation
M. Unbundling
N. Upcoding
O. Use

Let's Check It! Concepts

Choose the most appropriate answer for each of the following questions.

1. LO 40.4 The intent of HIPAA's Privacy Rule is to
   a. protect an individual's privacy.

1210   PART VI | REIMBURSEMENT, LEGAL, AND ETHICAL ISSUES

b. not interfere with the flow of information necessary for care.
   c. restrict health care professionals from doing their jobs.
   d. protect an individual's privacy and not interfere with the flow of information necessary for care.
2. LO 40.4 Protected health information (PHI) is
   a. any health information that can be connected to a specific individual.
   b. a listing of diagnosis codes.
   c. current procedural terminology.
   d. covered entity employee files.
3. LO 40.4 According to HIPAA, covered entities include all *except*
   a. health care providers.
   b. health plans.
   c. health care computer software manufacturers.
   d. health care clearinghouses.
4. LO 40.4 The term *use* per HIPAA's Privacy Rule refers to the exchange of information between health care personnel
   a. and health care personnel in other health care facilities.
   b. and family members.
   c. in the same office.
   d. and the pharmacist.
5. LO 40.4 The term *disclosure* per HIPAA's Privacy Rule refers to the exchange of information between health care personnel
   a. and health care personnel in other covered entities.
   b. and family members.
   c. in the same office.
   d. and the patient.
6. LO 40.4 Which of the following is *not* a covered entity under HIPAA?
   a. County hospital
   b. BlueCross BlueShield Association
   c. Physician Associates medical practice
   d. Computer technical support
7. LO 40.6 There are two premier trade organizations for professional coding specialists. Each organization has a code of ethics to guide members on the best professional way to conduct themselves. These two organizations are
   a. AHIMA and OFR.
   b. GPO and AAPC.
   c. AHIMA and AAPC.
   d. HIPAA and EEO.
8. LO 40.4 According to HIPAA's rules and regulations, a covered entity's workforce includes
   a. only paid, full-time employees.
   b. only licensed personnel working in the office.
   c. volunteers, trainees, and employees, part time and full time.
   d. business associates' employees.
9. LO 40.4 HIPAA's Privacy Rule has been carefully crafted to
   a. protect a patient's health care history.
   b. protect a patient's current medical issues.
   c. protect a patient's future health considerations.
   d. all of these.
10. LO 40.4 A written form to release PHI should include all *except*
    a. specific identification of the person who will be receiving the information.
    b. the specific information to be released.
    c. legal terminology so it will stand up in court.
    d. an expiration date.

CHAPTER 40 REVIEW

11. **LO 40.4** Those who are permitted to file an official complaint with DHHS are
    a. health care providers.
    b. any individual.
    c. health plans.
    d. clearinghouses.

12. **LO 40.4** Penalties for violating any portion of HIPAA apply to
    a. patients.
    b. patients' families.
    c. all covered entities.
    d. health care office managers.

13. **LO 40.3** An individual who files a false claim can be charged for violations by
    a. federal law.
    b. state law.
    c. both federal and state law.
    d. Filing a false claim is not a violation of law.

14. **LO 40.1** DHHS stands for
    a. Department of Home and Health Services.
    b. Division of Health and Health Care Sciences.
    c. Department of Health and Human Services.
    d. District of Health and HIPAA Systems.

15. **LO 40.2** Changing a code from one that is most accurate to one you know the insurance company will pay for is called
    a. coding for coverage.
    b. coding for packaging.
    c. unbundling.
    d. double billing.

16. **LO 40.2** Unbundling is an illegal practice in which coders
    a. bill for services never provided.
    b. bill for services with no documentation.
    c. bill using several individual codes instead of one combination code.
    d. bill using a code for a higher level of service than what was actually provided.

17. **LO 40.2** Upcoding is an illegal practice in which coders
    a. bill for services never provided.
    b. bill for services with no documentation.
    c. bill using several individual codes instead of one combination code.
    d. bill using a code for a higher level of service than what was actually provided.

18. **LO 40.2** Medicare's CCI investigates claims that include
    a. unbundling.
    b. the improper use of mutually exclusive codes.
    c. unacceptable reporting of CPT codes.
    d. all of these.

19. **LO 40.5** During fiscal year 2014, the federal government won or negotiated approximately _____ billion from those who submitted fraudulent claims.
    a. $1.3
    b. $1.75
    c. $2.3
    d. $2.5

20. **LO 40.7** According to the federal sentencing guidelines manual, all of the following are components of the seven steps to due diligence for an effective compliance program *except*
    a. establish compliance standards and procedures.
    b. assign overall responsibility to specific high-level individual(s).
    c. utilize monitoring and auditing system to detect noncompliant conduct.
    d. cease disciplinary sanctions.

Let's Check It! Rules and Regulations

Please answer the following questions from the knowledge you have gained after reading this chapter.

1. LO 40.4 Why was HIPAA's Privacy Rule written?
2. LO 40.2 Explain double billing. Is it permissible practice for a professional coding specialist?
3. LO 40.1 Explain civil law in relation to the health care industry.
4. LO 40.3 What is the False Claims Act's definition of a claim and what is the knowledge requirement?
5. LO 40.7 What are the federal sentencing guidelines manual's seven steps to due diligence for an effective compliance program? *Pg. 1209*

YOU CODE IT! Application

Following are some health care scenarios. Determine the best course of action that you, as the health information management professional for the facility, should take. Identify any legal and/or ethical issues that may need to be considered and explain how you would deal with the situation.

PRADER, BRACKER, & ASSOCIATES

A Complete Health Care Facility

159 Healthcare Way • SOMEWHERE, FL 32811 • 407-555-6789

PATIENT: HOLLAND, FELECIA

ACCOUNT/EHR #: HOLLFE001

DATE: 04/26/18

Attending Physician: Oscar R. Prader, MD

This 31-year-old female is 32 weeks pregnant. She presents today in tears. She is suffering from hemorrhoids and cannot stand it anymore. The pain and itching are making life difficult for her, as it hurts to sit for any length of time, and she cannot sleep. As it is difficult for her to lie on her stomach, due to the pregnancy, she can only find some comfort by either walking around or lying on her side. She is asking (more like begging) for a hemorrhoidectomy—a simple surgical procedure that can be done in the office and will almost immediately provide her with complete relief.

The correct CPT code for the treatment of Felecia's condition is

46260   Hemorrhoidectomy, internal and external, 2 or more columns/groups

However, Felecia's insurance carrier will not pay for a hemorrhoidectomy with a diagnosis that indicates there are no complications. According to the insurance customer service representative, it will only pay in full for the procedure

46250   Hemorrhoidectomy, external, 2 or more columns/groups

Felecia's husband, Ben, is a civilian who works for a defense contractor and is currently in Iraq supporting the troops. Money is tight for the family because Ben's paycheck has been delayed due to a mix-up in paperwork when he was transferred to the Middle East. There is no way they can afford to pay cash for the hemorrhoidectomy.

All you need to do is change the one number of the code and Felecia can have the relief she so desperately needs. As the professional coding specialist in this office, what should you do?

CHAPTER 40 REVIEW

PRADER, BRACKER, & ASSOCIATES

A Complete Health Care Facility

159 Healthcare Way • SOMEWHERE, FL 32811 • 407-555-6789

PATIENT: OKONEK, MARC

ACCOUNT/EHR #: OKONMA001

DATE: 08/12/18

Attending Physician: Andrew Bracker, MD

As the coding specialist for this facility, you are given the chart for this patient after his recent encounter with Dr. Bracker. On the face sheet you notice that Dr. Bracker has indicated the procedure provided to this patient to be Excision dermoid cyst, nose; simple, skin, subcutaneous. However, there is nothing at all in the rest of the documentation, including the encounter notes and lab reports, to support medical necessity for this procedure.

As a professional coding specialist in this office, what should you do?

PRADER, BRACKER, & ASSOCIATES

A Complete Health Care Facility

159 Healthcare Way • SOMEWHERE, FL 32811 • 407-555-6789

PATIENT: RIALS, ELIZABETH

ACCOUNT/EHR #: RIALEL001

DATE: 12/08/18

Attending Physician: Oscar R. Prader, MD

Today, Tonya Baliga comes into your office. She states that she is Elizabeth Rials's sister and that she has been asked by her sister to collect a copy of her complete medical record. Ms. Baliga tells you that her sister has moved to another town and needs the records for an upcoming medical appointment with her new doctor. She hands you a printout of an e-mail, supposedly from Ms. Rials, to serve as documentation that she should have the records.

As a professional coding specialist in this office, what should you do?

PRADER, BRACKER, & ASSOCIATES

A Complete Health Care Facility

159 Healthcare Way • SOMEWHERE, FL 32811 • 407-555-6789

PATIENT: SINGELTON, SANDRA

ACCOUNT/EHR #: SINGSA001

DATE: 03/13/18

Attending Physician: Andrew Bracker, MD

The patient is a 17-year-old female who came in for counseling on birth control.

Today, Angela Thurman came into the office. She stated that she is Sandra's mother and found an appointment card for this facility in her daughter's jeans. She demands to know why her daughter came to see the physician. She is angry and frustrated and states that she will not leave until she is told why her daughter saw the doctor.

As a professional coding specialist in this office, what should you do?

PRADER, BRACKER, & ASSOCIATES

A Complete Health Care Facility

159 Healthcare Way • SOMEWHERE, FL 32811 • 407-555-6789

PATIENT: EVERFIELD, CARL

ACCOUNT/EHR #: EVERCA001

DATE: 06/28/18

Attending Physician: Oscar R. Prader, MD

The patient came to see the physician because he hates his nose. His self-esteem is very low and, as a teenage boy, he has developed severe social anxiety. His family does not have the money to pay for a rhinoplasty (nose job) and the only way that the insurance company will pay for this cosmetic surgery is for medical necessity, such as a deviated septum.

You have been told to code the diagnosis of deviated septum to support medical necessity for the rhinoplasty. The doctor and office manager both tell you that this is the "right" thing to do.

As a professional coding specialist in this office, what should you do?

APPENDIX

E/M Coding Rubric Worksheet

Begin by narrowing down the entire E/M chapter to the appropriate subsection:

Step 1. Location	New Patient/Initial	Established /Subsequent
Office/Outpatient	99201–99205	99211–99215
Hospital—Observation	99218–99220	99224–99226
Hospital—Inpatient	99221–99223	99231–99233
Emergency Department	99281–99285	
Nursing Facility	99304–99306	99307–99310
Domiciliary (Assisted Living)	99324–99328	99334–99337
Home Services	99341–99345	99347–99350

Step 2. Key Components	New Patient/ Initial	Established/ Subsequent
History		
Problem-Focused: Chief complaint; brief history of present illness or problem.		
Expanded Problem-Focused: Chief complaint; brief history of present illness; problem-pertinent system review		
Detailed: Chief complaint; extended history of present illness; problem-pertinent system review extended to include a review of a limited number of additional systems; pertinent past, family, and/or social history directly related to patient's problem(s).		
Comprehensive: Chief complaint; extended history of present illness; review of systems that are directly related to the problem(s) identified in the history of the present illness plus a review of all additional body systems; complete past, family, and social history.		

CodePath: For more information on determining level of history, see *Let's Code It!* Chapter 23, Section 23.4 *Types of E/M Services – Level of Patient History* (beginning on page 648).

Step 3. Key Components	New Patient/ Initial	Established/ Subsequent
Physical Examination		
Problem-Focused: A limited exam of the affected body area or organ system		
Expanded Problem-Focused: A limited exam of the affected body area or organ system and other symptomatic or related organ system(s)		
Detailed: An extended exam of the affected body area(s) and other symptomatic or related organ system(s)		
Comprehensive: A general multisystem exam -or- a complete exam of a single organ system		

CodePath: For more information on determining level of Physical Examination, see *Let's Code It!* Chapter 23, Section 23.4 *Types of E/M Services – Level of Physical Examination* (beginning on page 650).

Step 4. Key Components	New Patient/ Initial	Established/ Subsequent
Medical Decision-Making		
Straightforward: Minimal number of possible diagnoses and/or treatment options; minimal quantity of information to be obtained, reviewed, and analyzed; and minimal risk of significant complications, morbidity, and/or mortality		
Low Complexity: Limited number of possible diagnoses and/or treatment options; limited quantity of information to be obtained, reviewed, and analyzed; and limited risk of significant complications, morbidity, and/or mortality		
Moderate Complexity: Multiple number of possible diagnoses and/or treatment options; moderate quantity of information to be obtained, reviewed, and analyzed; and moderate risk of significant complications, morbidity, and/or mortality		
High Complexity: Extensive number of possible diagnoses and/or treatment options; extensive quantity of information to be obtained, reviewed, and analyzed; and high risk of significant complications, morbidity, and/or mortality		

CodePath: For more information on determining level of Medical Decision-Making, see *Let's Code It!* Chapter 23, Section 23.4 *Types of E/M Services – Level of Medical Decision-Making* (beginning on page 652).

Combining Multiple Levels in One Code

Once you have determined what level of history was taken, what level of physician exam was performed, and what level of MDM was provided by the physician as documented in the case notes, this all needs to be put together into one code. When all three key components point to the same code, this is a piece of cake. But what about when the three levels point toward different E/M codes? How do you mesh them all into one code? The CPT guidelines state, "... *must meet or exceed the stated requirements to qualify for a particular level of E/M service."*

You must find the one level that is satisfied by ALL THREE levels of care when you are reporting for a NEW patient, or TWO out of THREE for established patients. Find the only code that has ALL THREE levels equal to or greater than the code's key component descriptors, as identified on your above worksheets, to determine which one E/M code should be reported.

CodePath: For new Patients ... You can only code as high as your lowest key component.

GLOSSARY

A

Ablation The destruction or eradication of tissue.

Abnormal Findings Test results that indicate a disease or condition may be present.

Abortifacient A drug used to induce an abortion.

Abortion The end of a pregnancy prior to or subsequent to the death of a fetus.

Abstracting The process of identifying the relevant words or phrases in health care documentation in order to determine the best, most appropriate code(s).

Abuse Regular consumption of a substance with manifestations.

Abuse This term is used in different manners: (a) extreme use of a drug or chemical; (b) violent and/or inappropriate treatment of another person (child, adult, elder).

Accessory Organs Organs that assist the digestive process and are adjacent to the alimentary canal: the gallbladder, liver, and pancreas.

Accommodation Adaptation of the eye's lens to adjust for varying focal distances.

Acute Severe; serious.

Administration To introduce a therapeutic, prophylactic, protective, diagnostic, nutritional, or physiological substance.

Administrative Laws Also known as rules and regulations, these are created and adjudicated by administrative agencies given authority by Congress.

Advanced Life Support (ALS) Life-sustaining, emergency care provided, such as airway management, defibrillation, and/or the administration of drugs.

Adverse Effect An unexpected bad reaction to a drug or other treatment.

Agglutination The process of red blood cells combining together in a mass or lump.

Allogeneic The donor and recipient are of the same species, e.g., human → human, dog → dog (also known as an *allograft*).

Allotransplantation The relocation of tissue from one individual to another (both of the same species) without an identical genetic match.

Alphabetic Index The section of a code book showing all codes, from A to Z, by the short code descriptions.

alphanumeric Containing both letters and numbers.

Ambulatory Surgery Center (ASC) A facility specially designed to provide surgical treatments without an overnight stay; also known as a *same-day surgery center*.

AMCC Automated Multi-Channel Chemistry—Automated organ disease panel tests performed on the same patient, by the same provider, on the same day.

Anatomical Site A specific location within the anatomy (body).

Anemic Any of various conditions marked by deficiency in red blood cells or hemoglobin.

Anesthesia The loss of sensation, with or without consciousness, generally induced by the administration of a particular drug.

Anesthesiologists Physicians specializing in the administration of anesthesia.

Angina Pectoris Chest pain.

Angiography The imaging of blood vessels after the injection of contrast material.

Anomaly An abnormal, or unexpected, condition.

Antibodies Immune responses to antigens.

Antigen A substance that promotes the production of antibodies.

Anus The portion of the large intestine that leads outside the body.

Anxiety The feelings of apprehension and fear, sometimes manifested with physical manifestations such as sweating and palpitations.

Approach The path the physician took to access the body part upon which the treatment or procedure was targeted.

Arthrodesis The immobilization of a joint using a surgical technique.

Arthrography The recording of a picture of an anatomical joint after the administration of contrast material into the joint capsule.

Arthropathy Disease or dysfunction of a joint [plural: arthropathies].

Articulation A joint.

Ascending Colon The portion of the large intestine that connects the cecum to the hepatic flexure.

Assume Suppose to be the case, without proof; guess the intended details.

Asymptomatic No symptoms or manifestations.

Atherosclerosis A condition resulting from plaque buildup on the interior walls of the arteries, causing reduced blood flow; also known as *arteriosclerosis*.

Atrium A chamber that is located in the top half of the heart and receives blood.

Audiology The study of hearing, balance, and related disorders.

Autologous The donor tissue is taken from a different site on the same individual's body (also known as an *autograft*).

Automobile Insurance Auto accident liability coverage will pay for medical bills, lost wages, and compensation for pain and suffering for any person injured by the insured in an auto accident.

Avulsion Injury in which layers of skin are traumatically torn away from the body.

Axis of Classification A single meaning within the code set; providing a detail.

B

Bacteria Single-celled microorganisms that cause disease.

Basic Life Support (BLS) The provision of emergency CPR, stabilization of the patient, first aid, control of bleeding, and/or treatment of shock.

Basic Personal Services Services that include washing/bathing, dressing and undressing, assistance in taking medications, and assistance getting in and out of bed.

Behavioral Disturbance A type of common behavior that includes mood disorders (such as depression, apathy, and euphoria), sleep disorders (such as insomnia and hypersomnia), psychotic symptoms (such as delusions and hallucinations), and agitation (such as pacing, wandering, and aggression).

Benign Nonmalignant characteristic of a neoplasm; not infectious or spreading.

Benign Prostatic Hyperplasia (BPH) Enlarged prostate that results in depressing the urethra.

Biofeedback Training to gain voluntary control of automatic bodily functions.

Bladder Cancer Malignancy of the urinary bladder.

Blepharitis Inflammation of the eyelid.

Blister A bubble or sac formed on the surface of the skin, typically filled with a watery fluid or serum.

Blood Fluid pumped throughout the body, carrying oxygen and nutrients to the cells and wastes away from the cells.

Blood Type A system of classifying blood based on the antigens present on the surface of the individual's red blood cells; also known as *blood group*.

Body Part The anatomical site upon which the procedure was performed.

Body System The physiological system, or anatomical region, upon which the procedure was performed.

Bulbar Conjunctiva A mucous membrane on the surface of the eyeball.

Bulla A large vesicle that is filled with fluid.

Burn Injury by heat or fire.

C

Capitation Plans Agreements between a physician and a managed care organization that pay the physician a predetermined amount of money each month for each member of the plan who identifies that provider as his or her primary care physician.

Carbuncle A painful, pus-filled boil due to infection of the epidermis and underlying tissues, often caused by staphylococcus.

Carcinoma A malignant neoplasm or cancerous tumor.

Care Plan Oversight Services E/M of a patient, reported in 30-day periods, including infrequent supervision along with preencounter and postencounter work, such as reading test results and assessment of notes.

Carrier An individual infected with a disease who is not ill but can still pass it to another person; an individual with an abnormal gene that can be passed to a child, making the child susceptible to disease.

Cataract Clouding of the lens or lens capsule of the eye.

Category I Codes The codes listed in the main text of the CPT book, also known as CPT codes.

Category II Codes Codes for performance measurement and tracking.

Category II Modifiers Modifiers provided for use with Category II CPT codes to indicate a valid reason for a portion of a performance measure to be deleted from qualification.

Category III Codes Codes for emerging technology.

Catheter A thin, flexible tube, inserted into a body part, used to inject fluid, to extract fluid, or to keep a passage open.

Cecum A pouchlike organ that connects the ileum with the large intestine; the point of connection for the vermiform appendix.

Centers for Medicare & Medicaid Services (CMS) The agency under the Department of Health and Human Services (DHHS) in charge of regulation and control over services for those covered by Medicare and Medicaid.

Cerebral Infarction An area of dead tissue (necrosis) in the brain caused by a blocked or ruptured blood vessel.

Cerebrovascular Accident (CVA) Rupture of a blood vessel causing hemorrhaging in the brain or an embolus in a blood vessel in the brain causing a loss of blood flow; also known as *stroke*.

Certified Registered Nurse Anesthetist (CRNA) A registered nurse (RN) who has taken additional, specialized training in the administration of anesthesia.

Character A letter or number component of an ICD-10-PCS code.

Chelation Therapy The use of a chemical compound that binds with metal in the body so that the metal will lose its toxic effect. It might be done when a metal disc or prosthetic is implanted in a patient, eliminating adverse reactions to the metal itself as a foreign body.

Chief Complaint (CC) The primary reasons why the patient has come for this encounter, in the patient's own words.

Cholelithiasis Gallstones.

Chondropathy Disease affecting the cartilage [plural: chondropathies].

Choroid The vascular layer of the eye that lies between the retina and the sclera.

Chronic Long duration; continuing over an extended period of time.

Chronic Kidney Disease (CKD) Ongoing malfunction of one or both kidneys.

Chronic Obstructive Pulmonary Disease (COPD) An ongoing obstruction of the airway.

Ciliary Body The vascular layer of the eye that lies between the sclera and the crystalline lens.

Civil Law Laws that govern the relationships between people, and between businesses.

Class A Finding Nontraumatic amputation of a foot or an integral skeletal portion.

Class B Finding Absence of a posterior tibial pulse; absence or decrease of hair growth; thickening of the nail, discoloration of the skin, and/or thinning of the skin texture; and/or absence of a posterior pedal pulse.

Class C Finding Edema, burning sensation, temperature change (cold feet), abnormal spontaneous sensations in the feet, and/or limping.

Classification Systems The term used in health care to identify ICD-10-CM, CPT, ICD-10-PCS, and HCPCS Level II code sets.

Clinical Laboratory Improvement Amendment (CLIA) Federal legislation created for the monitoring and regulation of clinical laboratory procedures.

Clinically Significant Signs, symptoms, and/or conditions present at birth that may impact the child's future health status.

Closed Treatment The treatment of a fracture without surgically opening the affected area.

Coagulation Clotting; the change from a liquid into a thickened substance.

Coding for Coverage Choosing a code on the basis of what the insurance company will cover (pay for) rather than accurately reflecting the truth.

Coding Process The sequence of actions required to interpret physician documentation into the codes that accurately report what occurred during a specific encounter between health care professional and patient.

Common Bile Duct The juncture of the cystic duct of the gallbladder and the hepatic duct from the liver.

Common Law Also known as case law, this is created by judicial decisions made during court trials.

Co-morbidity A separate diagnosis existing in the same patient at the same time as an unrelated diagnosis.

Complex Closure A method of sealing an opening in the skin involving a multilayered closure and a reconstructive procedure such as scar revision, debridement, or retention sutures.

Complication An unexpected illness or other condition that develops as a result of a procedure, service, or treatment provided during the patient's hospital stay.

Computed Tomography (CT) A specialized computer scanner with very fine detail that records imaging of internal anatomical sites; also known as computerized axial tomography (CAT).

Computed Tomography Angiography (CTA) A CT scan using contrast materials to visualize arteries and veins all over the body.

Concurrent Coding System in which coding processes are performed while a patient is still in the hospital receiving care.

Condition The state of abnormality or dysfunction.

Cone A receptor in the retina that is responsible for light and color.

Confirmed Found to be true or definite.

Congenital A condition existing at the time of birth.

Conjunctivitis Inflammation of the conjunctiva.

Conscious Sedation The use of a drug to reduce stress and/or anxiety.

Consultation An encounter for purposes of a second physician's opinion or advice, requested by another physician, regarding the management of a patient's specific health concern. A consultation is planned to be a short-term relationship between a health care professional and a patient.

Cornea Transparent tissue covering the eyeball; responsible for focusing light into the eye and transmitting light.

Corneal Dystrophy Growth of abnormal tissue on the cornea, often related to a nutritional deficiency.

Corrosion A burn caused by a chemical; chemical destruction of the skin.

Covered Entities Health care providers, health plans, and health care clearinghouses—businesses that have access to the personal health information of patients.

CPT Code Modifier A two-character code that may be appended to a code from the main portion of the CPT book to provide additional information.

Criminal Law Laws governing the behavior of the actions of the population related to health and well-being.

Critical Care Services Care services for an acutely ill or injured patient with a high risk for life-threatening developments.

Cushing's Syndrome A condition resulting from the hyperproduction of corticosteroids, most often caused by an adrenal cortex tumor or a tumor of the pituitary gland.

Cyst A fluid-filled or gas-filled bubble in the skin.

Cytology The investigation and identification of cells.

D

Dacryocystitis Lacrimal gland inflammation.

Decubitus ulcer A bedsore, or wound created by lying in the same position, on the same irritant without relief.

Deformity A size or shape (structural design) that deviates from that which is considered normal.

Demographic Demographic details include the patient's name, address, date of birth, and other personal details, not specifically related to health.

Densitometry The process used to measure bone density, most often done to assess the patient's risk for osteopenia or osteoporosis.

Dependence Ongoing, regular consumption of a substance with resulting significant clinical manifestations, and a dramatic decrease in the effect of the substance with continued use, therefore requiring an increased quantity of the substance to achieve intoxication.

Dependents Individuals who are supported, either financially or with regard to insurance coverage, by others.

Depressive An emotional state that includes sadness, hopelessness, and gloom.

Dermis The internal layer of the skin; the location of blood vessels, lymph vessels, hair follicles, sweat glands, and sebum.

Descending Colon The segment of the large intestine that connects the splenic flexure to the sigmoid colon.

Detoxification The process of removing toxic substances or qualities.

Device The identification of any materials or appliances that may remain in or on the body after the procedure is completed.

Diabetes Mellitus (DM) A chronic systemic disease that results from insulin deficiency or resistance and causes the body to improperly metabolize carbohydrates, proteins, and fats.

Diagnosis A physician's determination of a patient's condition, illness, or injury.

Diagnosis-Related Group (DRG) An episodic care payment system basing reimbursement to hospitals for inpatient services upon standards of care for specific diagnoses grouped by their similar usage of resources for procedures, services, and treatments.

Differential Diagnosis When the physician indicates that the patient's signs and symptoms may closely lead to two different diagnoses; usually written as "diagnosis A vs. diagnosis B."

Disability Compensation A plan that reimburses a covered individual a portion of his or her income that is lost as a result of being unable to work due to illness or injury.

Disclosure The sharing of information between health care professionals working in separate entities, or facilities, in the course of caring for the patient.

Discounted FFS An extra reduction in the rate charged to an insurer for services provided by the physician to the plan's members.

Dislocation The movement of a muscle away from its normal position.

DMEPOS Durable medical equipment, prosthetic, and orthotic supplies.

Donor Area (Site) The area or part of the body from which skin or tissue is removed with the intention of placing that skin or tissue in another area or body.

Dorsopathy Disease affecting the back of the torso [plural: dorsopathies].

Double Billing Sending a claim for the second time to the same insurance company for the same procedure or service, provided to the same patient on the same date of service.

Duodenum The first segment of the small intestine, connecting the stomach to the jejunum.

Duplex Scan An ultrasonic scanning procedure to determine blood flow and pattern.

Durable Medical Equipment (DME) Apparatus and tools that help individuals accommodate physical frailties, deliver pharmaceuticals, and provide other assistance that will last for a long time and/or be used to assist multiple patients over time.

Durable Medical Equipment Regional Carrier (DMERC) A company designated by the state or region to act as the fiscal intermediary for all DME claims.

Dyslipidemia Abnormal lipoprotein metabolism.

E

Early and Periodic Screening, Diagnostic, and Treatment (EPSDT) A Medicaid preventive health program for children under 21.

Ectopic Out of place, such as an organ or body part.

Edema An overaccumulation of fluid in the cells of the tissues.

Edentulism Absence of teeth.

Electronic Media Claim (EMC) A health care claim form that is transmitted electronically.

Electronic Remittance Advice (ERA) Remittance advice that is sent to the provider electronically.

Elevated Blood Pressure An occurrence of high blood pressure; an isolated or infrequent reading of a systolic blood pressure above 140 mmHg and/or a diastolic blood pressure above 90 mmHg.

Eligibility Verification The process of confirming with the insurance carrier that an individual is qualified for benefits that would pay for services provided by your health care professional on a particular day.

Embolus A thrombus that has broken free from the vessel wall and is traveling freely within the vascular system.

End-Stage Renal Disease (ESRD) Chronic, irreversible kidney disease requiring regular treatments.

Enteral Within, or by way of, the gastrointestinal tract.

Epidermis The external layer of the skin, the majority of which is squamous cells.

Episodic Care An insurance company pays a provider one flat fee to cover the entire course of treatment for an individual's condition.

Eponym A disease or condition named for a person.

Esophagus The tubular organ that connects the pharynx to the stomach for the passage of nourishment.

Established Patient A person who has received professional services within the last 3 years from either this provider or another provider of the same specialty belonging to the same group practice.

Etiology The original source or cause for the development of a disease; also, the study of the causes of disease.

Evaluation and Management (E/M) Specific components of a meeting between a health care professional and a patient.

Exacerbation An increase in the severity of a disease or its symptoms.

Excision The full-thickness removal of a lesion, including margins; includes (for coding purposes) a simple closure.

Executive Orders Official policies issued by the president of the United States.

Experimental A procedure or treatment that has not yet been accepted by the health care industry as the standard of care.

Explanation of Benefits (EOB) Another type of remittance advice, more typically sent to the policyholder. However, some in the industry use the term *EOB* interchangeably with *RA*.

Extent The percentage of the body that has been affected by the burn or corrosion.

External Cause An event, outside the body, that causes injury, poisoning, or an adverse reaction.

Extra-Articular Located outside a joint.

Extracorporeal Outside of the body.

Extraocular Muscles The muscles that control the eye.

F

Fee-for-Service (FFS) Plans Payment agreements that outline, in a written fee schedule, exactly how much money the insurance carrier will pay the physician for each treatment and/or service provided.

First-Degree Burn Redness of the epidermis (skin).

First-Listed "First-listed diagnosis" is used, when reporting outpatient encounters, instead of the term "principal diagnosis."

Fluoroscope A piece of equipment that emits x-rays through a part of the patient's body onto a fluorescent screen, causing the image to identify various aspects of the anatomy by density.

Fornix The conjunctival fornix is the area between the eyelid and the eyeball. The superior fornix is between the upper lid and eyeball; the inferior fornix is between the lower lid and the eyeball. Plural: *fornices*

Fracture Broken cartilage or bone.

Full-Thickness A measure that extends from the epidermis to the connective tissue layer of the skin.

Functional Activity Glandular secretion in abnormal quantity.

Fundus The section of an organ farthest from its opening.

Fungi Group of organisms, including mold, yeast, and mildew, that cause infection; fungus (singular).

Furuncle A staphylococcal infection in the subcutaneous tissue; commonly known as a *boil*.

G

Gallbladder A pear-shaped organ that stores bile until it is required to aid the digestive process.

Gangrene Necrotic tissue resulting from a loss of blood supply.

Gatekeeper A physician, typically a family practitioner or an internist, who serves as the primary care physician for an individual. This physician is responsible for evaluating and determining the course of treatment or services, as well as for deciding whether or not a specialist should be involved in care.

General Anesthesia The administration of a drug in order to induce a loss of consciousness in the patient, who is unable to be aroused even by painful stimulation.

Genetic Abnormality An error in a gene (chromosome) that affects development during gestation; also known as a *chromosomal abnormality*.

Gestation The length of time for the complete development of a baby from conception to birth; on average, 40 weeks.

Gestational Diabetes Mellitus (GDM) Usually a temporary diabetes mellitus occurring during pregnancy; however, such patients have an increased risk of later developing type 2 diabetes.

Gestational Hypertension Hypertension that develops during pregnancy and typically goes away once the pregnancy has ended.

Glands of Zeis Altered sebaceous glands that are connected to the eyelash follicles.

Glaucoma The condition that results when poor draining of fluid causes an abnormal increase in pressure within the eye, damaging the optic nerve.

Global Period The length of time allotted for postoperative care included in the surgical package, which is generally accepted to be 90 days for major surgical procedures and up to 10 days for minor procedures.

Global Surgical Package A group of services already included in the code for the operation and not reported separately.

Glomerular Filtration Rate (GFR) The measurement of kidney function; used to determine the stage of kidney disease. GFR is calculated by the physician using the results of a creatinine test in a formula with the patient's gender, age, race, and other factors; normal GFR is 90 and above.

Gross Examination The visual study of a specimen (with the naked eye).

Gynecologist (GYN) A physician specializing in the care of the female genital tract.

H

Hair A pigmented, cylindrical filament that grows out from the hair follicle within the epidermis.

Hair Follicle A saclike bulb containing the hair root.

Harvesting The process of taking skin or tissue (on the same body or another).

HCPCS Level II Modifier A two-character alphabetic or alphanumeric code that may be appended to a code from the main portion of the CPT book or a code from the HCPCS Level II book.

Health Care The total management of an individual's well-being by a health care professional.

Health Maintenance Organization (HMO) A type of health insurance that uses a primary care physician, also known as a gatekeeper, to manage all health care services for an individual.

Hematopoiesis The formation of blood cells.

Hemoglobin (hgb or Hgb) The part of the red blood cell that carries oxygen.

Hemolysis The destruction of red blood cells, resulting in the release of hemoglobin into the bloodstream.

Hemorrhage Excessive or severe bleeding.

Hemostasis The interruption of bleeding.

Hernia A condition in which one anatomical structure pushes through a perforation in the wall of the anatomical site that normally contains that structure.

High Osmolar An ionic water-soluble iodinated contrast medium.

HIPAA's Privacy Rule A portion of HIPAA that ensures the availability of patient information for those who should see it while protecting that information from those who should not.

History of Present Illness (HPI) The collection of details about the patient's chief complaint, the current issue that prompted this encounter: duration, specific signs and symptoms, etc.

Hospice An organization that provides services to terminally ill patients and their families.

Hospital-Acquired Condition (HAC) A condition, illness, or injury contracted by the patient during his or her stay in an acute care facility; also known as *nosocomial condition*.

Human Immunodeficiency Virus (HIV) A condition affecting the immune system.

Hyperglycemia Abnormally high levels of glucose.

Hypertension High blood pressure, usually a chronic condition; often identified by a systolic blood pressure above 140 mmHg and/or a diastolic blood pressure above 90 mmHg.

Hypoglycemia Abnormally low glucose levels.

Hypoglycemics Prescription, non-insulin medications designed to lower a patient's glycemic level.

Hypotension Low blood pressure; systolic blood pressure below 90 mmHg and/or diastolic measurements of lower than 60 mmHg.

Hypothyroidism A condition in which the thyroid converts energy more slowly than normal, resulting in an otherwise unexplained weight gain and fatigue.

I

Ileum The last segment of the small intestine.

Immunization To make someone resistant to a particular disease by vaccination.

Index to External Causes The alphabetic listing of the external causes that might cause a patient's injury, poisoning, or adverse reaction.

Infarction Tissue or muscle that has deteriorated or died (necrotic).

Infection The invasion of pathogens into tissue cells.

Infectious A condition that can be transmitted from one person to another.

Inflammation The reaction of tissues to infection or injury; characterized by pain, swelling, and erythema.

Influenza An acute infection of the respiratory tract caused by the influenza virus.

Infusion The introduction of a fluid into a blood vessel.

Injection Compelling a fluid into tissue or cavity.

Inpatient An individual admitted for an overnight or longer stay in a hospital.

Inpatient Facility An establishment that provides health care services to individuals who stay overnight on the premises.

Insurance Premium The amount of money, often paid monthly, by a policyholder or insured, to an insurance company to obtain coverage.

Intermediate Closure A multilevel method of sealing an opening in the skin involving one or more of the deeper layers of the skin. Single-layer closure of heavily contaminated wounds that required extensive cleaning or removal of particulate matter also constitutes intermediate closure.

Interpret Explain the meaning of; convert a meaning from one language to another.

Interval The time measured between one point and another, such as between physician visits.

Intervertebral Disc A fibrocartilage segment that lies between vertebrae of the spinal column and provides cushioning and support.

Intravascular Optical Coherence A high-resolution, catheter-based imaging modality used for the optimized visualization of coronary artery lesions.

Iris The round, pigmented muscular curtain in the eye.

Isogeneic The donor and recipient individuals are genetically identical (i.e., monozygotic twins).

J

Jejunum The segment of the small intestine that connects the duodenum to the ileum.

K

Keratitis An inflammation of the cornea, typically accompanied by an ulceration.

L

Laboratory A location with scientific equipment designed to perform experiments and tests.

Laceration Damage to the epidermal and dermal layers of the skin made by a sharp object.

Lacrimal Apparatus A system in the eye that consists of the lacrimal glands, the upper canaliculi, the lower canaliculi, the lacrimal sac, and the nasolacrimal duct

Laminaria Thin sticks of kelp-related seaweed, used to dilate the cervix, that can induce abortive circumstance during the first 3 months of pregnancy.

Laminectomy The surgical removal of a vertebral posterior arch.

Laterality The right or left side of anatomical sites that have locations on both sides of the body; e.g., right arm or left arm; *unilateral* means one side and *bilateral* means both sides.

Lens A transparent, crystalline segment of the eye, situated directly behind the pupil, that is responsible for focusing light rays as they enter the eye and travel back to the retina.

Level of Patient History The amount of detail involved in the documentation of patient history.

Level of Physical Examination The extent of a physician's clinical assessment and inspection of a patient.

Liability Insurance A policy that covers loss or injury to a third party caused by the insured or something belonging to the insured.

Linking Confirming medical necessity by pairing at least one diagnosis code to at least one procedure code.

Liters per Minute (LPM) The measurement of how many liters of a drug or chemical are provided to the patient in 60 seconds.

Liver The organ, located in the upper right area of the abdominal cavity, that is responsible for regulating blood sugar levels; secreting bile for the gallbladder; metabolizing fats, proteins, and carbohydrates; manufacturing some blood proteins; and removing toxins from the blood.

Local Anesthesia The injection of a drug to prevent sensation in a specific portion of the body; includes local infiltration anesthesia, digital blocks, and pudendal blocks.

Locum Tenens Physician A physician who fills in, temporarily, for another physician.

Low Birth Weight (LBW) A baby born weighing less than 5 pounds 8 ounces, or 2,500 grams.

Low Osmolar A non-ionic water-soluble iodinated contrast medium.

M

Macule A flat lesion with a different pigmentation (color) when compared with the surrounding skin.

Magnetic Resonance Arthrography (MRA) MR imaging of an anatomical joint after the administration of contrast material into the joint capsule.

Magnetic Resonance Imaging (MRI) A three-dimensional radiologic technique that uses nuclear technology to record pictures of internal anatomical sites.

Main Section The section of the CPT code book listing all of the codes in numeric order.

Major Complication and Co-morbidity (MCC) A complication or co-morbidity that has an impact on the treatment of the patient and makes care for that patient more complex.

Malformation An irregular structural development.

Malignant Invasive and destructive characteristic of a neoplasm; possibly causing damage or death.

Malunion A fractured bone that did not heal correctly; healing of bone that was not in proper position or alignment.

Managed Care A type of health insurance coverage that controls the care of each subscriber (or insured person) by using a primary care provider as a central health care supervisor.

Manic An emotional state that includes elation, excitement, and exuberance.

Manifestation A condition that develops as the result of another, underlying condition.

Manipulation The attempted return of a fracture or dislocation to its normal alignment manually by the physician.

Mass Abnormal collection of tissue.

Measurement To determine a level of a physiological or physical function.

Medical Decision Making (MDM) The level of knowledge and experience needed by the provider to determine the diagnosis and/or what to do next.

Medical necessity The assessment that the provider was acting according to standard practices in providing a procedure or service for an individual with a specific diagnosis.

Meibomian Glands Sebaceous glands that secrete a tear film component that prevents tears from evaporating so that the area stays moist.

Mesentery A fold of a membrane that carries blood to the small intestine and connects it to the posterior wall of the abdominal cavity.

Metastasize To proliferate, reproduce, or spread.

Microscopic Examination The study of a specimen using a microscope (under magnification).

Modifier A two-character code that affects the meaning of another code; a code addendum that provides more meaning to the original code.

Moll's Glands Ordinary sweat glands.

Monitored Anesthesia Care (MAC) The administration of sedatives, anesthetic agents, or other medications to relax but not render the patient unconscious while under the constant observation of a trained anesthesiologist; also known as "twilight" sedation.

Morbidity Unhealthy.

Morphology The study of the configuration or structure of living organisms.

Mortality Death.

Mutually Exclusive Codes Codes that are identified as those that are not permitted to be used on the same claim form with other codes.

Myalgia Pain in a muscle.

Myocardial Infarction (MI) Malfunction of the heart due to necrosis or deterioration of a portion of the heart muscle; also known as a *heart attack*.

Myopathy Disease of a muscle [plural: myopathies].

N

Neoplasm Abnormal tissue growth; tumor.

Neoplasm Table The Neoplasm Table lists all possible codes for benign and malignant neoplasms, in alphabetic order by anatomical location of the tumor.

Nevus An abnormally pigmented area of skin. A birthmark is an example.

New Patient A person who has not received any professional services within the past 3 years from either the provider or another provider of the same specialty who belongs to the same group practice.

Nodule A tissue mass or papule larger than 5 mm.

Nonessential Modifiers Descriptors whose inclusion in the physician's notes are not absolutely necessary and that are provided simply to further clarify a code description; optional terms.

Non-physician A non-physician can be a nurse practitioner, certified registered nurse anesthetist, certified registered nurse, clinical nurse specialist, or physician assistant.

Nonunion A fractured bone that did not heal back together; no mending or joining together of the broken segments.

Nosocomial A hospital-acquired condition; a condition that develops as a result of being in a health care facility.

Not Elsewhere Classifiable (NEC) Specifics that are not described in any other code in the ICD-10-CM book; also known as *not elsewhere classified*.

Not Otherwise Specified (NOS) The absence of additional details documented in the notes.

Notations Alerts and warnings that support more accurate use of codes in a specific code set.

NSTEMI A nontransmural elevation myocardial infarction—a heart event during which the coronary artery is partially occluded (blocked).

Nuclear Medicine Treatment that includes the injection or digestion of isotopes.

Nursing Facility A facility that provides skilled nursing treatment and attention along with limited medical care for its (usually long-term) residents, who do not require acute care services (hospitalization).

O

Obstetrics (OB) A health care specialty focusing on the care of women during pregnancy and the puerperium.

Obstruction A blockage or closing.

Official Guidelines A listing of rules and regulations instructing how to use a specific code set accurately.

Open Treatment Surgically opening the fracture site, or another site in the body nearby, in order to treat the fractured bone.

Ophthalmologist A physician qualified to diagnose and treat eye disease and conditions with drugs, surgery, and corrective measures.

Optometrist A professional qualified to carry out eye examinations and to prescribe and supply eyeglasses and contact lenses.

Oral Cavity The opening in the face that begins the alimentary canal and is used for the input of nutrition; also known as the *mouth*.

Orbit The bony cavity in the skull that houses the eye and its ancillary parts (muscles, nerves, blood vessels).

Orthotic A device used to correct or improve an orthopedic concern.

Other Specified Additional information the physician specified that isn't included in any other code description.

Otorhinolaryngology The study of the human ears, nose, and throat (ENT) systems.

Outpatient An **outpatient** is a patient who receives services for a short amount of time (less than 24 hours) in a physician's office or clinic, without being kept overnight. An **outpatient facility** includes a hospital emergency room, ambulatory care center, same-day surgery center, or walk-in clinic.

Outpatient Services Health care services provided to individuals without an overnight stay in the facility.

Overlapping Boundaries Multiple sites of carcinoma without identifiable borders.

P

Palpebrae The eyelids; singular *palpebra*.

Palpebral Conjunctiva A mucous membrane that lines the palpebrae.

Pancreas A gland that secretes insulin and other hormones from the islet cells into the bloodstream and manufactures digestive enzymes that are secreted into the duodenum.

Pancreatic Islets Cells within the pancreas that secrete insulin and other hormones into the bloodstream.

Papule A raised lesion with a diameter of less than 5 mm.

Parasites Tiny living things that can invade and feed off other living things.

Parathyroid Glands Four small glands situated on the back of the thyroid gland that secrete parathyroid hormone.

Parenteral By way of anything other than the gastrointestinal tract, such as intravenous, intramuscular, intramedullary, or subcutaneous.

Parenteral Enteral Nutrition (PEN) Nourishment delivered using a combination of means other than the gastrointestinal tract (such as IV) in addition to via the gastrointestinal tract.

Past, Family, and Social History (PFSH) Collection of details, related to the chief complaint, regarding possible signs, symptoms, behaviors, genetic connection, etc.

Patch A flat, small area of differently colored or textured skin; a large macule.

Pathogen Any agent that causes disease; a microorganism such as a bacterium or virus.

Pathology The study of the nature, etiology, development, and outcomes of disease.

Percutaneous Skeletal Fixation The insertion of fixation instruments (such as pins) placed across the fracture site. It may be done under x-ray imaging for guidance purposes.

Perforation An atypical hole in the wall of an organ or anatomical site.

Perinatal The time period from before birth to the 28th day after birth.

Personnel Modifier A modifier adding information about the professional(s) attending to the provision of this procedure or treatment to the patient during this encounter.

Phalanges Fingers and toes [singular: phalange or phalanx].

Phobia Irrational and excessive fear of an object, activity, or situation.

Physical Status Modifier A two-character alphanumeric code used to describe the condition of the patient at the time anesthesia services are administered.

***Physicians' Desk Reference* (PDR)** A series of reference books identifying all aspects of prescription and over-the-counter medications, as well as herbal remedies.

Placement To put a device in or on an anatomical site.

Plasma The fluid part of the blood.

Platelets (PLTs) Large cell fragments in the bone marrow that function in clotting; also known as *thrombocytes*.

Pneumonia An inflammation of the lungs.

Pneumothorax A condition in which air or gas is present within the chest cavity but outside the lungs.

Point-of-Service (POS) A type of insurance plan that will allow an HMO enrollee to choose his or her own nonmember physician at a lower benefit rate, costing the patient more money out-of-pocket.

Polydipsia Excessive thirst.

Polyuria Excessive urination.

Preferred Provider Organization (PPO) A type of health insurance coverage in which physicians provide health care services to members of the plan at a discount.

Prematurity Birth occurring prior to the completion of 37 weeks gestation.

Prenatal Prior to birth; also referred to as *antenatal*.

Present-On-Admission (POA) A one-character indicator reporting the status of the diagnosis at the time the patient was admitted to the acute care facility.

Pressure Ulcer An open wound or sore caused by pressure, infection, or inflammation.

Preventive A type of action or service that stops something from happening or from getting worse.

Preventive Care Health-related services designed to stop the development of a disease or injury.

Principal Diagnosis The condition, after study, that is the primary, or main, reason for the admission of a patient to the hospital for care; the condition that requires the largest amount of hospital resources for care.

Problem-Pertinent System Review The physician's collection of details of signs and symptoms, as per the patient, affecting only those body systems connected to the chief complaint.

Procedure Action taken, in accordance with the standards of care, by the physician to accomplish a predetermined objective (result); a surgical operation.

Products of Conception The zygote, embryo, or fetus, as well as the amnion, umbilical cord, and placenta.

Proptosis Bulging out of the eye; also known as *exophthalmos*.

Prostatitis Inflammation of the prostate.

Prosthetic Fabricated artificial replacement for a damaged or missing part of the body.

Protected Health Information (PHI) Any patient-identifiable health information regardless of the form in which it is stored (paper, computer file, etc.).

Psychotherapy The treatment of mental and emotional disorder through communication or psychologically rather than medical means.

Puerperium The time period from the end of labor until the uterus returns to normal size, typically 3 to 6 weeks.

Pupil The opening in the center of the iris that permits light to enter and continue on to the lens and retina.

Push The delivery of an additional drug via an intravenous line over a short period of time.

Pustule A swollen area of skin; a vesicle filled with pus.

Q

Qualifier Any additional feature of the procedure, if applicable.

Qualitative The determination of character or essential element(s).

Quantitative The counting or measurement of something.

Query To ask.

R

Radiation The high-speed discharge and projection of energy waves or particles.

Recipient Area The area, or site, of the body receiving a graft of skin or tissue.

Rectum The last segment of the large intestine, connecting the sigmoid colon to the anus.

Red Blood Cells (RBCs) Cells within the blood that contain hemoglobin responsible for carrying oxygen to tissues; also known as *erythrocytes*.

Regional Anesthesia The administration of a drug in order to interrupt the nerve impulses without loss of consciousness.

Rehabilitation Health care that is committed to improving, maintaining, or returning physical strength, cognition, and mobility.

Reimbursement The process of paying for health care services after they have been provided.

Relationship The level of familiarity between provider and patient.

Release of Information (ROI) The form (either on paper or electronic) that a patient must sign to give legal permission to a covered entity to disclose that patient's PHI.

Remittance Advice (RA) Notification identifying details about a payment from the third-party payer.

Respiratory Disorder A malfunction of the organ system relating to respiration.

Retina A membrane in the back of the eye that is sensitive to light and functions as the sensory end of the optic nerve.

Retinal Detachment A break in the connection between the retinal pigment epithelium layer and the neural retina.

Retinopathy Degenerative condition of the retina.

Rh (Rhesus) Factor An antigen located on the red blood cell that produces immunogenic responses in those individuals without it.

Risk Factor Reduction Intervention Action taken by the attending physician to stop or reduce a behavior or lifestyle that is predicted to have a negative effect on the individual's health.

rod An elongated, cylindrical cell within the retina that is photosensitive in low light.

Root Operation Term The category or classification of a particular procedure, service, or treatment.

Rule of Nines A general division of the whole body into sections that each represents 9%; used for estimating the extent of a burn.

S

Salivary Glands Three sets of bilateral exocrine glands that secrete saliva: parotid glands, submaxillary glands, and sublingual glands.

Saphenous Vein Either of the two major veins in the leg that run from the foot to the thigh near the surface of the skin.

Scale Flaky exfoliated epidermis; a flake of skin.

Schizophrenia A psychotic disorder with no known cause.

Sclera The membranous tissue that covers all of the eyeball (except the cornea); also known as *the white of the eye*.

Screening An examination or test of a patient who has no signs or symptoms that is conducted with the intention of finding any evidence of disease as soon as possible, thus enabling better patient outcomes.

Second-Degree Burn Blisters on the skin; involvement of the epidermis and the dermis layers.

Secondary Diabetes Mellitus Diabetes caused by medication or another condition or disease.

Secondary Hypertension The condition of hypertension caused by another condition or illness.

Self-Administer To give medication to oneself, such as a diabetic giving herself an insulin injection.

Sepsis Condition typified by two or more systemic responses to infection; a specified pathogen.

Septic Shock Severe sepsis with hypotension; unresponsive to fluid resuscitation.

Septicemia Generalized infection spread through the body via the bloodstream; blood infection.

Sequela A cause-and-effect relationship between an original condition that has been resolved with a current condition; also known as a late effect.

Service The provision of care for a patient using advice, recommendations, or discussion.

Service-Related Modifier A modifier relating to a change or adjustment of a procedure or service provided.

Services Spending time with a patient and/or family about health care situations.

Severe Sepsis Sepsis with signs of acute organ dysfunction.

Severity The level of seriousness.

Sigmoid Colon The dual-curved segment of the colon that connects the descending colon to the rectum; also referred to as the *sigmoid flexure*.

Signs Measurable indicators of a patient's health status.

Simple Closure A method of sealing an opening in the skin (epidermis or dermis), involving only one layer. It includes the administration of local anesthesia and/or chemical or electrocauterization of a wound not closed.

Site The specific anatomical location of the disease or injury.

Skin The external membranous covering of the body.

Somatic Related to the body, especially separate from the brain or mind.

Somatoform Disorder The sincere belief that one is suffering an illness that is not present.

Sonogram The use of sound waves to record images of internal organs and tissues; also called an *ultrasound*.

Specialty Care Transport (SCT) Continuous care provided by one or more health professionals in an appropriate specialty area, such as respiratory care or cardiovascular care, or by a paramedic with additional training.

Specimen A small part or sample of any substance obtained for analysis and diagnosis.

Sphincter A circular muscle that contracts to prevent passage of liquids or solids.

Spondylopathy Disease affecting the vertebrae [plural: spondylopathies].

Standard of Care The accepted principles of conduct, services, or treatments that are established as the expected behavior.

Status Asthmaticus The condition of asthma that is life-threatening and does not respond to therapeutic treatments.

Statutory Laws Laws that are enacted by federal and state legislature.

STEMI An ST elevation myocardial infarction—a heart event during which the coronary artery is completely blocked by a thrombus or embolus.

Stomach A saclike organ within the alimentary canal designed to contain nourishment during the initial phase of the digestive process.

Subcutaneous The layer beneath the dermis; also known as the *hypodermis*.

Supplemental Report A letter or report written by the attending physician or other health care professional to provide additional clarification or explanation.

Supporting documentation The paperwork in the patient's file that corroborates the codes presented on the claim form for a particular encounter.

Surgical Approach The methodology or technique used by the physician to perform the procedure, service, or treatment.

Surgical Pathology The study of tissues removed from a living patient during a surgical procedure.

Symbols Marks, similar to emojis, that provide additional direction to use codes correctly and accurately.

Symptom A subjective sensation or departure from the norm as related by the patient.

Systemic Spread throughout the entire body.

Systemic Condition A condition that affects the entire body and virtually all body systems, therefore requiring the physician to consider this in his or her medical decision making for any other condition.

Systemic Inflammatory Response Syndrome (SIRS) A definite physical reaction, such as fever, chills, etc., to an unspecified pathogen.

T

Table of Drugs and Chemicals The section of the ICD-10-CM code book listing drugs, chemicals, and other biologicals that may poison a patient or result in an adverse reaction.

Tables The section of the ICD-10-PCS code book listing all of the codes in alphanumeric order, based on the first three characters of the code.

Tabular List of Diseases and Injuries The section of the ICD-10-CM code book listing all of the codes in alphanumeric order.

Teeth Small, calcified protrusions with roots in the jaw. (singular: Tooth)

Third-Degree Burn Destruction of all layers of the skin, with possible involvement of the subcutaneous fat, muscle, and bone.

Third-Party Payer An individual or organization that is not directly involved in an encounter but has a connection because of its obligation to pay, in full or part, for that encounter.

Thrombus A blood clot in a blood vessel; plural = *thrombi*.

Thyroid Gland A two-lobed gland located in the neck that reaches around the trachea laterally and connects anteriorly by an isthmus. The thyroid gland produces hormones used for metabolic function.

Topical Anesthesia The application of a drug to the skin to reduce or prevent sensation in a specific area temporarily.

Topography The classification of neoplasms primarily by anatomical site.

Tracer An official request for a third-party payer to search its system to find a missing health claim form. It is also a term used for a replacement health claim form resubmitted to replace one that was lost.

Transfer of Care When a physician gives up responsibility for caring for a patient, in whole or with regard to one specific condition, and another physician accepts responsibility for the care of that patient.

Transfusion The provision of one person's blood or plasma to another individual.

Transplantation The transfer of tissue from one site to another.

Transverse Colon The portion of the large intestine that connects the hepatic flexure to the splenic flexure.

Treatment The provision of medical care for a disorder or disease.

TriCare A government health plan that covers medical expenses for the dependents of active-duty service members, CHAMPUS-eligible retirees and their families, and the dependents of deceased active-duty members.

Tuberculosis An infectious condition that causes small rounded swellings on mucous membranes throughout the body.

Type 1 Diabetes Mellitus A sudden onset of insulin deficiency that may occur at any age but most often arises in childhood and adolescence; also known as *insulin-dependent diabetes mellitus (IDDM)*, *juvenile diabetes*, or *type I*.

Type 2 Diabetes Mellitus A form of diabetes mellitus with a gradual onset that may develop at any age but most often occurs in adults over the age of 40; also known as *non-insulin-dependent diabetes mellitus (NIDDM)* or *type II*.

U

Ulcer An erosion or loss of the full thickness of the epidermis.

Unbundling Coding individual parts of a specific procedure rather than one combination, or bundle, that includes all the components.

Underlying Condition One disease that affects or encourages another condition.

Uniform Hospital Discharge Data Set (UHDDS) A compilation of data collected by acute care facilities and other designated health care facilities.

Unlisted Codes Codes shown at the end of each subsection of the CPT used as a catch-all for any procedure not represented by an existing code.

Unspecified The absence of additional specifics in the physician's documentation.

Upcoding Using a code on a claim form that indicates a higher level of service than that which was actually performed.

Urea A compound that is excreted in urine.

Urea Reduction Ratio (URR) A formula to determine the effectiveness of hemodialysis treatment.

Urinary System The organ system responsible for removing waste products that are left behind in the blood and the body.

Urinary Tract Infection (UTI) Inflammation of any part of the urinary tract: kidney, ureter, bladder, or urethra.

Use The sharing of information between people working in the same health care facility for purposes of caring for the patient.

Usual, Customary, and Reasonable (UCR) The process of determining a fee for a service by evaluating the *usual* fee charged by the provider, the *customary* fee charged by most physicians in the same community or geographical area, and what is considered *reasonable* by most health care professionals under the specific circumstances of the situation.

Uveal Tract The middle layer of the eye, consisting of the iris, ciliary body, and choroid.

V

Vascular Referring to the vessels (arteries and veins).

Venography The imaging of a vein after the injection of contrast material.

Ventricle A chamber that is located in the bottom half of the heart and receives blood from the atrium.

Vermiform Appendix A long, narrow mass of tissue attached to the cecum; also called *appendix*.

Vertebra A bone that is a part of the construction of the spinal column [plural: vertebrae].

Viruses Microscopic particles that initiate disease, mimicking the characteristics of a particular cell; viruses can reproduce only within the body of the cell that they have invaded.

Vitreous Chamber The interior segment of the eye that contains the vitreous body.

W

White Blood Cells (WBCs) Cells within the blood that help to protect the body from pathogens; also known as *leukocytes*.

Workers' Compensation An insurance program that covers medical care for those injured or for those who become ill as a consequence of their employment.

X

Xenogeneic The donor and recipient are of different species, e.g., bovine cartilage → human (also known as a *xenograft* or *heterograft*).

INDEX

Note: Page numbers followed by *f* and *t* indicate figures and tables, respectively. Page numbers in **boldface** indicate definitions of terms.

A

AAPC (American Academy of Professional Coders), 1207–1208
Abbreviations, 56, 285
ABCDE method for melanoma detection, 395, 398
Abnormal findings, **522**
Abortions, **499**
Abrasions, 73, 82–83, 436*f*
Abstracting
  in clinical documentation, 23–25, 39
  defined, **23**
  neoplasm details, 149–151
Abuse, 233, **344**, **457**–458
Acanthocephalins, 117
Accessory organs (digestive), **370**–373, 370*f*
Accidental poisoning, 445–446
Accommodation, **271**
ACE (angiotensin-converting enzyme) inhibitors, 205
Achilles tendon contracture, 415–416
Acquired (secondary) immunodeficiency conditions, 122
ACTH (adrenocorticotropic hormone), 211
Actinomyces, 266
Active-duty service members (ADSMs), 1160–1161
Activity codes, 430
Acute conditions, coding guidelines for, 66, **67**
Acute infections, **102**
Acute myocardial infarction (AMI), 299, 300
Acute pain, **251**
Acute renal failure (ARF), 476
Acute stress disorder (ASD), 242
Acute tubular necrosis (ATN), 476
Acute tubulointerstitial nephritis (ATIN), 476

Adaptive immunity, 133
Addison's keloid, 392
Additional characters required, 63
Adenovirus, 330
ADH (antidiuretic hormone), 210, 471
Administrative laws, **1187**, 1189*f*
Adolescent idiopathic scoliosis, 413
Adrenocorticotropic hormone (ACTH), 211
ADSMs (active-duty service members), 1160–1161
Advanced Alternative Payment Models (APMs), 1165
Adverse effects, 5, **77**, 444–446
Affective (mood) disorders, 230, 236–238
Affordable Care Act. *See* Patient Protection and Affordable Care Act of 2010
Aftercare codes, 440, 525–527
Agammaglobulinemia, 189
Agglutination, **184**
AHIMA (American Health Information Management Association), 1206–1207
AIDS. *See* HIV/AIDS
Airborne exposure to infection, 102
Akathisia, 240
Alcohol-related disorders
  digestive, 372, 373–374
  mental and behavioral, 232–235
Aldosterone, 471
Alimentary canal. *See also* Digestive disorders
  esophagus, 360–361, 360*f*
  large intestine, 367–369, 367*f*
  oral cavity, 356–359, 357*f*
  salivary glands, 359
  small intestine, 364–366
  stomach, 361–364, 361*f*, 365*f*
Allergic contact dermatitis, 383
Allergies, 189
Allergy lists, 24
Allocation of resources, 3
Allogeneic, 15, **527**, 527*t*
Alopecia mucinosa, 389
Alpha-1 antitrypsin deficiency, 330
Alphabetic Index (CPT), 10, 11*f*, **41**

Alphabetic Index (HCPCS Level II), 17, 17*f*, **41**
Alphabetic Index (ICD-10-CM), 4–5, 4*f*, **41**, 72–76*f*
Alphabetic Index (ICD-10-PCS), 12, **41**, 45
Alphanumeric order, **43**
Alphanumeric Section (HCPCS Level II), 17, 18*f*, **43**, 45
Alymphocytosis, 122
Alzheimer's disease, 245–246
American Academy of Professional Coders (AAPC), 1207–1208
American Health Information Management Association (AHIMA), 1206–1207
American Medical Association (AMA), 16
AMI (acute myocardial infarction), 299, 300
Amnestic disorder, 229–230
Amniocentesis, 506
Amphetamine-related disorders, 234
AMR (antimicrobial resistance), 133–136, 528–531
Anatomical site, defined, **62**
"And" notation, 61
Anemia, 162, 174–177, **474**–475, 507
Angina pectoris, **303**
Angiostrongyliasis, 117*f*
Angiotensin-converting enzyme (ACE) inhibitors, 205
Angiotensin receptor blockers (ARBs), 205
Anhidrosis, 390
Animal bites, 437–438
Ankylosing spondylitis (AS), 413
Annual physicals, 521
Anomaly, defined, **505**
Anorexia, 214
Antepartum (prenatal) care, 489–490
Antibiotics, 133, 332
Antibodies, **182**, **188**
Antidepressants, 236, 308
Antidiuretic hormone (ADH), 210, 471
Antigens, **182**, **188**
Antilipemics, 303

1229

Antimicrobial resistance (AMR), 133–136, 528–531
Antipsychotics, 236, 239–240
Anus, 367, **368**
Anxiety, **234**
Anxiolytics, **233**
Apgar test, 509
Aplastic anemia, 176
APMs (Advanced Alternative Payment Models), 1165
Apocrine glands, 390, 391
Appendix, 365f, **367**, 367f
Aqueductal stenosis, 247
Aqueous humor, 269
ARBs (angiotensin receptor blockers), 205
ARF (acute renal failure), 476
Arrhythmias, 294, 296
Arteries, **301**, 302–303
Arteriosclerotic heart disease (ASHD), 302
Arthritis, 406–407
Arthropathies, **406**–410
Articulations, **419**
AS (ankylosing spondylitis), 413
Ascariasis, 117
Ascending colon, 365f, 367, 367f
ASD (acute stress disorder), 242
ASHD (arteriosclerotic heart disease), 302
Aspergillus, 118, 121
Aspiration pneumonia, 119, 337
Aspirin, 283
Assault, 446
Assuming, **23**
Asthma, 341–342
Asymptomatic infections, 102, **124**
Atherosclerosis, **302**
Athlete's foot (tinea pedis), 118
ATIN (acute tubulointerstitial nephritis), 476
Atlas, 411
ATN (acute tubular necrosis), 476
Atopic conjunctivitis, 267–268
Atopic dermatitis, 382–383
Atrial fibrillation, 296–297
Atrium, 295f, **296**
Atypical pneumonia, 119
Atypical schizophrenia, 239
Audiology-related abbreviations, 285
Auditory dysfunctions, 278–284
    endolymphatic hydrops, 278
    hearing loss, 280–283
    labyrinthitis, 280
    otitis media, 278
    otosclerosis, 279
    perichondritis, 278
    tumors of ear canal, 279

Aura, 247
Auscultation, 307
Autologous, **527**, 527t
Automobile insurance, **1163**
Autosomal recessive agammaglobulinemia, 189
Autosomal recessive inherited diseases, 507
Avulsion fractures, 433
Avulsions, **437**

B

Bacilli, 104, 104f
Background retinopathy, 205
Bacteremia, 128
Bacteria and bacterial infections, **104**–108, 104f, 106t
Bacterial meningitis, 105, 244–245
Bacterial pneumonia, 119, 332, 337
Bacterial vaginosis (BV), 482
Basal cell carcinoma, 149f, 395
Basal skull fractures, 435
Basophils, 185, 186
Beau's lines, 388
Bedsores. See Pressure ulcers
Behavioral disorders, 231, 232–236
Behavioral disturbances, **229**
Benign neoplasms, **149**, 151
Benign prostatic hyperplasia (BPH), **480**
Beta-hemolytic streptococci, 266
Bile, 370, 371
Biopsies, 147
Bipolar disorder, 230, 236–237
Birth defects, 505
Birth presentations, 492, 492f
Bites, 437–438
Bladder. See Gallbladder; Urinary bladder
Bladder cancer, **478**
Blepharitis, **264**
Blindness, 205, 275
Blisters, **384**
Blood. See also Blood disorders
    components of, 173
    defined, **173**
    formation of, 173–174
    role of, 174, 175f
    transfusions, 184
    types and Rh factor, 182–183
Blood cultures, 147
Blood disorders, 174–186
    anemia, 162, 174–177, 474–475, 507
    clotting disorders, 178–180
    hematologic malignancies, 178
    hemolytic disease of the newborn, 182
    leukocytosis, 147, 185

    leukopenia, 185
    neutropenia, 185
    sickle cell disease, 177–178
    thrombocytopenia, 181, 183–184
    of white blood cells, 185–186
Blood infections, 128–133
Blood loss anemia, 176
Blood pressure, 305–306, 305t
Blood types, **182**
Blood urea nitrogen (BUN), 471
Blowout fractures, 435
Body mass index (BMI), 213, 214
Boils, 393
Bone fractures. See Fractures
Bone marrow, 173, 174f, 185
Bowman's membrane, 268
Bowstring tears, 438
BPH (benign prostatic hyperplasia), **480**
Brachial plexus, 250
Brackets, 55
Bradycardia, 296
BRCA gene, 163
Breast cancer, 163
Bromhidrosis, 391
Bronchitis, 332
Bronchopulmonary dysplasia, 501
Bruises (contusions), 436, 436f, 438
Bucket-handle tears, 438
Buckle fractures, 434
Bulbar conjunctiva, 263, **264**
Bulla, **393**, 394f
BUN (blood urea nitrogen), 471
Burns, 450–457
    defined, **451**
    extent of, 453–456, 454f
    infections and, 456
    sequelae of, 457
    severity of, 450–451, 451f
    site of, 450, 451–453
    solar and radiation, 457
Bursitis, 415
Burst fractures, 433
BV (bacterial vaginosis), 482

C

CAD (coronary artery disease), 303
Caffeine, 234
Ca in situ, 151
Calcitonin, 198
Calcium channel blockers, 303
Campylobacter, 106t
Cancer. See also Neoplasms
    bladder, 478
    breast, 163
    cervical, 483
    chemotherapy and, 162
    colon, 163

leukemia, 122, 154, 178
liver, 372
lung, 332
metastasis of, 151
oral, 373
pancreatic, 371
skin, 149f, 394–396, 398
stages of, 148t
Cancer registries, 148, 149, 159, 165
Candida albicans, 118, 266
CAP (community-acquired pneumonia), 119, 332
Capitation plans, **1163**–1164
Carbapenem-resistant *Enterobacteriaceae* (CRE), 133, 134
Carboplatin, 283
Carbuncles, **393**
Carcinoma, **149**. *See also* Cancer
Cardiac arrest, 294–296, 295f, 297
Cardiac asthma, 298
Cardia region of stomach, 361
Cardiovascular disorders, 294–320. *See also* Heart conditions; Hypertension
angina pectoris, 303
atherosclerosis, 302
cerebral infarction, 316–318
cerebrovascular accident, 247, 303, 316, 317f, 318
cerebrovascular disease, 229, 315, 319–320
coronary artery disease, 303
deep vein thrombosis, 302
hypotension, 240, 305, 305t
Cardiovascular system, 301, 301f. *See also* Cardiovascular disorders
Carpal tunnel syndrome, 249
Carriers, **523**, 524
Case law, 1187, 1188f
Cataracts, 205, **271**, 276–277
Catatonic schizophrenia, 239
Category I codes (CPT), 11
Category II codes (CPT), 10, 11
Category III codes (CPT), 10, 11
Category notes, 60
Causalgia, 250
Cause of injury codes, 430
CBC (complete blood count), 174
CDC. *See* Centers for Disease Control and Prevention
Cecum, **365**, 365f, 367, 367f
Celiac disease, 373
Cellulitis, 107
Centers for Disease Control and Prevention (CDC)
on antimicrobial resistance, 133, 134
authority of, 1187
on congenital heart defects, 508

on exemptions from use of POA indicators, 550
formation of, 1160
growth charts from, 214
on hypertension, 306
on protection from ultraviolet rays, 396
on sexually transmitted diseases, 482
on viral hepatitis, 110, 111
Centers for Medicare and Medicaid Services (CMS)
defined, **1160**
documentation principles from, 24–25
National Correct Coding Initiative from, 1165–1166
on Present-On-Admission indicators, 545–546, 549
Central nervous system (CNS)
hereditary and degenerative diseases of, 245–246
hydrocephalus and, 247, 248
inflammatory conditions of, 244–245
migraine headaches and, 247–248, 253–254
Central pain syndrome, 253
Cerebral infarction, 316, **317**, 318
Cerebral palsy, 418
Cerebrospinal fluid (CSF), 247
Cerebrovascular accident (CVA), 247, 303, **316**, 317f, 318
Cerebrovascular disease, 229, 315, 319–320
Cerumen, 282
Cervical cancer, 483
Cervical Pap smears, 486
Cervical plexus, 250
Cervical vertebrae, 411, 412f
CF (cystic fibrosis), 217, 330, 505, 507
Chapter heads, in Tabular List, 78, 80f
Cheeks, 356
Chemical table. *See* Table of Drugs and Chemicals (ICD-10-CM)
Chemotherapy, 162
CHF (congestive heart failure), 298, 306, 311–312
Chickenpox (varicella), 102, 113, 115
Childbirth. *See* Pregnancy
Chlamydia, 482
Chlamydophila pneumoniae, 119
Cholangitis, 371
Cholecystitis, 371
Cholelithiasis, **371**
Cholera, 105
Chondropathies, **406**
Chorionic villus sampling, 506

Choroid, 268f, **272**, 273f
Christmas disease, 179
Chromhidrosis, 391
Chromosomal abnormalities, 506–507
Chronic conditions, coding guidelines for, 66, **67**
Chronic infections, **102**
Chronic kidney disease (CKD), 472–476
anemia in, 474–475
defined, **472**
diabetes mellitus with renal manifestations, 205, 474
dialysis for, 475
end-stage renal disease, 473
hypertensive, 313–314, 473
laboratory tests for, 472–473
transplantation for, 475–476
Chronic lung disease, 501
Chronic migraines, 248
Chronic obstructive pulmonary disease (COPD), **340**–341
Chronic pain, **251**
Chronic pain syndrome, 251
Ciliary body, 268f, **272,** 273f
Circulatory manifestations of diabetes mellitus, 206
Circulatory system, 301, 301f. *See also* Cardiovascular disorders
Cirrhosis, 372
Cisplatin, 283
Civil law, **1188**–1190
Civil penalties, 1204
CKD. *See* Chronic kidney disease
Classic hemophilia, 179
Classification systems, **2**
Cleft lip/cleft palate, 507
Clinical documentation, 22–35
abstracting in, 23–25, 39
assuming vs. interpreting in, 23
co-morbidities and, 29
diagnostic statement deconstruction in, 25–27
external cause reporting in, 30–31
manifestations and, 28–29
procedural statement deconstruction in, 31–32
professional services involved in, 22–23
queries in, 34–35, 39
sequelae and, 30
source documents for, 23–24
Clinically significant conditions, **500**–501
Closed angle glaucoma, 273
Closed (simple) fractures, 432–433, 433f
Clostridium difficile (*C. diff*), 133, 134
Clostridium perfringens, 106t
Clotting disorders, 178–180

INDEX 1231

CMS. *See* Centers for Medicare and Medicaid Services
CMV (cytomegalovirus), 120
CNS. *See* Central nervous system
Coagulation, **178**–180
Coal worker's pneumoconiosis, 332
Cocci, 104*f*, 105
Coccyx, 411, 412, 412*f*
Code also notation, 60
Code first notation, 58–59
Code sequencing, 66
Codes of ethics, 1206–1208
Coding, 2–17
    Alphabetic Indexes for, 41–43
    diagnostic, 4–9
    for equipment and supplies, 17
    full code descriptions for, 43–44
    guidelines for, 45–46
    procedural, 9–16
    process for, 39–40
    purposes of, 2–3
    symbols and notations used in, 43–45, 54–63
Coding for coverage, **1191**
Coding process, **39**–40
Co-insurance, 1164
Colds, 338
Colles' fractures, 433*f*
Colon (anatomy), 367–369, 367*f*
Colon cancer, 163
Colonization, 101, 135
Colonoscopy, 3
Colon (punctuation), 56
Combination codes, 61, 67, 135
Combined systolic and diastolic heart failure, 298
Comminuted fractures, 433, 433*f*
Common bile duct, **370**, 370*f*
Common law, **1187**
Common variable immunodeficiency (CVID), 122
Communicable diseases, 102–103. *See also* Infections
Communicating hydrocephalus, 247
Community-acquired pneumonia (CAP), 119, 332
Co-morbidities, **29**, 551–**552**
Complete blood count (CBC), 174
Complex fractures, 433*f*
Complex regional pain syndrome (CRPS), 250
Compliance programs, 1208–1209
Complications
    defined, **551**
    documentation of, 458
    endocrine disorders, 211–212
    major complications and co-morbidities, 551, 552

neoplasms and, 162
pain as, 459
of pregnancy, 495–499
Compound (open) fractures, 432–433, 433*f*
Computerized tomography (CT) scans, 471
Conception. *See* Pregnancy
Concurrent coding, **541**, 542*f*
Condition, defined, **4**, **73**
Cones, 272, **273**
Confidentiality, 122. *See also* HIPAA Privacy Rule
Confirmed diagnoses, **61**, 67
Congenital, defined, **505**
Congenital anomalies, 281, 329, 330, 505–506, 508
Congenital heart defects, 508
Congenital hernia, 508
Congenital hip dysplasia, 418
Congenital lactase deficiency, 218
Congenital myopathies, 418
Congenital nasolacrimal duct anomalies, 265–266
Congenital (primary) immunodeficiency conditions, 122
Congenital rubella syndrome (CRS), 114
Congestive heart failure (CHF), 298, 306, 311–312
Conjunctivitis, 75, 83–84, 265, **267**–268
Consultations, 24
Contact dermatitis, 383
Contact exposure to infection, 102
Contiguous boundaries, 159
Continuing care, 525–527
Contracts, 1189, 1190*f*
Contusions, 436, 436*f*, 438
Co-payments, 1164
COPD (chronic obstructive pulmonary disease), **340**–341
Cornea, 268–269*f*, **268**–270, 273*f*
Corneal dystrophy, **270**
Corneal ulcers, 269–270
Coronary artery disease (CAD), 303
Corrosions, 450, **451**, 457
Corticosteroids, 308
Corticotropin, 211
Covered entities, **1195**
CPT. *See* Current Procedural Terminology
Cramps, muscle, 416
Craniofacial dissociation, 435
Creatinine, 471, 472
CRE (carbapenem-resistant *Enterobacteriaceae*), 133, 134
Criminal law, **1187**–1188, 1189*f*
Criminal penalties, 1204
CRPS (complex regional pain syndrome), 250

CRS (congenital rubella syndrome), 114
CSF (cerebrospinal fluid), 247
CT (computerized tomography) scans, 471
Current conditions, 69
Current Procedural Terminology (CPT)
    Alphabetic Index, 10, 11*f*, 41
    Category I codes, 11
    Category II codes, 10, 11
    Category III codes, 10, 11
    conventions used in, 45
    format of codes in, 11–12
    guidelines for, 46
    Main Section, 43, 45
    organization of, 10, 11*f*
Cushing's syndrome, 204, **211**, 308
CVA. *See* Cerebrovascular accident
CVID (common variable immunodeficiency), 122
Cyanosis, 329
Cystic duct, 370, 370*f*
Cystic fibrosis (CF), 217, 330, 505, 507
Cystitis, 477
Cysts, **393**
Cytomegalovirus (CMV), 120

D

Dacryocystitis, **266**
Dacryops, 266
DDH (developmental dysplasia of the hip), 418
Deafness. *See* Hearing loss
Death/discharge summary, 541
Decubitus ulcers, **384**
Deductibles, 1165
Deep third-degree burns, 450
Deep vein thrombosis (DVT), 302
Deer ticks, 116*f*
Deformities, **507**
Dehydration, 162, 217
Delivery. *See* Labor and delivery
Dementia, 229, 231–232, 245–246
Demographics, **24**
Dendrites, 232
Dendritic corneal ulcer, 270
Dental services, 17
Dependence on substances, **233**, 344
Dependents, **1160**
Depressed fractures, 433
Depressed skull fractures, 435
Depression, 230, 237–238
Depressive episodes, **236**
Dermal papillae, 382
Dermatitis, 382–383
Dermatopolymyositis, 415
Dermis, **382**, 383*f*
Descemet's membrane, 269
Descending colon, 367*f*, **368**

Deutschlander's disease, 433
Developmental dysplasia of the hip (DDH), 418
Developmental lactase deficiency, 218
Diabetes insipidus (DI), 210
Diabetes mellitus (DM), 203–210
    cataracts and, 271
    conditions related to, 208–210
    defined, **203**
    diagnostic testing for, 204
    hypoglycemics for, 207
    insulin and insulin pumps for, 204, 206, 208–210
    manifestations of, 205–206, 275, 474
    metabolic process dysfunction in, 216
    signs and symptoms of, 203–204
    types of, 204
Diabetic nephropathy, 205
Diabetic neuropathy, 205, 249
Diabetic retinopathy, 205, 275
Diagnoses
    confirmed, 61, 67
    defined, **3**
    differential, 68
    first-listed, 71
    of neoplasms, 146–149, 148*t*
    postoperative, 88
    preoperative, 88
    principal, 66, 71, 551
    unconfirmed, 71–72
Diagnosis coding. *See* International Classification of Diseases–10th Revision–Clinical Modification (ICD-10-CM)
Diagnosis-related groups (DRGs), **550**–552, **1164**
Diagnostic statement deconstruction, 25–27
Dialysis, 475
Diaper dermatitis, 383
Diastolic heart failure, 298
Diastolic pressure (DP), 306
Differential diagnoses, **68**
Digestive disorders, 356–374
    of accessory organs, 370–373, 370*f*
    alcohol involvement in, 373–374
    celiac disease, 373
    cholecystitis, 371
    diverticular disease, 369
    edentulism, 357–358
    of esophagus, 360–361
    gastroesophageal reflux disease, 360–361, 374
    hepatitis, 101, 103, 109*f*, 110–112, 122, 372
    hernias, 363–364
    of large intestine, 367–369
    of oral cavity, 356–359
    pancreatitis, 371, 374
    of salivary glands, 359
    sialoadenitis, 359
    of small intestine, 364–366
    of stomach, 361–364
    ulcerative colitis, 368–369
    ulcers, 206, 361, 362–363, 365–366
Diphtheria, 104
Directives, 1185–1187
Disability compensation, **1162**
Discharge disposition, 541
Discharge instructions, 541
Discharge summaries, 24, 541, 542–543
Disclosure, **1197**–1198
Discounted fee-for-service plans, **1163**
Diseases. *See specific names and types of diseases*
Diseases classified elsewhere, 103
Dislocations, **430**
Disorganized schizophrenia, 239
Disseminated cancer, 151
Diuretics, 283, 330
Diverticular disease, 369
DM. *See* Diabetes mellitus
DMD (Duchenne's muscular dystrophy), 418
DME (durable medical equipment), 17
Documentation. *See* Clinical documentation
Dominant genetic disorders, 505
Dorsopathies, **406**, 412–415
Double billing, **1191**
Dowager's hump, 412
Down syndrome (trisomy 21), 506–507
DP (diastolic pressure), 306
DRGs (diagnosis-related groups), **550**–552, **1164**
Droplet exposure to infection, 102
Drug-related disorders, 232–235
Drug-resistant *Neisseria gonorrhoeae*, 133, 134–135
Drug table. *See* Table of Drugs and Chemicals (ICD-10-CM)
Drug therapy, 17, 525–526
Duchenne's muscular dystrophy (DMD), 418
Duodenum, 361*f*, **364**–365, 365*f*, 370*f*
Durable medical equipment (DME), 17
DVT (deep vein thrombosis), 302
Dyslipidemia, **204**
Dysphagia, 320, 361
Dysphasia, 320
Dyspnea, 330, 334
Dysrhythmias, 296
Dysthymic disorder, 230
Dystonia, 240

E

Ears. *See* Auditory dysfunctions
Earwax, 282
Eccrine glands, 390, 391*f*
ECG (electrocardiogram), 299, 307
Echocardiography, 299, 307
Ectoparasites, 118
Ectopic neoplasms, **159**–160
Ectromelia, 418
Edema, 298, 302, **306**
Edentulism, **357**–358
Electrocardiogram (ECG), 299, 307
Electronic health record (EHR), 23
Electronic media claims (EMCs), **1158**
Electronic remittance advice (ERA), **1173**
Elevated blood pressure, **306**
Eligibility verification, **1174**
Embolus, **299**, 300, 302, 316, 332, 334
Embryonic period, 488
EMCs (electronic media claims), **1158**
Emphysema, 330
Encephalitis, 244
Endocrine disorders, 199–218. *See also* Diabetes mellitus (DM)
    Cushing's syndrome, 204, 211, 308
    diabetes insipidus, 210
    metabolic, 216–218
    nutritional deficiencies related to, 212
    postprocedural complications, 211–212
    thyroid disorders, 199–202
    weight factors related to, 213–214
Endolymphatic hydrops, 278
Endometriosis, 486
Endothelial corneal dystrophy, 270
Endothelium, 269
End-stage renal disease (ESRD), 473
EOB (explanation of benefits), **1173**
Eosinophils, 185, 186
Epicondylitis, 415, 416
Epidermis, **382**, 383*f*
Epididymitis, 134
Epiglottis, 360, 360*f*
Episodic care, **1164**
Epithelial corneal dystrophy, 270
Epithelium, 268
Eponychium, 388, 388*f*
Eponyms, **4**, 31, **73**
Equipment and supplies, 17
ERA (electronic remittance advice), **1173**
Erectile dysfunction, 482
Erythrocytes. *See* Red blood cells (RBCs)
Erythromycin, 332

Erythropoiesis, 173
Escherichia coli (*E. coli*), 106t, 134, 479
Esophagus, **360**–361
ESRD (end-stage renal disease), 473
Essential hypertension, 307
Ethical and legal coding, 1185–1209
    codes of ethics, 1206–1208
    compliance programs, 1208–1209
    False Claims Act on, 1193–1195
    Health Care Fraud and Abuse Control Program, 1205
    HIPAA Privacy Rule, 1186, 1195–1205
    rules for, 1190–1193
    sources for legal guidance, 1185–1190
Etiology, **29**
Evolving pressure ulcers, 386
Exacerbation, defined, **341**
Excised malignancies, 160–161
Excludes1 notation, 57
Excludes2 notation, 57–58
Excretory urography, 308
Executive orders, **1187**
Exfoliative dermatitis, 383
Exophthalmos, 265
Explanation of benefits (EOB), **1173**
Exposure to tobacco, 343–344
Extent of burns, **453**–456, 454f
External causes
    activity codes, 430
    cause of injury codes, 430
    defined, **6, 78**
    Index to External Causes, 6–7, 7f, 31, 77–78, 78f
    patient status codes, 430
    place of occurrence codes, 430
    reporting, 30–31, 429–432
    respiratory disorders and, 345–347
External optical disorders, 263–266
Extraocular muscles, **267**
Eyelids, 263, 264, 264f
Eyes. *See also* Optical disorders
    abbreviations related to, 285
    exterior of, 263, 264f
    interior of, 267–269f, 268–269, 271–273, 273f
    lacrimal apparatus of, 265

F

False Claims Act of 1863 (FCA), 1193–1195, 1193f
Familial hypercholesterolemia, 505
Familial retinoblastoma, 505
Family history codes, 146, 163, 505, 523–524
Farsightedness, 271

Fatigue fractures, 433
FCA (False Claims Act of 1863), 1193–1195, 1193f
Federal Register, 1185, 1186f
Fee-for-service (FFS) plans, **1163**
Felonies, 1188
Femoral hernias, 364
Femur fractures, 440
Fertility testing, 487
Fertilization, 488
Fetal abnormalities, 497
Fevers, 102
FFS (fee-for-service) plans, **1163**
Fiber-type disproportion, 418
Fibromyalgia, 415
Fight or flight response, 242
Fingerprints, 382
First-degree burns, 450, **451**, 451f
First-listed diagnoses, **71**
Fissured (linear) fractures, 433
Flappers, 437
Flatworms, 117
Fleas, 118
Fleming, Alexander, 133
Flexibilitas cerea, 239
Flu. *See* Influenza
Fluoroscopy, 471
Focal hyperhidrosis, 390
Folic acid, 508
Food, exposure to infection through, 103
Foodborne illnesses, 105–106, 106t
Food poisoning, 105–106
Forearm fractures, 440
Fractures
    pathological, 419–421
    seventh characters for, 439–440
    traumatic, 432–435, 433f
Fragile X syndrome, 508
Frey's syndrome, 390
Fuchs' dystrophy, 270
Functional activity of neoplasms, **156**–157
Fundus, **361**, 361f
Fungal pneumonia, 121
Fungi and fungal infections, **118**
Furuncles, **393**

G

Gallbladder, **370**–371, 370f, 372f
Gangrene, 206, **363**, **386**
Gastric juices, 361
Gastric (peptic) ulcers, 361, 362–363
Gastritis, 374
Gastroenteritis, 338
Gastroesophageal reflux disease (GERD), 360–361, 374
Gastrojejunal ulcers, 365–366

Gatekeepers, 1158, **1159**
Gaucher's disease, 505
GDM (gestational diabetes mellitus), **204**
Generalized cancer, 151
Gene therapy, 506
Genetic abnormalities, **506**
Genetic conditions, 505–508
    autosomal recessive inherited diseases, 507
    chromosomal abnormalities, 506–507
    congenital malformations vs., 505
    multifactorial abnormalities, 507
    respiratory disorders and, 330
    testing for, 487, 506
    x-linked inherited diseases, 507–508
Genetics, defined, 505
Genetic susceptibility, 523–524
Genetic testing, 487, 506
Genital herpes, 482
Genitourinary disorders, 471–484. *See also* Chronic kidney disease (CKD)
    acute renal failure, 476
    bladder cancer, 478
    diagnostic tools for, 471
    of male genital organs, 479–482
    renal calculi, 477–478
    sexually transmitted diseases, 482–484
    urinary tract infections, 471, 477
Gentamicin, 283
Genu recurvatum, 408
GERD (gastroesophageal reflux disease), 360–361, 374
German measles (rubella), 114, 281
Gestation, **488**–489, 497
Gestational diabetes mellitus (GDM), **204**
Gestational hypertension, **310**–311
GFR (glomerular filtration rate), **472**, 473
Glands
    apocrine, 390, 391
    eccrine, 390, 391f
    of eyelids, 263, 264
    parathyroid, 198–199
    salivary, 359
    sebaceous, 389
    thyroid, 198, 199f
Glands of Zeis, 263, **264**
Glaucoma, **273**–274
Glomerular filtration rate (GFR), **472**, 473
Glucose tolerance test (GTT), 204
Gluten enteropathy, 373
Goiter, 200, 201
Golfer's elbow (medial epicondylitis), 415, 416
Gonorrhea, 105, 134–135, 483
Gout, 408, 409

Government insurance plans, 1159–1161
GPO (U.S. Government Printing Office), 1185
Graves' disease, 200, 265
Greater curvature, 361
Greater omentum, 365
Greenstick fractures, 433, 433f
Grippe. *See* Influenza
GTT (glucose tolerance test), 204
Gum (periodontal) disease, 373, 375
Guttate psoriasis, 384
Gynecologists and gynecologic care, **485**–488

H

HACs (hospital–acquired conditions), **546**–547
Hair, **389**, 390f
Hair disorders, 389
Hair follicles, **389**, 390f
HAIs (health care-acquired infections), 102
Hallucinogens, 234
H&P (history and physical) form, 24, 546, 546–547f
Hard palate, 356, 357f
Hashimoto's thyroiditis, 201
HCFACP (Health Care Fraud and Abuse Control Program), 1205
HCFA (Health Care Financing Administration), 1159–1160
HCPCS Level II codes. *See* Healthcare Common Procedure Coding System Level II codes
Headaches, 247–248, 253–254
Head of pancreas, 370f, 371
Healing pressure ulcers, 386
Health care, defined, **1157**
Health care–acquired infections (HAIs), 102
Health care clearinghouses, 1196
Healthcare Common Procedure Coding System (HCPCS) Level II codes
    Alphabetic Index, 17, 17f, 41
    Alphanumeric Section, 17, 18f, 43, 45
    conventions used in, 45
    for equipment and supplies, 17
    format of, 17
    overview, 15–16
Health Care Financing Administration (HCFA), 1159–1160
Health Care Fraud and Abuse Control Program (HCFACP), 1205
Health insurance, 1156–1167
    compensation methods, 1163–1165
    co-payments/co-insurance, 1164

    coverage determination, 1166, 1167f
    deductibles, 1165
    managed care, 1156, 1157
    out-of-pocket contributions, 1164–1165
    participants in, 1158
    plan types, 1158–1163
    premiums, 1156
    role of, 1156–1158
    third-party payers and, 3, 1158
Health maintenance organizations (HMOs), **1158**–1159
Hearing loss
    causes of, 281, 283
    degrees of, 281, 281t
    psychogenic, 282
    signs and symptoms of, 280–281
    sound levels and, 283, 284t
Hearing services, 17
Heart, anatomical components of, 294, 295f
Heart attack. *See* Myocardial infarction (MI)
Heartburn, 360–361
Heart conditions, 294–300
    arrhythmias/dysrhythmias, 294, 296
    atrial fibrillation, 296–297
    cardiac arrest, 294–296, 295f, 297
    congenital defects, 508
    heart failure, 298, 306, 311–312
    hypertensive heart disease, 311–312, 314
    mitral valve prolapse, 296
    myocardial infarction, 294, 299–300
Heart failure, 298, 306, 311–312
Heat rash, 390
Hebephrenic schizophrenia, 239
Helminths, 117
Hematologic malignancies, 178
Hematomas, 436
Hematopoiesis, **173**
Hemimelia, 418
Hemiparesis, 249, 418
Hemiplegia, 249, 418
Hemodialysis, 475
Hemoglobin, **174**
Hemolysis, **184**
Hemolytic anemia, 176
Hemolytic disease of the newborn, 182
Hemophilia, 179–180, 507–508
Hemophilus influenzae, 120
Hemorrhages, **362**
Hemorrhagic anemia, 176
Hemorrhagic attacks, 316, 317f
Hemostasis, **178**, 179f
Hemostatic disorders, 178–179

Hemothorax, 330, 334
Hepatic duct, 370, 370f
Hepatic encephalopathy, 111
Hepatic flexure, 367–368
Hepatitis, 101, 103, 109f, 110–112, 122, 372
Hepatopancreatic ampulla, 370, 370f
Hepatopancreatic sphincter, 364, 370, 370f
Hereditary hypogammaglobulinemia, 189
Hereditary transmission, 505
Hernias, **363**–364, 508
Herniated discs, 414–415
Herpes simplex virus (HSV), 102, 114–115, 270, 281, 482
Herpesviral keratitis, 270
Herpes zoster virus, 113, 115
Hiatal hernias, 364
High blood pressure. *See* Hypertension
High-risk pregnancy, 490
HIPAA Privacy Rule, 1195–1205
    covered entities under, 1195–1196
    defined, **1195**
    notices regarding, 1202
    protected health information under, 1196–1197
    refusals to release patient information, 1205
    Release of Information forms and, 1198, 1199f
    statutory laws regarding, 1186
    use and disclosure under, 1197–1198, 1200–1201
    violation of, 1198f, 1203–1204, 1203f
Hirsutism, 389
Histopathology, 147
Histoplasmosis, 118
History and physical (H&P) form, 24, 546, 546–547f
HIV/AIDS, 122–127
    case study, 124–125
    clinical manifestations of, 483
    confidentiality and, 122
    defined, **101**
    gonorrhea and, 134
    inconclusive tests, 124
    medical necessity of testing, 122–123
    negative tests, 123–124
    obstetrics and, 126–127
    pneumonia as manifestation of, 121, 337
    positive tests, 124
    spread of, 103
    tuberculosis and, 332
    with unrelated conditions, 126
HMOs (health maintenance organizations), **1158**–1159

Hookworms, 116
Hormones, 198, 199, 210, 211, 471
Hospital-acquired conditions (HACs), **546**–547
Hospital-acquired pneumonia, 119
Hospital coding. *See* Inpatient coding
Hospital course, 541
HPV (human papillomavirus), 483
HSV. *See* Herpes simplex virus
Human bites, 437
Human papillomavirus (HPV), 483
Huntington's chorea, 245
Hutchinson-Guilford progeria, 505
Hydrocele, 480
Hydrocephalus, 247, 248, 508
Hydrops fetalis, 183
Hypercapnic respiratory failure, 336
Hyperchloremia, 216
Hyperemesis gravidarum, 495
Hyperglycemia, **208**
Hyperhidrosis, 390
Hypersensitivity reactions, 189
Hypertension, 305–315
    blood pressure levels and, 305, 305*t*
    defined, **305**
    essential, 307
    gestational, 310–311
    heart failure and, 298
    hypertensive crisis, 309–310
    manifestations of, 311–315
    prevalence of, 306
    primary, 306–307
    pulmonary arterial, 330
    risk factors for, 306
    secondary, 298, 308
Hypertensive cerebrovascular disease, 315
Hypertensive chronic kidney disease, 313–314, 473
Hypertensive crisis, 309–310
Hypertensive heart disease, 311–312, 314
Hypertensive retinopathy, 275–276, 315
Hyperthyroidism, 200–201, 296
Hyphens, 63
Hypnotics, **233**
Hypochondria, 241
Hypodermis, 382
Hypoglycemia, **208**
Hypoglycemics, **207**
Hyponychium, 388
Hypoparathyroidism, 271
Hypopharynx, 360
Hypopyon, 269
Hypotension, 240, **305**, 305*t*
Hypothyroidism, **199**–200

Hypoxemic respiratory failure, 336
Hysterical (psychogenic) hearing loss, 282

I

ICD-10-CM. *See* International Classification of Diseases–10th Revision–Clinical Modification
ICD-O (International Classification of Diseases for Oncology), 158–159
ICD-10-PCS. *See* International Classification of Diseases–10th Revision–Procedure Coding System
IDDM (insulin-dependent diabetes mellitus), 204
Ileum, **365**, 365*f*, 367, 367*f*
Imaging reports, 24
Immune system, 188–189
Immunodeficiency disorders, 122–127, 189
Impacted fractures, 433, 433*f*
Impetigo, 105
Incidental pregnant state, 490
Incisional hernias, 364
Incisions, 436*f*
Includes notation, 57
Incomplete fractures, 433*f*
Index to Diseases and Injuries. *See* Alphabetic Index (ICD-10-CM)
Index to External Causes (ICD-10-CM), 6–7, 7*f*, 31, 77–**78**, 78*f*
Infantile idiopathic scoliosis, 412
Infants. *See* Neonatal conditions
Infarction, 316, **317**, 318
Infected fractures, 433
Infections, 101–136. *See also specific diseases*
    acute vs. chronic, 101–102
    antimicrobial resistance to, 133–136
    asymptomatic, 102, 124
    bacterial, 104–108, 104*f*, 106*t*
    of blood, 128–133
    burns and, 456
    communicable, 102–103
    defined, **101**, **109**
    fungal, 118
    immunodeficiency conditions, 122–127
    inflammation and, 102
    parasitic, 116–117, 137
    reporting, 103–104
    spread of, 101, 102–103
    systemic, 101, 102, 126
    viral, 109–110*f*, 109–115

Infertility, 481, 482
Inflammation, **102**
Influenza, 102, 109*f*, 112–113, 120, 332, **338**
Inguinal hernias, 364
Inhalants, 234
Inheritance patterns, 506
Injuries, 432–440. *See also specific injuries*
    fractures, 419–421, 432–435, 433*f*
    muscular, 438–439
    seventh characters for status of care reporting, 439–440
    wounds, 436–438, 436*f*
Inpatient, defined, **12**
Inpatient facilities, **72**
Inpatient (hospital) coding, 541–553
    complications and co-morbidities in, 551–552
    concurrent coding, 541, 542*f*
    confirming medical necessity in, 48
    diagnosis-related groups in, 550–552
    diagnostic statement deconstruction in, 26
    discharge coding, 541, 542–543
    Official Guidelines for, 71–72, 544–545
    Present-On-Admission indicators in, 545–550
    principal diagnoses in, 71, 551
    unconfirmed diagnoses in, 71–72
    Uniform Hospital Discharge Data Set in, 552–553
Inpatient Prospective Payment System (IPPS), 550, 551
Insect bites, 103
Insect bites, 437
Insulin and insulin pumps, 204, 206, 208–210
Insulin-dependent diabetes mellitus (IDDM), 204
Insurance. *See also* Health insurance
    automobile, 1163
    disability compensation, 1162
    liability, 1162
    workers' compensation, 429, 1161–1162
Integumentary conditions, 382–396
    glandular disorders, 390–391
    hair disorders, 389
    nail disorders, 388–389
    skin disorders, 382–387, 393–396
Interactions, 447–449
Internal optical disorders, 267–273
International Classification of Diseases for Oncology (ICD-O), 158–159

International Classification of Diseases–10th Revision–Clinical Modification (ICD-10-CM), 54–88. *See also* Z codes
  abbreviations in, 56
  Alphabetic Index, 4–5, 4*f*, 41, 72–76*f*
  case studies, 568–576
  conventions used in, 44–45, 54–63
  examples of, 8–9
  format of codes in, 7
  Index to External Causes, 6–7, 7*f*, 31, 77–78, 78*f*
  Introduction section of, 54
  Neoplasm Table, 5, 6*f*, 76–77, 76*f*, 151–152, 152*f*
  Official Guidelines for, 45, 61, 63–72, 544–545
  punctuation in, 55–56
  screenings and preventive services, 87–88
  systemic conditions and, 85–86
  Table of Drugs and Chemicals, 5–6, 6*f*, 77, 77*f*, 440–444
  Tabular List of Diseases and Injuries, 5, 5*f*, 43–45, 78–84, 79*t*, 80–81*f*, 83–84*f*
  unrelated conditions and, 84–85
International Classification of Diseases–10th Revision–Procedure Coding System (ICD-10-PCS)
  Alphabetic Index, 12, 41, 45
  conventions used in, 45
  format of codes in, 12–15
  Official Guidelines for, 46
  Tables section, 12, 13*f*, 43
Interpreting, **23**, 32
Interstitial pneumonia, 332
Intervertebral discs, **411**, 413–414
Intracranial abscess, 244
Intractable migraines, 247
Intravenous pyelogram (IVP), 471
IPPS (Inpatient Prospective Payment System), 550, 551
Iris, 264*f*, 268–269*f*, **272**, 273*f*
Iron deficiency anemia, 175
Irritant contact dermatitis, 383
Ischemic attacks, 316, 317*f*
Islets of Langerhans, 371
Isogeneic, **527**, 527*t*
Italicized brackets, 55
IVP (intravenous pyelogram), 471

J

Jaundice, 372, 501
Jejunum, **365**, 365*f*
Jock itch (tinea cruris), 118

Juvenile dermatomyositis (JDM), 415
Juvenile diabetes, 204
Juvenile idiopathic scoliosis, 413

K

Karyotypes, 506
Keratitis, **269**–270
Keratoconus, 270
Kidney disease, 205, 308. *See also* Chronic kidney disease (CKD)
Kidneys, 470, 471*f*
Kidney stones, 477–478
Kidney-ureter-bladder (KUB) radiography, 471
Klebsiella pneumoniae carbapenemase (KPC), 134
Klinefelter's syndrome, 507
Klippel-Feil syndrome, 418
Knowledge requirement, 1194
KPC *(Klebsiella pneumoniae carbapenemase)*, 134
KUB (kidney-ureter-bladder) radiography, 471
Kyphosis, 412

L

Labor and delivery, 131, 491–495, 492*f*
Laboratory reports, 24, 147
Labyrinthitis, 280
Lacerations, **436**, 436*f*
Lacrimal apparatus, **265**–266
Lactose intolerance, 218
Large intestine, 367–369, 367*f*
Late effects. *See* Sequelae
Latent tuberculosis infection (LTBI), 108
Lateral epicondylitis (tennis elbow), 415
Laterality, **420**
Lateral mass fractures, 434
Lattice dystrophy, 270
LBW (low birth weight), **501**
LCD (Local Coverage Determination), 1166
LeFort fractures, 435
Left heart failure, 298, 306
Legal coding. *See* Ethical and legal coding
Legends, in Tabular List, 80–81
Leg fractures, 440
Legionella pneumophila, 119
Legionnaires' disease, 331–332
Lens, 268–269*f*, **271**
Lesions, 393–395, 394*f*
Lesser curvature, 361
Letters of appeal for reimbursement, 1178–1179
Leukemia, 122, 154, 178

Leukocytes. *See* White blood cells (WBCs)
Leukocytosis, 147, 185
Leukopenia, 185
Leukopoiesis, 173
Levator palpebrae muscle superioris, 263
Liability insurance, **1162**
Lice, 118
Linear (fissured) fractures, 433
Lingual tonsils, 356
Linking, **47**
Lips, 356, 357*f*
Listeria, 106*t*
Liver, **371**–372, 372*f*
Liver cancer, 372
Local Coverage Determination (LCD), 1166
Lockjaw (tetanus), 104, 107–108
Loop diuretics, 283
Low birth weight (LBW), **501**
Lower canaliculi, 265
Lower esophageal sphincter, 360, 361, 361*f*
LTBI (latent tuberculosis infection), 108
Lumbar plexus, 250
Lumbar punctures, 147, 178
Lumbar vertebrae, 411, 412*f*
Lung cancer, 332
Lunula, 388
Lupus, 410
Lyme disease, 103, 137
Lymphocytes, 185
Lymphomas, 178

M

MACRA (Medicare Access and CHIP Reauthorization Act of 2015), 1165
Macular edema, 205, 275
Macules, **393**, 394*f*
Maculopathy, 205
Magnetic resonance imaging (MRI), 471
Main Section (CPT), **43**, 45
Maisonneuve's fracture, 434
Major complications and co-morbidities (MCCs), 551, **552**
Major depressive disorder, 230, 237–238
Malabsorption, 374
Male genital system, 479–482, 479*f*
Malformations, **505**
Malignancies
  defined, **149**
  diagnostic tests for, 147, 148*t*
  of ectopic tissue, 159–160
  excised, 160–161
  hematologic, 178
  lesions, 394–395

Malignancies—Cont.
  overlapping boundaries of, 159
  in pregnancy, 154
  primary, 150
  in remission or relapse, 154
  secondary, 151
Malignant melanoma, 149f, 394–395
Malignant neuroleptic syndrome, 240
Malignant primary, 150
Malignant secondary, 151
Malnutrition, 374
Maltreatment, 457–458
Malunion of fractured bone, **435**
Managed care, 1156, **1157**
Manic episodes, **236**
Manifestations, **28**–**29**, **58**–59
Map-dot-fingerprint dystrophy, 270
March fractures, 433
Marfan syndrome, 296
Mass, **149**
Mastectomy, 163
Maxillary fractures, 435
MCCs (major complications and co-morbidities), 551, **552**
M codes, 159
Meares and Stamey technique, 480
Measles (rubeola), 102, 113, 330
Medial epicondylitis (golfer's elbow), 415, 416
Medicaid program, 1160, 1161f
Medical care, 1156, 1157f
Medical insurance. *See* Health insurance
Medically unlikely edits (MUE), 1166
Medical necessity
  confirming, 40, 47–48
  defined, **3**
  denial of claims due to lack of, 1175–1176
  of HIV testing, 122–123
Medical records, 23–25
Medical supplies, 17
Medicare Access and CHIP Reauthorization Act of 2015 (MACRA), 1165
Medicare program, 1160, 1160f
Medicare-Severity Diagnosis-Related Groups (MS-DRGs), 551
Medication logs, 24
Medications, 17, 525–526
MedlinePlus online dictionary, 23, 102
Meibomian glands, 263, **264**
Melanoma, 149, 149f, 394–395, 398
Ménière's disease, 278
Meningitis, 101, 105, 121, 244–245
Meningococcal disease, 121, 137
Mental disorders, 228–243
  amnestic disorder, 229–230
  dementia, 229, 231–232, 245–246
  mood disorders, 230, 236–238
  overview, 228
  personality disorders, 231, 240
  phobias, 241, 255
  physiological conditions related to, 228–231
  psychoactive substance use and, 232–236
  psychotic disorders, 239–240
  somatoform disorders, 241
  stress-related disorders, 242–243
Merit-Based Incentive Payment System (MIPS), 1165
Merkel cell carcinoma, 395
Mesentery, **365**, 365f
Metabolic disorders, 216–218
Metabolization, 216
Metastasis, **151**
Methicillin-resistant *Staphylococcus aureus* (MRSA), 105, 135–136
Migraine headaches, 247–248, 253–254
Miliaria, 390
MI (myocardial infarction), 294, **299**–300
Minicore disease, 418
MIPS (Merit-Based Incentive Payment System), 1165
Miscarriages, 499
Misdemeanors, 1187
Mites, 116f, 118
Mitral valve prolapse, 296
Mixed state bipolar disorder, 236
Modifiers
  format of, 11
  nonessential, 5, 55
  use of, 11–12
Moll's glands, 263, **264**
Monocytes, 185, 186
Monoplegia, 249
Mood (affective) disorders, 230, 236–238
Mooren's ulcer, 269
Morbidity, **502**
Morbid obesity, 213
Morning sickness, 495
Morphology, defined, **158**
Morphology codes (M codes), 159
Mortality, **502**
Mosaicism, 507
Mosquitoes, 116, 116f
Mouth, 356–359, 357f
MRI (magnetic resonance imaging), 471
MRSA (methicillin-resistant *Staphylococcus aureus*), 105, 135–136
MS-DRGs (Medicare-Severity Diagnosis-Related Groups), 551
Mucopurulent conjunctivitis, 267–268
MUE (medically unlikely edits), 1166
Multifactorial abnormalities, 507
Multiple-choice queries, 34, 35, 39
Multiple myeloma, 122, 154
Muscle cramps, 416
Muscle spasms, 416
Muscle tumors, 418
Muscular dystrophy, 418
Muscular injuries, 438–439
Muscular system, 406, 407f, 422
Musculoskeletal disorders, 406–421
  acquired conditions, 418
  arthropathies, 406–410
  congenital, 418
  fractures, 419–421, 432–435, 433f
  soft tissue disorders, 415–417
  spinal conditions, 412–415
Mutually exclusive codes, **1191**
Myalgia, **438**
Myasthenia gravis, 418
Mycoplasma pneumoniae, 119
Mycotic corneal ulcer, 269
Myelitis, 244
Myocardial infarction (MI), 294, **299**–300
Myofibrositis, 415
Myopathies, **406**, 418
Myositis, 415
Myxedema, 201

N

Nail avulsions, 437
Nail disorders, 388–389
Nail plate, 388
Nails, 387–388, 388f
Nasolacrimal duct, 264f, 265–266
National Cancer Registrars Association (NCRA), 165
National Correct Coding Initiative (NCCI), 1165–1166, 1191
National Coverage Determination (NCD), 1166, 1167f
National Heart, Lung, and Blood Institute, 298, 303
National Institutes of Health Stroke Scale (NIHSS), 318
National Kidney Foundation, 472
National Pressure Ulcer Advisory Panel (NPUAP), 384
National Program of Cancer Registries (NPCR), 165
NCCI (National Correct Coding Initiative), 1165–1166, 1191
NCD (National Coverage Determination), 1166, 1167f
NCRA (National Cancer Registrars Association), 165

NDM (*New Delhi Metallo-beta-lactamase*), 134
Nearsightedness, 271
Necessity. *See* Medical necessity
NEC (not elsewhere classifiable), **56**
Necrotizing enterocolitis (NEC), 501
Needlestick injuries, 103
Neglect, 457–458
Neisseria gonorrhoeae, 133, 134–135
Nemaline myopathy, 418
Neonatal conditions, 499–508
    clinically significant, 500–501
    congenital anomalies, 505–506, 508
    genetic, 505–508
    hemolytic disease, 182
    hydrops fetalis, 183
    lacrimal duct obstruction, 206
    maternal conditions affecting, 501–502
    pulmonary hypoplasia, 329
    respiratory distress syndrome, 329, 501, 502
    respiratory syncytial virus, 335
    sepsis, 131
    well-baby checks, 503, 521
    Z codes for, 499
Neoplasm-related pain, 253
Neoplasms, 145–163. *See also* Cancer; Malignancies
    abstracting details regarding, 149–151
    admissions related to treatment for, 160–163
    benign, 149, 151
    Ca in situ, 151
    chapter notes, 156–159
    chemotherapy and radiation therapy treatments, 162
    complications related to, 162
    defined, **149**
    diagnosis confirmation, 146–149, 148*t*
    of ear canal, 279
    ectopic, 159–160
    excised, 160–161
    functional activity of, 156–157
    grading and staging of, 147, 148*t*
    morphology (histology) of, 158–159
    muscle-related, 418
    overlapping boundaries, 159
    pathology reports on, 147–149
    prophylactic organ removal, 163
    reporting diagnoses for, 151–154, 152*f*
    screenings for, 145–146
    terms used for identification of, 149–150
    uncertain, 151
    unspecified behavior for, 151

Neoplasm Table (ICD-10-CM), 5, 6*f*, **76**–77, 76*f*, 151–152, 152*f*
Nephrogenic diabetes insipidus, 210
Nephropathy, 205
Nerve plexuses, 250
Nervous system. *See also* Neurological disorders
    central, 244–248, 253–254
    peripheral, 249–250
Neuroendocrine carcinoma, 395
Neuroleptic drugs, 239–240
Neurological disorders, 244–254
    of central nervous system, 244–248
    pain management for, 251–254
    of peripheral nervous system, 249–250
Neurologic manifestations of diabetes mellitus, 205
Neuropathy, 205, 249
Neutropenia, 185
Neutrophils, 185
Nevus, **393**
Newborns. *See* Neonatal conditions
New Delhi Metallo-beta-lactamase (NDM), 134
Nicotine dependence, 234–235
NIDDM (noninsulin-dependent diabetes mellitus), 204
NIHSS (National Institutes of Health Stroke Scale), 318
"N" indicator, 548
Nodules, **393**, 394*f*
Noncommunicating hydrocephalus, 247
Noncompliance of patients, 446
Nonessential modifiers, **5**, 55
Non-insulin-dependent diabetes mellitus (NIDDM), 204
Nonmood (psychotic) disorders, 239–240
Nontoxic goiter, 201
Nonunion of fractured bone, **435**
Normal pressure hydrocephalus (NPH), 247
NOS (not otherwise specified), 35, **56**
Nosocomial infections, **102**
Notations
    additional characters required, 63
    and, 61
    category notes, 60
    Code also, 60
    Code first, 58–59
    defined, **43**
    Excludes1, 57
    Excludes2, 57–58
    Includes, 57
    not elsewhere classifiable, 56
    not otherwise specified, 35, 56
    other specified, 61
    plus sign, 62–63

    see, 62
    see also, 62
    see condition, 62–63
    unspecified, 62
    Use additional code, 44–45, 59–60
    "with," 61
Not elsewhere classifiable (NEC), **56**
Notices of Privacy, 1202
Not otherwise specified (NOS), 35, **56**
NPCR (National Program of Cancer Registries), 165
NPH (normal pressure hydrocephalus), 247
NPUAP (National Pressure Ulcer Advisory Panel), 384
NSTEMI (nontransmural ST elevation myocardial infarction), **299**
Nummular psoriasis, 384
Nutritional anemia, 175
Nutritional deficiencies, 212

O

OA (osteoarthritis), 407, 408–409
Obesity, 213
Oblique fractures, 434
Obliterative bronchiolitis, 330
Observation periods, 524–525
Obstetrics (OB), 126–127, **486**
Obstructions, **364**
Obstructive hydrocephalus, 247
Ocular disorders. *See* Optical disorders
Office of Civil Rights (OCR), 1190
Office of the Federal Register (OFR), 1185
Office of the Inspector General (OIG), 1192, 1205, 1208
Official Guidelines (ICD-10-CM), 63–72
    acute and chronic conditions, 66
    chapter-specific guidelines, 70–71
    combination codes, 61, 67
    conventions and general guidelines, 65–70
    current conditions, 69
    differential diagnoses, 68
    excerpt from, 64*f*
    on hypertensive heart and chronic kidney disease, 314
    inpatient services, 71–72, 544–545
    multiple and additional codes, 65–66
    outpatient services, 71
    overview, 45, 63–64
    placeholder characters, 70
    Present-On-Admission indicators, 72
    principal and additional diagnoses, 71
    seventh characters, 70

Official Guidelines (ICD-10-PCS), 46
OFR (Office of the Federal Register), 1185
OIG (Office of the Inspector General), 1192, 1205, 1208
Oligospermia, 481
-Oma (suffix), 150
"1" indicator, 549
Onychogryphosis, 388–389
Onycholysis, 388
Onychomycosis, 118
Open angle glaucoma, 273
Open (compound) fractures, 432–433, 433*f*
Open-ended queries, 34, 35, 39
Operative reports, 24
Ophthalmic manifestations of diabetes mellitus, 205, 275
Ophthalmoscopy, 271, 307
Opportunistic pneumonia, 332
Optical disorders, 264–277.
    See also Eyes
    blepharitis, 264
    blindness, 205, 275
    cataracts, 205, 271, 276–277
    conjunctivitis, 75, 83–84, 265, 267–268
    corneal dystrophy, 270
    dacryocystitis, 266
    exophthalmos, 265
    external, 264–266
    glaucoma, 273–274
    internal, 267–273
    keratitis, 269–270
    of lacrimal apparatus, 265–266
    retinal detachment, 273
    retinopathy, 205, 275–276, 315, 501
Oral cancer, 373
Oral cavity, **356**–359, 357*f*
Oral hygiene, 375
Orbit, **263**
Organ donation, 527–528, 527*t*, 532
Organ transplants, 459, 475–476
Orthostatic hypotension, 240
Orthotics, 17
Osgood-Schlatter disease, 417
Osteitis deformans, 417
Osteoarthritis (OA), 407, 408–409
Osteochondrosis, 417
Osteoporosis, 417, 419, 432
Other specified notation, **61**
Otitis externa, 278
Otitis media, 278
Otological disorders. *See* Auditory dysfunctions
Otosclerosis, 279
Ototoxic medications, 283
Outpatient, defined, **10, 71**

Outpatient coding
    confirming medical necessity in, 47–48
    diagnostic statement deconstruction in, 26
    first-listed diagnoses in, 71
    Official Guidelines for, 71
    unconfirmed diagnoses in, 71
Outpatient facilities, **10, 71**
Overdose of insulin, 210
Overlapping boundaries, **159**
Overweight, 213

P

Paget's disease, 417
Pain
    as complication, 459
    management of, 251–254
    pelvic, 486
    rating scale for, 251, 252*t*
Palatine tonsils, 356, 357*f*
Palpebrae (eyelids), **263**, 264
Palpebral conjunctiva, **263**, 267
Palpitations, 296
Pancreas, **371**
Pancreatic cancer, 371
Pancreatic duct, 370, 370*f*, 371
Pancreatic islets, **371**
Pancreatitis, 371, 374
Pap smears, 486
Papules, **393**, 394*f*
Paralytic syndromes, 418
Paranoid schizophrenia, 239
Paraplegia, 418
Parasites and parasitic infections, **116**–117, 137
Parastrongylus cantonensis, 117*f*
Parathyroid glands, **198**–199
Parathyroid hormone (PTH), 199
Parentheses, 55–56
Parkinsonism, 240, 245
Parotitis, 359
Paroxysmal atrial tachycardia (PAT), 296
Patches on skin, **393**, 394*f*
Patent ductus arteriosus (PDA), 501
Pathogens, **101**. *See also* Infections
Pathological fractures, 419–421
Pathology reports, 24, 147–149
Patient noncompliance, 446
Patient Protection and Affordable Care Act of 2010, 519, 532–533, 1208
Patient registration forms, 24
Patient status codes, 430
PCPs (primary care physicians), 1158–1159
PDA (patent ductus arteriosus), 501

PDR (*Physician's Desk Reference*), 134, **442**
Pedigree, 506
Pelvic inflammatory disease (PID), 134, 483
Pelvic pain, 486
Penicillin, 133
Peptic (gastric) ulcers, 361, 362–363
Percentage of body surface, 453
Percutaneous transluminal coronary angioplasty (PTCA), 303
Perforations, **362**
Perichondritis, 278
Perinatal period, **501**
Periodontal (gum) disease, 373, 375
Periosteal fractures, 434
Peripartum conditions, 497–498
Peripheral nervous system (PNS), 249–250
Peripheral ulcerative keratitis, 269
Peripheral vascular disease, 206
Peritoneal dialysis, 475
Pernicious anemia, 175
Personal history codes, 146, 160, 319
Personality disorders, 231, 240
Phalanges, **387**
Pharmaceuticals, 17, 525–526
Pharyngeal tonsils, 356
Phenylketonuria (PKU), 507
PHI (protected health information), **1196**–1197
Phobias, **241,** 255
Physician notes, 24
Physician's Desk Reference (PDR), 134, **442**
PID (pelvic inflammatory disease), 134, 483
Pilon fractures, 434
Pink eye. *See* Conjunctivitis
Pinworms, 116
Pituitary diabetes insipidus, 210
PKU (phenylketonuria), 507
Placeholder characters, 70
Place of occurrence codes, 430
Place-of-Service (POS) codes, 1167–1171
Plague, 103
Plaque, 302–303
Plaque psoriasis, 384
Plasma, **173**
Plaster ulcers. *See* Pressure ulcers
Platelets (PLTs), **173,** 174, 178, 181
Platyhelminths, 117
Pleural disorders, 330, 333–334
Pleural effusion, 334
Pleurisy, 330, 333
Plexus disorders, 249–250
PLTs. *See* Platelets

Pneumocystis jiroveci, 121
Pneumonia, 119–121, 135, 332, **336**–338
Pneumothorax, 330, **334**
PNS (peripheral nervous system), 249–250
POA indicators. *See* Present-On-Admission indicators
Point-of-service (POS) plans, **1159**
Poisoning, 445–446
Polydipsia, **203**
Polymyositis, 415
Polyuria, **203**
POS (Place-of-Service) codes, 1167–1171
POS (point-of-service) plans, **1159**
Posthemorrhagic anemia, 176
Postherpetic neuralgia (herpes zoster), 113, 115
Postoperative care, 88
Postpartum care, 497–498
Postpartum sepsis, 131
Postpartum thyroiditis, 201
Postprocedural pain, 253
Post-thoracotomy pain, 253
Post-traumatic hydrocephalus, 247
Post-traumatic osteoporosis, 417
Post-traumatic stress disorder (PTSD), 242–243
Preexisting conditions, 1176–1177
Preferred provider organizations (PPOs), **1159**
Pregnancy, 488–499
   abortions, 499
   anatomical sites of, 491*f*
   complications of, 495–499
   diabetes mellitus and, 204
   embryonic period, 488
   fertilization and gestation, 488–489, 497
   fetal abnormalities, 497
   high-risk, 490
   hypertension and, 310–311
   incidental pregnant state, 490
   labor and delivery, 131, 491–495, 492*f*
   malignancies during, 154
   normal, 489–490
   peripartum conditions, 497
   postpartum care, 497–498
   preexisting conditions affecting, 496
   prenatal care, 489–490
   sequelae of complications, 498
   seventh characters for, 497
   tests for, 487, 488
   trimesters of, 488–489
Premature births, **501**
Premature rupture of the membranes (PROM), 501

Premiums, **1156**
Prenatal care, **489**–490
Preoperative care, 88
Presbycusis, 282
Prescription drugs, 17, 525–526
Present-On-Admission (POA) indicators
   conditions exempt from, 549–550
   defined, **545**
   in inpatient coding, 545–550
   Official Guidelines for, 72
   reporting guidelines, 546–547
   types of, 548–549
Pressure ulcers, **384**–387
Preterm labor, 495
Preventive services, **519**–522, 532–533, 1156, 1157*f*
Primary care physicians (PCPs), 1158–1159
Primary (congenital) immunodeficiency conditions, 122
Primary hypertension, 306–307
Primary lactase deficiency, 218
Principal diagnoses, **66, 71,** 551
Privacy. *See* HIPAA Privacy Rule
Procedural statement deconstruction, 31–32
Procedure coding. *See* Current Procedural Terminology (CPT); Healthcare Common Procedure Coding System (HCPCS) Level II codes; International Classification of Diseases–10th Revision–Procedure Coding System (ICD-10-PCS)
Procedures, defined, **3**
Procedure-to-procedure (PTP) edits, 1165–1166
Procreative management, 487
Proliferative retinopathy, 205
PROM (premature rupture of the membranes), 501
Prophylactic organ removal, 163
Proptosis, **265**
Prostate gland, 479–480, 479*f*
Prostatitis, **479**–480
Prosthetics, 17, **527,** 527*t*
Protected health information (PHI), **1196**–1197
Protozoal diseases, 117
Protozoan pneumonia, 337
Psoriasis, 384
Psychoactive substance use, 232–236
Psychogenic (hysterical) hearing loss, 282
Psychotic (nonmood) disorders, 239–240
PTCA (percutaneous transluminal coronary angioplasty), 303
PTH (parathyroid hormone), 199

PTP (procedure-to-procedure) edits, 1165–1166
PTSD (post-traumatic stress disorder), 242–243
Puerperal sepsis, 131
Puerperium, **486**
Pulmonary arterial hypertension, 330
Pulmonary edema, 298, 306
Pulmonary embolism, 332, 334
Pulmonary fibrosis, 335
Pulmonary hypoplasia, 329
Punctuation conventions, 55–56
Puncture fractures, 434
Puncture wounds, 436–437, 436*f*
Pupil, 264*f*, 268–269*f*, **271**
Pustules, **393,** 394*f*
Pyelogram, 471
Pyloric sphincter, 361, 361*f*, 364, 370*f*

Q

Q fever, 121
Quadriplegia, 418
Quality Payment Program, 1165
Queries, **34**–35, 39
Quinine, 283
Quinolones, 134
Qui tam provision, 1194

R

Radiation burns, 457
Radiation therapy, 162
RBCs (red blood cells), **173,** 174, 177–178, 182
RDS (respiratory distress syndrome), 329, 501, 502
Recessive genetic disorders, 505, 507
Rectum, 367, 367*f*, **368**
Red blood cells (RBCs), **173,** 174, 177–178, 182
Referrals, 24
Reflex sympathetic dystrophy syndrome, 250
Reimbursement
   coverage determination, 1166, 1167*f*
   defined, **3**
   denial of claims, 1173–1177
   information required for, 429
   letters of appeal for, 1178–1179
   methods of, 1163–1165
   National Correct Coding Initiative and, 1165–1166
   organization of claims, 1172–1180
   paid claims, 1173
   Place-of-Service codes for, 1167–1171
   resubmission of claims, 1180
   Type-of-Service codes for, 1171–1172

Relapse, malignancies in, 154
Release of Information (ROI) forms, **1198,** 1199*f*
Remission, 154, 236
Remittance advice, **1173**
Renal calculi, 477–478
Renal disease, 205, 308. *See also* Chronic kidney disease (CKD)
Renal manifestations of diabetes mellitus, 205, 474
Renovascular hypertension, 308
Residual schizophrenia, 239
Resistance to antimicrobial drugs, 133–136, 528–531
Resource allocation, 3
Respiratory disorders, 329–347
    alpha-1 antitrypsin deficiency, 330
    asthma, 341–342
    bronchitis, 332
    chronic obstructive pulmonary disease, 340–341
    coal worker's pneumoconiosis, 332
    congenital anomalies and, 329
    defined, **329**
    dyspnea, 330, 334
    emphysema, 330
    environmental influences and, 331–332
    external cause codes for, 345–347
    genetics and, 330
    influenza, 102, 109*f*, 112–113, 120, 332, 338
    Legionnaires' disease, 331–332
    lifestyle behaviors and, 332
    manifestations of, 330
    obliterative bronchiolitis, 330
    pleural disorders, 330, 333–334
    pneumonia, 119–121, 135, 332, 336–338
    pulmonary embolism, 332, 334
    pulmonary fibrosis, 335
    pulmonary hypoplasia, 329
    respiratory distress syndrome, 329, 501, 502
    respiratory failure, 336
    respiratory syncytial virus, 335
    tobacco involvement in, 343–344
    trauma-related, 330
    tuberculosis, 101, 103–104, 108, 137, 330, 332
    underlying causes of, 329–332
Respiratory distress syndrome (RDS), 329, 501, 502
Respiratory failure, 336
Respiratory syncytial virus (RSV), 335
Restzustand, 239
Retina, 268*f*, **272**–273, 273*f*, 275–276
Retinal detachment, **273**

Retinopathy, 205, **275**–276, 315, 501
Retrograde pyelogram, 471
Rheumatic fever, 121, 296
Rheumatoid arthritis, 406–407
Rh (Rhesus) factor, **182**–183
Rickets, 408
Right heart failure, 298, 306
Rods, 272, **273**
ROI (Release of Information) forms, **1198,** 1199*f*
Rosenthal's disease, 180
Roundworms, 117
RSV (respiratory syncytial virus), 335
Rubella (German measles), 114, 281
Rubeola (measles), 102, 113, 330
Rule of nines, **454**–455, 454*f*
Ruptures, 438

S

Sacral plexus, 250
Sacrum, 412, 412*f*
Salivary glands, **359**
Salmonella, 106*t,* 137
Salter-Harris physeal fractures, 434
Sarcoidosis, 189
Scales on skin, **393,** 394*f*
Scarlet fever, 105
SCD (sickle cell disease), 177–178
Schistosomiasis, 121
Schizoid personality disorder, 240
Schizophrenia, **239**–240
Schizophrenic catalepsy, 239
SCID (severe combined immunodeficiency), 122
Sclera, 264*f,* **268,** 268–269*f,* 273*f*
Scleroderma, 308
Scoliosis, 412–413
Screenings
    for neoplasms, 145–146
    for skin disorders, 396
    Z codes for, 87, 522
Sebaceous glands, 389
Seborrheic dermatitis, 383
Sebum, 389
Secondary (acquired) immunodeficiency conditions, 122
Secondary diabetes mellitus, **204**
Secondary hemophilia, 180
Secondary hypertension, **298, 308**
Secondary lactase deficiency, 218
Secondary normal pressure hydrocephalus, 247
Secondary pneumonia, 121
Second-degree burns, 450, **451,** 451*f*
Sedatives, **233**
See also notation, 62
See condition notation, 62–63

See notation, 62
Segmental fractures, 434
Self-harm, 446
Sensory diabetic neuropathy, 205
Sensory nerves, 392
Sepsis, **129**–132
Septicemia, **128,** 135
Septic shock, **130**–131
Sequelae (late effects)
    of burns, 457
    of cerebrovascular disease, 319–320
    defined, **30, 60**
    of fractures, 435
    of obstetric complications, 498
    of rickets, 408
Sequencing pain codes, 253
Services, defined, **9**
Seventh characters, 70, 439–440, 497
Severe combined immunodeficiency (SCID), 122
Severe sepsis, **129**–131
Severity of burns, 450–**451,** 451*f*
Sexually transmitted diseases (STDs), 482–484. *See also* HIV/AIDS
Sharps injuries, 103
Shigella, 106–107, 106*t*
Shingles, 113, 115
Sialoadenitis, 359
Sickle cell anemia, 177, 507
Sickle cell disease (SCD), 177–178
Sickle cell trait, 178
Sigmoid colon, 367*f,* **368**
Signs, defined, **26**
Simple (closed) fractures, 432–433, 433*f*
SIRS (systemic inflammatory response syndrome), **128,** 132–133
Site, defined, **420, 451**
Site-specific pain codes, 253
Skeletal disorders. *See* Musculoskeletal disorders
Skeletal fractures, 440
Skeletal system, 419, 420*f*
Skin, **382,** 383*f*
Skin cancer, 149*f,* 394–396, 398
Skin disorders
    cancer, 149*f,* 394–396, 398
    dermatitis, 382–383
    lesions, 393–395, 394*f*
    pressure ulcers, 384–386
    prevention and screenings, 396
    psoriasis, 384
Skull fractures, 435
Slanted brackets, 55
SLE (systemic lupus erythematosus), 410
Slit-lamp examinations, 271
Small intestine, 364–366
Soft palate, 356, 357*f*

Soft tissue disorders, 415–417
Somatic sensory system, 392
Somatoform disorders, **241**
Sonograms (ultrasound), 471
Spasms, muscle, 416
Sphincter
    defined, **360**
    esophageal, 360, 361, 361*f*
    hepatopancreatic, 364, 370, 370*f*
    pyloric, 361, 361*f*, 364, 370*f*
Sphygmomanometer, 305
Spina bifida, 418, 508
Spinal ankylosis, 413
Spinal tap (lumbar puncture), 147, 178
Spine, 411–412
Spiral fractures, 434
Spirilla, 104–105, 104*f*
Splenic dysfunction, 186
Splenic flexure, 368
Spondylopathies, **406,** 412–415
Sprains, 438, 439
SP (systolic pressure), 305
Squamous blepharitis, 264
Squamous cell carcinoma, 149*f*, 395
Stages of pressure ulcers, 384–385, 386*f*
Staphylococcal bacteria, 105, 107, 133
Staphylococcal blepharitis, 264
Staphylococcus aureus, 105, 135–136, 266
Statistical analysis, 3
Status asthmaticus, **341**–342
Status migrainosus, 248
Status of care reporting, 439–440
Statutory laws, **1186**
STDs (sexually transmitted diseases), 482–484. *See also* HIV/AIDS
Stellate fractures, 435
STEMI (ST elevation myocardial infarction), **299**–300
Stents, 302
Stomach, **361**–364, 361*f*, 365*f*
Strains, 438
Streptococcal bacteria, 105, 107
Streptococcus pneumoniae, 119, 266
Stress fractures, 433
Stress-related disorders, 242–243
Stroke. *See* Cerebrovascular accident (CVA)
Stroma, 268
Subclinical infections, 102
Subcutaneous layer of skin, **382,** 383*f*
Subsequent encounters, 440
Subsequent myocardial infarction, 300
Substance interactions, 447–449
Substance use, 232–235
Sudeck's atrophy, 417
Suicide, 446
Sunburns, 457

Sun protection, 396
Superconfidential information, 122
Superficial wounds, 436
Supplies, 17
Supporting documentation, **1190**
Surgical procedures
    septic condition resulting from, 131–132
    transplantations, 459, 475–476
Sweat disorders, 390–391
Symbols, **43**–45, 63
Symptoms, defined, **26**
Syngeneic, **15**
Syphilis, 105, 483–484
Systemic conditions, **85**–86, 307
Systemic infections, 101, **102,** 126
Systemic inflammatory response syndrome (SIRS), **128,** 132–133
Systemic lupus erythematosus (SLE), 410
Systolic heart failure, 298
Systolic pressure (SP), 305

T

Table of Drugs and Chemicals (ICD-10-CM), 5–6, 6*f*, 77, 77*f*, 440–444
Tables section (ICD-10-PCS), 12, 13*f*, **43**
Tabular List of Diseases and Injuries (ICD-10-CM), 5, 5*f*, **43**–45, **78**–84, 79*t*, 80–81*f*, 83–84*f*
Tachycardia, 296
Tailbone. *See* Coccyx
Tanning beds, 396
Tape worms, 116, 116*f*, 117
Tay-Sachs disease, 507
TB. *See* Tuberculosis
TBI (traumatic brain injury), 231, 247
TBSA (total body surface area), 453
Tears, 265
Tears, muscle, 438
Teeth, **356**–359
Tennis elbow (lateral epicondylitis), 415
Tetanus (lockjaw), 104, 107–108
Third-degree burns, 450, **451,** 451*f*
Third-party payers, 3, **1158**
Thoracic outlet syndrome, 249–250
Thoracic vertebrae, 411, 412*f*
Thrombocytopenia, 181, 183–184
Thrombophilia, 179
Thrombotic disorders, 179
Thrombus, **299,** 300, 302, 316, 332
Throxine (T$_4$), 198
TH (thyroid hormone), 198, 199
Thyroid disorders, 199–202
Thyroid gland, **198,** 199*f*

Thyroid hormone (TH), 198, 199
Thyroiditis, 200–201
Thyroid nodules, 200
Thyroid-stimulating hormone (TSH), 198, 199
Thyroid-stimulating immunoglobulin (TSI), 200
Thyrotoxicosis, 200–201
Ticks, 116*f*, 118
Tinea cruris (jock itch), 118
Tinea pedis (athlete's foot), 118
Tissue biopsies, 147
Tobacco use, 234, 343–344
Tongue, 356, 357*f*
Tonsillitis, 105
Tonsils, 356, 357*f*
Topography, **158**
Torticollis, 416
Torus fractures, 434
TOS (Type-of-Service) codes, 1171–1172
Total body surface area (TBSA), 453
Touch exposure to infection, 102
Tourette's disorder, 73, 81–82
Toxic effects, 446–447
Toxoplasmosis, 281
Tracers, **1180**
Trachea, 360, 360*f*
Transcondylar fractures, 434
Transfusions, **184**
Transplantations, 459, 475–476
Transportation services, 17
Transverse colon, 367*f*, **368**
Transverse fractures, 434
Trauma-related disorders, 242–243, 330
Traumatic brain injury (TBI), 231, 247
Traumatic fractures, 432–435, 433*f*
Traumatic spondylolisthesis, 416
Traumatic wounds, 436–438, 436*f*
Treatments, defined, **9**
TriCare, **1160**–1161, 1161*f*
Trichinella, 116*f*
Trichomoniasis, 484
Trichorrhexis nodosa, 389
Triiodothyronine (T$_3$), 198
Trimesters of pregnancy, 488–489
TSH (thyroid-stimulating hormone), 198, 199
TSI (thyroid-stimulating immunoglobulin), 200
Tuberculosis (TB), **101,** 103–104, 108, 137, 330, 332
Tumors. *See* Neoplasms
Turbulent flow, 307
Type I bipolar disorder, 236
Type I diabetes mellitus, **204**
Type II bipolar disorder, 236
Type II diabetes mellitus, **204**

Type III traumatic spondylolisthesis, 416
Type-of-Service (TOS) codes, 1171–1172

U

UCR (usual, customary, and reasonable), **1164**
UHDDS (Uniform Hospital Discharge Data Set), **552**–553
"U" indicator, 548–549
Ulcerative blepharitis, 264
Ulcerative colitis, 368–369
Ulcerative keratitis, 269
Ulcers
    corneal, 269–270
    decubitus, 384
    defined, 362, **393**
    on foot, 206
    gastric, 361, 362–363
    gastrojejunal, 365–366
    pressure, 384–387
    skin, 393, 394f
Ultrasounds (sonography), 471
Umbilical hernias, 364
Unbundling, **1191**
Uncertain neoplasms, 151
Unconfirmed diagnoses, 71–72
Underdosing, 208–209, 446
Underlying conditions, 28–29, **58,** 59, 229
Underweight, 214
Undifferentiated schizophrenia, 239
Uniform Hospital Discharge Data Set (UHDDS), **552**–553
Unintentional poisoning, 445–446
Universal donors, 184
Universal recipients, 184
Unrelated conditions, 84–85
Unspecified behavior for neoplasms, 151
Unspecified diagnosis codes, 35
Unspecified notation, **62**
Upcoding, **1191**
Upper canaliculi, 265
Upper esophageal sphincter, 360
Urea, **470**
Ureters, 470, 471f
Urethra, 470, 471f
Urethritis, 477
Uric acid, 408, 471
Urinalysis, 308, 471
Urinary bladder, 470, 471f
Urinary system, **470**–471, 471f. See also Genitourinary disorders
Urinary tract infections (UTIs), **471,** 477
Urosepsis, 129
U.S. Food and Drug Administration, 508
U.S. Government Printing Office (GPO), 1185
U.S. National Library of Medicine, 247
Use, defined, **233,** 344, **1197**
Use additional code notation, 44–45, 59–60
Usual, customary, and reasonable (UCR), **1164**
Uterine fibroids, 486
UTIs (urinary tract infections), **471,** 477
Uveal tract, **272**
Uvula, 356, 357f

V

Vaginal Pap smears, 486
VAP (ventilator-associated pneumonia), 338
Varicella (chickenpox), 102, 113, 115
Vascular, defined, **306**
Vascular dementia, 229
Vascular disease, 206
Vasodilators, 303, 330
Vectors, 506
Veins, **301,** 302
Ventilator-associated pneumonia (VAP), 338
Ventricles, 295f, **296**
Vermiform appendix, **367,** 367f
Vernal conjunctivitis, 268
Vertebrae, **411**–412
Vertigo, 279, 280
Vibrio, 104f, 106t
Viral conjunctivitis, 267
Viral hepatitis, 109f, 110–112, 122
Viral pneumonia, 120, 332, 337
Viral warts, 109–110f, 110
Viruses and viral infections, 109–110f, **109**–115
Vision services, 17
Vitamin deficiencies, 212
Vitreous chamber, 268f, **271**

W

Walking pneumonia, 119
Warts, 109–110f, 110
Water, exposure to infection through, 103
WBCs (white blood cells), **173,** 174, 178, 185–186
Wedge compression fractures, 435
Weight considerations, 213–214
Well-baby checks, 503, 521
Well-woman exams, 521
Whistleblower Statute, 1194
White blood cells (WBCs), **173,** 174, 178, 185–186
WHO (World Health Organization), 133
Widely metastatic cancer, 151
"W" indicator, 549
Wiskott-Aldrich syndrome, 189
"With" notation, 61
Workers' compensation, 429, **1161**–1162
World Health Organization (WHO), 133
Wounds
    avulsions, 437
    bites, 437–438
    contusions and hematomas, 436, 436f, 438
    lacerations, 436, 436f
    puncture, 436–437, 436f

X

Xenogeneic, **527,** 527t
X-linked agammaglobulinemia (XLA), 122
X-linked inherited diseases, 507–508

Y

Yellow nail syndrome, 388
"Y" indicator, 548

Z

Z codes, 519–532
    antimicrobial resistance, 528–531
    continuing care and aftercare, 525–527
    as first-listed/principal diagnosis, 531
    genetic susceptibility, 523–524
    HIV testing, 122
    neonatal care, 499
    observation, 524–525
    organ donation, 527–528, 532
    postpartum care, 498
    prenatal care, 489–490
    preventive services, 519–522
    screenings, 87, 522
Zika virus, 103, 115
Zooplastic, **15**
Zygotes, 488